# Handbook of Detection of Enzymes on Electrophoretic Gels

# Handbook of Detection of Enzymes on Electrophoretic Gels

## Gennady P. Manchenko

**CRC Press**
Boca Raton   Ann Arbor   London   Tokyo

**Library of Congress Cataloging-in-Publication Data**

Manchenko, Gennady P.
   A Handbook of detection of enzymes on electrophoretic gels
Gennady P. Manchenko.
      p.   cm.
   Includes bibliographical references.
   ISBN 0-8493-8935-6
   1. Enzymes--Purification--Handbooks, manuals, etc.   2. Gel
electrophoresis--Handbooks, manuals, etc.   I. Title.
QP601.M314   1994
574.19$\cent$25--dc20                                    94-11112
                                          CIP

No claim to original U.S. Government works
International Standard Book Number 0-8493-8935-6
Library of Congress Card Number 94-11112
Printed in the United States of America  1  2  3  4  5  6  7  8  9  0
Printed on acid-free paper

# Preface

Gel electrophoresis of enzymes is a very powerful analytical method which is at present widely used in various fields of biological and medical sciences and successfully applied in different fields of practical human activity. The tremendous expansion of the method is mainly due to its simplicity and its ability to separate isozymes and allozymes, which have proven to be very useful genetic markers.

The key step of enzyme electrophoresis is the detection of enzymes on electrophoretic gels, i.e., the procedure of obtaining enzyme electropherograms, or zymograms. Within about 35 years since the first adaptations of histochemical methods for purposes of electrophoretic zymography there were many significant advances in this field, which was extremely active in respect to development of new techniques. Information on enzyme-detection techniques, which is contained in some well-known handbooks and manuals, does not reflect these new developments and in this respect is out of date.

The purpose of this book is to bring together descriptions of numerous enzyme-detection techniques, which have been developed during the last three and a half decades, in one special volume. This book should be useful not only for those who work professionally in the field but also for those who are only starting to master techniques of electrophoretic zymography. Therefore, the book includes detailed descriptions of numerous enzyme-specific methods suitable for detection of more than 300 different enzymes, as well as descriptions of the general principles of enzyme detection on electrophoretic gels.

# The Author

Gennady P. Manchenko, Ph.D., is Senior Researcher at the Laboratory of Genetics at the Institute of Marine Biology of Russian Academy of Sciences at Vladivostok.

Dr. Manchenko graduated from Novosibirsk State University in 1973 with the qualification of a cytogeneticist. As a Probationer, he joined the Institute of Marine Biology at Vladivostok in 1973 and was promoted to Junior Researcher in 1975. He obtained his Ph.D. in 1981 from the Leningrad State University. From 1983 he was employed as the Senior Researcher at the Laboratory of Genetics of the Institute of Marine Biology at Vladivostok.

Dr. Manchenko was a member of the American Genetic Association from 1978 to 1983 and is a member of Vavilov Society of Geneticists and Breeders in Russia, and a member of the Scientific Council of the Institute of Marine Biology at Vladivostok.

He has been the recipient of research support from the George Soros Foundation and International Science Foundation. Current research interests focus on biochemical genetics and systematics of marine invertebrates.

# Acknowledgments

I should like to thank Dr. Alexander I. Pudovkin (Institute of Marine Biology, Vladivostok) and Dr. Robert P. Higgins (Smithsonian Institution, Washington) for reading some parts of the manuscript and correcting my English. I should also like to thank my Russian colleagues for their encouragement and my foreign colleagues for reprints of original papers, which are referred to in the book. However, the first and most honorable position in the list of acknowledgments must be given to my first teacher in isozymology, Dr. Oleg L. Serov (Institute of Cytology and Genetics, Novosibirsk), who introduced me to this exciting field of molecular genetics two decades ago when I was still an undergraduate at the State University at Novosibirsk.

Preparation of the manuscript was partially supported by the George Soros Foundation.

# Table of Contents

---

\*   More than 300 different enzymes are considered in this section, presented in numerical order according to their Enzyme Commission numbers. For convenience, the enzyme numbers are given at the beginning of each enzyme sheet headline. An alphabetical list of the enzymes is also given as Appendix B.

*To Clement L. Markert*

# I ——————— Introduction

Detection of enzymes on electrophoretic gels means visualization of gel areas occupied by specific enzyme molecules after their electrophoretic separation.

Electrophoresis is the migration of charged particles (e.g., protein molecules) in electrolyte under the influence of an electric field. Tiselius may be considered the father of protein electrophoresis. He developed the "moving boundary" method to separate serum proteins in solution.[1] As the result of further developments, a modified method called "zone" electrophoresis was devised in which different protein molecules were separated into distinct zones in stabilized media. In 1955 Smithies introduced starch gel as a stabilized (or supporting) medium for electrophoretically separated proteins.[2] In 1957 Kohn reported the use of cellulose acetate as a very useful supporting medium.[3] Polyacrylamide gel was introduced two years later by Ornstein and Davis[4] and Raymond and Weintraub.[5] At present these supporting media are the most widely used for electrophoretic separation of proteins. The pore size of starch and polyacrylamide gel matrices is of the same order of magnitude as the size of protein molecules. This results in the "molecular sieving" effect, which allows more effective electrophoretic separation of similarly charged protein molecules that differ in their size and shape. Thus, during zone electrophoresis molecules of each protein type move at different rates along the gel according to their specific properties. Using different concentrations of polyacrylamide or starch (this influences the pore size of the gel matrix) and different electrophoretic buffer systems (this influences the net charge of the protein molecule) discrete zones on electrophoretic gels may be obtained almost for each protein type. It is beyond the scope of this book to give a full theoretical treatment to the principles underlying protein electrophoresis. This was done extremely well by Andrews.[6]

The basis for the specific enzyme detection was set in 1939 by the pioneering efforts of Gomori, who developed histochemical methods for visual identification of sites of alkaline phosphatase activity in animal tissues.[7] Further developments have led to the foundation of enzyme histochemistry as a separate field of biological investigation.[8-10]

In 1957 Hunter and Markert first applied histochemical staining procedures to starch gel after electrophoresis of crude tissue extracts for the visualization of gel areas containing esterase activity.[11] As a result, the position of the enzyme was marked by a band (or zone) of stain directly in the gel. This visual display of enzymes on electrophoretic gels has been termed a "zymogram".[12] Since that time methods of detection of enzymes on electrophoretic gels are also known as zymographic (or zymogram) techniques.

The term "isozymes" (or "isoenzymes") was introduced in 1959 by Markert and Möller to designate different molecular forms of the same enzyme occurring either in a single individual or in different members of the same species.[12] Numerous studies of different enzymes have shown that there are three main causes of formation of multiple molecular forms of enzymes. These are (1) the presence of more than one gene locus coding for the enzyme, (2) the presence of more than one allele at a single gene locus coding for the enzyme, and (3) the posttranslation modifications of the formed enzymatic polypeptides resulting in formation of nongenetic or so-called "secondary" isozymes.[13-19] According to the recommendations of the Commission on Biological Nomenclature of IUPAC-IUB, isozymes are defined as genetically determined multiple molecular forms of an enzyme.[20] The term isozymes is usually used to denote multiple molecular forms deriving from different genetic loci, whereas the term "allozymes" is used to denote multiple molecular forms deriving from different alleles of the same genetic locus. The term "allelic isozymes" is also used by some isozymologists.

Since the advent of the zymogram method and the discovery of isozymes, enzyme electrophoresis has been used increasingly to provide useful information in a wide range of biological and biochemical fields and in different fields of practical human activities. The use of isozymes and allozymes as gene markers significantly advanced our knowledge in such areas as population and evolutionary genetics, developmental genetics, molecular evolution, and enzymology. Isoenzymes and allozymes are widely used for solving numerous problems of systematics as well as for reconstruction of phylogenetic relationships between related species. They are of considerable importance for clinical and diagnostic medicine and medical genetics, breeding control of agricultural organisms, agricultural entomology, fishery management, genetic monitoring of environmental pollution, estimation of genetic resources, forensic science, etc.

For a long period of time the major limitation of enzyme electrophoresis was a relatively small number of enzymes for which specific zymogram methods were developed. By the middle of the 1970s, only about 50 enzymes were available for electrophoretic analysis.[21] The best manual for the enzyme detection technique, published by Harris and Hopkinson,[14] includes specific zymogram methods for only 80 of about 2500 enzymes that have been identified by the Nomenclature Committee of the International Union of Biochemistry up to 1983.[22] New zymographic methods (predominantly histochemical and autoradiographic) were developed from time to time for different purposes, but these accumulated at a slow rate and frequently were hidden in special journals, thus being not easily available for all those who work with isozymes. Since the late 1970s and early 1980s several, principally new, approaches were implemented which enriched electrophoresis and enzyme detection considerably. These were (1) bioautographic methods based on the use of a microbial reagent to locate specific enzyme activity after gel electrophoresis;[23] (2) two-dimensional spectroscopy of electrophoretic gels using special optical devices, which permitted one to analyze two-dimensional gels in a fashion analogous to one-dimensional spectroscopy of solutions;[24] and (3) immunoblotting, or the procedure for immunohistochemical visualization of an enzyme protein, which was based on the use of monoclonal antibodies specific to a certain enzyme.[25] Theoretically, these new methods permit the detection of isozymal patterns of almost all the known enzymes.

The combination of electrophoresis of DNA restriction fragments with the transfer of fragments onto hybridization membranes and subsequent visualization of fragments by hybridization with specific labeled DNA probes offers an exciting opportunity to detect directly the specific gene DNA on electrophoretic gels. These new methods have several advantages over enzyme detection methods; however, they are considerably more expensive and complex. Enzyme electrophoresis so far remains the most simple and quite powerful tool for separation and identification of the second-level structural gene products. This is especially true for population-level studies.[26]

The main purpose of this book is to bring together in one volume specific zymogram techniques developed during the last three and a half decades.

The general principles of visualization of enzymes on electrophoretic gels are outlined in Part II, which includes descriptions of histochemical, autoradiographic, bioautographic, two-dimensional spectroscopy, and immunoblotting methods.

Part III, which comprises the main part of the book, includes detailed descriptions of numerous zymogram techniques developed for more than 300 enzymes.

The book does not cover practical aspects of the procedure of enzyme electrophoresis and genetic interpretation of enzymatic patterns developed on gels. These areas are covered in detail in the *Handbook of Enzyme Electrophoresis in Human Genetics* by Harris and Hopkinson,[14] in *Allozyme Electrophoresis: a Handbook for Animal Systematics and Population Studies* by Richardson, Baverstock, and Adams,[18] and in some other more recent publications.[19,26,27] All publications cited above make excellent companion references for this book. This book should prove useful for all those who use enzyme electrophoresis and isozymes in their research or apply isozymes for solving numerous practical questions arising in various human activities.

# References for Part I

1. Tiselius, A., A new apparatus for electrophoretic analysis of colloidal mixtures, *Trans. Faraday Soc.*, 33, 524, 1937.

2. Smithies, O., Zone electrophoresis in starch gels: group variations in the serum proteins of normal human adults, *Biochem. J.*, 61, 629, 1955.

3. Kohn, J., A cellulose acetate supporting medium for zone electrophoresis, *Clin. Chim. Acta*, 2, 297, 1957.

4. Ornstein, L. and Davis, B. J., Disc Electrophoresis, Distillation Products Industries (Division of Eastman Kodak Co.), 1959.

5. Raymond, S. and Weintraub, L., Acrylamide gel as a supporting medium for zone electrophoresis, *Science*, 130, 711, 1959.

6. Andrews, A. T., *Electrophoresis: Theory, Techniques, and Biochemical and Clinical Applications*, Clarendon Press, Oxford, 1988.

7. Gomori, G., Microtechnical demonstration of phosphatase in tissue sections, *Proc. Soc. Exp. Biol. Med.*, 42, 23, 1939.

8. Pearse, A. G. E., *Histochemistry. Theoretical & Applied, Volume I*, Williams & Wilkins Co., Baltimore, 1968.

9. Pearse, A. G. E., *Histochemistry. Theoretical & Applied, Volume II*, Williams & Wilkins Co., Baltimore, 1972.

10. Burstone, M. S., *Enzyme Histochemistry*, Academic Press, New York, 1962.

11. Hunter, R. L. and Markert, C. L., Histochemical demonstration of enzymes separated by zone electrophoresis in starch gels, *Science*, 125, 1294, 1957.

12. Markert, C. L. and Möller, F., Multiple forms of enzymes: tissue, ontogenetic, and species specific patterns, *Proc. Natl. Acad. Sci. U.S.A.*, 45, 753, 1959.

13. Kenney, W. C., Molecular nature of isozymes, *Horizons Biochem. Biophys.*, 1, 38, 1974.

14. Harris, H. and Hopkinson, D. A., *Handbook of Enzyme Electrophoresis in Human Genetics*, North-Holland, Amsterdam (Loose leaf, with supplements in 1977 and 1978), 1976.

15. Korochkin, L. I., Serov, O. L., and Manchenko, G. P., Definition of isoenzymes, in *Genetics of Isoenzymes*, Beljaev, D. K., Ed., Nauka, Moscow, 1977, 5 (in Russian).

16. Rothe, G. M., A survey on the formation and localization of secondary isozymes in mammalian, *Hum. Genet.*, 56, 129, 1980.

17. Moss, D. W., *Isoenzymes*, Chapman and Hall Ltd, London, 1982.

18. Richardson, B. J., Baverstock, P. R., and Adams, M., *Allozyme Electrophoresis: A Handbook for Animal Systematics and Population Studies*, Academic Press, Sydney, 1986.

19. Buth, D. G., Genetic principles and the interpretation of electrophoretic data, in *Electrophoretic and Isoelectric Focusing Techniques in Fisheries Management*, Whitmore, D. H., Ed., CRC Press, Boca Raton, 1990, 1.

20. IUPAC-IUB Commission on Biochemical Nomenclature, Nomenclature of multiple forms of enzymes: recommendations (1976), *J. Biol. Chem.*, 252, 5939, 1977.

21. Siciliano, M. J. and Shaw, C. R., Separation and visualization of enzymes on gels, in *Chromatographic and Electrophoretic Techniques, Vol. 2, Zone Electrophoresis*, Smith, I., Ed., Heineman, London, 1976, 185.

22. Nomenclature Committee of the International Union of Biochemistry, *Enzyme Nomenclature*, Academic Press, Orlando, 1984.

23. Naylor, S. L. and Klebe, R. L., Bioautography: a general method for the visualization of enzymes, *Biochem. Genet.*, 15, 1193, 1977.

24. Klebe, R. J., Mancuso, M. G., Brown, C. R., and Teng, L., Two-dimensional spectroscopy of electrophoretic gels, *Biochem. Genet.*, 19, 655, 1981.

25. Vora, S., Monoclonal antibodies in enzyme research: present and potential applications, *Anal. Biochem.*, 144, 307, 1985.

26. Morizot, D. C. and Schmidt, M. E., Starch gel electrophoresis and histochemical visualization of proteins, in *Electrophoretic and Isoelectric Focusing Techniques in Fisheries Management*, Whitmore, D. H., Ed., CRC Press, Boca Raton, 1990, 23.

27. Murphy, R. W., Sites, J. W., Jr., Buth, D. G., and Haufler, C. H., Proteins I: Isozyme electrophoresis, in *Molecular Systematics*, Hillis, D. M. and Moritz, C., Eds., Sinauer, Sunderland, 1990, 45.

# II ——— General Principles of Enzyme Detection on Electrophoretic Gels

The objective of this part is to describe the general principles involved in visualization of gel areas containing specific enzymes separated during gel electrophoresis. These principles may be classified as resulting in positive or negative zymograms, as chemical or physical, as chromogenic or fluorogenic, as based on chemical coupling or enzymatic coupling, etc. It seems, however, that the mixed operational classification will be preferable for purely practical consideration. According to this classification, the main principles of enzyme visualization on electrophoretic gels are defined as

1. Based on chromogenic reactions
2. Based on fluorogenic reactions
3. Autoradiography
4. Bioautography
5. Two-dimensional gel spectroscopy
6. Immunoblotting

Two-dimensional spectroscopy of electrophoretic gels and immunohistochemical methods have good perspectives and are of great value for further developments in electrophoretic zymography. However, the great majority of zymographic techniques so far developed are based on the use of chromogenic and fluorogenic reactions.

## Section 1
## Chromogenic Reactions

Chromogenic reactions are those which result in formation of a chromophore at sites of enzyme activities. The great majority of these reactions were adopted from well-tried histochemical or colorimetric enzyme assay methods. In a simple one-step chromogenic reaction a colorless substrate is enzymatically converted into a colored product. In a broad sense, the class of chromogenic reactions includes any reactions or set of reactions that reveal visible at day light discrete zones (or bands) of enzyme activity. In most cases the primary product(s) of an enzyme reaction is not readily detectable, and supplementary reagent(s) is added to the reaction mixture which somehow reacts with the primary product(s) to form a visible secondary product(s). These secondary products can be formed as the result of spontaneous reactions or so-called chemical coupling. In some cases, however, none of the primary products can be detected by chemical coupling, and an additional enzymatic reaction(s) is needed in order to reach a detectable product(s). This procedure is called enzymatic coupling, and supplementary exogenous enzymes that are added to reaction mixtures are known as linking or auxiliary enzymes. The resultant zymogram is positively stained (colored bands on achromatic background) if the color is formed by a reaction with the product of the enzyme activity. A negatively stained zymogram (achromatic bands on colored background) is obtained if the color is formed by a reaction with the substrate.

Many different enzymes produce the same molecules (e.g., NADH, NADPH, orthophosphate, ammonia, hydrogen peroxide, etc.) or different molecules with essentially the same chemical properties (e.g., aldehydes, ketones, reducing sugars, thiols, etc.). This means that very similar or identical chromogenic reactions can be used to detect different enzymes. Thus, classification of chromogenic reactions based on properties of

products that are detected seems to be the more useful and practical approach. Such classification is advantageous because it allows one to choose an adequate chromogenic reaction to visualize activity bands even of those enzymes that have not yet been detected on electrophoretic gels.

## PRODUCTS REDUCING TETRAZOLIUM SALTS

The first histochemical method for the detection of enzyme activity using a tetrazolium salt was developed in 1951 by Seligman and Rutenberg.[1] Markert and Möller[2] were the first to adopt this histochemical procedure for detection of NAD(P)-dependent dehydrogenases on electrophoretic gels. These dehydrogenases produce reduced NADH or NADPH which are the electron donors for reduction of tetrazolium salts, which are especially good electron acceptors. Reduction of a tetrazolium salt results in formation of intensely colored, water-insoluble precipitate, formazan. The reductive reaction proceeds rapidly in the presence of some electron carrier intermediaries. Initially, the diaphorase/methylene blue system was used for the transfer of electrons from NAD(P)H to a tetrazolium salt.[2] Further, it was found that phenazine methosulfate (PMS) is preferable as an intermediary catalyst. Molecules of PMS can accept electrons from NAD(P)H and reduce a tetrazolium salt, repeating the cycle and thus being very effective even at low concentrations. Many NAD(P)-dependent dehydrogenases are detected on electrophoretic gels using the PMS/tetrazolium system (e.g., see 1.1.1.1 — ADH, Method 1; 1.1.1.37 — MDH, Method 1; 1.1.1.40 — ME; 1.1.1.42 — IDH, Method 1, etc.).*

The enzymes that are FMN- or FAD-containing flavoproteins (e.g., many oxidases) can also be detected using the PMS/tetrazolium system by a mechanism similar to that described above for NAD(P)-dependent dehydrogenases. In an oxidase detection system PMS molecules accept electrons from a reduced flavine group of an enzymatic flavoprotein and transfer them to a tetrazolium salt (e.g., see 1.1.3.15 — GOX, Method 1; 1.1.3.22 — XOX). Being the prosthetic groups, FMN and FAD are tightly bound to the enzyme molecules and are not dissociated during electrophoresis, so they can be omitted from staining solutions used to detect oxidase activities.

Different tetrazolium salts that vary in their reduction potentials are now commercially available. Tetrazolium salts with high reduction potential are reduced with greater ease than those with low reduction potential. Among tetrazolium salts commonly used in electrophoretic zymography, MTT (methyl thiazolyl blue) is usually preferable for NAD(P)H detection because of its high reduction potential and photostability. Tetranitro blue tetrazolium (TNBT) possesses somewhat lower reduction potential than MTT but higher than NBT (nitro blue tetrazolium). The lowest reduction potential is characteristic for TTC (triphenyltetrazolium chloride).

The products of enzymatic reactions containing free sulfhydryl groups (e.g., CoA-SH) can also reduce tetrazolium salts (usually NBT and MTT are preferable) in the presence of PMS or another intermediary catalyst, DCIP (dichlorophenol indophenol). An example is the detection method of citrate synthase (4.1.3.7. — CS).

---

* Referenced enzymes and methods can be found in Part III, Section 3, where they are listed in numerical order according to the EC numbers recommended by the Nomenclature Committee of the International Union of Biochemistry.

When DCIP is substituted for PMS, NAD(P)H cannot effectively reduce MTT but sulfhydryls (e.g., glutathione) can do this by the use of DCIP as intermediary catalyst. This property of DCIP is used in detection methods developed for NAD(P)H-dependent glutathione reductase (1.6.4.2 — GSR, Method 2) and NAD(P)H diaphorases [1.6.99.1. — DIA(NADPH); 1.8.1.4 — DIA(NADH)].

Such products of enzymatic reactions as 4-imidazolone-5-propionate and β-sulfinylpyruvate can also reduce tetrazolium salts (*viz.* NBT) in the presence of PMS (2.6.1.1 — GOT, Method 3; 4.2.1.49 — UH). 5-Bromo-4-chloro-3-indoxyl can directly reduce NBT at room temperature without any intermediary catalyst (3.1.3.1 — ALP, Method 2).

Reducing sugars cause reduction of TTC in alkaline medium at room temperature (ketohexoses) or at 100°C (aldohexoses). Many enzymes producing ketosugars (e.g., D-fructose) and aldohexoses (e.g., D-mannose) are detected using this tetrazolium salt (2.4.1.7 — SP; 4.2.1.46 — TDPGD; 3.2.1.24 — α–MAN, Method 3; 3.2.1.26 — FF, Method 4).

Some nonenzymatic proteins containing sulfhydryl groups may be nonspecifically stained on dehydrogenase zymograms obtained using the PMS/NBT or MTT system at alkaline pH. This nonspecific staining of –SH-rich proteins is sometimes erroneously attributed to so-called "nothing dehydrogenases" (1.X.X.X — NDH). Unlike real "nothing dehydrogenases", however, –SH-rich proteins can also be stained in alkaline tetrazolium solutions lacking PMS.

The ability of free –SH groups to reduce NBT (or MTT) in alkaline medium is used to detect some enzymes generating alkaline products (for details see below, *Products that Cause a pH Change*).

Many enzymes generate products that are the substrates for certain NAD(P)-dependent dehydrogenases. These enzymes can be detected using exogenous dehydrogenases as linking enzymes in couple with the PMS/MTT or NBT systems. For example, the stains for hexokinase (2.7.1.1 — HK), phosphoglucomutase (5.4.2.2 — PGM, Method 1), and glucose-6-phosphate isomerase (5.3.1.9 — GPI) all use glucose-6-phosphate dehydrogenase as linking enzyme; the stain for fumarate hydratase (4.2.1.2 — FH, Method 1) uses exogenous malate dehydrogenase; the stain for aconitase (4.2.1.3 — ACON, Method 1) uses auxiliary isocitrate dehydrogenase (1.1.1.42 — IDH, Method 1), etc. Similarly, xanthine oxidase in couple with the PMS/MTT system is used as linking enzyme in enzyme-linked stain for purine-nucleoside phosphorylase (2.4.2.1 — PNP).

For the detection of some enzymes, one or even more linked enzymatic reactions are used in order to reach a product detectable via dehydrogenase or oxidase. For example, mannose-6-phosphate isomerase (5.3.1.8 — MPI) is detected using two linked reactions sequentially catalyzed by auxiliary glucose-6-phosphate isomerase and glucose-6-phosphate dehydrogenase. Similarly, the stain for adenosine deaminase (3.5.4.4 — ADA, Method 1) uses exogenous purine-nucleoside phosphorylase to produce hypoxanthine, which is then detected by xanthine oxidase coupled with the PMS/NBT or MTT system. The detection system of mannokinase (2.7.1.7 — MK) includes three linked enzymatic reactions sequentially catalyzed by auxiliary mannose-6-phosphate isomerase, glucose-6-phosphate isomerase, and glucose-6-phosphate dehydrogenase. Three linking enzymes are also used in the detection system of dextransucrase (2.4.1.5 — DS, Method 3).

It should be noted that staining solutions containing PMS and a tetrazolium are light-sensitive. Thus, incubation of gels in PMS/ tetrazolium solutions should be carried out in the dark.

Until now, the tetrazolium dyes remain of central importance in enzyme staining methods. A great majority of zymographic techniques described in Part III of this handbook is based on the use of the PMS/ tetrazolium system.

## PRODUCTS CAPABLE OF COUPLING WITH DIAZONIUM SALTS

Many hydrolytic enzymes (e.g., aminopeptidases, esterases, glycosidases, phosphatases) are visualized on electrophoretic gels using artificial substrates which are naphthol or naphthylamine derivatives. When naphthol or naphthylamine is liberated enzymatically, it immediately couples with a diazonium salt. An insoluble colored precipitate (an azo dye) is formed as a result of the coupling reaction in gel areas where specific hydrolase activity is located.

There are two main components of the azo coupling system. The first one is the diazonium ion. The diazonium ions are not stable and need to be in a salt form for prolonged storage.[3] A number of different stabilized diazonium salts are now commercially available. Usually these are salts or double salts of zinc chloride (e.g., Fast Blue B salt, Fast Blue BB salt, Fast Blue RR salt, Fast Violet B salt), tetrafluoroborate or sulfate (e.g., Fast Garnet GBC salt), naphthalenedisulfonate (e.g., Fast Red B salt), etc.[4] For further stabilization such inert additives as aluminum, magnesium, sodium and zinc sulfates, magnesium oxide and bicarbonate, and some others can also be added to commercial diazonium salt preparations.

It should be taken into account that some enzymes may be inhibited by these additives. When the diazonium salt acts as an enzyme inhibitor, a two-step, or so-called postcoupling, staining procedure is recommended. In this procedure, the gel is initially incubated in substrate solution for an essential period of time (usually 30 min) and only then diazonium salt is added. However, the one-step azo coupling procedure is usually preferable because it considerably reduces diffusion of enzymatically liberated naphthols and naphthylamines and results in development of more sharp and distinct activity bands.

Dissolved diazonium salts give very unstable ions, so solutions should be prepared immediately before use. The stability of diazonium ions depends on the pH of the staining solution. For example, Fast Black K salt is stable in acidic pH while Fast Blue RR salt is recommended for use at neutral and alkaline pH. High temperature also contributes to decreasing stability of diazonium salts. When the azo coupling system is used to detect the enzyme, a compromise should be achieved between the pH-optimum of the enzyme activity and diazonium salt stability. If pH values extreme for diazonium salt stability must be used, it is recommended that the diazonium salt solution be replaced as often as necessary, depending on the total period of gel incubation. Because diazonium ions can themselves act as enzyme inhibitors, the use of optimal concentrations of 1 mg/ml is recommended.[3]

The second component of the azo coupling system is an enzyme-specific artificial substrate which is an amide, an ester, or a glucoside of the coupling agent (naphthol or naphthylamine). The substrates that are derivatives of substituted naphthol (e.g., 6-bromo-2-naphthol) or substituted naphthylamine (e.g., 1-metoxy-3-naphthylamine) may be preferable; this is because some substituted naphthols being coupled with diazonium ions give azo dyes of greater insolubility. The use of derivatives of 1-metoxy-3-naphthylamine, which complexes much more quickly with diazonium ions than does 2-naphthylamine, reduces the problem of product diffusion during color formation.

Examples of the use of the azo coupling system in electrophoretic zymography are the detection of esterases (3.1.1... — EST, Method 1) and acid phosphatase (3.1.3.2 — ACP, Method 3), with α-naphthol as coupling agent; the detection of β-glucuronidase (3.2.1.31 — β-GUS, Method 2), with naphthol-AS-BI and 6-bromo-2-naphthol as coupling agents; the detection of leucine aminopeptidase (3.4.11.1 — LAP, Method 1), with 2-naphthylamine as coupling agent; and the detection of some proteinases (3.4.21-24... — PROT, Visualization Procedures), with 1-metoxy-3-naphthylamine as coupling agent.

Diazonium ions also couple with such enzymatic products as oxaloacetate, which serves as a coupling agent of the azo coupling system in the detection of some nonhydrolytic enzymes, e.g., glutamic–oxaloacetic transaminase (2.6.1.1 — GOT, Method 1), phospho-enolpyruvate carboxylase (4.1.1.31 — PEPC), and pyruvate carboxylase (6.4.1.1 — PC).

The azo coupling system was the first enzyme-staining system successfully adopted from histochemistry for purposes of electrophoretic zymography.[5] A great number of zymographic techniques described in Part III are based on the use of this staining system.

## PRODUCTS THAT CAUSE A pH CHANGE

Local acidic–alkaline pH change takes place in areas of acid electrophoretic gels where enzymes producing ammonia ions are localized. These enzymes are detected by incubation of electrophorized gels in staining solutions containing the substrate and an appropriate pH indicator dye, e.g., Phenol Violet, which is light orange at acidic pH and becomes dark blue at alkaline pH. Examples are the detection of urease (3.5.1.5 — UR, Method 1), adenosine deaminase (3.5.4.4 — ADA, Method 3), and AMP deaminase (3.5.4.6 — AMPDA, Method 3).

The local pH increase due to enzymatic production of ammonia ions is used in catalyzing silver deposition from neutral nitrate solution in the presence of photographic developers, 4-hydroxyphenol and 4-hydroxyaniline and the reducing thiol reagent 2-mercaptoethanol.[6] 2-Mercaptoethanol is used to increase the difference of the reduction potential between ammonia-producing enzyme bands and gel background. In the absence of this reducing agent the intensity of the enzyme activity bands is sensibly decreased and the gel background increased. Optimal contrast between enzymatic bands and background is due to 4-hydroxyaniline, which reduces the initially oxidized 4-hydroxyphenol, and this last reduces faster and with more contrast the silver ions to the black metallic form. The photographic developers initiate silver deposition, which further proceeds in an autocatalyzed way. Thus, the method is based on the faster deposition of metallic silver from a neutral silver solution in gel areas where the ammonia-producing enzyme is localized than in enzyme-free gel areas. The example of successful application of the silver deposition method is urease (3.5.1.5 — UR, Method 2).

Tetrazolium salts may also be used to detect enzymes that produce ammonia ions and so elevate pH in those gel areas where they are localized. In these cases the elevated pH increases the rate of reduction of tetrazolium salt by the sulfhydryl compound dithiothreitol, which is included in the staining solution along with the substrate and a tetrazolium salt. The slightly less-sensitive NBT is recommended for use in these stains in preference to MTT.[7] Examples of applications of this detection system are staining methods for arginase (3.5.3.1 — ARG, Method 1) and cytidine deaminase (3.5.4.5 — CDA, Method 1).

Local alkaline–acidic pH changes can also occur in electrophoretic gels as a result of the catalytic activity of some enzymes. These local pH changes are detected using such pH indicator dyes as Bromothymol Blue (blue at pH >7.6; yellow at pH <6.0) or Phenol Red (red at pH >8.2; yellow at pH <6.8). Examples of this are the detection of trypsin (3.4.21.4 — T; Other Methods, A), esteroprotease (3.4.21.40 — EP, Method 2), and carbonic anhydrase (4.2.1.1 — CA, Method 1). The orthophosphate, liberated by enzymatic activity, being treated with calcium ions, liberates protons during the formation of calcium phosphate gel. So, phosphatase activity bands can also be detected by the color change of the pH indicator dye. The example is alkaline phosphatase (3.1.3.1 — ALP, Method 6).

The following conditions should be kept when any method of the local pH change detection is applied: (1) nonbuffered staining solutions should be used, and (2) gel buffers should be of minimal concentrations

and desirable pH values to allow the pH change to occur as the result of an enzyme action.

The main disadvantage of all staining methods using pH indicator dyes is the diffused character of developed enzyme activity bands. This is not the case, however, for the NBT/dithiothreitol method, which results in formation of practically nondiffusable formazan.

## ORTHOPHOSPHATE

Many enzymes liberate orthophosphate as the reaction product. Several different methods were developed for the visualization of phosphate-liberating enzymes. These include the lead sulfide method and its reduced modification, the calcium phosphate method, the acid phosphomolybdate method and its malachite green modification, the pH indicator method (described above) and the enzymatic method. All these methods may be applied only when electrophoresis and gel staining are carried out in phosphate-free buffers.

Gomori[8] was the first to use calcium ions to precipitate orthophosphate released by the action of phosphate-liberating enzymes. Calcium phosphate precipitate, however, is soluble in acidic solution and so cannot be used for the detection of some phosphate-liberating enzymes with acidic pH-optimum, e.g., acid phosphatase. In order to avoid this drawback, a lead is used which forms insoluble lead phosphate.[9] This phosphate salt is colorless and therefore not easily recognizable; however, treating it with sulfide results in the formation of a brownish-black insoluble precipitate of lead sulfide. Examples of the application of the lead sulfide method in electrophoretic zymography are the detection methods for alkaline phosphatase (3.1.3.1 — ALP, Method 7) and acylphosphatase (3.6.1.7 — AP). The main disadvantage of the method is the need for sequential treatment of electrophorized gel with several solutions in order to achieve a colored end product. When this method is used, it should be remembered that lead also precipitates borate ions. So, borate-containing buffers should not be used for electrophoresis or staining. The silver nitrate may be used to form silver phosphate, which is then reduced by sodium hydroxide treatment to black metallic silver. This method has some advantages over the lead sulfide method. The example of application of this method is aldolase (4.1.2.13 — ALD, Other Methods).

The reduced Gomori method can be applied to transparent electrophoretic gels (e.g., polyacrylamide gel, PAG). It is based on the formation of white calcium phosphate precipitate which is insoluble in alkaline conditions. The white bands of calcium phosphate precipitation are clearly visible when stained gel is viewed against a dark background.[10] For example, this method is used to detect fructose bisphosphatase (3.1.3.11 — FBP, Method 2), dehydroquinate synthase (4.6.1.3 — DQS), and chorismate synthase (4.6.1.4 — CHOS). When more opaque electrophoretic gels are used (e.g., starch or acetate cellulose), calcium phosphate may be subsequently stained with Alizarin Red S.

The acid phosphomolybdate method is based on the formation of phosphomolybdate and its subsequent reduction by aminonaphthol sulfonic acid[11] or ascorbic acid,[12] which results in a blue stain. The example is the detection method for inorganic pyrophosphatase (3.6.1.1 — PP, Method 1). The phosphomolybdate method, however, suffers from the diffusion of both orthophosphate and phosphomolybdate. Isozyme patterns visualized by this method fade quickly. To reduce diffusion of the colored end product, the use of an additional stain ingredient, malachite green, is recommended.[13] The malachite green–phosphomolybdate complex formed is almost fully insoluble, so zymograms obtained by this method may be stored for several months (for details see 3.6.1.1 — PP, Method 1, Notes).

The enzymatic method[14] has proven to be the most sensitive for the detection of phosphate-liberating enzymes. The principle of the method involves employing the phosphate-requiring phosphorolytic cleavage of inosine catalyzed by auxiliary purine-nucleoside phosphorylase to produce hypoxanthine, which is then detected using a second linking enzyme, xanthine oxidase, coupled with the PMS/NBT or MTT system. The colored end product is blue formazan. The enzymatic method, compared to other methods for the detection of orthophosphate, is advantageous due to its high sensitivity and generation of a nondiffusible formazan. The example of this method is the detection of alkaline phosphatase (3.1.3.1 — ALP, Method 8).

Other enzymatic methods for detection of orthophosphate exist which use linked enzymatic reactions involving either the glyceraldehyde-3-phosphate dehydrogenase[15] or the phosphorylase[16] reactions. Both these methods include readily reversible enzymatic reactions. In addition, the first one requires glyceraldehyde-3-phosphate, which is unstable, while the other involves three enzymatic steps subsequently catalyzed by auxiliary phosphorylase, phosphoglucomutase, and glucose-6-phosphate dehydrogenase and so is very complex. Because of these disadvantages, neither enzymatic method is in wide use.

Some enzymes which produce phosphorus-containing compounds also can be detected by appropriate phosphate-detecting methods described above after the cleavage of orthophosphate by auxiliary alkaline phosphatase (e.g., see 3.1.4.17 — CNPE, Method 2; 3.1.4.40 — CMP-SH; 3.6.1.X — NDP). In these cases, however, it should be taken into account that auxiliary alkaline phosphatase must not cleave orthophosphate from phosphorous-containing substrates.

Orthophosphate can also be cleaved from glucose-1-phosphate and ribose-1-phosphate by treatment with $H_2SO_4$ and subsequently detected by the acid phosphomolybdate method or malachite green phosphomolybdate modification of this method. As a result, the positively stained zymograms are obtained for enzymes that produce these phosphosugars (5.4.2.7 — PPM, Method 3), whereas negative zymograms are obtained when these phosphosugars are used as substrates (5.4.2.2 — PGM, Method 2). Orthophosphate can be liberated from glycerone phosphate and glyceraldehyde-3-phosphate by treatment with iodacetamide or iodacetate and then detected by a suitable phosphate-detecting method. For example, see aldolase (4.1.2.13 — ALD, Other Methods).

Since many enzymes liberate orthophosphate as the reaction product or produce phosphorus-containing products from which orthophosphate can be readily cleaved chemically or enzymatically, the phosphate-detecting methods are of great importance for electrophoretic zymography.

## PYROPHOSPHATE

Pyrophosphate-liberating enzymes can be visualized by incubation of transparent electrophoretic gels with buffered solutions containing certain substrates and subsequently treating the gels with calcium ions.[10] As a result, white bands of calcium pyrophosphate precipitation are clearly visible when stained gel is viewed against a dark background. The examples are detection methods for DNA-directed RNA polymerase (2.7.7.6 — DDRP) and UDPglucose pyrophosphorylase (2.7.7.9 — UGPP, Method 3).

Manganese ions also can be used to detect the product pyrophosphate on transparent electrophoretic gels. The bands formed as a result of manganese pyrophosphate precipitation are not apparent when stained gel is placed directly on a dark background, but they are very distinct when gel is held a few inches from a dark background and lighted indirectly. An example is the detection method for hypoxanthine phosphoribosyltransferase (2.4.2.8 — HPRT, Method 3).

A coupled reaction catalyzed by auxiliary inorganic pyrophosphatase from yeast can be used to convert the product pyrophosphate into orthophosphate, which is then visualized by an appropriate phosphate-detecting method (see the section on

*Orthophosphate,* above). Yeast inorganic pyrophosphatase is a specific catalyst for the hydrolysis of pyrophosphate in the presence of magnesium ions and several organic pyrophosphates, such as ATP and ADP, are not attacked. This method may not be used for detection of pyrophosphate-releasing enzymes, which use substrates also hydrolyzed by auxiliary pyrophosphatase. An example of successful application of this method is sulfate adenylyltransferase (2.7.7.4 — SAT).

Pyrophosphate can also be detected using three coupled reactions sequentially catalyzed by auxiliary enzymes pyrophosphate-fructose-6-phosphate 1-phosphotransferase (PFPPT), aldolase, and NAD-dependent glyceraldehyde-3-phosphate dehydrogenase in couple with the PMS/MTT system. The use of bacterial PFPPT is recommended because the plant enzyme requires for its activity fructose-2,6-bisphosphate, which is very expensive. Triose-phosphate isomerase may be used as the fourth auxiliary enzyme to accelerate coupling reactions and to enhance intensity of colored bands. This enzymatic method is adopted from the detection method for PFPPT (2.7.1.90 — PFPPT). Fluorogenic modification of the method may also be found in the same place.

## HYDROGEN PEROXIDE

Hydrogen peroxide is the obligatory product of almost all oxidases that use oxygen as acceptor. It also serves as a proton-accepting substrate for peroxidase. So, a coupled peroxidase reaction is widely used to detect enzymes producing hydrogen peroxide. There are many redox dyes that can be used as proton donors in the peroxidase reaction. The more frequently used dyes are 3-amino-9-ethyl carbazole, o-dianisidine dihydrochloride, and tetramethyl benzidine (see also 1.11.1.7 — PER). When oxidized, these redox dyes change in both color and solubility. They are soluble when reduced but become insoluble upon oxidation. The former goes from a yellow or light-brown dye to a red or dark-brown compound, while the latter two change from colorless to orange and blue, respectively.

The chromogenic peroxidase reaction also is used as the last step in some enzyme-linked detection systems. The more widely used one is the staining method for peptidases (3.4.11 or 13... — PEP, Method 1) where the peroxidase reaction is used in couple with the first-step coupled reaction catalyzed by auxiliary L-amino acid oxidase. Another example is the enzyme-linked detection system for β-fructofuranosidase (3.2.1.26 — FF, Method 3), in which the chromogenic peroxidase reaction is used in couple with a hydrogen peroxide–generating reaction catalyzed by the other auxiliary enzyme glucose oxidase.

Hydrogen peroxide also takes part in chemical chromogenic reactions, which usually are used in detection methods for enzymes utilizing hydrogen peroxide as the substrate. In these cases, negatively stained zymograms are obtained. Two such chromogenic reactions are used to detect catalase (1.11.1.6 — CAT, Methods 1 and 2). The first one is based on the formation of a dark-green compound as a result of the chemical reaction between hydrogen peroxide and potassium ferricyanide in the presence of $Fe^{3+}$ ions. The second chromogenic reaction proceeds between potassium iodide and starch in the presence of hydrogen peroxide and thiosulfate. In areas of the starch gel (or PAG-containing starch) where CAT is localized, hydrogen peroxide is enzymatically destroyed. Upon exposure to potassium iodide, wherever hydrogen peroxide is not destroyed, the iodide is oxidized to iodine and intense blue starch–iodine chromatophore is formed. Thiosulfate is inactivated in gel areas where hydrogen peroxide is presented and remains active in areas of CAT activity where hydrogen peroxide is destroyed. The function of thiosulfate is to reduce any iodine that escapes into solution during the staining procedure and settles on the gel areas occupied by CAT.[17]

The highly sensitive lanthanide luminescence method has been developed based on the photoassisted oxidation of phenantroline dicarboxylic acid dihydrazide (PDAdh) by hydrogen peroxide. The resulting PDA interacts with europium ions and luminescent Eu:PDA complex forms, which can be observed under UV light (for more details see Section 2, *Products that Form Luminescent Lanthanide Chelates*).

## CARBONATE IONS

Carbon dioxide–producing enzymes are visualized using the calcium carbonate method.[10] This method is based on the formation of a white calcium carbonate precipitate in gel areas where the enzyme producing carbon dioxide is localized. The method is applicable only for transparent gels and is applied as a one-step procedure using buffered staining solution containing the enzyme-specific substrate(s) and $Ca^{2+}$ ions. After an appropriate period of incubation in staining solution the gel is viewed against a dark background for white bands of calcium carbonate precipitation. The examples are detection methods for isocitrate dehydrogenase (1.1.1.42 — IDH, Method 2) and pyruvate decarboxylase (4.1.1.1 — PDC, Method 1).

The calcium carbonate method is essentially the same as the calcium phosphate and calcium pyrophosphate methods (see above), but about 10 times less sensitive. An enzymatic method for detection of carbon dioxide–producing enzymes also exists. This method uses a linked enzymatic reaction catalyzed by auxiliary phosphoenolpyruvate carboxylase to convert phosphoenolpyruvate and carbon dioxide into orthophosphate and oxaloacetate. Oxaloacetate is then coupled with diazonium salt to form insoluble azo dye (4.1.1.31 — PEPC).

The modification of this method is possible by the use of an additional linked reaction catalyzed by auxiliary malate dehydrogenase in place of the azo coupling reaction. In this modification oxaloacetate and NADH are converted by malate dehydrogenase into malate and NAD. Gel areas where NADH into NAD conversion occurs may be registered in long-wave UV light as dark (nonfluorescent) bands visible on a light (fluorescent) background. When bands are well developed, the gel may be treated with PMS/MTT to obtain a zymogram with achromatic bands on a blue background.

Further modification of the enzymatic method may consist of the application of different phosphate-detecting methods (see above) to visualize areas of orthophosphate production by linked-enzyme phosphoenolpyruvate carboxylase. The calcium phosphate method, however, may not be used because calcium carbonate precipitate will also form and block the linked reaction of phosphoenolpyruvate carboxylase.

The use of plant phosphoenolpyruvate carboxylase is preferable because it does not require acetyl-CoA for its activity.

## COLORED PRODUCTS

In some cases the products of enzymatic reactions are readily visible due to the acquisition of some properties not found in the substrates. For instance, chromogenic synthetic substrates which are derivatives of *para*-nitrophenol or *para*- nitroaniline are used to detect some hydrolytic enzymes. These substrates are colorless; however, hydrolytically cleaved *para*-nitrophenol and *para*-nitroaniline are yellow (e.g., 3.1.3.1 — ALP, Method 4; 3.4.21.5 — THR). Colored bands developed by the use of these chromogenic substrates may be too faint for visual quantitative analysis and are usually registered spectrophotometrically on transparent gels using a scanning spectrophotometer. The treatment of acidic gels with alkali enhances the band coloration caused by *para*-nitrophenol (3.1.16.1 — SE, Method 1). Yellow *para*-nitroaniline may be converted into a readily visible red azo dye after diazotation with

*N*-(1-naphtyl)ethylenediamine.[18] The examples are detection methods for trypsin (3.4.21.4 — T, Method 3) and chymotrypsin (3.4.21.4 — CT, Method 3).

Another example of the detection methods based on formation of colored product is the use of phenolphthalein phosphate as substrate for acid phosphatase (3.1.3.2 — ACP, Method 1). In this method, released phenolphthalein leads to the formation of pink zones after treatment of the gel with alkali.

Synthetic chromogenic substrates that are derivatives of the indoxyl are also used to detect different hydrolytic activities. When indoxyl derivatives (e.g., indoxyl esters) are hydrolyzed, the liberated indoxyl is oxidized by atmospheric oxygen to an intensely colored indigo dye. This oxidation, however, occurs very slowly, especially in acidic conditions. So, undesirable diffusion of soluble indoxyl may be significant. Derivatives of 5-bromo-4-chloro-3-indoxyl, ammonium 5-indoxyl, and 5-bromoindoxyl are usually used in place of simple indoxyl derivatives (e.g., 3.1.3.1 — ALP, Method 2; 3.1.4.1 — PDE-1, Method 2; 3.2.1.31 — β-GUS, Method 3). Hydrolytically cleaved 5-bromo-4-chloro-3-indoxyl forms a ketone, which dimerizes under alkaline conditions into dehydroindigo and releases hydrogen ions. If NBT is added, it is reduced by these ions to blue formazan. Thus, the formation of insoluble formazan and an indigo dye occurs simultaneously, resulting in development of sharp colored bands. An example is the detection method for alkaline phosphatase (3.1.3.1 — ALP, Method 2).

## PRODUCTS BEARING REDUCED THIOL GROUPS

There are at least three different methods for the detection of products bearing reduced thiol groups. The disulfide 5,5′-dithio-bis(2-nitrobenzoic acid), DTNB, reacts with a free thiol at pH 8.0 and yields a compound of yellow color. This reaction is used in the detection method for glutathione reductase (1.6.4.2 — GSR, Method 3). DTNB attached to polyacrylamide was synthesized and shown to be useful for detection of thiol-producing enzymes after PAG electrophoresis (3.1.1.7 — ACHE, Method 2; 3.1.3.1 — ALP, Method 9).[19]

The products bearing free thiol groups reduce ferricyanide to ferrocyanide which further reacts with mercury and yields a reddish-brown precipitating complex. For instance, this reaction is used to detect acetyl-CoA hydrolase (3.1.2.1 — ACoAH) and malate synthase (4.1.3.2 — MS).

Free thiol groups can also reduce tetrazolium salts via the intermediary catalyst dichlorophenol indophenol, resulting in formation of insoluble formazan (see also *Products Reducing Tetrazolium Salts*, above). Examples include the detection methods for glutathione reductase (1.6.4.2 — GSR, Method 2) and citrate synthase (4.1.3.7 — CS).

A starch–iodine chromogenic reaction also can be used to detect enzymes that use or produce compounds bearing reduced thiol groups (for details see the next section).

## PRODUCTS THAT INFLUENCE THE STARCH–IODINE REACTION

The starch–iodine chromogenic reaction has been known for more than a century. However, iodine ($I_2$) is insoluble in water. Its solubility increases considerably in the presence of iodide ($I^-$), so KI is usually included in iodine solutions. Some compounds influence the starch–iodine reaction due to their ability to reduce iodine to iodide, which fails to react with starch. Such reductive properties toward iodine are displayed by some compounds bearing free thiol groups, e.g., by reduced glutathione. On the contrary, oxidized glutathione does not preclude the formation of the starch–iodine chromophore. Thus, positively stained zymograms can be obtained after starch gel electrophoresis (or electrophoresis in PAG containing soluble starch) by the use of the starch–iodine reaction for those enzymes that convert reduced glutathione into its oxidized form. The examples are detection methods for glutathione transferase (2.5.1.18 — GT, Method 1) and glyoxalase 1 (4.4.1.5 — GLO, Method 3). Using the starch–iodine reaction negatively stained zymograms will be obtained for enzymes that convert oxidized glutathione into its reduced form. In principle, glutathione reductase can serve as a good candidate for application of the starch–iodine detection method; however, several more sensitive and practical methods are available for detection of this enzyme (1.6.4.2 — GSR).

Hydrogen peroxide influences the starch–iodine reaction due to its ability to oxidize iodide in acid conditions into iodine, which then takes part in formation of the starch–iodine colored complex. This property of hydrogen peroxide is used to obtain negatively stained zymograms of catalase (for details see *Hydrogen Peroxide,* above).

Enzymes that release iodine can be detected after electrophoresis in starch-containing gels using acid peroxide reagent.[20] The only enzyme detected by this method is glutathione transferase (2.5.1.18 — GT, Method 2). In this case the detection depends on the release of iodine from synthetic substrate (which is the iodide derivative) as a result of its conjugation with reduced glutathione and subsequent oxidation of the iodide to iodine. In gel areas where iodide is enzymatically liberated, blue staining develops due to starch–iodine complex formation.

## PRODUCTS OF POLYMERIZING ENZYMES

Some enzymes catalyze reactions of polymerization using specific polymeric molecules as primers. Detection of these enzymes is based on the elevation of concentration of polymeric molecules in those gel areas where polymerizing enzymes are located. The use of stains specific to polymeric molecules usually results in the appearance of intensely stained bands visible on a less intensely stained background. For instance, iodine solution is used as a specific stain for detection of starch or glycogen synthesized by phosphorylase (2.4.1.1 — PHOS, Method 1). Methylene Blue and Pyronin B are used as specific stains for poly(A)ribonucleotide molecules synthesized by polyribonucleotide nucleotidyltransferase (2.7.7.8 — PNT) and mRNA replicas produced by RNA-directed RNA polymerase (2.7.7.48 — RNAP).

In some cases when direct chromogenic staining of polymeric products is not possible, additional chemical treatments may be needed to visualize polymerase activity bands (e.g., see 2.4.1.5 — DS, Method 2).

## PRODUCTS OF DEPOLYMERIZING ENZYMES

There are many hydrolytic enzymes that display depolymerizing activity toward such polymeric molecules as polypeptides, RNA, DNA, polysaccharides, and mucopolysaccharides. The general principle of the methods used to detect depolymerizing enzymes is the incorporation of a specific polymeric substrate into a reactive agarose plate, which is held in contact with an electrophorized gel. After incubation of this "sandwich" for a sufficient period of time, a substrate-containing agarose plate is treated with a substrate-precipitating agent, washed to remove the low-molecular weight-products of depolymerization, and specifically stained for general proteins, nucleic acids, polysaccharides, or mucopolysaccharides. Depolymerase activity areas appear as achromatic bands on colored backgrounds. Examples of the "sandwich" method are detection procedures for endopeptidases (3.4.21-24... — PROT), endonucleases (3.1.21.1 — DNASE; 3.1.27.5 — RNASE, Method 1), and endoglucanases (3.2.1.6 — EG).

In some cases depolymerase activity bands become visible just after treatment with a substrate-precipitating agent, so that no addi-

tional staining of substrate-containing gel is needed. The example is the detection method for polygalacturonase (3.2.1.15 — PG).

Different modifications of the "sandwich" method have been developed. Some of them consist of methods using colored substrates and are based on decoloration of the substrate-containing agarose gels in those areas that are in contact with areas of depolymerizing enzyme located in separating gels. The examples are detection methods for cellulase and endoxylanase (3.2.1.4 — CEL, Method 2; 3.2.1.8 — EX). The inclusion of polymeric substrates into the separating gel matrix may be preferable for detection of depolymerizing enzymes, which may be renatured after electrophoresis in sodium dodecyl sulfate (SDS)-containing gels, where SDS is used to inactivate depolymerizing enzymes and prevent substrate hydrolysis during the run. This modification is advantageous because separated enzymes do not need to diffuse out of the separating gel and, therefore, isozymes with slight differences in electrophoretic mobility can be readily differentiated (e.g., 3.2.1.4 — CEL, Method 2, Notes; 3.1.21.1 — DNASE, Notes).

The separating starch gel itself serves as a substrate for amylase (3.2.1.1 — α-AMY, Method 1) and phosphorylase (2.4.1.1 — PHOS, Method 3).

All methods described above are "negative" in the sense that color is formed by a chromogenic reaction with the substrate. These methods are usually used in a two-step procedure. The exceptions are those methods where colored substrates are used.

# Section 2
# Fluorogenic Reactions

Fluorogenic reactions are those that result in formation of a fluorochrome at sites of enzymatic activities in electrophoretic gels. Fluorochromes are molecules that, being irradiated by UV light, reradiate with emission of light of a longer wavelength. "Positive" fluorescent methods depend on the generation of a highly fluorescent product by an enzyme action on a nonfluorescent substrate(s). On the contrary, "negative" fluorescent methods depend on the generation of a nonfluorescent product from a fluorescent substrate.

The more widely used in electrophoretic zymography are the natural fluorochromes NADH and NADPH, which lose their fluorescent properties upon oxidation. There is also a diverse group of artificial fluorochromes. Among these, 4-methylumbelliferon is the most widely used.

## NADH AND NADPH

Positive fluorescent zymograms may be obtained for almost all NAD(P)-dependent dehydrogenases that generate NAD(P)H from NAD(P). These dehydrogenases are usually detected using the tetrazolium method, which is more convenient because it results in the development of dehydrogenase activity bands visible in daylight (see Section 1, *Products Reducing Tetrazolium Salts*). However, positive fluorescent stains are less expensive than tetrazolium stains because they do not require PMS and a tetrazolium salt. These stains are valuable for detection of some dehydrogenases that are inhibited by PMS or require reduced glutathione for their activity, which causes nonspecific formation of formazan (1.1.1.205 — IMPDH; 1.2.1.1 — FDH; 2.4.2.8 — HPRT, Method 2). For some dehydrogenases activated by manganese ions the positive fluorescent stains may be more sensitive than the tetrazolium stains because of the inhibitory effect of manganese ions on the action of PMS as electron carrier intermediary (1.1.1.40 — ME, Notes; 1.1.1.42 — IDH, General Notes).

Negative fluorescent stains are less sensitive and less convenient than positive ones. This is because the concentration of fluorescent substrates (NADH or NADPH) needs to be adjusted very carefully so as to enable detection of nonfluorescent products (NAD or NADP) against a fluorescent background. If NADH or NADPH concentrations are too low, the fluorescence of the gel background may not be sufficiently intense to detect nonfluorescent bands of NAD or NADP generated by backward dehydrogenase reactions. On the contrary, if NADH or NADPH concentrations are too high, dehydrogenase isozymes of low activity may not be able to oxidize all NADH or NADPH molecules and, thus, to be detected as nonfluorescent bands on a fluorescent background. Nevertheless, negative fluorescent stains are important and valuable for detection of the NADH- and NADPH-dependent activities of some reductases [e.g., 1.1.1.1 — ADH, Method 2; 1.1.1.2 — ADH(NADP), Method 2 and General Notes; 1.6.4.2 — GSR, Method 1]. These stains are very useful for detecting some dehydrogenases using backward reactions if the substrates for the forward reactions are not available or are too expensive (e.g., see 1.1.1.17 — M-1-PDH, Method 2; 1.5.1.17 — ALPD, Method 2 and General Notes). Finally, the backward NADH- or NADPH-dependent reactions of exogenous dehydrogenases are widely used as the end-point reactions in enzyme-linked detection methods. In these cases the negative fluorescent zymograms are also obtained. Many different enzymes are detected by enzyme-linked negative fluorescent methods. For example, lactate dehydrogenase is used as the linking enzyme to detect pyruvate-producing enzymes. The stains for those enzymes depend on detection of nonfluorescent NAD against a background of fluorescent NADH (e.g., 2.6.1.2 — GPT, Method 1; 2.7.1.40 — PK, Method 1). Exogenous lactate dehydrogenase in combination with exogenous pyruvate kinase is widely used for negative fluorescent detection of ADP-producing enzymes (e.g., 2.7.1.6 — GALK, Method 2; 2.7.1.30 — GLYCK, Method 3; 2.7.1.35 — PNK; 2.7.3.2 — CK, Method 1; 2.7.3.3 — ARGK, Method 2; 2.7.4.3 — AK, Method 2).

In general, when the backward NADH- or NADPH-dependent reaction of any exogenous dehydrogenase is used to detect the end product, negative fluorescent zymograms are obtained. Many different dehydrogenases are used as linking enzymes in negative fluorescent stains. These are glycerol-3-phosphate dehydrogenase (e.g., 2.2.1.2 — TALD, Method 1), glyceraldehyde-3-phosphate dehydrogenase (e.g., 2.7.2.3 — PGK), malate dehydrogenase (e.g., 2.6.1.1 — GOT, Method 2), octopine dehydrogenase (e.g., 2.7.3.3 — ARGK, Method 3), saccharopine dehydrogenase (e.g., 4.1.1.20 — DAPD), glutamate dehydrogenase (e.g., 4.3.2.1 — ASL, Method 1).

## 4-METHYLUMBELLIFERONE

The positive fluorescent stains that are based on the use of the artificial fluorochrome, 4-methylumbelliferone, are very sensitive and especially valuable for the detection of hydrolytic enzymes. Such derivatives of this fluorochrome as esters and glycosides do not fluoresce. However, being freed upon hydrolytic cleavage of the ester or glycosidic linkages, 4-methylumbelliferone restores its fluorescent properties. 4-Methylumbelliferone exhibits optimum fluorescence in alkaline conditions, while the great majority of hydrolases exhibit optimal activity in acid conditions. Thus, the positive fluorescent stains that employ derivatives of 4-methylumbelliferone as substrates usually are applied in two-step procedures. The first step is the incubation of electrophorized gel with acid substrate solution, and the second step is making the surface of the gel alkaline by using ammonia vapor or an alkaline buffer. The examples of positive fluorescent stains based on the use of 4-methylumbelliferone derivatives are the detection methods for esterases (3.1.1... — EST, Method 2), phosphatases (3.1.3.1 — ALP, Method 3; 3.1.3.2 — ACP, Method 2), phosphodiesterase I (3.1.4.1 — PDE-I, Method 1), arylsulfatase (3.1.6.1 — ARS, Method

1), cellulase (3.2.1.4 — CEL, Method 3), sialidase (3.2.1.18 — SIA), α-glucosidase (3.2.1.20 — α-GLU, Method 1), β-galactosidase (3.2.1.23 — β-GAL, Method 1), etc.

## PRODUCTS THAT FORM LUMINESCENT LANTHANIDE CHELATES

Luminescent lanthanide chelates are compounds that consist of a lanthanide ion (e.g., $Tb^{3+}$ or $Eu^{3+}$) bound to an organic chelating molecule capable of absorbing ultraviolet light and then transferring the excitation energy to the bound lanthanide ion, which emits luminescence in the green-to-red region of the spectrum.[21]

Artificial substrates were synthesized for alkaline phosphatase, β-galactosidase, and xanthine oxidase, which are converted by enzymatic action into the product salicylic acid, which then forms the luminescent lanthanide chelate after treatment with $Tb^{3+}$ ions and ethylene diamine tetraacetate (EDTA) in alkaline conditions (3.2.1.23 — β-GAL, Method 5). The lanthanide chelate luminescence is easily visible to the naked eye under a UV lamp emitting in the mid-ultraviolet range (300 to 340 nm) and can be photographed on Polaroid instant film using a time-resolved photographic camera.[22]

The hydrogen peroxide molecules produced by numerous oxidases cannot interact directly with a lanthanide ion and form a luminescent lanthanide chelate. However, in the presence of light and hydrogen peroxide the 1,10-phenantroline-2,9-dicarboxylic acid dihydrazide (PDAdh) is converted into the product, 1,10-phenantroline-2,9-dicarboxylic acid (PDA), which forms a luminescent lanthanide chelate in the presence of $Eu^{3+}$ ions. This conversion is due to photoassisted oxidation of PDAdh to PDA by hydrogen peroxide followed by formation of the Eu:PDA luminescent complex. In principle, the use of this phenomenon allows detection of numerous oxidases that produce hydrogen peroxide (see Section 1, on *Hydrogen Peroxide*). This approach, however, is not widely used now because PDAdh is not yet commercially available and should be synthesized under laboratory conditions.[22] Glucose oxidase (1.1.3.4 — GO, Method 2) is the only enzyme that can be detected by this method at present.

The lanthanide luminescent methods have several disadvantages that restrict their wide application. The first one is that the luminescent products readily diffuse in a solution. To minimize undesirable diffusion, the staining solutions should be applied as 1% agar overlays. The problem of diffusion of a lanthanide chelate product was solved for alkaline phosphatase (3.1.3.1 — ALP, Method 10) by the use of the 5-*tert*-octyl- substituent of the substrate salicyl phosphate. The bulky, hydrophobic nature of this substituent minimizes diffusion of the product 5-*tert*-octylsalicylic acid, especially when alkaline phosphatase transferred on a nylon membrane is detected.[21] Another disadvantage of the lanthanide luminescent methods is that some of the substrates involved in luminescent detection are not yet commercially available and should be synthesized under laboratory conditions (3.2.1.23 — β-GAL, Method 5, Notes). Finally, the detection of enzyme activity by this method cannot be carried out in a one-step procedure when derivatives of salicylic acid are used as substrates. This is because highly alkaline conditions (pH 12.5) are required for optimal formation of the luminescent ternary complex salicylic acid:$Tb^{3+}$:EDTA. These conditions are not compatible with those required for normal action of any enzyme under analysis. Fortunately, this is not the case for enzymes producing hydrogen peroxide, where formation of the luminescent lanthanide complex occurs at considerably lower pHs so that the enzyme detection can be carried out in a one-step procedure (1.1.3.4 — GO, Method 2).

The main advantage of the lanthanide chelate luminescent methods is their high sensitivity, which in some cases is comparable to or even higher than that obtained with radioisotopic detection methods.[21] Again, these methods are of good perspective because they can be used for detection of a great number of hydrolases and oxidoreductases after synthesis of convenient substrates suitable for formation of luminescent lanthanide chelates.[22]

## MISCELLANY

There is also a heterogeneous group of natural and artificial fluorochromes that are used in positive fluorescent stains of separate enzymes. These are oxidized homovanilinic acid and bieugenol (1.11.1.7 — PER, Notes), 5-dimethylaminonaphthalene-1-sulfonyl (2.3.2.13 — PGGT, Other Methods; 2.8.1.1 — TST, Method 2; 2.8.1.3 — TTST; 4.2.1.1 — CA, Other Methods, B), fluorescein (3.1.1... — EST, Method 3; 4.2.1.1 — CA, Method 2, Notes), Bromocressol Blue (4.2.1.1 — CA, Method 1, Notes), naphthylamine (3.4.19.3 — OPP; 3.4.21-24... — PROT), antranilate (4.1.3.27 — AS), uroporphyrin (4.3.1.8 — UPS), and flavanone (5.5.1.6 — CI, Notes).

Ethidium bromide is the only fluorochrome that is used in negative fluorescent stains (3.1.21.1 — DNASE, Notes; 3.1.27.5 — RNASE, Method 1, Notes).

# Section 3
# Autoradiography

There is a group of positive zymographic methods that depend on the detection of radioactive products by conventional autoradiography on X-ray film. These methods are based on separation of the radioactively labeled products from their labeled precursors. There are several different approaches to separate radioactive substrates and products.

The first approach is to precipitate the radioactive product in a gel matrix and wash away the substrate. Lanthanum chloride is used to precipitate such phosphorylated products as phosphosugars (e.g., 2.4.2.3 — UP; 2.7.1.6 — GALK, Method 1), glycerone phosphate (2.7.1.30 — GLYCK, Method 1), and nucleoside monophosphates (e.g., 2.7.1.20 — ADK, 2.7.1.74 — DCK; 2.7.1.113 — DGK). Such products as phosphoproteins and aminoacyl tRNAs are precipitated using trichloroacetic acid (e.g., 2.7.1.37 — PROTK; 6.1.1.2 — TRL), and DNA is precipitated by streptomycin (2.7.7.7 — DDDP).

Another approach is to use an ion exchange process to bind the radioactive products to special papers that incorporate an ion exchanger and wash away the radioactive substrates. The ion exchange papers used for this purpose are acetate cellulose (e.g., 2.1.1.6 — CMT), DEAE cellulose (e.g., 2.4.2.7 — APRT), and nitrocellulose (e.g., 3.4.21.31 — UK, Method 1).

Radioactively labeled streptavidin is used as a specific probe to detect enzymes that are biotinyl-proteins. This method is specific for plant acetyl-CoA carboxylase (6.4.1.2 — ACC), which is the only known biotinyl-protein in plants.

The ability of some enzymes to transfer the product molecules to its own molecules gives a good opportunity to detect their activity in electrophoretic gels using radioactively labeled substrates. Separation of a labeled substrate from a labeled product is achieved by precipitations of the enzyme–product complex with trichloracetic acid (e.g., 2.4.2.30 — NART).

Perhaps only one negative enzyme-detecting method based on precipitation of the radioactively labeled substrate and washing away the labeled product is now in practical use (3.1.3.5 — 5′-N, Method 1), though in the past such methods were used for detection of some depolymerizing enzymes.

As Harris and Hopkinson[7] have pointed out, the radioactive methods can be applied to the analysis of a variety of enzymes. They are of good resolution and sensitivity. However, they are disadvantageous because there is inevitably a time lag of a week or more between carrying out electrophoresis and seeing the results. At present, the radioactive methods are usually used only for those enzymes which cannot be detected by any other more practical procedure.

# Section 4
# Bioautography

The term "bioautography" was introduced for the first time to designate a detection system used to identify vitamins after paper chromatography.[23] After separation of vitamins, chromatographic paper was placed in contact with an agar layer containing mutant bacteria requiring certain vitamins for their growth and proliferation. The areas of bacterial proliferation were easily visible on a transparent agar layer.

A similar bioautographic procedure was developed for visualization of enzymes on electrophoretic gels using bacterial stocks with different auxotrophic mutations and naturally occurring stocks of fastidious yeast.[24,25] Deficient bacteria or yeast that cannot utilize the substrate of the enzyme to be detected and require the product of the enzyme reaction for growth are used. After indicator agar containing mutant bacteria, minimal medium, and a certain substrate(s) is placed in contact with electrophorized gel and incubated for a sufficient period of time, the areas of a certain enzyme being detected become visible as opaque bands on a translucent background of indicator agar.

The most important step in the application of the bioautographic method for the detection of certain enzymes is the selection of an appropriate auxotrophic mutant. A strain of bacteria deficient in a particular enzyme is the logical choice to detect corresponding plant or animal enzymes. However, the substrate of the enzyme under study must not be metabolized by alternative pathways in the bacterium. Another requirement is that the end product of the enzyme reaction must be transported into the bacteria (e.g., some phosphorylated products do not penetrate the bacterial cell wall). Finally, the bacterial strain must have a low frequency of reverse mutations that lead to prototrophy.

In order to test whether or not a bioautographic procedure can be developed with a given bacterial strain, the following test is recommended.[25] About $10^7$ bacteria should be inoculated into 5 ml of each of the following media: (1) medium lacking the nutrient, i.e., the end product of the enzyme reaction; (2) medium lacking the nutrient but containing the substrate for the enzyme; (3) medium containing the nutrient, and (4) medium containing both the substrate and the nutrient. The bacteria are suitable for bioautography if they grow only in the medium containing nutrient. The compositions of media for E. coli and P. cerevisiae are presented in Appendix A-1 and Appendix A-2, respectively.

Enzymes detected by bioautography, the stocks of bacteria used, and related information are presented in the Table on the next page.

It should be pointed out that bioautographic methods are not in wide use. This is because bioautography is not practical and because visualized bands of enzymatic activities usually are not sufficiently sharp due to diffusion of enzymatic products. However, bioautography is of great value for visualization of enzymes that are difficult or impossible to detect using other methods.

# Section 5
# Two-Dimensional Gel Spectroscopy

An optical technique termed "two-dimensional gel spectroscopy" has been developed which permits one to analyze two-dimensional electrophoretic gels in a fashion that is essentially identical to the routine spectrophotometric or fluorometric methods of analysis of enzymes in solution.[26] The principle of two-dimensional gel spectroscopy involves the irradiation of electrophorized PAG (or translucent agarose replica) at a desired wavelength and subsequent analysis of the gel at a desired wavelength for absorption or fluorescent bands that arise as a result of enzymatic conversion of a substrate to an optically detectable product.

Special optical apparatus may be constructed from commercially available optics.[26] The apparatus can both generate and detect monochromatic light at any wavelength from 200 nm in the ultraviolet to greater than 4500 nm in the infrared. Highly monochromatic light of a particular wavelength is selected by the proper choice of interference filters. This light is of spectral purity comparable to that obtained with a spectrophotometer that utilizes a grating monochromator. The light emanating from the gel is analyzed using a catadioptric lens, which has a spectral transmission from 200 to 4500 nm and utilizes first surface mirrors in order to image objects on the film plane. The use of mirrors permits the transmission of ultraviolet and infrared light that would be absorbed by glass lenses. A standard f/1.2, 55-mm camera lens is used at wavelengths above 400 nm.

Photographic films suitable for recording signals from approximately 200 to 1100 nm are commercially available.[27,28] For the recording of fluorescence Kodak Tri-X (ASA 400) film is employed. A high-contrast image is obtained with Kodak Technical Pan 2415 film in situations in which light is not a limiting factor. Exposure times are determined empirically. This is because each filter combination requires a different amount of light for proper exposure.

By means of two-dimensional gel spectroscopy, enzymes can be detected in transparent gels under conditions that are identical to those employed in spectrophotometric and fluorometric methods under which enzymes are operationally defined. The choice of the proper

interference filter(s) depends on the spectral characteristics of the substrates and products and the intensity of mercury lines in the desired area of the spectrum. Thus, the conditions to be employed in the detection of a certain enzyme are predictable either from the literature or from routine spectrophotometric assays.

At present, the method is not widely used because the apparatus needed for two-dimensional gel spectroscopy is not commercially available. Only three enzymes have so far been detected by two-dimensional gel spectroscopy. These are lactate dehydrogenase (1.1.1.27 — LDH, Other Methods, C), monoamine oxidase (1.4.3.4 — MAOX, Other Methods, A), and trypsin (3.4.21.4 — T, Other Methods, C). However, since many published spectrophotometric or fluorometric methods can be used virtually without change, two-dimensional gel spectroscopy is of great potential value for electrophoretic zymography of many previously undetectable enzymes.

# Section 6
# Immunoblotting

In the present context, immunoblotting refers to techniques for transferring separated zones of proteins from electrophoretic gels to immobilization matrices and subsequent detection of certain immobilized proteins using specific antibodies and anti-antibodies that are radiolabeled or linked with an indicator enzyme (see *The Flowchart for Immunoblotting* on the next page).[29-31]

## IMMOBILIZATION MATRICES

One of the most widely used immobilizing matrices is nitrocellulose (NC). A nitrocellulose membrane with 0.45-μm pore size is most commonly employed. However, NC membranes with other porosities also may be of value. For example, material with 0.22 μm pore size may be preferable for low-molecular-weight proteins. In addition to the NC the nylon-based membrane "Zetabind" (ZB) available from AMF Cuno Division (Meriden, Connecticut) has been introduced for protein blotting. This material is also marketed as "Zeta Probe" by Bio-Red Lab (Richmond, California) and "Hybond-N" by Amersham (Arlington Heights, Illinois). The ZB membrane possesses several advantages. It is as thin and fine-grained as a NC membrane but mechanically

**DEFICIENT BACTERIA EMPLOYED IN BIOAUTOGRAPHY OF SOME ENZYMES**[24-26]

| Enzyme to be detected | Bacterial stock[a] | Bacterial mutation | Bacterial enzyme defect | Nutritional requirement[b] |
|---|---|---|---|---|
| 2.4.2.7 — APRT | *E. coli* (PC 0273) | pur A⁻ | Adenylosuccinate synthase | Adenine |
| 3.5.4.4 — ADA | *E. coli* (PC 0273) | pur A⁻ | Adenylosuccinate synthase | Adenine |
| 6.3.4.5 — AS | *E. coli* (AB 1115) | arg G⁻ | Argininosuccinate synthase | Arginine |
| 4.3.2.1 — ASL | *E. coli* (AT 753) | arg H⁻ | Argininosuccinate lyase | Arginine |
| | *P. cerevisiae* (ATCC 8081) | —[c] | Arginine biosynthesis | Arginine |
| 3.4.21.4 — T | *E. coli* (AT 753) | arg H⁻ | Argininosuccinate lyase | Arginine |
| 1.1.1.27 — LDH | *E. coli* (CB 482) | lct⁻ | L-Lactate dehydrogenase | Pyruvate |
| 3.5.1.14 — AA | *P. cerevisiae* (ATCC 8081) | —[c] | Aminoacylase | Methionine |
| 2.6.1.42 — BCT | *P. cerevisiae* (ATCC 8081) | —[c] | Branched chain amino acid biosynthesis | Isoleucine (or leucine or valine) |
| 1.5.1.3 — DHFR | *P. cerevisiae* (ATCC 8081) | —[c] | Dihydrofolate reductase | Folinic acid |

[a]  *E. coli* K12 stocks from the *E. coli* Genetic Stock Center at Yale University Medical School; *P. cerevisiae* ATCC 8081 (American Type Culture Collection, strain 8081).

[b]  Each bacterial stock may have other requirements.

[c]  Naturally occurring auxotroph.

stronger and has about a sixfold higher protein-binding capacity. In addition, the highly charged cationic nature of the ZB matrix results in better transfer of proteins from SDS-containing gels in which proteins are present as complexes with anionic SDS molecules.

A number of other immobilizing matrices were also introduced, but they are not in such wide use for protein blotting as are NC and ZB membranes.[32]

## TRANSFER OF PROTEINS

There are two main ways of transferring proteins from electrophoretic gels onto the immobilizing matrix: )1) capillary blotting and (2) electroblotting.

Capillary blotting consists in transferring of proteins by means of solvent flow.[33] In this method the transfer is achieved by placing the gel onto several thicknesses of filter paper or Whatman 3MM paper wetted with transfer buffer and supported on a piece of sponge with the same buffer. A sheet of transfer membrane is placed on top of the gel, then several pieces of dry filter paper and paper towels are placed above the transfer membrane and held together with a light weight (usually 0.5 to 1.0 kg). The buffer flows from the sponge and wet filter paper through the gel carrying the protein molecules onto the transfer membrane, through which the buffer passes and is absorbed by dry filter papers. Overnight blotting is usually enough to transfer sufficient amounts of proteins to be detected.

Electroblotting employs electrophoretic elution of the proteins.[29] The procedure consists of wetting a sheet of transfer membrane and placing it on the gel, which is supported by a porous pad (e.g., foam sponge or layers of wet filter paper) mounted on a stiff plastic grid. No air bubbles should be trapped between the gel and transfer membrane. A second porous pad and plastic grid are placed above the transfer membrane. The "sandwich" is then strengthened with rubber bands and placed in a tank of transfer buffer between two electrodes.

Electrophoretic gel buffers of low ionic strength are usually used as transfer buffers for capillary blotting and electroblotting. The voltage gradients of 5 to 10 V/cm enable transfers to be essentially complete in 1 to 3 h. The use of lower gradients requires longer times for complete transfer. For transfer of proteins from SDS-containing gels, neutral or weakly basic buffers are used. In these conditions the proteins migrate as anions and the NC membrane must be on the anode side. In general, it is important to know the net charge of the proteins to be transferred under the conditions used to choose the correct side of the gel on which the transfer membrane must be placed.

One reason for the increased effectiveness of ZB membranes in protein transfer relates to the lack of requirement for methanol in the transfer buffer. Methanol was introduced because it was found to increase the binding capacity of NC membranes for proteins. However, methanol also reduces the efficiency with which proteins are eluted from gels, and electroblotting must therefore be carried out for at least 12 h to obtain efficient transfer of high-molecular-weight proteins, especially when 10% PAG is used. When ZB membranes are used, methanol need not be present in the transfer buffer. This

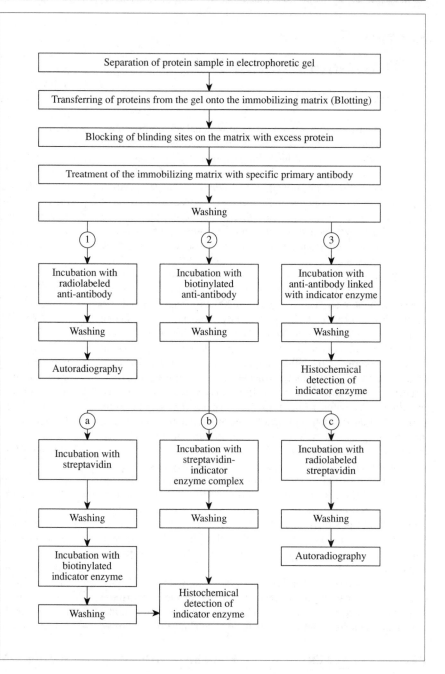

*The Flowchart for Immunoblotting.*

increases the detection sensitivity and reduces diffusion of protein molecules because the time of electroblotting can be reduced considerably.

## SPECIFIC ANTIBODIES AND LABELED ANTI-ANTIBODIES

Specific primary antibodies against certain enzymes can be obtained by routine immunization procedures using pure enzyme preparations and subsequent separation of immunoglobulins, which are essentially polyclonal antibodies specific to different immunogenic determinants of the same enzyme molecule.

Monoclonal primary antibodies specific to certain enzymes are of special value and good perspective for immunohistochemical or immunoautoradiographic detection of enzymes immobilized on NC or ZB membranes.[34] Monoclonal antibodies specific to certain proteins are produced by specific hybridomas.[35] The construction of specific hybridoma includes the following steps:

1. Immunization of the mouse with crude protein preparation
2. Separation of lymphocytes from the spleen of the immunized mouse
3. Hybridization of lymphocytes with myeloma cells (the malignant cells of the immune system)
4. Cloning of somatic cell hybrids
5. Selection of the clone(s) that produces antibodies specific to certain enzymes or isozymes

Among all the known advantages of monoclonal antibodies, the feasibility of using unpurified protein preparations to produce monospecific antibodies is very useful for specific detection of the enzyme proteins immobilized on the supporting matrix.

Species-specific second antibodies, or anti-antibodies, can be obtained by routine immunization of sheep, goat, rabbit, or donkey with species-specific immunoglobulins. When monoclonal antibodies produced by hybridomas are used as primary antibodies, anti-antibodies specific to mouse immunoglobulins should be used as second antibodies. Different species-specific anti-antibodies are now commercially available, e.g., from Sigma Chemical Company or from Amersham. These are (1) radiolabeled anti-antibodies, (2) biotinylated anti-antibodies, and (3) anti-antibodies linked with indicator enzyme (see the Flowchart). Biotinylated anti-antibodies are used in couple with (a) streptavidin and biotinylated indicator enzyme, (b) streptavidin–indicator enzyme complex, or (c) radiolabeled streptavidin or protein A. Peroxidase, β-galactosidase, and alkaline phosphatase are usually used as indicator enzymes.

## DETECTION OF TRANSFERRED PROTEINS ON BLOTS

After blotting, any given protein can be visualized on immobilizing membrane by the methods pictured in the Flowchart. An important step in immunological detection of transferred proteins is the blocking of all additional binding sites on the matrix with immunologically neutral protein. Usually 1 to 5% bovine serum albumin, ovalbumin, hemoglobin, or fish skin gelatin dissolved in buffered saline solution is used to saturate excess protein-binding sites. This process was termed "quenching". Buffered Tween 20 was also shown to be a very useful agent for quenching NC membranes.[36] After quenching, an immobilizing membrane is incubated with the appropriate dilution of specific primary antibody in quenching solution and rinsed in quenching solution. After this treatment three different methods may be used to visualize antigen–primary antibody complex (Flowchart). The most direct ways (as designated on the Flowchart) are (1) the treatment of the membrane with radiolabeled anti-antibody, and subsequent washing and autoradiography; or (3) the treatment of the membrane with anti-antibody linked with an indicator enzyme, washing, and subsequent histochemical detection of an indicator enzyme using appropriate histochemical procedures described in Part III for peroxidase, β-galactosidase, or alkaline phosphatase, which are commonly used as indicator enzymes in immunoblotting procedures. Another, more complex way (2) includes the treatment of the membrane with biotinylated anti-antibody and subsequent washing of the membrane. After this, three different procedures may be employed. The first one includes incubation of the membrane with streptavidin to form a streptavidin bridge, washing the membrane, incubation with biotinylated indicator enzyme, a second washing, and histochemical detection of an indicator enzyme. The second method includes treatment of the membrane with streptavidin–indicator enzyme complex, washing and subsequent histochemical detection of an indicator enzyme. The third method includes incubation of the membrane with radiolabeled streptavidin, washing, and autoradiography.

Immunoblotting in conjunction with the use of monoclonal antibodies is valuable for the detection of specific enzymatic and nonenzymatic proteins on electrophoretic gels. At present, however, considerable time, energy, and expense are involved in the production of hybridoma antibodies. This is perhaps the main reason why the diversity of commercially available protein-specific monoclonal antibodies is not very rich and why immunoblotting is not widely used in electrophoretic zymography. The near-absence of commercially available monoclonal antibodies specific to enzymes is also the main reason why immunoblotting methods are not given in this handbook in details but are cited in Part III as "Other Methods" only for those enzymes for detection of which more practical alternative methods are also available. The examples are carbonic anhydrase (4.2.1.1 — CA, Other Methods, C), 6-phosphofructokinase (2.7.1.11 — PFK, Other Methods, A), and pyruvate kinase (2.7.1.40 — PK, Other Methods). Nevertheless, the growing body of information on successful construction of hybridomas producing monoclonal antibodies specific to different enzymes allows one to be optimistic in respect to future wide applications of immunoblotting methods in electrophoretic zymography.[34] Moreover, a relatively simple and rapid method of immunization that gives polyclonal antibodies of high specificity has been developed recently.[37] This method includes the following steps: (1) separation of proteins by two-dimensional gel electrophoresis, (2) transfer of proteins onto NC membrane by blotting technique, and (3) immunization of rabbits by specific proteins bound to a NC matrix after cutting out of corresponding protein spots on the NC membrane and powdering of the membrane pieces by sonication.

# References for Part II

1. Seligman, A. M. and Rutenberg, A. M., The histochemical demonstration of succinic dehydrogenase, *Science*, 113, 317, 1951.
2. Markert, C. L. and Möller, F., Multiple forms of enzymes: tissue, ontogenetic, and species specific patterns, *Proc. Natl. Acad. Sci. U.S.A.*, 45, 753, 1959.
3. Pearse, A. G. E., *Histochemistry. Theoretical and Applied, Volume I*, Williams & Wilkins Co., Baltimore, 1968.
4. Burstone, M. S., *Enzyme Histochemistry*, Academic Press, New York, 1962.
5. Hunter, R. L. and Markert, C. L., Histochemical demonstration of enzymes separated by zone electrophoresis in starch gels, *Science*, 125, 1294, 1957.
6. Martin de Llano, J. J., Garcia-Segura, J. M., and Gavilanes, J. G., Selective silver staining of urease activity in polyacrylamide gels, *Anal. Biochem.*, 177, 37, 1989.
7. Harris, H. and Hopkinson, D. A., *Handbook of Enzyme Electrophoresis in Human Genetics*, North-Holland, Amsterdam (Loose leaf with supplements in 1977 and 1978), 1976.
8. Gomori, G., Microtechnical demonstration of phosphatase in tissue sections, *Proc. Soc. Exp. Biol. Med.*, 42, 23, 1939.
9. Gomori, G., Distribution of acid phosphatase in the tissues under normal and under pathologic condition, *Arch. Pathol.*, 32, 189, 1941.
10. Nimmo, H. G. and Nimmo, G. A., A general method for the localization of enzymes that produce phosphate, pyrophosphate, or $CO_2$ after polyacrylamide gel electrophoresis, *Anal. Biochem.*, 121, 17, 1982.
11. Fiske, C. H. and Subbarow, Y., The colorimetric determination of phosphorus, *J. Biol. Chem.*, 66, 375, 1925.
12. Fisher, R. A., Turner, B. M., Dorkin, H. L., and Harris, H., Studies on human erythrocyte inorganic pyrophosphatase, *Ann. Hum. Genet.*, 37, 341, 1974.
13. Zlotnick, G. W. and Gottlieb, M., A sensitive staining technique for the detection of phosphohydrolase activities after polyacrylamide gel electrophoresis, *Anal. Biochem.*, 153, 121, 1986.

14. Klebe, R. J., Schloss, S., Mock, L., and Link, C. R., Visualization of isozymes which generate inorganic phosphate, *Biochem. Genet.*, 19, 921, 1981.

15. Cornell, N. W., Leadbetter, M. G., and Veech, R. L., Modifications in the enzymatic assay for inorganic phosphate, *Anal. Biochem.*, 95, 524, 1979.

16. Lowry, O. H., Schulz, D. W., and Passoneau, J. V., Effects of adenylic acid on the kinetics of muscle phosphorylase a, *J. Biol. Chem.*, 239, 1947, 1964.

17. Thorup, O. A., Strole, W. B., and Leavell, B. S., A method for the localization of catalase on starch gels, *J. Lab. Clin. Med.*, 58, 122, 1961.

18. Ohlsson, B. G., Weström, B. R., and Karlsson, B. W., Enzymoblotting: a method for localizing proteinases and their zymogens using *para*-nitroanilide substrates after agarose gel electrophoresis and transfer to nitrocellulose, *Anal. Biochem.*, 152, 239, 1986.

19. Harris, R. B. and Wilson, I. B., Polyacrylamide gels which contain a novel mixed disulfide compound can be used to detect enzymes that catalyze thiol-producing reactions, *Anal. Biochem.*, 134, 126, 1983.

20. Clark, A. G., A direct method for the visualization of glutathione S-transferase activity in polyacrylamyde gels, *Anal. Biochem.*, 123, 147, 1982.

21. Templeton, E. F. G., Wong, H. E., Evangelista, R. A., Granger, T., and Pollak, A., Time-resolved fluorescence detection of enzyme-amplified lanthanide luminescence for nucleic acid hybridization assays, *Clin. Chem.*, 37, 1506, 1991.

22. Evangelista, R. A., Pollak, A., and Templeton, E. F. G., Enzyme-amplified lanthanide luminescence for enzyme detection in bioanalytical assays, *Anal. Biochem.*, 197, 213, 1991.

23. Usdin, E., Shockman, G. D., and Toennies, G., Tetrazolium bioautography, *Appl. Microbiol.*, 2, 29, 1954.

24. Naylor, S. L. and Klebe, R. J., Bioautography: a general method for the visualization of enzymes, *Biochem. Genet.*, 15, 1193, 1977.

25. Naylor, S. L., Bioautographic visualization of enzymes, in *Isozymes: Current Topics in Biological and Medical Research, Volume 4*, Rattazzi, M. C., Scandalios, J. G., and Whitt, G. S., Eds., Alan R. Liss, New York, 1980, 69.

26. Klebe, R. J., Mancuso, M. G., Brown, C. R., and Teng, L., Two-dimensional spectroscopy of electrophoretic gels, *Biochem. Genet.*, 19, 655, 1981.

27. Kodak, *Kodak Plates and Films for Scientific Photography*, Kodak Tech. Publ. P-315. Eastman Kodak Co., Rochester, New York, 1973.

28. West, W., The spectral sensitivity of emulsions spectral sensitization, desensitization and other photographic effects of dyes, in *Neblette's Handbook of Photography and Reprography*, Sturge, J. M., Ed., Van Nostrand & Reinhold, New York, 1977, 73.

29. Towbin, H., Staehelin, T., and Gordon, J., Electrophoretic transfer of proteins from polyacrylamide gels to nitrocellulose sheets: procedure and some applications, *Proc. Natl. Acad. Sci. U.S.A.*, 76, 4350, 1979.

30. Burnette, W. N., "Western blotting": electrophoretic transfer of proteins from sodium dodecyl sulfate-polyacrylamide gels to unmodified nitrocellulose and radiographic detection with antibody and radiolabeled protein A, *Anal. Biochem.*, 112, 195, 1981.

31. Gershoni, J. M. and Palade, G. E., Protein blotting: principles and applications, *Anal. Biochem.*, 131, 1, 1983.

32. Andrews, A. T., *Electrophoresis: Theory, Techniques, and Biochemical and Clinical Applications*, Clarendon Press, Oxford, 1988.

33. Southern, E. M., Detection of specific sequences among DNA fragments separated by gel electrophoresis, *J. Mol. Biol.*, 98, 503, 1975.

34. Vora, S., Monoclonal antibodies in enzyme research: present and potential applications, *Anal. Biochem.*, 144, 307, 1985.

35. Köhler, G. and Milstein, C., Continuous cultures of fused cells secreting antibody of predefined specificity, *Nature*, 256, 495, 1975.

36. Blake, M. S., Johnston, K. H., Russell-Jones, G. J., and Gotschlich, E. C., A rapid, sensitive method for detection of alkaline phosphatase-conjugated anti-antibody on Western blots, *Anal. Biochem.*, 136, 175, 1984.

37. Diano, M., Le Bivic, A., and Hirn, M., A method for the production of highly specific polyclonal antibodies, *Anal. Biochem.*, 166, 224, 1987.

# III ——————— Methods of Detection of Specific Enzymes

This part is central for the book. It contains detailed descriptions of more than 500 enzyme-specific zymogram techniques suitable for visualization on electrophoretic gels of more than 300 different enzymes. The information presented therein is traditionally arranged around the "enzyme sheet", which includes basic information required for the detection of a particular enzyme. At the beginning of this part, additional information of general relevance to the enzyme sheets is given. It includes a description of the structure of an enzyme sheet, general considerations, comments and recommendations concerning application of zymogram techniques, as well as resource-saving strategies, troubleshooting, and safety measures. Abbreviations commonly used in the enzyme sheets are also given there.

## Section 1
## The Structure
## of Enzyme Sheets

The enzymes considered in this part are presented in numerical order according to the EC numbers recommended by the Nomenclature Committee of the International Union of Biochemistry.[1] Each enzyme sheet is presented in a set format and includes information on enzyme reaction, enzyme source, specific zymogram methods (with four types of information given for each method: visualization scheme, staining solution, procedure, and notes), additional methods, general notes, and references.

As a rule, the recommended enzyme name is given in the enzyme sheet headline while additional enzyme names are presented for cross-reference purposes in the section "Other Names". The enzyme symbols used are the same as the enzyme abbreviations most commonly encountered in the literature. Some symbols (while absent from the literature) are constructed as upper-case abbreviations in accordance with specific recommendations.[2,3] Thus, the enzyme sheet heading includes the EC number, and full and abbreviated names of the enzyme, for example, "**1.1.1.1 — Alcohol dehydrogenase; ADH**". An alphabetical list of all the enzymes considered is given for convenience in Appendix B.

The enzyme reaction adapted from the enzyme list published by the Nomenclature Committee of the International Union of Biochemistry[1] is given in each enzyme sheet under the subheading "Reaction".

Groups of living organisms that are sources of the specific enzyme are listed in the section "Enzyme Source" to address more directly the application of specific zymogram methods to the certain groups of organisms. This information was selected from the book *Enzymes* by Dixon and Webb,[4] current literature, current reference books, and catalogs of several chemical companies.

More than one principally different zymogram techniques are given for many enzymes. Information on each separate technique is given in the section "Method", which is subdivided into four subsections.

The diagram of the reaction sequence involved in the enzyme detection is schematically pictured in the subsection "*Visualization Scheme*". A general principle was used to construct such diagrams for the great majority of the enzyme-detection methods described in this book. According to this principle, arrows indicate the direction of the reactions leading to visualization of the enzyme activity bands on the electrophoretic gels. All the participants of the enzyme-detection reactions are given. Reagents included in the staining solution are given in bold type. All enzyme names are abbreviated, with the abbreviated names of the linking enzymes deciphered in the recipe of the staining solution. The abbreviated name of the enzyme being detected is enclosed in a box. The final product that enables the enzyme to be visualized is indicated by UV when registered in ultraviolet light or VIS when registered in daylight; for those compounds that change color during the reaction, VIS′ indicates the initial color and VIS indicates the color after the change. When the visualization procedure is a compound process that should be carried out sequentially step by step, different stages of the procedure are indicated on the reaction diagram. In some cases (e.g., when the scheme of autoradiographic procedure is given) different stages depicted on the diagram are supplied with additional information for convenience (e.g., "*Stage 1: Enzyme reaction*", "*Stage 2: Washing the gel*", etc).

The subsection "*Staining Solution*" ("*Reaction Mixture*" and "*Indicator Agar*" for autoradiographic and bioautographic methods, respectively) gives the recipe for the reaction mixture used to visualize areas occupied by the enzyme on electrophoretic gel. The reference for the given recipe is also presented. Efforts have been made to obtain the recipes from the original articles in which they were first published. This goal, however, was not always achieved because many of the original recipes were modified throughout the years and the accumulated changes were not always well documented. The recipe may include several subrecipes, designated A, B, C, etc., when the compound-visualization procedure should be carried out in a step-by-step fashion or when the preparation of the staining solution should be carried out by successive mixing of solutions prepared separately according to subrecipes. As a rule, the recipes are given in the form in which they are presented in the cited paper. As a consequence, in some recipes the involved reagents are given in absolute quantities while in others they are given in concentrations. Each of the two modes of presentation of reagents in a recipe has its own advantages and disadvantages, therefore no attempt has been made for overall standardization of the recipe presentation.

The subsection "*Procedure*" contains a detailed description of sequential procedures leading to the development of enzyme activity bands on an electrophoretic gel and, thus, represents a peculiar "know-how" of the method. It may be subdivided when a compound procedure of the enzyme visualization is described. The information on the mode of documentation of results obtained and some peculiarities of preservation of stained gels is also given there.

Diverse information that is of value for more successful application of the method and more adequate interpretation of obtained results is given under the subheadline "*Notes*". This information (if any) includes remarks concerning possible artifacts generated by the method and recommendations on control gel stainings, when they are needed. It also includes recommendations concerning possible counterstaining procedures used to make stained bands more contrasting and clearly visible, highlights some important details of the mechanism involved in the enzyme-detection system, etc.

The section "Other Methods" initially included those methods for which the author had information concerning only general principles of the enzyme visualization. However, during the writing of the book this section was filled with methods that seemed supplementary or not widely used. For example, such detection methods as bioautography, two-dimensional spectroscopy, and immunoblotting were referred to as "Other Methods" when more simple and practical or commonly used zymogram methods were available for the enzyme under consideration. Methods that seemed adequate but had not been used so far to detect the enzyme under consideration were also given under "Other Methods", as recommended for application. It is not excluded for some enzymes that such methods may prove even more useful in comparison with the methods given in the section "Method".

"General Notes" are given after description of all the main zymogram methods developed for the enzyme under consideration. These notes give additional information that is of value for all the methods described for the enzyme. These are remarks on the enzyme substrate specificity, specific inhibitors and activators, comparative analysis of different detection methods, etc.

The list of "References" is given for each enzyme at the end of the enzyme sheet. The original papers are included in the list when possible to indicate the priority in development of the enzyme detection methods. In some cases where there are many references, those which contain reviews are preferred.

## REFERENCES

1. Nomenclature Committee of the International Union of Biochemistry, *Enzyme Nomenclature*, Academic Press, Orlando, 1984.
2. Shows, T. B., and 24 coauthors, Guidelines for human gene nomenclature. An international system for human gene nomenclature (ISGN), 1987), *Cytogenet. Cell Genet.*, 46, 11, 1987.
3. Shaklee, J. B., Allendorf, F. W., Morizot, D. C., and Whitt, G. S., Gene nomenclature for protein-coding loci in fish, *Trans. Am. Fish. Soc.*, 119, 2, 1990.
4. Dixon, M. and Webb, E. C., *Enzymes*, Academic Press, San Diego, 1979.

# Section 2
# General Considerations, Comments, and Recommendations

## THE CHOICE OF SUPPORT MEDIUM FOR ENZYME ELECTROPHORESIS AND DETECTION

The principles of detection of enzymes on electrophoretic gels are not dependent upon the type of support medium used for enzyme separation. However, in practice, the adequate choice of support medium is of great importance. This is because

1. The quality of zymograms obtained via enzyme-detection methods depends upon characteristics that differ significantly in different support media.
2. A certain support medium may be preferable, when a certain biological object is used as the source of the enzyme.
3. The choice of a certain support medium may depend upon the question to be answered and the resources available to the researcher.
4. A number of zymographic methods are adapted or are recommended to be preferably applied to a certain support medium.

At present the most popular support media are starch, cellulose acetate, and polyacrylamide. Many of the characteristics that should be taken into account during the choice of support medium have been discussed by many authors.[1-5] The most important of them are considered below.

## Cellulose Acetate Gel

The cellulose acetate gel requires only 0.5 to 2 µl per sample per enzyme run and, thus, is the medium of preference when many enzymes must be detected from single small samples. The use of cellulose acetate may be highly desirable when small samples are more easily obtained than large ones (e.g., such a situation is usual for isozyme studies of cell cultures or cultures of microorganisms). It is also preferable when enzyme stains containing very expensive ingredients should be used. This is because the 30 by 15 cm cellulose acetate sheets usually require not more than 3 ml of the staining solution. Cellulose acetate gels are commercially available and are ready for loading with samples after 10 min of soaking in an appropriate electrophoretic buffer. Only 1 h is usually needed to run cellulose acetate gels using relatively low run voltages. This allows, if necessary, the electrophoretic separation of enzymes to be carried out at room temperature without special cooling devices. Enzyme activity bands develop on cellulose acetate gels quickly because of the high porosity of the gel matrix and since the ingredients of the staining solution easily diffuse into the gel. This advantage is especially valuable when the procedure for the enzyme detection involves exogenous linking enzyme(s) of high molecular weight(s). Electrophorized cellulose acetate gels can be frozen before or after the completion of the staining and thus can be available for further reference. Finally, cellulose acetate gels are durable and flexible, allowing the stained gel to be handled without unnecessary caution.

On the other hand, cellulose acetate gels cannot be sliced into a number of thin gels in the fashion of starch gel blocks. They are more expensive than equivalent starch or polyacrylamide gels, not translucent, and so cannot be quantified by densitometric methods without additional treatment. Cellulose acetate gels display reduced stain intensity for isozymes with low activity because only small volumes of samples can be applied to the gel. This support medium does not have the ability to cause a molecular sieving effect because of its coarse pore structure. So it separates proteins primarily on charge, with little or no separation on size. Finally, electroendosmosis does occur to an appreciable extent with just this support medium. In practice, however, at least some of these disadvantages are not critical. Indeed, the electroendosmosis usually does not affect the relative mobility of allozymes and isozymes. Again, it may be reduced by the use of relatively more concentrated electrophoretic buffers. The absence of the molecular sieving effect does not play any important role in separation of allozymes, which usually do not differ markedly in molecular weight or shape. The gel slicing may offer no advantage in peculiar situations that commonly occur during biochemical systematic studies. For example, during interspecific comparisons, each compared locus may require specimens from different species to be applied to a gel in a locus-specific order, placing side by side just those allozymes that need to be tested for identity or difference. As to the relatively high cost of the cellulose acetate gels, it should be pointed out that equivalent starch or polyacrylamide gels are actually more costly when labor costs are included. If densitometric scanning is desired, stained cellulose acetate gels can be cleared by washing them in 5% acetic acid, treating with 95% ethanol for 1 min, and immersing in 10% acetic acid and 90% ethanol mixture for 5 min. Before scanning, the gel should be dried and heated on a glass plate at 60 to 70°C for 20 min.

It should also be kept in mind that the use of cellulose acetate strips (i.e., the nongel form) does not give as good resolution of allozymes and isozymes as cellulose acetate gels do. Cellulose acetate gels are produced by a number of manufacturers; the most popular is "Cellogel" made by Chemetron (Milan, Italy).

The excellent handbook by Richardson et al.[4] contains comprehensive information on the application of cellulose acetate gels for isozyme and allozyme analysis and is recommended for more detailed consultation.

## Polyacrylamide Gel

This support medium is formed by the vinyl polymerization of acrylamide monomers and cross-linking of the formed long polyacrylamide chains by the bifunctional co-monomer $N,N'$-methylene-bis-acrylamide in anaerobic conditions in the presence of such catalysts as ammonium persulfate and $N,N,N',N'$-tetramethylethylenediamine, or 3-dimethylaminopropionitrile. The main advantages of polyacrylamide gels are as follows:

1. The composition of the gel can be modified in a controlled way to achieve the best separation of the isozymes under question due to optimal molecular sieving effect.
2. The gel matrix is highly homogeneous.
3. The gel is clear and can be directly subjected to quantification of enzyme activity bands by densitometry.
4. The results obtained with polyacrylamide gels are highly reproducible.
5. The use of this support medium allows detection of enzymes after electrophoresis of very dilute samples (e.g., some biological fluids, extracts of algal tissues, etc.).
6. The denaturing SDS-polyacrylamide gel system is the only electrophoretic medium suitable for analysis of many nonwater-soluble monomeric enzymes that can be renatured after appropriate treatments.
7. The sharpest protein bands are obtained with this support medium.
8. The polyacrylamide gels are rigid and thus are convenient for handling.

It is commonly acknowledged at present that polyacrylamide gel is the best medium for separation of different classes of nonenzymatic proteins. This is, however, not always true for enzymatic proteins because of at least several pronounced disadvantages of this gel towards electrophoretic analysis of enzymes.

The first and the most critical disadvantage is the formation of nongenetic secondary isozymes as a result of the action of residual nonreacted persulfate, an oxidizing agent, which can cause structural modifications of enzyme molecules or the loss of their catalytic activity. Polyacrylamide gels always contain a small residual fraction of unpolymerized acrylamide monomers, which also can react with enzymatic molecules. This drawback may be eliminated by pre-electrophoresis treatment, but only if continuous electrophoretic buffer systems are used. When the use of discontinuous buffer systems is needed, the polymerized gel should be soaked for a period of days in several changes of an appropriate gel buffer. This diminishes the value of polyacrylamide gel in large-scale electrophoretic analysis of enzymes.

The next disadvantage of polyacrylamide gel is the almost total impossibility to slice gel blocks into thin gel plates. This considerably limits the multilocus analysis from one electrophoretic run.

When vertical polyacrylamide gels are used, only isozymes moving towards one electrode (usually anode) are detected. Hence, two separate runs are needed to detect both anodally and cathodally moving isozymes. This problem can be avoided by the use of horizontal gel slabs, which allows the placing of samples anywhere in the slab. Positioning samples in the middle of the gel causes isozymes migrating towards either one or both electrodes to be observed on the same gel. The use of horizontal gel blocks, however, does not allow exploitation of the most important advantage of vertical polyacrylamide gels, i.e., its value for analysis of very dilute samples with low enzyme concentration.

A problem with detection of some enzymes on polyacrylamide gels can occur when visualization mechanisms involve linking enzymes of large molecular weight. This is because of the slow diffusion of such enzymes into the polyacrylamide gel matrix. Indeed, most separations of enzymes are carried out with 5 to 12% polyacrylamide gels, which optimally separate proteins with a molecular weight range of 20,000 to 150,000.[5] So, diffusion of such routine linking enzymes as, for example, xanthine oxidase from milk (mol wt 290,000), or glutamate dehydrogenase from liver (mol wt 1,000,000) into commonly used 7.5% gels will be very slow if at all.

Finally, both acrylamide and bis-acrylamide are highly toxic, and even very dilute solutions of these monomers can cause skin irritation and disturbance of the central nervous system. Polymerized gel, however, is relatively nontoxic and can be handled safely.

## Starch Gel

At present starch gel is the most popular support medium for enzyme electrophoresis in population genetics and biochemical systematics studies. This is due to some critical advantages of starch gel over other support media.

The main advantage of this support medium is that starch gel blocks can be easily sliced into several gel slices. As many as eight to ten slices can be obtained from a gel block 1 cm thick. This affords a researcher the ability to reveal the genotype of an individual for a much larger number of genic loci in one run than is possible with any other support medium. This characteristic of starch gel is especially valuable for large-scale isozyme and allozyme screenings. It allows rapid assessment of the genetic composition of a population, and (or) the multilocus identity of individuals.

Being a natural biological product, starch does not contain any undesirable admixtures capable of inactivating enzymes or causing *in vitro* generation of nongenetic secondary isozymes, as is characteristic of polyacrylamide gel. This simplifies isozymal patterns displayed on zymograms and makes them more easily interpretable in genetic terms, especially for those enzymes that are represented by multiple isozymal forms. The degree of resolution attainable by electrophoresis on starch gel is exceeded only by that attainable with polyacrylamide gel. Starch gel works well with samples the size of a fruit fly. Some zymographic techniques (e.g., those based on the use of the starch–iodine chromogenic reaction) were developed specifically for starch gel.

At the same time, starch gel has some disadvantages, which are, however, not critical and do not considerably diminish its value for large-scale isozyme and allozyme surveys. When compared with polyacrylamide and cellulose acetate the following disadvantages of starch gel are usually listed:

1. Different lots of commercially available hydrolyzed starch supplied by different (and even the same) manufacturers usually differ in composition and may contain differing proportions of amylose and amylopectin, which can affect gelling ability and resolution. Thus, it is essential that each new lot of starch be thoroughly tested in order to calibrate it before use.
2. Starch gel is not translucent and so not suitable for direct quantitative measurement by densitometry. However, it can be relatively easily rendered transparent by soaking it in hot (70°C) glycerol for a few minutes, or by soaking it first in water:glycerol:acetic acid (5:5:1 by volume) and then overnight in pure glycerol. The lack of uniformity of the starch gel matrix also makes it less suitable for densitometric quantitation in comparison with polyacrylamide gel. Again, this disadvantage is not critical for population genetics surveys because the great majority of electrophoretically detectable intra- and interspecific allozymic and isozymal differences are qualitative rather than quantitative.
3. Conventional starch gel stains usually involve volumes of 25 to 50 ml, which is about one order more than is required for staining of cellulose

acetate gels of the same size. The amount of staining solution, however, can be reduced considerably by the use of an appropriate procedure for stain application. For example, only 6 ml of the stain is just enough to cover the cut surface of the gel (30 × 20 cm) if applied dropwise with a Pasteur pipette.

4. Starch gel is more friable than polyacrylamide or cellulose acetate gels and is not easy to handle; however, there are usually no serious problems with handling starch gel for those who have spent a day for special practice.

The choice of the most appropriate support medium is a very important step in any survey that uses enzyme electrophoresis. Usually no single support medium is *a priori* superior to any other. Each of the three media discussed above has its own particular characteristics that should be taken into account depending on the problem to be solved, the biological object to be used as the enzyme source, the battery of enzymes to be analyzed, the resources available to the researcher, and other factors and circumstances. The correct choice of support medium will allow one to save time and money and to obtain more adequate data for solving the problem under investigation.

## STRATEGIES OF GEL STAINING

Several important questions which should be optimally resolved usually arise in connection with staining electrophoretic gels. The main ones are

1. The choice of a more appropriate zymogram method, when more than one detection method is available for the enzyme under question
2. The choice of procedure for the faster and more correct preparation of functional staining solution
3. The choice of the mode of application of staining solution to electrophoretic gel
4. The choice of methods allowing an increase in the staining intensity of the enzyme activity bands
5. The choice of the adequate staining of control gels for the assurance that the chosen zymogram method is specific for the enzyme under analysis

Unfortunately, each choice depends on many factors that may not be predicted with certainty beforehand. The most important characteristics of these factors are given below, with the purpose of allowing one to choose an optimal strategy of gel staining depending on the circumstances.

### The Choice of Zymogram Method

This book comprises about 500 different zymogram methods developed for more than 300 different enzymes. Thus, for many enzymes two or more principally different zymogram methods are available. Different methods developed for the same enzyme may differ in

- Their applicability to a certain support medium
- Sets of reagents and special equipment needed
- Sensitivity
- Stain compatibility in double staining of the same gel
- Time and labor demands
- Methods of quantification of the resulting zymograms
- Sharpness and stability of stained bands
- Modes of band registration and zymogram preservation
- The cost of information obtained, etc.

These differences should be taken into account when making the choice of the more optimal zymogram method, depending on species and tissues that are thought to be used as the enzyme source, the support medium that is planned to be used or which has already been chosen,

the problem under study, the resources available, the kind and quality of information that must be obtained, etc. It is obvious that in each situation the choice of an optimal zymogram method will be the result of a complex compromise.

### Preparation of Staining Solution

Each staining solution is buffered with the staining buffer at a specific pH. The pH value of the staining buffer used for the enzyme stain is a compromise between (1) the pH-optimum of the enzyme activity, (2) the pH-optimum of the staining reaction(s) used in the detection method, (3) the pH value of the buffer used for preparation of the gel, and (4) the pH-optimum of the linking enzymes, if those are involved in staining reaction(s).

Many substrates (e.g., those used by dehydrogenases) are acids. In such cases stronger buffering capacity is required. Therefore, the use of high-concentration staining buffers is recommended. In some cases the substrates are such strong acids that their solutions must be prepared and brought to neutral pH before being added to staining solutions. Some commercially available substrates are unstable or very expensive. Solutions of such substrates can be prepared enzymatically in the laboratory. An example is glyceraldehyde-3-phosphate (see 1.2.1.12 —GA-3-PD, Method 1). It is a good practice to add substrates and other ingredients to staining buffers but not vice versa. This prevents the possible sharp decrease of the pH value of the staining mixture to a level at which the enzyme under analysis will not function or other ingredients of the stain will be inactivated. For example, the reduced forms of NAD and NAD(P) cofactors denature in acid conditions very quickly. Dry chemicals should be taken out of the refrigerator or freezer about half an hour before preparation of staining solutions. This lets them warm up and prevents condensation. It is a general rule to add ingredients to the staining buffer in the sequence given in the recipe of the stain. The intermediate and final pH values should be checked for staining solutions that include acids or that are prepared for the first time.

For large-scale population surveys of isozymes the preparation of stock solutions of reagents that are used regularly is recommended. The use of stock solutions allows one to prepare staining solutions quickly and accurately, to use only minimal quantities of expensive reagents, and to reduce the number of times the refrigerated chemicals are opened. This mode of stain preparation is especially valuable when large numbers of samples are being run for only a few enzymes. On the contrary, when as large as possible a number of enzymes are needed to be stained only once, the use of dry reagents is preferable. Many workers with much experience in stain preparation use "analytical spatula" and simple eye control to weigh most dry reagents, unless they are very expensive or proportions of the stain ingredients are critical. For example, the amounts of NADH or NADPH added to the negative fluorescent stains are critical. If too little amounts are added, the background will not fluoresce sufficiently, but when too much is added, the detected enzyme [or NAD(P)H-dependent linking enzyme] will not be able to convert sufficient quantities of NAD(P)H into NAD(P) for nonfluorescent bands to become visible. Substrates at a high concentration can sometimes inhibit enzymatic activity. An example is the brain isozyme of octopine dehydrogenase in cuttlefish. When a negative fluorescent method is used to detect this enzyme, the use of pyruvate concentration higher than 2 m$M$ is not recommended (see 1.5.1.11 — ONDH, Method 2, Notes). Again, special care should be taken with some couplers and dyes that can display inhibitory effects on catalytic activity of some enzymes when they are above certain critical concentrations or even at relatively low levels. Examples are some diazo dyes, which have inhibitory effects on acid phosphatase (see 3.1.3.2 — ACP, Method 3, Notes) and the PMS/MTT system, which inhibits some dehydrogenases [e.g., see 1.1.1.22 — UGDH and

1.1.1.138 — MD(NADP)]. Many of the staining mixtures tolerate, to some extent, variations in the amounts of their ingredients. It should be remembered, however, that use of substrate concentrations that are only somewhat lower than saturation levels can cause weak staining of enzymatic bands. On the other hand, substrate concentrations that are sufficiently higher than saturation levels usually do not reduce the staining intensity of enzymatic bands. Therefore, when unique and precious material is analyzed or when the optimal substrate concentration for the enzyme under analysis is not known, the use of higher substrate concentrations is recommended. The same is true for linking enzymes. The concentration of linking enzymes should also be increased when their activity is decreased as a result of storage. However, when a particular staining solution is used regularly the possibility of reduction of the quantity of expensive ingredients usually exists. The recipes of staining solutions presented in this part often involve the addition of excess amounts of reagents. Thus, it is usually possible to reduce the amounts of the more expensive reagents and thus the total costs of stains.

As a rule the use of allozymes and isozymes as genic markers does not require quantitative measurements. Thus, the exact quantitative standardization is usually not necessary when preparing the same staining solution to detect allele frequencies or to compare isozyme patterns in different populations or in samples taken from the same population at different times.

It is a general rule to prepare staining solutions as quickly as possible and just before use. The speed of the stain preparation is often more important than the precision. This is especially true for large-scale surveys in which many enzymes are to be stained. The speed of stain preparation may in some cases be the most important limiting condition, essential for the production of functional staining solutions.

The main limitation of the use of reagents as stock solutions is their instability. The stock solutions usually involve only those reagents that are stable in solutions for at least several weeks. When two or more reagents have been mixed in a solution, the stain should be further prepared as quickly as possible. On the other hand, the mixtures of dry reagents essential for visualization of some enzymes can be stored in a refrigerator for a long time while being desiccated. The use of dry reagent mixtures is advantageous for electrophoretic enzyme assays that are to be carried out under field conditions. At present some producers are beginning to supply enzyme-detection kits that are ready for use. For example, Innovative Chemistry, Inc. (P.O. Box 90, Marshfield, MA 02050) supplies kits suitable for detection of 18 different human enzymes. The only thing that must be done with the kit is to reconstitute one vial of enzyme reagent with a certain volume of deionized water and to pour the resulting staining solution over the surface of the electrophoretic gel.

It should always be remembered that the use of reagents (especially substrates and linking enzyme preparations) of high purity will allow one to avoid many problems caused by the use of low-quality reagents containing concomitants, which can interfere with other compounds and make the staining mixture nonfunctional or result in development of artifactual or nonspecifically stained bands. In many cases the cost of high-quality reagents is of secondary concern, because the most expensive "ingredients" in enzyme electrophoretic surveys are labor, time, and the precious collected material.

Amounts of staining solutions sufficient for gel staining vary considerably depending on the size of the gel to be stained and the mode of application of the staining solution to the gel.

## Modes of Application of Staining Solutions

Staining solutions can be applied directly to the surface of electrophoretic gels or used as filter paper or agar overlays. A standard staining solution method is the earliest and the most widely used. It consists of placing electrophoretic gel (or gel slice) in a special staining tray, adding the staining solution until the gel is completely covered by fluid, and incubation of the gel at room temperature or 37°C (usually in the dark) until enzyme activity bands are visible. Specifically designed staining trays made of glass or plexiglass are usually used for this purpose. It is better to use a staining tray that exactly fits the size of the gel to be stained. If the trays for gel staining are larger than the gel, the amount of staining solution will have to be increased. This is not desirable because stains are usually expensive. For the staining tray that exactly fits the size of the 300 cm² gel, only about 50 ml of staining solution is needed to cover the top surface of the gel with fluid. However, this method is not always practical since many stains include reagents that are too expensive to be maintained at effective concentrations in large volumes. The problem can be overcome by preparing the concentrated staining solution in a small total volume which is just enough to flood the gel surface if applied dropwise with a pipette. Automatic adjustable-volume pipettes with disposable plastic tips or simple Pasteur pipettes are usually used for this purpose. The stain diffuses directly into the gel where the visualization reaction takes place. When the dropwise application method is used, only about 3 ml of staining solution is needed to stain a gel of 300 cm² size. Another method of application may also be recommended. It comprises placing a glass rod on the edge of the gel, pouring the staining solution on the gel above the glass rod, and spreading the solution evenly over the gel surface with the glass rod. When dealing with cellulose acetate gels, small amounts of staining solution can be applied by spreading it evenly on the glass plate to the width of the gel and subsequent spreading of the stain over the gel surface by placing the gel, with the porous side down, onto the solution, avoiding the formation of air bubbles between gel and glass plate. Methods that use small amounts of concentrated staining solutions are applicable to cellulose acetate gels and cut surfaces of starch and (less frequently) polyacrylamide gels. It is important to point out that application and spreading of small amounts of staining solutions should be done as quickly as possible to prevent uneven entrapping of the fluid by the gel matrix and subsequent uneven staining intensity of the enzyme activity bands in different parts of the gel. After the stain is absorbed (usually after 1 to 5 min) the gel should be covered with a sheet of plastic wrap sufficiently large to fully enclose the gel and protect it from drying during incubation.

Many stains, predominantly those which are based on positive or negative fluorescence, are applied to the gel using the filter-paper overlay method. This method requires considerably less stain than the standard staining solution method based on the use of staining trays and requiring the immersion of the whole gel into the staining solution. When the period of time of gel incubation is expected to be longer than 30 min, the paper–gel sandwich should be covered with a sheet of plastic wrap of appropriate size. Filter and chromatographic paper (Whatmann No. 1 and 3MM) are usually used in this method. Cellulose acetate strips are also used sometimes and work even better than filter paper, but they are more expensive. The filter-paper overlay method is useful for negative staining of enzymatic bands using negative fluorescent stains containing NAD(P)H in couple with subsequent counterstaining of the gel with a PMS/MTT mixture. In this case the areas of the gel occupied by the enzyme are indicated by achromatic bands on a blue background of the gel and paper. Moreover, the precipitation of blue formazan in the paper is preferential. Thus, the stained paper may be easily washed, fixed, dried, and stored for a permanent record.

Staining solutions can also be applied as a 1:1 mixture with 2% molten agar (or agarose) cooled to 50 to 60°C. After preparation the mixture is quickly poured uniformly over the gel and allowed to cool and solidify. It should be remembered when using this method that if the agar solution is too hot it can inactivate some reagents, e.g., linking enzymes, but if it is too cold it can solidify just in the process of mixing with the staining solution. The agar overlay method has the advantage of bringing the reagents into intimate contact with the enzyme molecules to be stained for, and it also prevents diffusion of the stained bands, especially when the final product of the enzyme visualizing reaction is soluble or when coupled enzymatic reactions generating soluble intermediates are involved in the enzyme visualizing mechanism. Usually, the bands of enzymatic activity are well visible on the transparent agar layer. It can easily be taken off from the electrophoretic gel and the developed bands quantified by scanning densitometer. Placed on a sheet of filter paper and dried, the developed agar layer may be stored for a long time and used as a permanent record of the zymogram. The agar overlay method is the only method suitable for detection of enzymes on nontransparent gels by two-dimensional gel spectroscopy. At present this method is one of the most popular methods of stain application in starch gel electrophoresis of enzymes.

The reactive agarose plate method is a modification of the agar overlay method. In this method 1% agarose solution containing all reagents needed for visualization of the enzyme activity is poured into a tray that fits the size of the electrophoretic gel to be stained. After agarose solidification the electrophoretic gel is laid over the agarose in order to expose the reactive agarose to the gel-entrapped enzyme. This method is used for visualization of enzymes by bioautography. Thin substrate-containing agarose plates are also widely used for detection of many hydrolases with depolymerizing activity.

Each of the three main methods of application of staining solutions described above has its own advantages and disadvantages that depend on the type of support medium used for enzyme electrophoresis, the zymogram method chosen for visualization of the enzyme activity bands, the character and quality of information desired, and financial resources available. In general, however, the agar overlay technique gives better results than any other method and is always preferable when isozymes with high and low activity are presented on the same gel.

## Modes of Enhancement of Staining Intensity of Enzyme Activity Bands

These modes can be divided into two main groups. The first group is represented by methods that are applicable before the procedure of detection of enzyme activity bands. It includes methods of protection and activation of enzymes during preparation of enzyme-containing samples and their electrophoretic run. Some modifications of the sample application procedure can increase the sample amount applied onto the gel and, thus, increase the enzyme amount in the gel and the staining intensity of enzymatic bands on zymograms. These methods, however, have no direct relation to the procedure and mechanisms of the enzyme visualization and so are beyond the scope of this book. If interested, the reader may find more detailed information on the matter in other manuals on enzyme electrophoresis.[1,2,4,6-9]

The second group comprises methods that are applied during or after the procedure of visualization of enzyme activity bands. One of these methods is the so-called "post-coupling" technique. It is recommended for use when the staining solution contains a particular reagent(s) that inhibits catalytic activity of the enzyme to be stained. For example, acid phosphatase is inhibited by some "Fast" diazo dyes (see 3.1.3.2 — ACP, Method 3, Notes) while some dehydrogenases [see 1.1.1.22 — UGDH and 1.1.1.138 — MD(NADP)] are supposed to be inhibited by PMS or MTT, or both. In such cases all reagents except the potential inhibitor should be applied to the gel at the first step in the usual way. After incubation for an appropriate period of time (depending on the expected activity of the detected enzyme), the remaining reagent should be added to the stain. The main disadvantage of the post-coupling technique is that it is not always possible to monitor the intensity of the visualizing reaction over time. Indeed, the product of the phosphatase reaction, naphthol, becomes visible only

after coupling with diazo dye. Fortunately, the reaction catalyzed by NAD(P)-dependent dehydrogenases can be monitored under a UV lamp because the reaction products NADH or NADPH fluoresce in long-wave UV light. Thus, when the bands of NAD(P)H fluorescence are well developed, PMS/MTT mixture should be added to the stain to make dehydrogenase activity bands visible in daylight. Another disadvantage of the post-coupling technique is the diffuse character of the developed enzymatic bands. This is because of relatively small sizes of enzyme product molecules, which readily diffuse through the gel matrix before insoluble colored precipitates are formed.

Some NAD(P)-dependent dehydrogenases are activated by manganese ions. When the PMS/MTT system is used to detect such enzymes, weak staining intensity of the enzymatic bands can be observed because of the inhibitory effect of manganese ions towards PMS as electron acceptor (e.g., see 1.1.1.42 — IDH, Method 1, Notes). To overcome this problem diaphorase should be used in place of PMS (see 2.4.1.90 — AGS, Method 1, Notes), or the amount of PMS included in the stain should be increased several times. Another way is to observe the enzyme activity bands in long-wave UV light after incubation of the gel in staining solution lacking PMS and MTT. When applying PMS/tetrazolium stains it should also be kept in mind that PMS is not stable at high-alkaline pHs.[10] This can cause weak staining intensity of activity bands of dehydrogenases with high pH-optima or when staining solutions with erroneously high pHs are used. The positive fluorescent methods may be preferable over PMS/tetrazolium methods when the endogenous enzyme superoxide dismutase (also known as tetrazolium oxidase) comigrates with NAD(P)-dependent dehydrogenases and considerably reduces or even fully prevents development of their bands via PMS/tetrazolium stain.[11]

It may sometimes be desirable to increase the concentration of certain reagents (usually substrates, cofactors, and linking enzymes) in order to enhance the intensity of staining of the enzyme activity bands. The use of the agar overlay method for detection of weak-activity enzymes on cellulose acetate gels is preferable because it allows not only increasing the quantities of reagents applied but also prolonging the time of gel incubation.

In some cases weak staining of enzyme activity bands may be the consequence of inhibitory action of the enzyme reaction product towards the detected enzyme. To increase the speed of the enzyme reaction the product of enzymatic reaction should be trapped. An auxiliary enzyme that utilizes the product of the detected enzyme as its own substrate can be used for this purpose (see 2.6.1.1 — GOT, Method 4, Notes). Some original zymographic methods are based on the same mechanism (e.g., see 5.4.2.4 — BPGM). In some cases the excess products may be trapped and the intensity of band staining enhanced by the use of specific reagents. For example, such carbonyl-trapping reagents as hydrazine hydrate and aminooxiacetic acid are used to trap 2-oxoglutarate with the purpose of displacing the glutamate dehydrogenase reaction toward the production of NAD(P)H, which serves as a fluorescent indicator of the enzyme reaction.[12] As a result, the accelerated production of NAD(P)H intensifies the staining of glutamate dehydrogenase bands by the tetrazolium method (see 1.4.1.2-4 — GDH, Method 1, Notes).

The apparent activity of some enzymes can be doubled by linking it to two sequential reactions or to dehydrogenase 1/isomerase/dehydrogenase 2 sequential reactions, which produce two molecules of reduced or oxidized dehydrogenase cofactor. For example, two NADP-dependent sequentially acting dehydrogenases — glucose-6-phosphate dehydrogenase and 6-phosphogluconate dehydrogenase — are used to double the production of fluorescent NADPH in the positive fluorescent method developed for detection of galactokinase (see 2.7.1.6 — GALK, Method 3). Another example is the glycerol-3-phosphate dehydrogenase/triosephosphate-isomerase/glyceraldehyde-

3-phosphate dehydrogenase system of sequentially acting auxiliary enzymes, which can work in both directions and may be used to double the production of NADH (the forward direction) or NAD (the backward direction). Examples of the use of this linking enzyme system are detection methods for glycerol kinase (2.7.1.30 — GLYCK, Method 2), phosphoglycerate mutase (5.4.2.1 — PGLM, Method 1), and phosphoglycerate kinase (2.7.2.3 — PGK).

Fluorescence of 4-methylumbelliferone, which is the product of hydrolytic cleavage of 4-methylumbelliferone derivatives by numerous hydrolases, may be enhanced considerably by treating the developed acidic gels with an alkaline buffer (pH 9 to 10) or ammonia vapor.

The miniaturization of developed polyacrylamide gels by treatment with hot (70°C) 50% (w/v) polyethyleneglycol (PEG 2000) increases the sensitivity of enzyme-detection methods five to ten times.[13] Methanol-containing fixatives may be used to miniaturize (although to a less extent) developed starch gels (for details see *Recording and Preservation of Zymograms,* below).

## Specificity of Zymogram Methods and Some Related Problems

Most of the zymogram methods presented in this part are enzyme-specific. However, some methods can detect more than one enzyme. This results from the ability of some enzymes to utilize one or more of the applied reagents, or to use certain buffer constituents in couple with the applied staining solution reagents. Another reason for the development of unexpected enzymatic bands is the combined effect of two comigrating endogenous enzymes, one of which acts as a linking enzyme for the other in the presence of certain necessary reagents contained in the applied staining solution. Some enzymes can form complexes with cofactors and/or substrates that are stable during electrophoresis, or can use residual amounts of their substrates that are contained in some reagents as concomitants. Therefore, when other reagents needed for visualization reactions of such enzymes are available from applied staining solutions, the nonspecifically stained additional bands will appear. Finally, several cases are known when nonenzymatic protein bands or even nonprotein bands are developed by the use of certain stains.

Thus, when a new enzyme-detection method is developed or when an approved method is used to detect a certain enzyme from a new enzyme source, it should be tested for its specificity for the enzyme under analysis. This is especially necessary for complex methods involving one or more reactions catalyzed by exogenous linking enzymes. A standard procedure for testing specificity of the method to be used includes a series of experimental stainings in which each individual constituent of the stain is omitted one at a time in order to determine if any stained bands appear after treating control gels with incomplete stains. The specificity of the enzyme-detection method can also be tested by the use of alternative methods, if they are available for the enzyme under investigation, or if they may be devised by using a backward reaction, or by using a principally different mechanism of visualization, which involves different substrates, cofactors, sets of linking enzymes, etc.

Nonspecific staining of additional unexpected bands on zymograms of some enzymes is illustrated by the following examples.

Bands of adenylate kinase (see 2.7.4.3 — AK, Method 1) can develop on zymograms of pyruvate kinase (2.7.1.40 — PK, Method 2), creatine kinase (2.7.3.2 — CK, Method 2), and arginine kinase (2.7.3.3 — ARGK, Method 1). This is because all the reagents needed for AK detection (i.e., ADP, glucose, NADP, MTT, PMS, hexokinase, and glucose-6-phosphate dehydrogenase) are contained in staining solutions used to detect the enzymes listed above.

It is well established that adenylate kinase molecules have a monomeric subunit structure which is highly conserved during organismal evolution.[14] In this connection, the description of unusual allozymic polymorphisms of "dimeric" adenylate kinase revealed in some invertebrate and vertebrate animals[15-17] is rather the consequence of misleading interpretation of allozymic variation of nonspecifically stained bands of dimeric glucose dehydrogenase (see 1.1.1.47 — GD), which is widely distributed among different animal groups. To be developed, this dehydrogenase requires just those reagents (i.e., glucose, NADP, MTT, and PMS) that are present in the adenylate kinase stain.

When negative fluorescent methods are used to detect octopine dehydrogenase (1.5.1.11 — ONDH, Method 2) and alanopine dehydrogenase (1.5.1.17 — ALPDH, Method 2), the bands caused by lactate dehydrogenase activity also develop in some invertebrate species containing all these dehydrogenases.

Some phosphatases of invertebrates and vertebrates can use phosphoenolpyruvate as substrate and thereby produce pyruvate. Thus, the bands of phosphoenolpyruvate phosphatase activity can develop on pyruvate kinase zymograms obtained by a negative fluorescent method (2.7.1.40 — PK, Method 1, Note) and on zymograms of many other enzymes obtained using detection methods involving pyruvate kinase and lactate dehydrogenase as linking enzymes (e.g., see 2.7.3.2 — CK, Method 1; 2.7.3.3 — ARGK, Method 2; 2.7.4.3 — AK, Method 2; 2.7.4.4 — NPK; 2.7.4.8 — GUK, Method 1; 2.7.6.1 — RPPPK, Method 1).

It has been found that human aconitase isozymes can sometimes appear on zymograms obtained using staining solution lacking both the enzyme substrate, *cis*-aconitate, and the linking enzyme, isocitrate dehydrogenase.[2] This unexpected phenomenon was shown to occur only when electrophoresis was carried out using a citrate-containing buffer. It is known that aconitase is capable of catalyzing two reactions:

1. citrate = *cis*-aconitate + $H_2O$
2. *cis*-aconitate + $H_2O$ = isocitrate (see 4.2.1.3 — ACON).

Thus, aconitase can use citrate from a citrate-containing gel buffer as a substrate and thereby produce isocitrate. When aconitase comigrates with isocitrate dehydrogenase, staining occurs at those gel sites where two endogenous enzymes occur together. When one or both of these enzymes are polymorphic the individual differences in development of unexpected additional bands may be observed, because under these conditions both enzymes migrate to overlapping positions only in some individuals.

When a standard staining solution method is used to detect hexokinase (see 2.7.1.1 — HK), bands of 6-phosphogluconate dehydrogenase (1.1.1.44 — PGD) may also develop, especially when the gel is subjected to prolonged incubation. This is because the linking enzyme glucose-6-phosphate dehydrogenase utilizes the glucose-6-phosphate generated by endogenous hexokinase and produces glucono-1,5-lactone 6-phosphate, which spontaneously turns into 6-phosphogluconate, the substrate of 6-phosphogluconate dehydrogenase. The molecules of this substrate freely diffuse in the liquid stain and become available for endogenous 6-phosphogluconate dehydrogenase, for which bands may further develop in the presence of NADP, PMS, and MTT involved in the hexokinase stain. Of course, this is the case only when NADP-dependent glucose-6-phosphate dehydrogenase preparation is used in the hexokinase stain.

Additional unexpected bands are frequently observed on zymograms of NAD(P)-dependent dehydrogenases. These bands develop even when staining solutions lacking any dehydrogenase substrates are used. This effect has been referred to as "nothing dehydrogenase" (see I.X.X.X — NDH). Two main reasons are known to cause the NDH phenomenon: (1) binding of endogenous substrates by some dehydrogenase molecules, and (2) contamination of some commercial preparations with substances that serve as substrates for some dehydrogenases.

Two enzymes — alcohol dehydrogenase and lactate dehydrogenase — usually are the most probable candidates for NDH. The bands of NDH activity may be easily identified by their repetitive occurrence on gels stained for different dehydrogenases or other enzymes detected using linked dehydrogenase reactions.

Some nonenzymatic proteins can also cause the development of false bands on gels specifically stained for some enzymatic activities. At least four examples are known. The first one concerns SH-rich proteins, which are capable of reducing a tetrazolium salt even in the absence of NAD(P) and PMS.[18,19] The second example is the interference of albumins with the starch–iodine color reaction, resulting in the development of false amylase bands on zymograms obtained by the negative starch–iodine method.[20] Albumins are also known to be able to cause the appearance of additional artifactual bands on acid phosphatase[21] and alkaline phosphatase[22] zymograms obtained with the azo coupling methods. In the last case it is shown that the alkaline phosphatase–like activity in the albumin zone is an artifact due to a bilirubin/albumin complex that nonspecifically couples with a diazo compound.

When the samples used for electrophoresis contain high levels of endogenous reduced glutathione or other sulfhydryl compounds (e.g., 2-mercaptoethanol or dithiothreitol) added to the samples prior to electrophoresis to stabilize or activate the enzyme under analysis, the appearance of additional stained bands should be expected on zymograms obtained by the use of MTT/PMS-containing staining solutions. The bands caused by electrically neutral 2-mercaptoethanol and dithiothreitol molecules are usually detected in the cathodal part of starch gels because of the effect of electroendosmosis. Negatively charged molecules of reduced glutathione usually migrate to the very anodal part of the gel. The bands caused by all these thiol reagents are monomorphic, diffuse, and stained fairly weakly, and are observed on zymograms of different enzymes detected for the same samples by tetrazolium methods.

Two different enzymes with overlapping substrate specificity are able to catalyze the same reaction and thus to display their activity bands on the same zymogram. For example, it was shown that some isozymes of alcohol dehydrogenase from *Drosophila melanogaster* also oxidize L(+)-lactate or D(–)-lactate with NAD as cofactor and intraspecific electrophoretic variation observed on lactate dehydrogenase zymograms could be attributed to the presence of alcohol dehydrogenase.[23] This phenomenon was called "pseudopolymorphism". Another example is the existence of some isozymes in the snail *Cepaea nemoralis* that can utilize either malate or lactate as a substrate, converting both into pyruvate.[24] A special study has shown[25] that there are many enzymes that are listed in the enzyme list[26] under different code numbers although they are coded by one and the same gene in a wide range of organisms that represent phylogenetically distinct groups. As to dehydrogenases, identical allozymic patterns were revealed on zymograms of octanol dehydrogenase (1.1.1.73 — ODH), formaldehyde dehydrogenase (1.2.1.1 — FDH) and D-lactaldehyde dehydrogenase (1.1.1.78 — DLADH) from the sipunculid *Phascolosoma japonicum*. Identical allozymic variations were observed on zymograms of ODH and FDH in each of four bivalve species of the genus *Macoma* that were examined. In the phoronid *Phoronopsis harmeri* the allozymic pattern of ODH-1 isozyme was found to be identical with those of DLADH, while the allozymic pattern of ODH-2 isozyme was identical with that observed on the FDH zymogram. The same allozymic patterns were revealed on ODH, FDH (FDH-2 isozyme), and DLADH zymograms in the mushroom *Boletus edulis*. All these examples are evidence that certain dehydrogenases that are believed to be different proteins are really a single enzyme protein with broad substrate specificity. The same bands can also be observed on zymograms of acid and alkaline phosphatases, and on zymograms of different peptidases.

It was shown, for example, that numerous phosphatases from the sipunculid intestine display identical allozymic patterns in the same sample of conspecific individuals.[27] Similar results were obtained with hexokinase (2.7.1.1 — HK) and fructokinase (2.7.1.4 — FK) from mushroom, nemertine, domestic fly, starfish, and sea urchin.[25] Thus, a number of cases are known where enzymes that are believed to be different are encoded by a single genic locus, and the possibility exists to erroneously score the same locus twice or even more.

## RECORDING AND PRESERVATION OF ZYMOGRAMS

There are at least three different methods of recording the enzyme patterns developed on electrophoretic gels: (1) schematic recording of zymograms, (2) photography of zymograms, and (3) the tracing of band position on paper overlays or cellulose acetate gels. After recording, zymograms can be stored in special fixative solutions or dried.

Schematic recording of zymograms involves a two-dimensional representation of the banding patterns observed on developed gels. Although such representation suggests some degree of simplification and subjectivity, it can be excused during routine surveys of well-known enzyme polymorphisms.

Another technique that allows keeping a permanent record of the results of each electrophoretic experiment is photography. The main advantage of photographs is their objectivity. They are relatively rapidly produced and easy to store. Stained cellulose acetate and starch gels are photographed with uniform lighting from above, while stained translucent agar overlays and polyacrylamide gels are photographed on a light box with lighting transmitted from below. Sometimes special conditions are required for photographing stained gels. For example, polyacrylamide gels stained using the method of calcium phosphate precipitation should be photographed by reflected light against a dark background. In order to produce permanent records of indicator agar plates developed by the method of bioautography, an indirect lighting system is used which is a large version of the lighting system employed for photography of immunodiffusion plates. For photographing fluorescent bands (or nonfluorescent bands on fluorescent background) reflected UV light is used in combination with yellow filter (e.g., Wratte Gelatin Filter No. 2E, Eastman Kodak Company). The exposure for fluorescent gels is usually 20 to 30 s. The use of an automatic-exposure camera considerably facilitates the photographing of such gels. The use of a yellow filter also enhances contrast of blue bands and is routinely employed in photographing all gels stained with tetrazolium stains. Black-and-white films such as Kodak Panatomic-X, Kodak Plus-X, or Technical Pan are recommended for photographing bands visible in daylight. For photographing fluorescent bands (or nonfluorescent bands on fluorescent background), high-speed films such as Polaroid film type 55 or 57 or regular film ASA 400 are recommended. Color slides of good quality can be obtained with Kodachrome ASA 25.[28,29]

Another, more rapid way of photorecording is direct photocopying of the stained gels using a photocopier. This method does not possess the lag time between taking a photograph and obtaining usable information. It is less expensive than the photography techniques. The main disadvantage of this method is that it gives photocopies of slightly inferior quality as compared to photographs.[4]

The position of stained bands can be traced directly on cellulose acetate gels and filter-paper overlays or on transparent protective coverings (e.g., polyethylene sheets) by careful tracing over the bands with a ball-point pen or a marker. This technique is especially useful for recording electrophoretic patterns obtained using fluorescent detection methods or for recording bands that fade after a short period of time.

Stained gels can be fixed and stored for a permanent record or dried after appropriate treatments. Cellulose acetate gels are usually fixed in 5% formalin or 10% acetic acid for 10 to 15 min and then stored in 10% glycerol or placed in airtight plastic bags for convenient handling. Starch gels are usually fixed in 7% acetic acid or 50% ethanol and then stored in special trays filled with a 5:5:1 (v/v) mixture of methanol:water:acetic acid. This fixative toughens and shrinks the gels and makes them opaque. The "alcohol gel wash" recommended for starch gels consists of a 5:4:2:1 (v/v) mixture of ethanol:water:acetic acid:glycerol.[30] It not only stops the staining but also toughens the gel and helps bleach out some of the background. The use of 50 to 100% glycerol does not harden the starch gel as the alcohol-containing fixatives do; however, it helps to maintain gel integrity and makes the gel translucent and suitable for densitometric measurements. A 5% glycerol–7% acetic acid mixture is also frequently used for fixing and storing stained starch gels. Fixed gels can also be stored in airtight plastic bags. Stained polyacrylamide gels are usually fixed in 7% acetic acid or glycerol–acetic acid mixtures. The fixed gels can then be stored in a refrigerator for several months.

The method that gives a more permanent record of isozyme patterns is gel drying. For example, a simple method was developed for the preparation of fully transparent, flexible, dry sheets of stained starch gels.[31] In this method the stained gel is kept in 7% acetic acid, washed twice with water to remove excess reagents, and kept in 5% glycerol for 15 to 30 min. The gel is then placed on a glass plate of appropriate size, previously covered with a second cellophane sheet. Both sheets must be sufficiently large to allow at least a 2-cm margin on all sides of the glass plate. Both cellophane sheets must be soaked in 5% glycerol solution for 15 to 30 min before use. The formation of air bubbles between the gel and the sheets should be avoided. The four edges of the double cellophane are then folded over the back of the glass plate, the excess amount of glycerol solution removed by filter paper, and the processed plate dried at room temperature or at 60 to 80°C. After the gel and cellophane have been dried, the cellophane sheets are cut with a razor blade, about 1 cm from the border of the gel. The dried transparent and flexible gel covered with cellophane can then easily be stripped off the glass plate. This method allows storage of stained starch gels up to 9 years with full preservation of isozyme patterns. A similar procedure may be used to obtain dried polyacrylamide slab gels, except 65% methanol containing 0.5% glycerol should be substituted for the 5% glycerol solution. Dry polyacrylamide slab gels suitable for autoradiographic detection of [$^{14}$C]- and [$^3$H]-labeled zones can also be obtained by placing the thin slab onto a glass plate large enough to allow the formation of at least a 2-cm margin all around the gel, subsequent covering of the gel with 2% agarose solution, and drying the "sandwich" slowly and evenly, at first using an infrared lamp and then at room temperature. The stained polyacrylamide slab gels pretreated for 1 h with a 7.5% acetic acid–1.5% glycerol solution also can be dried after being covered with a 5% aqueous solution of gelatin or sprinkled with aquacide I, II, or III.[5,32] The instruction for a treatment that converts cellulose acetate gel into a film similar to cellophane is supplied with Cellogel by the producer.

## RESOURCE-SAVING STRATEGIES

The cost of information obtained by enzyme detection methods can be a limiting factor in some electrophoretic surveys of enzymes, e.g., in large-scale population studies. Several different ways exist to overcome this problem.

As was outlined above, the choice of adequate and less-expensive zymogram methods, the reduction of quantities of the most expensive reagents in the staining solutions used, and use of the most economical modes of stain application can help one to decrease expenses considerably. For example, when detecting glutamate–oxaloacetate transaminase (see 2.6.1.1 — GOT) in a population survey there is no need

to use quantitative enzymatic Method 4 because the routine diazo coupling Method 1 gives quite satisfactory results and is about two orders less expensive than the former one. For many histochemical detection methods the expenditure of staining solutions can be decreased more than ten times when applied on a filter-paper overlay or dropwise.

Some other specific tactics also can be used to save resources during electrophoretic studies of enzymes. The most important of them are (1) simultaneous detection of two or even more enzymes on the same gel, (2) successive detection of different enzymes on the same gel, (3) reusing of staining solutions, (4) the use of several origins on the same gel, (5) multiple replication of running gels by electroblotting, and (6) the use of semipreparative gels as the sources of linking enzymes.

**Simultaneous Detection of Several Enzymes on the Same Gel**
Theoretically, any two or more different enzymes can be simultaneously stained on the same gel when their detection methods are based on the same visualizing mechanism.[4] In practice, however, the combined stains are applicable only to those enzymes displaying nonoverlapping isozymal spectra under the electrophoretic conditions used.

Good examples of stain compatibility based on identity of the detection mechanisms involved are many NAD(P)-dependent dehydrogenase stains involving the PMS/tetrazolium system and some other stains using any NAD(P)-dependent dehydrogenase as a linking enzyme to catalyze the last step in the visualizing reaction, i.e., the production of colored formazan.

Different dehydrogenase stains are also compatible when positive or negative fluorescent detection of their bands is based on NAD(P) into NAD(P)H or NAD(P)H into NAD(P) conversion mechanism, respectively, or when detection of some nondehydrogenase enzymes is based on this same mechanism implemented through a linked reaction catalyzed by an appropriate NAD(P)-dependent dehydrogenase.

Combination of stains for different hydrolases that use 4-methylumbelliferone derivatives as substrates is possible and can be successful, especially when hydrolases with similar pH-optima are combined.

The main disadvantage of the stain combinations listed above and of some other possible combinations is that different sets of bands displayed by different enzymes are of the same color and hence may be confused. Thus, before being combined, different enzymes should be stained on separate gels electrophorized under the same conditions or stained on different gel slices obtained from the same gel block to identify relative positions of bands displayed by enzymes, the stainings of which are supposed to be combined. However, when compatible stains of polymorphic enzymes with different subunit structure of their molecules are combined, there is no need to stain enzymes separately because allozymic patterns displayed by different enzymes can be easily identified through the number of allozymes displayed in heterozygous individuals.[2,33]

Combination of compatible enzyme stains is particularly suited to large-scale population surveys where the range of expected genotypes is known. This tactic also allows staining of more enzymes when only extremely small sample volumes are available which are not sufficient for loading several different gels. It not only saves expensive reagents involved in the process of enzyme staining but also decreases the gel and time expense.

Simultaneous staining of different enzymes on the same gel is possible even when their detection methods are incompatible. This can be achieved through application of incompatible staining solutions in different strips of agar overlays applied to different parts of the gel. The tactic of by-strip application is justifiable only when gel areas occupied by different enzymes to be detected were identified as a result of previous stainings of enzymes on separate gels. The use of the by-strip application method prevents mixing of incompatible stains, and interaction or interference of ingredients from different stains can occur only in narrow contact zone where ingredients from different stains are mixing due to restricted diffusion.

## Successive Detection of Different Enzymes on the Same Gel

This approach can be implemented not only when the stain compatibility of different enzymes is based upon identity of mechanisms of their detection (i.e., in situations described above) but also when compatibility is based upon tolerance of different detection mechanisms.[4] The latter situation assumes that none of the reagents from the first stain interacts or interferes with any reagent from the next one. In this case the activity bands caused by different enzymes usually are of different colors and so can be readily distinguished. A particular sequence of applied stains may not be reversible. For example, successful double stains are purine-nucleoside phosphorylase tetrazolium stain (see 2.4.2.1 — PNP) followed by glutamate–oxaloacetate transaminase stain based on the diazo coupling mechanism (see 2.6.1.1 — GOT, Method 1), and esterase fluorescent stain (see 3.1.1... — EST, Method 2), followed by a peptidase stain involving L-amino acid oxidase and peroxidase as linking enzymes (see 3.4.11 or 13... — PEP, Method 1). In both these cases the reverse sequence of stain application will not be successful simply because the products of the first-step staining reactions will mask the products of the second-step staining reactions.

In some cases different stains are incompatible because an ingredient of one stain is able to react with an ingredient in another one. Examples are glycerol-3-phosphate dehydrogenase tetrazolium stain (see 1.1.1.8 — G-3-PD) followed by glycerol kinase tetrazolium stain (see 2.7.1.30 — GLYCK, Method 2), or glucose-phosphate isomerase stain (see 5.3.1.9 — GPI) followed by mannose-phosphate isomerase stain (see 5.3.1.8 — MPI), where the substrates of the first stains will react with linking enzymes of the following ones. The same is true for negative fluorescent stains involving NAD(P)H followed by a tetrazolium stain where NAD(P)H of the first stain will interact with the PMS/tetrazolium system of the following one and, thus, will result in formation of colored formazan across the whole gel surface. The problem of stain incompatibility can be overcome by careful washing of the gel after the first staining, with the purpose of removing soluble ingredients capable of interaction with ingredients in the following stain.[4] This tactic, however, is applicable only when undesirable compounds of the first stain are soluble. Most suitable for implementation of this tactic are coarse-pored cellulose acetate gels, thin slices of starch gel blocks, and thin blocks of low-percentage polyacrylamide gel. The use of just those gels allows small molecules of undesirable reagents to diffuse readily into the washing solution while large enzyme molecules remain in their final run position, being incorporated into the gel matrix. In some cases this tactic may be the only possible one for detecting different enzymes on the same gel when incompatible detection mechanisms are involved in different stains. The example is a situation when banding patterns produced by different incompatible stains overlap and thus the by-strip application method cannot be used.

The successive detection of different enzymes using compatible stains may also sometimes be preferable because it does not require preliminary identification staining of different enzymes on separate gels. An example is the situation when the final detected products of successive stains are of the same color, and banding patterns displayed by different enzymes cannot be identified on the basis of differences of

their subunit structure (e.g., when all enzymes are monomorphic or when their molecules are of the same subunit structure).

When compatibility of successive stains is based on the identity of the detection mechanisms involved, both reagent and gel saving may be achieved because only the addition of a specific substrate is needed for detection of each following enzyme. Only gel saving is achieved through double staining of the same gel if different detection mechanisms are involved in different successive stains. Again, successive double stainings are of great value when extremely small volumes of samples, which are not sufficient for loading more than one gel, are available, and gel areas occupied by different enzymes overlap.

## Reusing of Staining Solutions

When a large-scale population survey is carried out using the standard staining solution method of enzyme detection, some staining solutions may be used repeatedly immediately after the first use, after 1 d of storage in a refrigerator, or after several days of storage frozen. The staining solutions that easily endure this tactic are those used for tetrazolium detection of numerous NAD(P)-dependent dehydrogenases and many other enzymes that are detected through the use of dehydrogenases as linking enzymes to produce a final visible product, the formazan. The repeated addition of MTT or NBT and a linking enzyme (if involved) to the previously used staining solution is sometimes desirable. The tactic of reusing tetrazolium-containing stains is of great value, especially when expensive substrates and cofactors are involved in visualizing reactions. The potential reagent savings make this tactic a desirable addition to the resource-saving strategies of a laboratory.

## The Use of Several Origins on One Gel

Two or more different sets of samples may be loaded in different origin positions on the same gel.[4] This is a very useful tactic, especially when large-scale population screening of single-locus enzyme polymorphisms is carried out. The use of multiple origins is most effective for polymorphic enzymes with a small number of allelic variants of low electrophoretic mobility. Preliminary test runs may be needed to find optimal relative positions of origins to be sure that allozyme sets from different origins do not overlap. It should be taken into consideration that separation of the same allozymes started from different origins may be different. This disadvantage is especially pronounced when discontinuous buffer systems are used for electrophoresis. However, there are usually no problems with genetic interpretation of enzyme polymorphisms with known genotypes. The multiple-origin tactic is the most effective one in a search for rare electrophoretic variants. The advantages of this tactic are the obvious cost savings in gel media, fine biochemicals, and time.

## Multiple Replication of Electrophoretic Gels by Electroblotting

Electrophoretic transfer of enzymes from a single running gel onto immobilizing matrices (e.g., "Zeta Pore" or "Hybond-N" membranes and Whatman "DE" 81 paper) allows one to obtain multiple replicas, which can then be developed separately using different enzyme stains.[34] It is important to remember when using this tactic that the faster-migrating enzymes should be detected on the first replica, while the slower-migrating ones should be on the last replica. Thus, use of the replication tactic requires preliminary knowledge of relative positions of isozymal sets displayed by different enzymes under analysis. Multiple replication and multiple successive staining tactics may be combined, resulting in a considerable increase in the number of different enzymes analyzed through one gel electrophoretic run. Electrophoretic transfer of enzymes requires additional expensive materials, special designs, and time. Thus, it is not as practical as some other resource-saving tactics described above. At the same time it may be potentially very valuable when only extremely small volumes of each sample are available and obtaining additional material is very labor- and time-consuming, or impossible.

## The Use of Semipreparative Gels for Production of Preparations of Linking Enzymes

A great number of enzyme-visualizing methods listed below in this part involve exogenous linking enzymes, some of which are not yet commercially available. Again, in some cases the purchase of even one vial of very expensive enzyme preparation may not be reasonable, e.g., when only one or a few gel stainings are supposed to be carried out. In such situations the semipreparative gel electrophoresis presents a good opportunity to obtain the enzyme needed in small but sufficient amounts and purity. In principle, all the enzymes that can be detected through any visualizing methods and thus located on electrophoretic gels may be used as linking enzymes. One critical condition must be fulfilled threat: the preparation of the enzyme to be used as the linking one must be free of the enzyme to be detected. The use of the linking-enzyme preparation contaminated with the enzyme under detection will result in background staining without any distinctly visible bands. The tactic of using semipreparative gels for production of linking enzyme preparations was tested by the author and proved to be a good addition to his zymographic "cookery".

The starch gel blocks routinely used for analytic electrophoresis may be easily adapted for semipreparative enzyme electrophoresis. After completion of electrophoretic separation the position of a desired enzyme on the gel is located by an appropriate detection method, and the gel area occupied by the enzyme is cut out. The use of starch gel as supporting medium is preferable because a simple "freezing–squeezing" procedure may be used to remove the enzyme from the gel matrix. This procedure, for example, was successfully used by the author to obtain preparation of isocitrate dehydrogenase involved as a linking enzyme in aconitase stain (see 4.2.1.3 — ACON). A more effective method, electrophoretic elution, may also be used to remove enzymes from a gel matrix, but it is more time-consuming and requires an additional device.[5]

An electrophoretic procedure very similar to that used for electrophoretic transfer of proteins may sometimes be even more effective than that described above. In this case proteins move in the transverse direction after being applied on the upper surface of a starch gel block by the agar overlay method. After an appropriate period of time electrophoresis is stopped. The position of the desired linking enzyme within the gel block is located by a specific detection method. For this purpose the gel slice obtained by transverse slicing through the gel block is used. A longitudinal slice is then made through the zone occupied by the enzyme, and two reactive gel plates with enzyme-containing cut surfaces are obtained. The staining solution containing all necessary ingredients except the linking enzyme is applied dropwise to the surface of the gel to be stained. The reactive gel plates are then placed above, the cut surfaces down, avoiding formation of air bubbles. The linking enzyme molecules embedded in the gel matrix of the reactive plates usually work sufficiently well due to the diffusion of small molecules of reagents involved in the stain and those produced by the enzyme under detection. This variant of the method, for example, was successfully used by the author to obtain the reactive starch gel plates containing glucose-phosphate isomerase involved in the mannose-phosphate isomerase stain (see 5.3.1.8 — MPI) as the linking enzyme.

Of course, the use of semipreparative gel electrophoresis for production of auxiliary enzymes is not appropriate for large-scale isozyme survey; however, it provides a good opportunity for new developments in electrophoretic zymography. This tactic should not be considered now as an effective resource-saving one. It can, rather, help

to develop and test new enzyme-detection methods and, thus, is of great potential value.

## TROUBLESHOOTING

During practical application of enzyme-detection methods some problems concerning the enzyme staining originate from time to time. One may hope that a good knowledge of the detection mechanisms given in Part II will help to solve these problems. Nevertheless, some useful advice concerning stain troubleshooting is given below. These pieces of advice are organized into a list including the most common causes of stain failures and recommendations for their avoidance:

- **Some reagents are erroneously omitted from the staining solution:** Check the recipe. Add missing reagents or prepare new solution.
- **Unstable reagents deteriorated during storage under inappropriate conditions**: First of all, check the reactivity of the linking enzymes, if involved, by a rough qualitative enzyme assay using appropriate staining solutions. Replace linking-enzyme preparations if they have deteriorated. If the stain still does not work, check which reagents of the stain other than linking enzymes are not functional. This may be done through simple analysis of functioning of other stains that include reagents common to the stain under question or through one-by-one replacement of suspected reagents with fresh ones. If reserve vials of suspect reagents are not available, try to use suitable enzyme preparations and substrates to produce suspect reagents enzymatically. If available, use any alternative detection method to be sure that the enzyme under detection is active in your samples. Use control samples that show activity of the enzyme under detection with certainty. Follow storage instructions depicted on containers. Store most chemicals in a refrigerator or freezer in a special airtight box with a desiccant. Do not leave refrigerated chemicals open at room temperature. Hydrolysis following water condensation is particularly damaging to many compounds. To prevent condensation, take the chemicals out of the refrigerator about half an hour before use or warm the containers in your hands before opening. On the contrary, keep linking-enzyme preparations at room temperature for as short a time as possible. Remember that some reagents are light-sensitive and that high temperature also contributes to breakdown of many reagents.
- **Intermediate or final pH value of staining solution deviates from that recommended in the recipe**: Check intermediate pHs during preparation of the staining solution and final pH before application. Prepare new staining buffer if it has deteriorated. Use sodium or other salts rather than free strong acids or bases if they are involved in the stain. Always add reagents in the sequence given in the recipe of staining solution.
- **Enzyme inhibitors are present in used water**: If the stain works well in laboratory conditions and does not work under field conditions, the bad quality of the water used is the first candidate for the reason of a stain failure. Use filtered rain or thawed snow water in the field and bidistilled or deionized water in the laboratory.

It also should be kept in mind that many errors that have been made during former stages of enzyme electrophoretic analysis (e.g., storage, preparation, and electrophoretic run of samples) manifest themselves only during the stage of enzyme detection. For example, the enzyme to be detected may be inactivated during tissue storage under inappropriate conditions (e.g., after freezing–thawing events) or may run off the anodal or cathodal end of the gel (e.g., when the enzyme moves quickly towards anode or cathode and/or running time is too long).

Some other hints for troubleshooting, especially for stages other than enzyme staining, may be found in the excellent handbook for allozyme electrophoresis by Richardson et al.[4]

## SAFETY REGULATIONS

A large array of compounds is used in enzyme-visualizing procedures. A number of these compounds are known to be carcinogens, skin irritants, or poisons. Many of these compounds even have not yet been tested for their long-term effects on human health and heredity. Thus, it is good practice for those dealing with such a diverse group of chemicals to follow the general safety codex given below:

- Treat all chemicals as potentially hazardous to your health.
- Wear gloves and a dust mask when handling chemicals.
- Do not breathe dust and vapors; mix stains in a vented hood.
- Avoid contaminating other things with the chemicals being used.
- Read all labels on containers and follow the prescribed safety measures.
- Be careful when handling stained gels and disposing of used staining solutions.
- Thoroughly clean up any spills on your chemical table.
- Wash your hands after each handling.
- Do not keep food in a refrigerator together with chemicals.

## REFERENCES

1. Brewer, G. J., *An Introduction to Isozyme Techniques*, Academic Press, New York, 1970.
2. Harris, H. and Hopkinson, D. A., *Handbook of Enzyme Electrophoresis in Human Genetics*, North-Holland, Amsterdam (Loose leaf with supplements in 1977 and 1978), 1976.
3. Gordon, A. H., *Electrophoresis of Proteins in Polyacrylamide and Starch Gels*, North-Holland, Amsterdam, 1980.
4. Richardson, B. J., Baverstock, P. R., and Adams, M., *Allozyme Electrophoresis: A Handbook for Animal Systematics and Population Studies*, Academic Press, Sydney, 1986.
5. Andrews, A. T., *Electrophoresis: Theory, Techniques, and Biochemical and Clinical Applications*, Clarendon Press, Oxford, 1988.
6. Conkle, M. T., Hodgskiss, P. D., Nunnally, L. B., and Hunter, S. C., *Starch Gel Electrophoresis of Conifer Seeds: a Laboratory Manual*, Pacific Southwest Forest and Range Experiment Station, Berkeley, California, General Technical Report PSW-64, 1982.
7. Cheliak, W. M. and Pitel, J. A., *Techniques for Starch Gel Electrophoresis of Enzymes from Forest Tree Species*, Petawawa National Forestry Institute, Canadian Forestry Service, Agriculture Canada, Chalk River, Ont. Information Report PI-X-42, 1984.
8. Morizot, D. C. and Schmidt, M. E., Starch gel electrophoresis and histochemical visualization of proteins, in *Electrophoretic and Isoelectric Focusing Techniques in Fisheries Management*, Whitmore, D. H., Ed., CRC Press, Boca Raton, 1990, 23.
9. Murphy, R. W., Sites, J. W., Jr., Buth, D. G., and Haufler, C. H., Proteins I: Isozyme electrophoresis, in *Molecular Systematics*, Hillis, D. M. and Moritz, C., Eds., Sinauer, Sunderland, MA, 1990, 45.
10. Ghosh, R. and Quayle, J. R., Phenazine ethosulfate as a prefered electron acceptor to phenazine methosulfate in dye linked enzyme assays, *Anal. Biochem.*, 99, 112, 1980.
11. Andersen, E. and Christensen, K., Superoxide dismutase (E.C. 1.15.1.1) polymorphism in various breeds of dogs, *Anim. Blood Groups Biochem. Genet.*, 8 (Suppl. 1), 27, 1977.
12. Pérez-de la Mora, M., Méndez-Franco, J., Salceda, R., and Riesgo-Escovar, J. R., A glutamate dehydrogenase-based method for the assay of L-glutamic acid: formation of pyridine nucleotide fluorescent derivatives, *Anal. Biochem.*, 180, 248, 1989.
13. Mohamed, M. A., Lerro, K. A., and Prestwich, G. D., Polyacrylamide gel miniaturization improves protein visualization and autoradiographic detection, *Anal. Biochem.*, 177, 287, 1989.
14. Manchenko, G. P., Subunit structure of enzymes: allozymic data, *Isozyme Bull.*, 21, 144, 1988.
15. Ahmad, M., Skibinsky, D. O. F., and Beardmore, J. A., An estimate of genetic variation in the common mussel *Mytilus edulis*, *Biochem. Genet.*, 15, 833, 1977.
16. Fujio, Y. and Kato, Y., Genetic variation in fish populations, *Bull. Jpn. Soc. Sci. Fish.*, 45, 1169, 1979.
17. Fujio, Y., Yamanaka, R., and Smith, P. J., Genetic variation in marine molluscs, *Bull. Jpn. Soc. Sci. Fish.*, 49, 1809, 1983.
18. Somer, H., "Nothing dehydrogenase" reaction as an artefact in serum isoenzyme analyses, *Clin. Chim. Acta*, 60, 223, 1975.
19. Sri Venugopal, K. S. and Adiga, P. R., Artifactual staining of proteins on polyacrylamide gels by nitro blue tetrazolium chloride and phenazine methosulfate, *Anal. Biochem.*, 101, 215, 1980.
20. Zimniak-Przybylska, Z. and Przybylska, J., Interference of *Pisum* seed albumins with detecting amylase activity on electropherograms: an apparent relationship between protein patterns and amylase zymograms, *Genet. Pol.*, 17, 133, 1976.
21. Zimniak-Przybylska, Z. and Przybylska, J., Relationships between electrophoretic seed protein patterns and zymograms of amylases and acid phosphatases in *Pisum*, *Genet. Pol.*, 15, 435, 1974.
22. Hardin, E., Passey, R. B., and Fuller, J. B., Artifactual alkaline phosphatase isoenzyme band, caused by bilirubin, on cellulose acetate electropherograms, *Clin. Chem.*, 24, 178, 1978.
23. Onoufriou, A. and Alahiothis, S. N., Enzyme specificity: "pseudopolymorphism" of lactate dehydrogenase in *Drosophila melanogaster*, *Biochem. Genet.*, 19, 277, 1981.
24. Gill, P. D., Nongenetic variation in isoenzymes of lactate dehydrogenase of *Cepaea nemoralis*, *Comp. Biochem. Physiol.*, 59B, 271, 1978.
25. Manchenko, G. P., unpublished data, 1994.
26. Nomenclature Committee of the International Union of Biochemistry, *Enzyme Nomenclature*, Academic Press, Orlando, 1984.
27. Manchenko, G. P., Allozymic variation and substrate specificity of phosphatase from sipunculid *Phascolosoma japonicum*, *Isozyme Bull.*, 21, 168, 1988.
28. Vallejos, C. E., Enzyme activity staining, in *Isozymes in Plant Genetics and Breeding, Part A*, Tanskley, S. D. and Orton, T. J., Eds., Elsevier, Amsterdam, 1983, 469.
29. Shaklee, J. B. and Keenan, C. P., *A Practical Laboratory Guide to the Techniques and Methodology of Electrophoresis and Its Application to Fish Fillet Identification*, CSIRO Marine Laboratories, Report 177, Hobart, Australia, 1986.
30. Siciliano, M. J. and Shaw, C. R., Separation and visualization of enzymes on gels, in *Chromatographic and Electrophoretic Techniques, Vol. 2, Zone Electrophoresis*, Smith, I., Ed., Heineman, London, 1976, 185.
31. Numachi, K.-I., A simple method for preservation and scanning of starch gels, *Biochem. Genet.*, 19, 233, 1981.
32. Remtulla, M. A. and Boyde, T. R. C., Method for the preservation of polyacrylamide slabs after electrophoresis, *Lab. Practice*, 23, 484, 1974.
33. Buth, D. G., Genetic principles and the interpretation of electrophoretic data, in *Electrophoretic and Isoelectric Focusing Techniques in Fisheries Management*, Whitmore, D. H., Ed., CRC Press, Boca Raton, 1990, 1.
34. McLellan, T. and Ramshaw, J. A. M., Serial electrophoretic transfers: a technique for the identification of numerous enzymes from single polyacrylamide gels, *Biochem. Genet.*, 19, 647, 1981.

# Section 3
## Enzyme Sheets

### ABBREVIATIONS COMMONLY USED
### IN THE ENZYME SHEETS

| | |
|---|---|
| ADP | Adenosine 5'-diphosphate |
| AMP | Adenosine 5'-monophosphate |
| ATP | Adenosine 5'-triphosphate |
| CDP | Cytidine 5'-diphosphate |
| CMP | Cytidine 5'-monophosphate |
| CoA | Coenzyme A |
| CTP | Cytidine 5'-triphosphate |
| DNA | Deoxyribonucleic acid |
| EDTA | Ethylenediaminetetraacetic acid |
| FAD | Flavin-adenine dinucleotide |
| FMN | Flavin mononucleotide |
| GDP | Guanosine 5'-diphosphate |
| GMP | Guanosine 5'-monophosphate |
| GTP | Guanosine 5'-triphosphate |
| IMP | Inosine 5'-monophosphate |
| INT | *p*-Iodonitrotetrazolium Violet |
| ITP | Inosine 5'-triphosphate |
| MTT | Methyl thiazolyl tetrazolium (Thiazolyl blue) |
| NAD | Nicotinamide–adenine dinucleotide (oxidized) |
| NADH | Nicotinamide–adenine dinucleotide (reduced) |
| NADP | Nicotinamide–adenine dinucleotide phosphate (oxidized) |
| NADPH | Nicotinamide–adenine dinucleotide phosphate (reduced) |
| NBT | Nitro blue tetrazolium |
| PAG | Polyacrylamide gel |
| PMS | Phenazine methosulfate |
| RNA | Ribonucleic acid |
| SDS | Sodium dodecyl sulfate |
| TRIS | Tris(hydroxymethyl) aminomethane |
| UDP | Uridine 5'-diphosphate |
| UMP | Uridine 5'-monophosphate |
| UTP | Uridine 5'-triphosphate |
| UV | Ultraviolet |

# 1.1.1.1 — Alcohol Dehydrogenase; ADH

OTHER NAMES     Aldehyde reductase

REACTION     Alcohol + NAD = aldehyde or ketone + NADH

ENZYME SOURCE     Bacteria, fungi, plants, protozoa, invertebrates, vertebrates

## METHOD 1

### Visualization Scheme

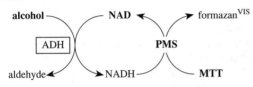

### Staining Solution[1] (modified)

| | |
|---|---|
| 0.05 $M$ Tris–HCl buffer, pH 8.5 | 50 ml |
| Ethanol | 2 ml |
| NAD | 40 mg |
| MTT | 10 mg |
| PMS | 1 mg |

### Procedure

Incubate the gel in staining solution in the dark at 37°C until dark blue bands appear. Rinse stained gel in water and fix in 50% ethanol.

*Notes:*   A large number of primary and secondary straight- and branched-chain, aliphatic and aromatic alcohols and hemiacetals may be used as substrates to examine additional ADH isozymes. The animal enzyme acts on cyclic secondary alcohols while the yeast enzyme does not.

Some ADH isozymes from various invertebrate and vertebrate species display high substrate specificity to octanol. These ADH forms were included in the enzyme list under the separate name "octanol dehydrogenase" (see 1.1.1.73 — ODH).[2]

ADH bands often appear on other NAD-dependent dehydrogenase zymograms (see 1.X.X.X — NDH). Pyrazole is usually used as a specific inhibitor of mammalian ADH. The addition of pyrazole (final concentration 1 to 2 mg/ml) does not interfere with any of the stains so far tested.[3]

## METHOD 2

### Visualization Scheme

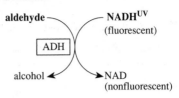

### Staining Solution[4]

| | |
|---|---|
| A.   0.05 $M$ Tris–phosphate buffer, pH 7.0 | 25 ml |
|      Acetaldehyde | 0.1 ml |
|      NADH | 10 mg |
| B.   2% Agar solution (60°C) | 25 ml |

### Procedure

Mix A and B components of the staining solution and pour the mixture over the surface of the gel. Incubate the gel at 37°C and view under long-wave UV light after 10 min to about 1 h. When dark bands are clearly visible on a light (fluorescent) background, photograph gel using a yellow filter.

To make these bands visible in daylight (white bands on blue background), cover processed gel with a second 1% agar overlay containing MTT (or NBT) and PMS.

*Notes:*   If too much NADH is added to the staining solution, the enzyme should not be able to convert enough NADH into NAD for nonfluorescent bands to become visible.

Many different aldehydes may be used as substrates to examine NADH-dependent aldehyde reductase activity of ADH.

## GENERAL NOTES

Some ADH isozymes may utilize both NAD(H) and NADP(H) as cofactors and some of them catalyze the reaction only in one direction [see 1.1.1.2 — ADH(NADP), General Notes].

## REFERENCES

1. Brewer, G. J., *An Introduction to Isoenzyme Techniques*, Academic Press, New York, 1970, 117.
2. Nomenclature Committee of the International Union of Biochemistry, *Enzyme Nomenclature*, Academic Press, Orlando, 1984.
3. Richardson, B. J., Baverstock, P. R., and Adams, M., *Allozyme Electrophoresis: A Handbook for Animal Systematics and Population Studies*, Academic Press, Sydney, 1986, 221.
4. Smith, M., Hopkinson, D. A., and Harris, H., Studies on the properties of the human alcohol dehydrogenase isozymes determined by the different loci $ADH_1$, $ADH_2$, $ADH_3$, *Ann. Hum. Genet.*, 37, 49, 1973.

OTHER NAMES     Aldehyde reductase (NADPH)

REACTION     Alcohol + NADP = aldehyde + NADPH

ENZYME SOURCE     Bacteria, invertebrates, vertebrates

## METHOD 1

### Visualization Scheme

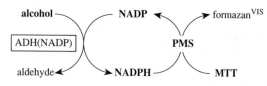

### Staining Solution[1]

| | |
|---|---|
| 0.1 $M$ Glycine–NaOH buffer, pH 9.5 | 50 ml |
| NADP | 20 mg |
| NBT | 20 mg |
| PMS | 2 mg |
| 1,2-Propanediol | 5 ml |

### Procedure

Incubate the gel in staining solution in the dark at 37°C until dark blue bands appear. Rinse stained gel in water and fix in 50% ethanol.

*Notes:*  Many different alcohols may be used as substrates for ADH(NADP). Bacterial enzymes oxidize only primary alcohols while others act also on secondary alcohols. Some ADH(NADP) isozymes of invertebrate and vertebrate species display relatively high specificity towards certain alcohols and aldehydes and are included in the enzyme list under separate names (see 1.1.1.19 — GLR; 1.1.1.72 — GLYD; 1.1.1.80 — IPDH).

## METHOD 2

### Visualization Scheme

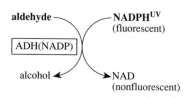

### Staining Solution[2]

| | | |
|---|---|---|
| A. | 0.2 $M$ Sodium-phosphate buffer, pH 7.0 | 8 ml |
| | 5 mg/ml NADPH | 5 ml |
| | 10 m$M$ $p$-Nitrobenzaldehyde | 5 ml |
| B. | 1.4% Agar solution (60°C) | 20 ml |

### Procedure

Mix A and B components of the staining solution and pour the mixture over the surface of the gel. Incubate the gel at 30°C and view under long-wave UV light. When dark bands are clearly visible on a light (fluorescent) background, photograph gel using a yellow filter. To make these bands visible in daylight (white bands on blue background), cover processed gel with a second 1% agar overlay containing MTT (or NBT) and PMS. Wash negatively stained gel in water and fix in 50% ethanol.

*Notes:*  Many different aldehydes may be used as substrates to examine the NADPH-dependent aldehyde reductase activity of ADH(NADP). Some NADPH-dependent aldehyde reductases catalyze the reaction only in one (reductase) direction. For example, it is the case for mouse liver enzyme highly specific to $p$-nitrobenzaldehyde. The amount of NADPH added to the staining solution is critical for the development of nonfluorescent bands of ADH(NADP). If too much NADPH is added to the staining solution, the enzyme should not be able to convert enough NADPH into NADP for nonfluorescent bands to become visible.

### GENERAL NOTES

Aldehyde reductase is a generic term used to describe the activities of a number of enzymes catalyzing the reduction of various aliphatic, aromatic, and biogenic aldehydes in the presence of NADPH. Much of the problem in identifying aldehyde reductase forms appears to lie in conflicts in terminology, arising from overlapping substrate specificity and an absence of agreement about the physiological roles of these enzymes. Clear classification of aldehyde reductases requires further biochemical and genetic studies.[2]

### REFERENCES

1.  Turner, A. J. and Tipton, K. F., The characterization of two reduced nicotinamide–adenine dinucleotide phosphate-linked aldehyde reductases from pig brain, *Biochem. J.*, 130, 765, 1972.
2.  Duley, J. A. and Holmes, R. S., Biochemical genetics of aldehyde reductase in the mouse: *Ahr-1* — a new locus linked to the alcohol dehydrogenase gene complex on chromosome 3, *Biochem. Genet.*, 20, 1067, 1982.

## 1.1.1.3 — Homoserine Dehydrogenase; HSDH

REACTION    L-Homoserine + NAD(P) = L-aspartate
4-semialdehyde + NAD(P)H

ENZYME SOURCE  Bacteria, fungi, plants

## METHOD

### Visualization Scheme

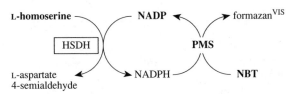

### Staining Solution[1]

100 mM Tris–HCl buffer, pH 8.9
50 mM L-Homoserine
1 mM NADP
0.25 mg/ml NBT
0.025 mg/ml PMS
400 mM KCl

### Procedure

Incubate the gel in staining solution in the dark at 37°C until dark blue bands appear. Wash developed gel in water and fix in 50% ethanol.

*Notes:*  The enzyme from some sources (e.g., yeast) acts most rapidly with NAD while from others (e.g., *Neurospora*) with NADP. The enzyme from *E. coli* catalyzes the phosphorylation of L-aspartate in addition to its dehydrogenase activity.

### REFERENCE

1. Ogilvie, J. M., Sightler, J. H., and Clark, R. B., Homoserine dehydrogenase of *Escherichia coli* K 12 λ. I. Feedback inhibition by L-threonine and activation by potassium ions, *Biochemistry*, 8, 3557, 1969.

## 1.1.1.8 — Glycerol-3-phosphate Dehydrogenase; G-3-PD

OTHER NAMES    α-Glycerophosphate dehydrogenase

REACTION    Glycerol-3-phosphate + NAD = glycerone phosphate + NADH

ENZYME SOURCE  Bacteria, fungi, protozoa, invertebrates, vertebrates

## METHOD

### Visualization Scheme

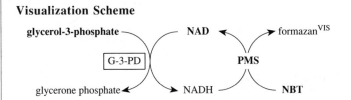

### Staining Solution[1]

| | |
|---|---:|
| 0.1 M Tris–HCl buffer, pH 8.0 | 85 ml |
| NAD | 50 mg |
| NBT | 30 mg |
| PMS | 2 mg |
| 1 M Glycerol-3-phosphate (pH 7.0) | 10 ml |
| 0.1 M NaCN | 5 ml |

### Procedure

Incubate the gel in staining solution in the dark at 37°C until dark blue bands appear. Wash developed gel in water and fix in 50% ethanol.

*Notes:*  NaCN is included in the stain to prevent development of superoxide dismutase (see 1.15.1.1 — SOD) bands, which can interfere with G-3-PD bands. Pyruvate and pyrazole may be added in a staining solution to final concentration 1 to 2 mg/ml of each to inhibit nonspecific NAD into NADH conversion by LDH and ADH, respectively. The enzyme activity is highly dependent on substrate concentration. When a low concentration of glycerol-3-phosphate is used, the product glycerone phosphate, which inhibits the forward G-3-PD reaction, should be taken away using two exogenous linking enzymes, triose-phosphate isomerase (5.3.1.1 — TPI) and glyceraldehyde-3-phosphate dehydrogenase (1.2.1.12 — GA-3-PD). The latter enzyme doubles NADH production and formation of the formazan. Only those preparations of the linking enzymes which are substantially free of G-3-PD impurity should be used for this purpose.

### REFERENCE

1. Shaw, C. R. and Prasad, R., Starch gel electrophoresis of enzymes: a compilation of recipes, *Biochem. Genet.*, 4, 297, 1970.

## 1.1.1.10 — L-Xylulose Reductase; XR

REACTION    Xylitol + NADP = L-xylulose + NADPH

ENZYME SOURCE  Vertebrates

## METHOD

### Visualization Scheme

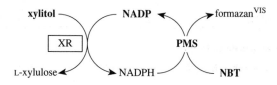

### Staining Solution[1]

| | |
|---|---|
| 0.1 $M$ Tris–HCl buffer, pH 8.0 | 50 ml |
| Xylitol | 150 mg |
| NADP | 10 mg |
| NBT | 10 mg |
| PMS | 1.5 mg |

### Procedure

Incubate the gel in staining solution in the dark at 37°C until dark blue bands appear. Wash stained gel in water and fix in 50% ethanol.

### REFERENCE

1. Bell, L. J., Moyer, J. T., and Numachi, K.-I., Morphological and genetic variation in Japanese populations of the anemonefish *Amphiprion clarkii*, *Mar. Biol.*, 72, 99, 1982.

## 1.1.1.14 — Sorbitol Dehydrogenase; SORDH

OTHER NAMES    L-Iditol dehydrogenase (recommended name), polyol dehydrogenase

REACTIONS    1. L-Iditol + NAD = L-sorbose + NADH
2. D-Sorbitol + NAD = D-fructose + NADH

ENZYME SOURCE  Bacteria, plants, invertebrates, vertebrates

## METHOD

### Visualization Scheme

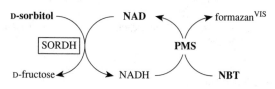

### Staining Solution[1]

| | |
|---|---|
| 0.05 $M$ Tris–HCl buffer, pH 8.0 | 100 ml |
| D-Sorbitol | 500 mg |
| NAD | 10 mg |
| NBT | 15 mg |
| PMS | 2 mg |

### Procedure

Incubate the gel in staining solution in the dark at 37°C until dark blue bands appear. Wash stained gel in water and fix in 50% ethanol.

*Notes:* Pyruvate and pyrazole may be included in a staining solution to final concentration 1 to 2 mg/ml of each to inhibit LDH and ADH, respectively, and to prevent appearance of nonspecifically stained bands. The enzyme from some sources (e.g., *Candida utilis*) is more active with xylitol. Many sugars may be used as substrates but NAD cannot be replaced by NADP. NADP-dependent SORDH activity has been reported only in *Drosophila melanogaster*.[2]

### REFERENCES

1. Lin, C. C., Schipmann, G., Kittrell, W. A., and Ohno, S., The predominance of heterozygotes found in wild goldfish of Lake Erie at the gene locus for sorbitol dehydrogenase, *Biochem. Genet.*, 3, 603, 1969.
2. Bischoff, W. L., Ontogeny of sorbitol dehydrogenases in *Drosophila melanogaster*, *Biochem. Genet.*, 16, 485, 1978.

REACTION    D-Mannitol-1-phosphate + NAD = D-fructose-6-phosphate + NADH

ENZYME SOURCE  Bacteria, fungi

## METHOD 1

### Visualization Scheme

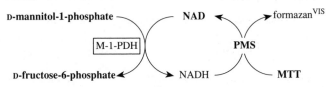

### Staining Solution[1]

| | |
|---|---:|
| 0.2 *M* Tris–HCl buffer, pH 8.0 | 50 ml |
| Mannitol-1-phosphate | 5 mg |
| NAD | 20 mg |
| MTT | 12.5 mg |
| PMS | 5 mg |

### Procedure

Incubate the gel in staining solution in the dark at 37°C until dark blue bands appear. Wash stained gel in water and fix in 50% ethanol.

## METHOD 2

### Visualization Scheme

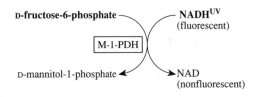

### Staining Solution*

| | |
|---|---:|
| A.  0.02 *M* Tris–HCl buffer, pH 8.0 | 25 ml |
| D-Fructose-6-phosphate (Ba salt) | 20 mg |
| NADH | 10 mg |
| B.  2% Agarose solution (60°C) | 25 ml |

### Procedure

Mix A and B components of the staining solution and pour over the surface of the gel. Incubate the gel at 37°C and view under long-wave UV light after 10 to 60 min. When dark bands are clearly visible on a light (fluorescent) background, photograph gel using a yellow filter. To make these bands visible in daylight (white bands on blue background), cover the processed gel with a second 1% agarose overlay containing MTT (or NBT) and PMS. Wash negatively stained gel in water and fix in 50% ethanol.

*Notes:*   The amount of NADH added to the staining solution is critical for development of M-1-PDH bands. If too much NADH is added, the enzyme should not be able to convert enough NADH into NAD for nonfluorescent bands to become visible.

The staining solution recommended in Method 2 is about 100 times less expensive than that in Method 1.

## GENERAL NOTES

The enzyme is highly specific to both the substrate and the cofactor.

## REFERENCE

1. Selander, R. K., Caugant, D. A., Ochman, H., Musser, J. M., Gilmour, M. N., and Whittam, T. S., Methods of multilocus enzyme electrophoresis for bacterial population genetics and systematics, *Appl. Environ. Microbiol.*, 51, 873, 1986.

*   New; recommended for use.

## 1.1.1.19 — Glucuronate Reductase; GLR

OTHER NAMES     Hexonate dehydrogenase

REACTION     L-Gulonate + NADP = D-glucuronate + NADPH

ENZYME SOURCE   Vertebrates

## METHOD

### Visualization Scheme

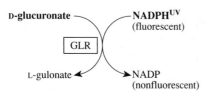

### Staining Solution[1]

| | |
|---|---|
| 0.03 $M$ Potassium phosphate buffer, pH 7.0 | 5 ml |
| D-Glucuronate (Na salt) | 5 mg |
| NADPH | 1.5 mg |

### Procedure

Apply the staining solution to gel on filter-paper overlay and after incubation at 37°C (30 to 60 min) view gel under long-wave UV light. Dark (nonfluorescent) bands of GLR are visible on the light (fluorescent) background of the gel. Photograph developed gel using a yellow filter.

    These bands may be made visible in daylight (white bands on blue background) after treating the processed gel with MTT/PMS solution applied as filter paper or 1% agarose overlay.

*Notes:*   The amount of NADPH added to the staining solution is critical for development of nonfluorescent GLR bands. If too much NADPH is added, the enzyme should not be able to convert enough NADPH into NADP for nonfluorescent bands to become visible.

    The enzyme also reduces D-galacturonate. Mammalian enzyme may be identical with NADP-dependent alcohol dehydrogenase [see 1.1.1.2 — ADH(NADP); Method 1, *Notes*; General Notes].

### REFERENCE

1. Baker, C. M. A. and Manwell, C., Heterozygosity of the sheep: polymorphism of "malic enzyme," isocitrate dehydrogenase (NADP⁺), catalase and esterase, *Aust. J. Biol. Sci.*, 30, 127, 1977.

## 1.1.1.22 — UDPglucose Dehydrogenase; UGDH

REACTION     UDPglucose + 2NAD + H$_2$O = UDP-glucuronate + 2NADH

ENZYME SOURCE   Invertebrates, vertebrates

## METHOD

### Visualization Scheme

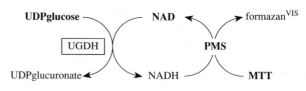

### Staining Solution[1]

| | |
|---|---|
| 0.03 $M$ Potassium phosphate buffer, pH 7.0 | 10 ml |
| UDPglucose | 2 mg |
| NAD | 4 mg |
| PMS | 1 mg |
| MTT | 10 mg |

### Procedure

Apply the staining solution to gel on filter-paper overlay and incubate at 37°C in a dark, moistened chamber until dark blue bands appear. Wash developed gel in water and fix in 50% ethanol.

*Notes:*   Staining solution lacking PMS and MTT may also be used to detect UGDH activity bands (fluorescent bands visible in long-wave UV light). The fluorescent detection system is more sensitive than the PMS/MTT system because of the presumed inhibitory effect of PMS and/or MTT on UGDH activity.[1]

    The reaction catalyzed by UGDH is essentially irreversible.

### REFERENCE

1. Baker, C. M. A. and Manwell, C., Heterozygosity of the sheep: polymorphism of "malic enzyme," isocitrate dehydrogenase (NADP⁺), catalase and esterase, *Aust. J. Biol. Sci.*, 30, 127, 1977.

## 1.1.1.23 — Histidinol Dehydrogenase; HISDH

REACTION        L-Histidinol + 2NAD = L-histidine + 2NADH (see *Notes*)

ENZYME SOURCE  Bacteria, fungi, plants

### METHOD

#### Visualization Scheme

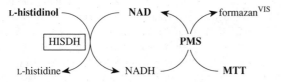

#### Staining Solution[1]

| | |
|---|---|
| 0.1 *M* Tris–HCl buffer, pH 8.0 | 50 ml |
| L-Histidinol | 40 mg |
| NAD | 20 mg |
| MTT | 10 mg |
| PMS | 1 mg |

#### Procedure

Incubate the gel in staining solution in the dark at 37°C until dark blue bands appear. Wash developed gel in water and fix in 50% ethanol.

*Notes:*  L-Histidinol is oxidized in two steps:

1. L-Histidinol + NAD = L-histidinal + NADH
2. L-Histidinal + NAD = L-histidine + NADH

### REFERENCE

1. Creaser, E. H., Bennett, D. J., and Drysdale, R. B., The purification and properties of histidinol dehydrogenase from *Neurospora crassa*, *Biochem. J.*, 103, 36, 1967.

## 1.1.1.25 — Shikimate Dehydrogenase; SHDH

REACTION        Shikimate + NADP = 3-dehydroshikimate + NADPH

ENZYME SOURCE  Bacteria, plants

### METHOD

#### Visualization Scheme

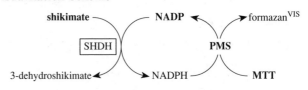

#### Staining Solution[1]

| | |
|---|---|
| 0.1 *M* Tris–HCl buffer, pH 7.1 | 30 ml |
| Shikimic acid | 25 mg |
| NADP | 5 mg |
| MTT | 6 mg |
| PMS (see Procedure) | 1 mg |

#### Procedure

Incubate the gel 30 min at 37°C in the dark in a staining solution lacking PMS, then add PMS and incubate until dark blue bands appear. Wash developed gel in water and fix in 4% formaldehyde or 50% ethanol.

### REFERENCE

1. Van Dijk, H. and Van Delden, W., Genetic variability in *Plantago* species in relation to their ecology. Part 1: Genetic analysis of the allozyme variation in *P. major* subspecies, *Theor. Appl. Genet.*, 60, 285, 1981.

OTHER NAMES        Lactic acid dehydrogenase

REACTION        L-Lactate + NAD = pyruvate + NADH

ENZYME SOURCE   Bacteria, fungi, plants, protozoa, invertebrates, vertebrates

## METHOD

### Visualization Scheme

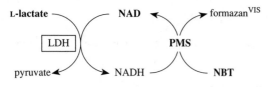

### Staining Solution[1]

| | |
|---|---|
| 0.2 M Tris–HCl buffer, pH 8.0 | 60 ml |
| 0.5 M L-Lactate (pH 8.0) | 12 ml |
| 10 mg/ml NAD | 2.7 ml |
| 1 mg/ml NBT | 6.7 ml |
| 1 mg/ml PMS | 6.7 ml |

### Procedure

Incubate the gel in staining solution in the dark at 37°C until dark blue bands appear. Wash developed gel in water and fix in 50% ethanol.

*Notes:*   The LDH activity bands can also be detected, though weakly, even in the absence of lactate from the staining solution.[2] This is the so-called "nothing dehydrogenase" (see 1.X.X.X — NDH) phenomenon, which is probably due to lactate bound to the enzyme molecules.

Mammalian LDH-X isozyme specific to postpubertal testis and sperm is relatively more active with α-hydroxybutyrate and α-hydroxyvaleriate than with lactate.[3]

## OTHER METHODS

A. The reverse reaction can also be used to detect LDH activity bands.[3] Staining solution includes 20 ml 0.05 M Tris–HCl buffer (pH 8.0), 100 mg sodium pyruvate and 10 mg NADH. Dark (nonfluorescent) bands of LDH activity are observed under long-wave UV light.

B. A bioautographic procedure for visualization of LDH activity bands was developed using *E. coli* strain CB482 deficient in LDH as the microbial reagent.[4] For growth and proliferation of *E. coli* (CB482), pyruvate is required as the source of carbon. An indicator agar for LDH bioautography contains $10^8$ microorganisms/ml, 2.5 mg/ml L-lactate, and 2.5 mg/ml NAD in minimal medium (see Appendix A-1) lacking a carbon source. When electrophoretic gel containing zones of LDH activity is placed in contact with indicator agar, bacteria proliferate at the regions where L-lactate is converted to pyruvate by exogenous LDH. Bands of bacterial proliferation are observed by transmitted light. Bioautographic detection of LDH is significantly more complex and time-consuming than the NBT/PMS method and therefore less appropriate for routine laboratory use.

C. Two-dimensional spectroscopy of electrophoretic gels also permits detection of LDH activity bands.[5] This procedure however, requires a special optical device which is not commercially available.

### REFERENCES

1. Whitt, G. S., Developmental genetics of the lactate dehydrogenase isozymes of fish, *J. Exp. Zool.*, 175, 1, 1970.
2. Falkenberg, F., Lehmann, F.-G., and Pfleiderer, G., LDH (lactate dehydrogenase) isozymes as cause of nonspecific tetrazolium salt staining in gel enzymograms ("nothing dehydrogenase"), *Clin. Chim. Acta*, 23, 265, 1969.
3. Harris, H. and Hopkinson, D. A., *Handbook of Enzyme Electrophoresis in Human Genetics*, North-Holland, Amsterdam (Loose leaf with supplements in 1977 and 1978), 1976.
4. Naylor, S. L. and Klebe, R. J., Bioautography: a general method for the visualization of isozymes, *Biochem. Genet.*, 15, 1193, 1977.
5. Klebe, R. J., Mancuso, M. G., Brown, C. R., and Teng, L., Two-dimensional spectroscopy of electrophoretic gels, *Biochem. Genet.*, 19, 655, 1981.

## 1.1.1.29 — Glycerate Dehydrogenase; G-2-DH

**OTHER NAMES**       Glycerate-2-dehydrogenase

**REACTION**        D-Glycerate + NAD = hydroxypyruvate + NADH

**ENZYME SOURCE**  Fungi, plants, invertebrates, vertebrates

## METHOD

### Visualization Scheme

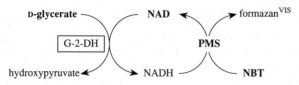

### Staining Solution[1]

| | |
|---|---|
| 0.04 $M$ Tris–HCl buffer, pH 8.0 | 50 ml |
| D,L-Glyceric acid (hemicalcium salt) | 100 mg |
| NAD | 25 mg |
| NBT | 15 mg |
| PMS | 1 mg |

### Procedure

Incubate the gel in staining solution in the dark at 37°C until dark blue bands appear. Wash developed gel in water and fix in 50% ethanol.

*Notes:*  Because LDH can also react with D-glycerate, an additional gel should be stained for LDH as a control.

G-2-DH activity in plants is an associated activity of glyoxylate reductase (EC 1.1.1.26) and is not a different protein moiety.

The rat liver enzyme is equally effective with reduced NAD or NADP in the reverse reaction, but in the forward reaction NAD is more effective than NADP.

### REFERENCE

1. Siciliano, M. J. and Shaw, C. R., Separation and visualization of enzymes on gels, in *Chromatographic and Electrophoretic Techniques, Vol. 2, Zone Electrophoresis*, Smith, I., Ed., Heinemann, London, 1976, 185.

## 1.1.1.30 — 3-Hydroxybutyrate Dehydrogenase; HBDH

**OTHER NAMES**       β-Hydroxybutyrate dehydrogenase

**REACTION**        D-β-Hydroxybutyrate + NAD = acetoacetate + NADH

**ENZYME SOURCE**  Bacteria, protozoa, invertebrates, vertebrates

## METHOD

### Visualization Scheme

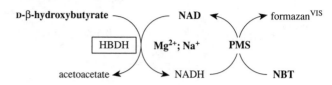

### Staining Solution[1] (modified)

| | |
|---|---|
| 0.1 $M$ Phosphate buffer, pH 7.4 | 90 ml |
| 1 $M$ D,L-β-Hydroxybutyrate | 10 mg |
| NAD | 30 mg |
| NBT | 25 mg |
| PMS | 2.5 mg |
| MgCl$_2$ (anhydrous) | 10 mg |
| NaCl | 575 mg |

### Procedure

Incubate the gel in staining solution in the dark at 37°C until dark blue bands appear. Wash developed gel in water and fix in 50% ethanol.

*Notes:*   The addition of NAD to electrophoretic gel is often beneficial. The addition of 1 to 2 mg/ml pyruvate and/or 1 to 2 mg/ml pyrazole to the staining solution may be desirable if the tissue chosen as the source of HBDH has high levels of LDH and/or ADH, respectively.

*Drosophila* enzyme may be identical to 1.1.1.45 — GUDH and 1.1.1.69 — GNDH (see below).

The beef heart mitochondrial enzyme has a specific and absolute requirement for lecithin.

### REFERENCE

1. Shaw, C. R. and Prasad, R., Starch gel electrophoresis of enzymes: a compilation of recipes, *Biochem. Genet.*, 4, 297, 1970.

OTHER NAMES     β-Hydroxyacyl dehydrogenase, β-keto-reductase

REACTION     L-3-Hydroxyacyl-CoA + NAD = 3-oxoacyl-CoA + NADH

ENZYME SOURCE   Vertebrates

## METHOD

### Visualization Scheme

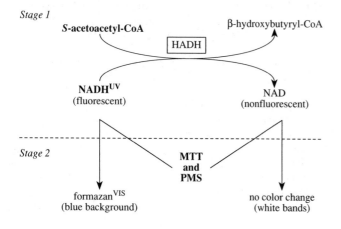

Stage 1

**S-acetoacetyl-CoA**      β-hydroxybutyryl-CoA

HADH

**NADH$^{UV}$** (fluorescent)      NAD (nonfluorescent)

Stage 2

**MTT and PMS**

formazan$^{VIS}$ (blue background)      no color change (white bands)

### Staining Solution[1]

A. 0.1 *M* Citrate–phosphate buffer, pH 5.3
    1.7 m*M* S-Acetoacetyl-CoA
    2 m*M* NADH

B. 0.1 *M* Citrate–phosphate buffer, pH 5.3
    2.5 mg/ml MTT
    0.02 mg/ml PMS

### Procedure

Apply solution A to the gel surface dropwise and incubate the gel at 37°C in a moist chamber. View the gel under long-wave UV light. Dark bands of HADH activity are visible on the light (fluorescent) background of the gel. When the bands are clearly visible, apply solution B to reveal HADH activity as white bands on a blue background. Rinse negatively stained gel under hot tap water for about 30 s to increase the intensity of the background color. Fix developed gel in 50% ethanol.

*Notes:* The enzyme also oxidizes L-3-hydroxyacyl-*N*-acylthioethanolamine and L-3-hydroxyacylhydrolipoate; HADH from some sources acts, more slowly, with NADP.

### REFERENCE

1. Craig, I., Tolley, E., and Bobrow, M., A preliminary analysis of the segregation of human hydroxyacyl coenzyme A dehydrogenase in human–mouse somatic cell hybrids, *Cytogenet. Cell Genet.*, 16, 114, 1976.

OTHER NAMES     Malic dehydrogenase

REACTION     L-Malate + NAD = oxaloacetate + NADH

ENZYME SOURCE     Bacteria, fungi, algae, plants, protozoa, invertebrates, vertebrates

## METHOD 1

### Visualization Scheme

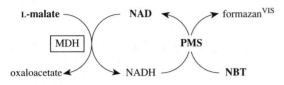

### Staining Solution[1]

| | |
|---|---:|
| 0.1 *M* Tris–HCl buffer, pH 8.0 | 100 ml |
| L-Malic acid (disodium salt) | 250 mg |
| NAD | 30 mg |
| NBT | 25 mg |
| PMS | 2 mg |

### Procedure

Incubate the gel in staining solution in the dark at 37°C until dark blue bands appear. Wash developed gel in water and fix in 50% ethanol.

*Notes:* The adding of 1 to 2 mg/ml pyruvate and/or 1 to 2 mg/ml pyrazole to the staining solution may be desirable if the tissue chosen as the source of MDH has high levels of LDH and/or ADH, respectively.

## METHOD 2

### Visualization Scheme

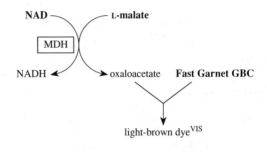

### Staining Solution[2]

| | |
|---|---:|
| 0.1 *M* Tris–HCl buffer, pH 8.0 | 50 ml |
| Fast Garnet GBC salt | 150 mg |
| L-Malic acid (sodium salt) | 125 mg |
| NAD | 60 mg |

### Procedure

Incubate the gel in staining solution in the dark at 37°C until light brown bands appear. Wash developed gel in water and fix in 50% glycerol.

*Notes:* Greater sensitivity of the method may be obtained using a post-coupling technique. All ingredients of the staining solution except Fast Garnet GBC (the potential inhibitor of MDH) are applied to the gel. The gel is incubated for a period of time and Fast Garnet GBC (dissolved in a minimal volume of stain buffer) is then added.

## GENERAL NOTES

Method 1 is more commonly used and more sensitive than Method 2. It does, however, allow the nonspecific staining of NAD-dependent "nothing dehydrogenase" bands (see 1.X.X.X — NDH), whereas Method 2 avoids this problem.

## REFERENCES

1. Shaw, C. R. and Prasad, R., Starch gel electrophoresis of enzymes: a compilation of recipes, *Biochem. Genet.*, 4, 297, 1970.
2. Richardson, B. J., Baverstock, P. R., and Adams, M., *Allozyme Electrophoresis: A Handbook for Animal Systematics and Population Studies*, Academic Press, Sydney, 1986, 201.

## 1.1.1.40 — Malate Dehydrogenase (NADP); ME

**OTHER NAMES**    "Malic" enzyme

**REACTION**    L-Malate + NADP = pyruvate + $CO_2$ + NADPH

**ENZYME SOURCE**    Bacteria, fungi, plants, protozoa, invertebrates, vertebrates

## METHOD

### Visualization Scheme

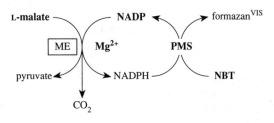

### Staining Solution[1]

| | |
|---|---|
| 0.05 $M$ Tris–HCl buffer, pH 8.0 | 50 ml |
| L-Malic acid (sodium salt) | 700 mg |
| NADP | 15 mg |
| NBT | 15 mg |
| PMS | 1 mg |
| $MgCl_2$ (anhydrous) | 50 mg |

### Procedure

Incubate the gel in staining solution in the dark at 37°C until dark blue bands appear. Rinse stained gel in water and fix in 50% ethanol.

*Notes:*  In some cases increased activity of ME can be obtained using $MnCl_2$ in place of $MgCl_2$ in the staining solution. It should be remembered, however, that in the presence of $Mn^{2+}$ ions PMS acts less effectively as an electron-carrier intermediary. When $Mn^{2+}$ ions are used, a "positive" fluorescent stain may be preferable. This stain uses a staining solution similar to that described above but lacking PMS and NBT and containing $MnCl_2$ in place of $MgCl_2$. After an appropriate period of time of incubating the gel with staining solution fluorescent bands of ME activity can be observed under long-wave UV light.

### REFERENCE

1. Siciliano, M. J. and Shaw, C. R., Separation and visualization of enzymes on gels, in *Chromatographic and Electrophoretic Techniques, Vol. 2, Zone Electrophoresis*, Smith, I., Ed., Heinemann, London, 1976, 185.

## 1.1.1.41 — Isocitrate Dehydrogenase (NAD); IDH(NAD)

**OTHER NAMES**    β-Ketoglutaric–isocitric carboxylase

**REACTION**    Isocitrate + NAD = 2-oxoglutarate + $CO_2$ + NADH

**ENZYME SOURCE**    Fungi, plants, invertebrates, vertebrates

## METHOD

### Visualization Scheme

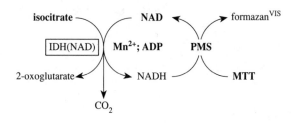

### Staining Solution[1]

| | |
|---|---|
| 0.1 $M$ Tris–HCl buffer, pH 8.4 | 100 ml |
| Isocitric acid | 125 mg |
| ADP | 7.5 mg |
| $MnCl_2$ | 65 mg |
| NAD | 6 mg |
| MTT | 8 mg |
| PMS | 2 mg |

### Procedure

Incubate the gel in staining solution in the dark at 37°C until dark blue bands appear. Rinse developed gel in water and fix in 50% ethanol.

*Notes:*  It is recommended to use $MgCl_2$ in place of $MnCl_2$ because $Mn^{2+}$ ions significantly lower the PMS action as electron-carrier intermediary. The enzyme is an allosteric one specifically activated by ADP. In the absence of ADP, activity of IDH(NAD) is very low.

### REFERENCE

1. Menken, S. B. J., Allozyme polymorphism and the speciation process in small ermine moths (Lepidoptera, Yponomeutidae), Ph.D. Thesis, University of Leiden, Leiden, The Netherlands, 1980.

OTHER NAMES    Oxalosuccinate decarboxylase

REACTION    Isocitrate + NADP = 2-oxoglutarate + $CO_2$ + NADPH

ENZYME SOURCE    Bacteria, fungi, plants, protozoa, invertebrates, vertebrates

## METHOD 1

### Visualization Scheme

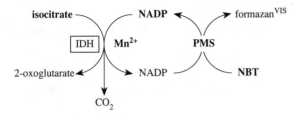

### Staining Solution[1]

| | |
|---|---:|
| 0.1 $M$ Tris–HCl buffer, pH 8.0 | 100 ml |
| 0.1 $M$ Isocitric acid (trisodium salt) | 3 ml |
| NADP | 20 mg |
| NBT | 10 mg |
| PMS | 3 mg |
| 0.25 $M$ MnCl$_2$ | 0.4 ml |

### Procedure

Incubate the gel in staining solution in the dark at 37°C until dark blue bands appear. Wash stained gel in water and fix in 50% ethanol.

*Notes:* Addition of NADP to the gel or acetate cellulose soaking buffer usually proves beneficial. It is recommended to use MgCl$_2$ instead of MnCl$_2$ because Mn$^{2+}$ ions significantly lower the PMS action as electron-carrier intermediary.

## METHOD 2

### Visualization Scheme

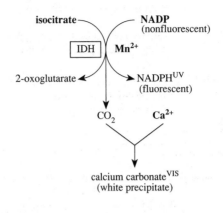

### Staining Solution[2]

100 m$M$ Tris–HCl buffer, pH 7.5
1 m$M$ Isocitrate
1 m$M$ NADP
100 m$M$ Mn$^{2+}$
100 m$M$ Ca$^{2+}$

### Procedure

Place electrophorized PAG in the stain buffer at 37°C. After 20 to 30 min transfer gel to staining solution and incubate at 37°C. View gel against a dark background and, when an activity stain of sufficient intensity is obtained, remove gel from the staining solution and store in 50 m$M$ glycine–KOH buffer (pH 10.0), 5 m$M$ Ca$^{2+}$ either at 5°C or at room temperature in the presence of an antibacterial agent. Under these conditions, stained gel can be stored for several months with little deterioration.

*Notes:* This method was developed for PAG. It is, however, also applicable to acetate cellulose and starch gels where IDH activity bands can be observed in long-wave UV light as fluorescent zones on a dark (nonfluorescent) background.

## GENERAL NOTES

Method 1 is more commonly used than Method 2. It does, however, allow the staining of NADP-dependent "nothing dehydrogenase" (see 1.X.X.X — NDH), whereas the use of Method 2 avoids this problem.

Manganese ions are the best activators of IDH; however, their use in tetrazolium stain is not effective because of inhibitory effect towards PMS. So, "positive" fluorescent stain using a staining solution similar to those presented in Methods 1 and 2, but lacking PMS/NBT or Ca$^{2+}$, respectively, may be preferable when preparations with low IDH activity are studied.

### REFERENCES

1. Henderson, N, S., Isozymes of isocitrate dehydrogenase: subunit structure and intracellular location, *J. Exp. Zool.*, 158, 263, 1965.
2. Nimmo, H.G. and Nimmo, G.A., A general method for the localization of enzymes that produce phosphate, pyrophosphate, or $CO_2$ after polyacrylamide gel electrophoresis, *Anal. Biochem.*, 121, 17, 1982.

## 1.1.1.44 — Phosphogluconate Dehydrogenase; PGD

OTHER NAMES Phosphogluconic acid dehydrogenase, 6-phosphogluconate dehydrogenase, 6-phosphogluconic dehydrogenase, 6-phosphogluconic carboxylase

REACTION 6-Phospho-D-gluconate + NADP = D-ribulose-5-phosphate + $CO_2$ + NADPH

ENZYME SOURCE Bacteria, green algae, fungi, plants, protozoa, invertebrates, vertebrates

## METHOD

### Visualization Scheme

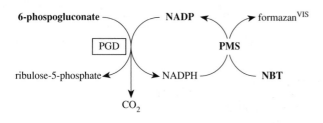

### Staining Solution[1]

| | |
|---|---|
| 0.05 $M$ Tris–HCl buffer, pH 8.0 | 100 ml |
| 6-Phosphogluconic acid (trisodium salt) | 200 mg |
| NADP | 20 mg |
| NBT | 25 mg |
| PMS | 2 mg |

### Procedure

Incubate the gel in staining solution in the dark at 37°C until dark blue bands appear. Wash developed gel in water and fix in 50% ethanol.

*Notes:* Addition of $MgCl_2$ to the staining solution (25 m$M$ final concentration) accelerates development of PGD activity bands. The amounts of substrate and cofactor in the staining solution may be decreased five and two times, respectively.

### REFERENCE

1. Shaw, C. R. and Prasad, R., Starch gel electrophoresis of enzymes: a compilation of recipes, *Biochem. Genet.*, 4, 297, 1970.

## 1.1.1.45 — L-Gulonate Dehydrogenase; GUDH

OTHER NAMES L-3-Aldonate dehydrogenase, L-gluconate dehydrogenase, β-L-hydroxyacid dehydrogenase, 3-oxoacid dehydrogenase

REACTION L-Gulonate + NAD = 3-keto-L-gulonate + NADH; also oxidizes other L-3-hydroxyacids

ENZYME SOURCE Invertebrates

## METHOD

### Visualization Scheme

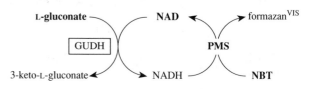

### Staining Solution[1]

| | |
|---|---|
| 0.05 $M$ Tris–phosphate buffer (pH 8.2) containing 40 m$M$ pyrazole | 100 ml |
| L-Gluconate | 200 mg |
| NAD | 20 mg |
| NBT | 10 mg |
| PMS | 0.4 mg |

### Procedure

Incubate the gel in staining solution in the dark at 37°C until dark blue bands appear. Wash stained gel in water and fix in 50% ethanol.

*Notes:* β-Hydroxybutyrate also may be used as substrate for *Drosophila* GUDH. D-Gluconate is also oxidized by *Drosophila* GUDH. *Drosophila* GUDH may be identical with 1.1.1.30 — HBDH (see above) and/or 1.1.1.69 — GNDH (see below).

### REFERENCE

1. Tobler, J. E. and Grell, E. H., Genetics and physiological expression of β-hydroxy acid dehydrogenase in *Drosophila*, *Biochem. Genet.*, 16, 333, 1978.

OTHER NAMES   Galactose-6-phosphate dehydrogenase, hexose-6-phosphate dehydrogenase

REACTIONS   1. β-D-glucose + NAD(P) = D-glucono-1,5-lactone + NAD(P)H

2. D-Galactose-6-phosphate + NADP = galactono-1,4-lactone-6-phosphate + NADPH (presumed reaction)

ENZYME SOURCE   Bacteria, fungi, invertebrates, vertebrates

## METHOD 1

### Visualization Scheme

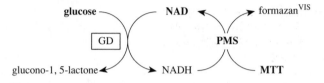

### Staining Solution[1] (modified)

| | |
|---|---|
| 0.05 *M* Phosphate buffer, pH 7.3 | 50 ml |
| D-Glucose | 5 g |
| NAD | 30 mg |
| MTT | 8 mg |
| PMS | 3 mg |

### Procedure

Incubate the gel in staining solution in the dark at 37°C until dark blue bands appear. Wash developed gel in water and fix in 50% ethanol.

*Notes:*   In some situations (e.g., when *Drosophila* male whole-body homogenates are used as the source of enzyme) glucose oxidase (see 1.1.3.4 — GO) bands are also visualized by Method 1.[2]

## METHOD 2

### Visualization Scheme

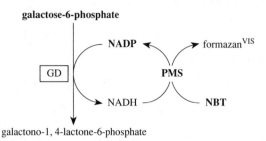

### Staining Solution[3] (modified)

| | |
|---|---|
| 0.05 *M* Tris–HCl buffer, pH 7.0 | 45 ml |
| 1 *M* Galactose-6-phosphate | 2.5 ml |
| NADP | 20 mg |
| NBT | 25 mg |
| PMS | 2 mg |

### Procedure

Incubate the gel in staining solution in the dark at 37°C until dark blue bands appear. Wash developed gel in water and fix in 50% ethanol.

*Notes:*   The enzyme is also capable of using glucose-6-phosphate as substrate in some taxa. It may appear as a stain artifact on hexokinase (2.7.1.1 — HK), adenylate kinase (2.7.4.3 — AK, Method 1), and glucose-6-phosphate dehydrogenase (1.1.1.49 — G-6-PD) zymograms.

## GENERAL NOTES

The addition of NAD(P) to electrophoretic gels and acetate cellulose soaking buffers often proves beneficial. D-Xylose also may be used as substrate for GD.

## REFERENCES

1. Harris, H. and Hopkinson, D. A., *Handbook of Enzyme Electrophoresis in Human Genetics*, North-Holland, Amsterdam (Loose leaf with supplements in 1977 and 1978), 1976.
2. Cavener, D. R., Genetics of male-specific glucose oxidase and the identification of other unusual hexose enzymes in *Drosophila melanogaster*, *Biochem. Genet.*, 18, 929, 1980.
3. Shaw, C. R. and Koen, A. L., Glucose-6-phosphate dehydrogenase and hexose-6-phosphate dehydrogenase of mammalian tissues, *Ann. NY Acad. Sci.*, 151, 149, 1968.

## 1.1.1.48 — Galactose Dehydrogenase; GALDH

REACTION       D-Galactose + NAD = D-galactono-1,4-lactone + NADH

ENZYME SOURCE  Bacteria, vertebrates

## METHOD

### Visualization Scheme

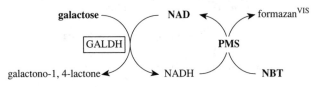

### Staining Solution[1]

| | |
|---|---:|
| 0.1 M Tris–HCl buffer, pH 8.4 | 100 ml |
| D(+)Galactose | 900 mg |
| NAD | 30 mg |
| NBT | 20 mg |
| PMS | 4 mg |

### Procedure

Incubate the gel in staining solution in the dark at 37°C until dark blue bands appear. Wash developed gel in water and fix in 50% ethanol.

### REFERENCE

1. Cuatrecasas, P. and Segal, S., Electrophoretic heterogeneity of mammalian galactose dehydrogenase, *Science*, 154, 533, 1966.

## 1.1.1.49 — Glucose-6-phosphate Dehydrogenase; G-6-PD

REACTION       D-Glucose-6-phosphate + NADP = D-glucono-1,5-lactone-6-phosphate + NADPH

ENZYME SOURCE  Bacteria, green algae, fungi, plants, protozoa, invertebrates, vertebrates

## METHOD

### Visualization Scheme

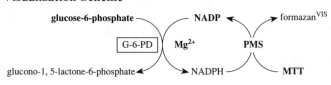

### Staining Solution[1] (modified)

| | |
|---|---:|
| 0.1 M Tris–HCl buffer, pH 8.0 | 45 ml |
| Glucose-6-phosphate (disodium salt) | 20 mg |
| NADP | 10 mg |
| MTT | 10 mg |
| PMS | 1 mg |
| 0.2 M MgCl$_2$ | 5 ml |

### Procedure

Incubate the gel in staining solution in the dark at 37°C until dark blue bands appear. Wash developed gel in water and fix in 50% ethanol.

*Notes:* The addition of NADP to electrophoretic gels and acetate cellulose soaking buffers often proves beneficial. The bands of glucose dehydrogenase (see 1.1.1.47 — GD, Method 2) also can develop on G-6-PD zymograms.[2] Thus, an additional slice of the same starch gel block, or additional acetate cellulose strip, should, in some situations, be stained for GD as controls.

### OTHER METHODS

The immunoblotting procedure (for details see Part II) based on the utility of monoclonal antibodies specific to rat[3] and human[4] G-6-PD can also be used to detect the enzyme protein on electrophoretic gels. This procedure is not as practical as that described above; however, it may be of great value in special (biochemical, immunological, phylogenetic, and genetic) analyses of G-6-PD.

### REFERENCES

1. Shaw, C. R. and Prasad, R., Starch gel electrophoresis of enzymes: a compilation of recipes, *Biochem. Genet.*, 4, 297, 1970.
2. Shaw, C. R. and Koen, A. L., Glucose-6-phosphate dehydrogenase and hexose-6-phosphate dehydrogenase of mammalian tissues, *Ann. NY Acad. Sci.*, 151, 149, 1968.
3. Dao, M. L., Johnson, B. C., and Hartman, P. E., Preparation of monoclonal antibody to rat liver glucose-6-phosphate dehydrogenase and the study of its immunoreactivity with native and inactivated enzyme, *Proc. Natl. Acad. Sci. U.S.A.*, 79, 2860, 1980.
4. Damiani, G., Frascio, M., Benatti, U., Morelli, A., Zocchi, E., Fabbi, M., Bargellesi, A., Pontremoli, S., and De Flora, A., Monoclonal antibodies to human erythrocyte glucose-6-phosphate dehydrogenase, *FEBS Lett.*, 119, 169, 1980.

## 1.1.1.53 — (R)-20-Hydroxysteroid Dehydrogenase; HSDH

OTHER NAMES    Cortisone reductase

REACTION        (20R)-17α,20,21-Trihydroxypregn-4-ene-3,11-dione + NAD = cortisone + NADH (see also *Notes*)

ENZYME SOURCE  Bacteria

### METHOD

#### Visualization Scheme

**(20R)-17α, 20, 21-trihydroxypregn-4-ENE-3, 11-dione**

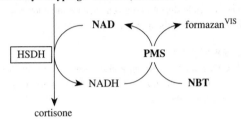

#### Staining Solution[1]
0.1 *M* Tris–HCl buffer, pH 7.1
0.5 m*M* NAD
0.02 mg/ml 5α-Pregnan-20β-ol-3-on (dissolved in minimal volume of isopropanol)
0.3 mg/ml NBT
0.02 mg/ml PMS

#### Procedure
Incubate the gel in staining solution in the dark at 37°C until dark blue bands appear. Fix stained gel in 50% ethanol.

*Notes:*  The enzyme also acts on other 20-keto-steroids containing different substituents of the steroid system.

    Alcohol dehydrogenase bands can also become apparent on HSDH zymograms obtained by this method. Thus, an additional gel should be stained for alcohol dehydrogenase (see 1.1.1.1 — ADH, Method 1) as a control.

#### REFERENCE
1. Blomquist, C. H., The molecular weight and substrate specificity of 20β-hydroxysteroid dehydrogenase from *Streptomyces hydrogenans*, *Arch. Biochem. Biophys.*, 159, 590, 1973.

## 1.1.1.67 — Mannitol Dehydrogenase; MD(NAD)

REACTION        D-Mannitol + NAD = D-fructose + NADH

ENZYME SOURCE  Bacteria, fungi

### METHOD

#### Visualization Scheme

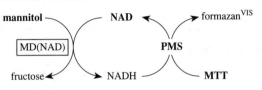

#### Staining Solution*
A.  0.1 *M* Tris–HCl buffer, pH 8.5    25 ml
    NAD    20 mg
    D-Mannitol    200 mg
    MTT    10 mg
    PMS    1 mg
B.  2% Agarose solution (60°C)    25 ml

#### Procedure
Mix A and B components and pour the mixture over the surface of the gel. Incubate the gel at 37°C in the dark until dark blue bands appear. Fix stained agarose plate in 50% ethanol.

*Notes:*  This method was used by the author to detect MD(NAD) from mushroom *Boletus edulis* (unpublished data).

---

*  New, recommended for use.

OTHER NAMES    5-Keto-D-gluconate reductase, D-gluconate dehydrogenase

REACTION    D-Gluconate + NAD(P) = 5-dehydro-D-gluconate + NAD(P)H

ENZYME SOURCE  Bacteria, invertebrates, vertebrates

## METHOD

### Visualization Scheme

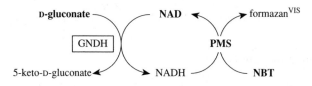

### Staining Solution[1]

| | |
|---|---|
| 0.2 $M$ Tris–HCl buffer, pH 8.0 | 25 ml |
| 80 mg/ml D-Gluconate (pH 8.0) | 25 ml |
| 10 mg/ml NAD | 1 ml |
| 10 mg/ml NBT | 0.5 ml |
| 10 mg/ml PMS | 0.5 ml |

### Procedure

Incubate the gel in staining solution in the dark at 37°C until dark blue bands appear. Wash stained gel in water and fix in 50% ethanol.

*Notes:* To prepare D-gluconate solution, dissolve 2.0 g D-gluconic acid lactone in 25 ml $H_2O$ and adjust the pH to 12.5 with sodium hydroxide pellets. After 30 min incubation at room temperature readjust the pH to 8.0 by adding HCl.

    *Drosophila* enzyme may be identical to 1.1.1.45 — GUDH (see above).

    D-2-Hydroxyacid dehydrogenase (EC 1.1.99.6) activity bands can also appear on GNDH zymograms as a result of the interchange between the oxidized and reduced states of D-2-hydroxyacid dehydrogenase flavoprotein. The reduced forms of this enzyme from some sources can chemically reduce NBT via PMS without the need for NAD.

### REFERENCE

1. Buth, D. G., Staining procedures for D-2-hydroxyacid dehydrogenase as applied to studies of lower vertebrates, *Isozyme Bull.*, 13, 115, 1980.

OTHER NAMES     Glyceraldehyde reductase

REACTION     Glycerole + NADP = D-glyceraldehyde + NADPH

ENZYME SOURCE   Fungi, invertebrates, vertebrates

## METHOD 1

### Visualization Scheme

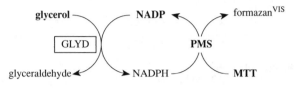

### Staining Solution[1]

| | |
|---|---|
| 0.1 *M* Tris–HCl buffer, pH 8.4 | 95 ml |
| Glycerol | 5 ml |
| NADP | 8 mg |
| MTT | 10 mg |
| PMS | 2 mg |

### Procedure

Incubate the gel in staining solution in the dark at 37°C until dark blue bands appear. Wash stained gel in water and fix in 50% ethanol.

*Notes:* Specificity of GLYD staining should be verified by exclusion of glycerol from staining solution.

## METHOD 2

### Visualization Scheme

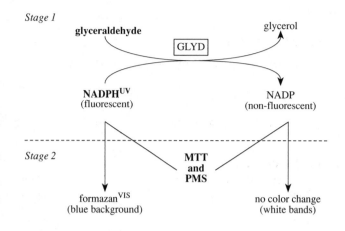

### Staining Solution[2]

A. 80 m*M* Sodium phosphate buffer, pH 7.0
    6 m*M* NADPH
    110 m*M* D-Glyceraldehyde
B. 260 m*M* Tris–HCl buffer, pH 8.0
    0.6 m*M* PMS
    1.8 m*M* MTT
C. 2% Agar solution (60°C)

### Procedure

Mix equal volumes of A and C solutions and pour the mixture over the gel surface. Incubate the gel 30 min at 37°C and view under long-wave UV light. Dark bands of GLYD activity are visible on a light (fluorescent) background. When the bands are clearly visible, lift away the agar overlay. Mix equal volumes of B and C solutions and pour over the gel surface. White bands clearly visible on a blue background appear almost immediately. Rinse stained gel under hot tap water for about 30 s to increase the intensity of the background color. Fix developed gel in 50% ethanol.

*Notes:* It should be kept in mind that the amount of NADPH added to the staining solution is critical for development of nonfluorescent GLYD bands. When too much NADPH is added, the enzyme should not be able to convert enough NADPH into NADP for nonfluorescent bands to become visible.

     After electrophoresis of mammalian tissue preparations some isozymes of NADP-dependent alcohol dehydrogenase [see 1.1.1.2 — ADH(NADP)], as well as glucuronate reductase (see 1.1.1.19 — GLR) bands, may also appear on GLYD zymograms obtained by this method.

### REFERENCES

1. Menken, S. B. J., Allozyme polymorphism and the speciation process in small ermine moths (Lepidoptera, Yponomeutidae), Ph.D. Thesis, University of Leiden, Leiden, The Netherlands, 1980.
2. Mather, P. B. and Holmes, R. S., Aldehide reductase isozymes in the mouse: evidence for two new loci and localization of *Ahr-3* on chromosome 7, *Biochem. Genet.*, 23, 483, 1985.

## 1.1.1.73 — Octanol Dehydrogenase; ODH

REACTION          Octanol + NAD = octanal + NADH

ENZYME SOURCE  Fungi, invertebrates, vertebrates

## METHOD

### Visualization Scheme

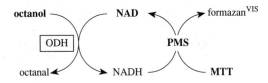

### Staining Solution[1]

| | |
|---|---|
| 0.1 $M$ Tris–HCl buffer, pH 8.4 | 100 ml |
| Octanol | 0.25 ml |
| NAD | 8 mg |
| MTT | 10 mg |
| PMS | 2 mg |

### Procedure

Incubate the gel in staining solution in the dark at 37°C until dark blue bands appear. Wash stained gel in water and fix in 50% ethanol.

*Notes:*  Usually octanol is dissolved in 1 to 2 ml of ethanol before being included in a staining solution. However, this requires control staining of an additional gel for alcohol dehydrogenase (see 1.1.1.1 — ADH, Method 1).

### REFERENCE

1. Menken, S. B. J., Allozyme polymorphism and the speciation process in small ermine moths (Lepidoptera, Yponomeutidae), Ph.D. Thesis, University of Leiden, Leiden, The Netherlands, 1980.

## 1.1.1.80 — Isopropanol Dehydrogenase (NADP); IPDH

REACTION          Isopropanol + NADP = acetone + NADPH

ENZYME SOURCE  Invertebrates

## METHOD

### Visualization Scheme

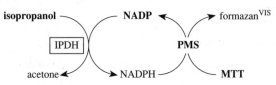

### Staining Solution[1]

| | |
|---|---|
| 0.1 $M$ Tris–HCl buffer, pH 8.4 | 100 ml |
| Isopropanol | 4 ml |
| NADP | 8 mg |
| MTT | 10 mg |
| PMS | 2 mg |

### Procedure

Incubate the gel in staining solution in the dark at 37°C until dark blue bands appear. Rinse stained gel in water and fix in 50% ethanol.

*Notes:*  The enzyme also acts on other short-chain secondary alcohols, and, slowly, on primary alcohols.

### REFERENCE

1. Menken, S. B. J., Allozyme polymorphism and the speciation process in small ermine moths (Lepidoptera, Yponomeutidae), Ph.D. Thesis, University of Leiden, Leiden, The Netherlands, 1980.

## 1.1.1.96 — Aromatic α-Keto Acid Reductase; AKAR

**OTHER NAMES**  Diiodophenylpyruvate reductase (recommended name), α-keto acid reductase

**REACTION**  *p*-Hydroxyphenylpyruvic acid + NADH = *p*-hydroxyphenyllactic acid + NAD

**ENZYME SOURCE**  Vertebrates

## METHOD

### Visualization Scheme

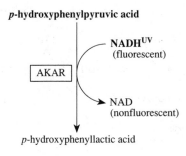

**p-hydroxyphenylpyruvic acid**

NADH[UV] (fluorescent)

AKAR

NAD (nonfluorescent)

*p*-hydroxyphenyllactic acid

### Staining Solution[1]

| | |
|---|---|
| A. 0.2 *M* Tris–HCl buffer, pH 7.6 | 25 ml |
| NADH | 10 mg |
| *p*-Hydroxyphenylpyruvic acid | 25 mg |
| L-Lactic acid | 25 mg |
| B. 2% Agar solution (60°C) | 25 ml |

### Procedure

Mix A and B components of the staining solution and pour the mixture over the gel surface. Incubate the gel at 37°C for 1 to 3 h. Dark (nonfluorescent) bands visible in long-wave UV light on a light (fluorescent) background indicate areas of AKAR localization. Record the zymogram or photograph using a yellow filter.

*Notes:*  If too much NADH is added, the enzyme should not be able to convert enough NADH into NAD for nonfluorescent bands to become visible.

A negative zymogram (white bands on blue background) visible in daylight may be obtained after treatment of the processed gel with the PMS/MTT solution.

Lactic acid is added to the staining solution to inhibit lactate dehydrogenase, which also displays low activity towards *p*-hydroxyphenylpyruvic acid.

The reverse reaction using *p*-hydroxyphenyllactic acid as substrate and NAD as cofactor results in bands similar to those seen with the forward reaction. However, lactate dehydrogenase is very prominent even in the presence of pyruvic acid (inhibitor of the forward LDH reaction), and the AKAR bands are poorly defined after prolonged incubation of the gel.

### REFERENCE

1. Donald, L. J., A description of human aromatic α-keto acid reductase, *Ann. Hum. Genet.*, 46, 299, 1982.

## 1.1.1.103 — L-Threonine 3-Dehydrogenase; TRDH

**REACTION**  L-Threonine + NAD = L-2-amino-3-oxobutanoate + NADH

**ENZYME SOURCE**  Bacteria, vertebrates

## METHOD

### Visualization Scheme

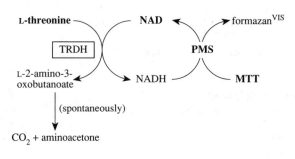

**L-threonine**  **NAD**  formazan[VIS]

TRDH  PMS

L-2-amino-3-oxobutanoate  NADH  MTT

(spontaneously)

$CO_2$ + aminoacetone

### Staining Solution[1]

| | |
|---|---|
| 0.015 *M* Sodium phosphate buffer, pH 7.0 | 50 ml |
| L-Threonine | 50 mg |
| 1.25% MTT | 1 ml |
| 1% PMS | 0.5 ml |
| 1% NAD | 2 ml |

### Procedure

Incubate the gel in staining solution in the dark at 37°C until dark blue bands appear. Rinse developed gel in water and fix in 50% ethanol.

### REFERENCE

1. Selander, R. K., Caugant, D. A., Ochman, H., Musser, J. M., Gilmour, M. N., and Whittam, T. S., Methods of multilocus enzyme electrophoresis for bacterial population genetics and systematics, *Appl. Environ. Microbiol.*, 51, 873, 1986.

## 1.1.1.105 — Retinol Dehydrogenase; RDH

**REACTION**  Retinol + NAD = retinal + NADH

**ENZYME SOURCE**  Vertebrates

## METHOD

### Visualization Scheme

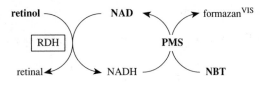

### Staining Solution[1]

| | |
|---|---|
| 0.01 $M$ Phosphate buffer, pH 7.0 | 100 ml |
| NAD | 66 mg |
| NBT | 35 mg |
| PMS | 2 mg |
| Retinol (dissolved in minimal volume of acetone) | 100 mg |

### Procedure

Incubate the gel in staining solution in the dark at 37°C until dark blue bands appear. Rinse developed gel in water and fix in 50% ethanol.

### REFERENCE

1. Koen, A. L. and Shaw, C. R., Retinol and alcohol dehydrogenases in retina and liver, *Biochim. Biophys. Acta*, 128, 48, 1966.

## 1.1.1.122 — L-Fucose Dehydrogenase; FUCDH

**OTHER NAMES**  D-*threo*-Aldose dehydrogenase (recommended name), (2$S$,3$R$)-aldose dehydrogenase

**REACTION**  D-*threo*-Aldose + NAD = D-*threo*-aldono-1,5-lactone + NADH

**ENZYME SOURCE**  Bacteria, invertebrates, vertebrates

## METHOD

### Visualization Scheme

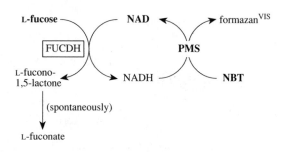

### Staining Solution[1]

10 m$M$ Tris–HCl buffer, pH 8.0
30 m$M$ L-Fucose
6 m$M$ NAD
0.08% NBT
0.014% PMS

### Procedure

Incubate the gel in staining solution in the dark at 37°C until dark blue bands appear. Wash stained gel in water and fix in 50% ethanol.

*Notes:*  The enzyme is reported to act on several other aldoses (D-arabinose, D-lyxose, L-xylose) but shows the fastest rate with L-fucose. Animal enzyme was also shown to act on L-arabinose and L-galactose. The enzyme from *Pseudomonas* also acts on L-glucose.

### REFERENCE

1. Schachter, H., Sarney, J., McGuire, E. J., and Roseman, S., Isolation of diphosphopyridine nucleotide-dependent L-fucose dehydrogenase from pork liver, *J. Biol. Chem.*, 244, 4785, 1969.

## 1.1.1.138 — Mannitol Dehydrogenase (NADP); MD(NADP)

**REACTION**      D-Mannitol + NADP = D-fructose + NADPH

**ENZYME SOURCE**   Fungi

## METHOD

### Visualization Scheme

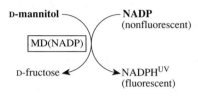

### Staining Solution[1]

| | |
|---|---:|
| 0.05 $M$ Tris–HCl buffer, pH 8.5 | 10 ml |
| NADP | 10 mg |
| D-Mannitol | 100 mg |

### Procedure

Lay a piece of filter paper saturated with the staining solution on top of the gel, and incubate at 37°C for 30 to 60 min. Remove the filter paper and view the gel under long-wave UV light. Fluorescent bands of MD(NADP) are visible on the dark (nonfluorescent) background of the gel. Record the zymogram or photograph using a yellow filter.

*Notes:* When a final zymogram easily visible in daylight is required, counterstain the processed gel with MTT/PMS solution. This will result in the appearance of dark blue bands of MD(NADP). The post-coupling technique is recommended because of the presumed inhibitory effect of PMS or MTT (or both) on MD(NADP) activity.

### REFERENCE

1. Royse, D. J. and May, B., Use of isozyme variation to identify genotypic classes of *Agaricus brunnescens*, *Mycologia*, 74, 93, 1982.

## 1.1.1.145 — 3β-Hydroxy-Δ⁵-Steroid Dehydrogenase; 3β-HSD

**OTHER NAMES**     Progesterone reductase

**REACTION**      3β-Hydroxy-$\Delta^5$-steroid + NAD = 3-oxo-$\Delta^5$-steroid + NADH

**ENZYME SOURCE**   Vertebrates

## METHOD

### Visualization Scheme

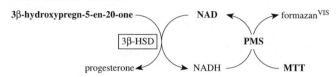

### Staining Solution[1]

| | |
|---|---:|
| 0.1 $M$ Tris–HCl buffer, pH 8.0 | 50 ml |
| 3β-Hydroxypregn-5-en-20-one (dissolved in minimal volume of ethanol or isopropanol) | 50 mg |
| NAD | 20 mg |
| MTT | 10 mg |
| PMS | 1 mg |

### Procedure

Incubate the gel in staining solution in the dark at 37°C until dark blue bands appear. Wash stained gel in water and fix in 50% ethanol.

*Notes:* An additional gel should be stained for alcohol dehydrogenase (see 1.1.1.1 — ADH) as a control. The enzyme also acts on 3β-hydroxyandrost-5-en-17-one to form androst-4-ene-3,17-dione.

### REFERENCE

1. Engel, W., Frowein, J., Krone, W., and Wolf, U., Induction of testis alcohol dehydrogenase in prepubertal rats. I. The effects of human chorion gonadotropine (HCG), theophylline, and dibutyryl cyclic AMP, *Clin. Gen.*, 3, 34, 1971.

## 1.1.1.179 — D-Xylose Dehydrogenase (NADP); XD(NADP)

REACTION        D-Xylose + NADP = D-xylono-1,5-lactone + NADPH

ENZYME SOURCE  Vertebrates

## METHOD

### Visualization Scheme

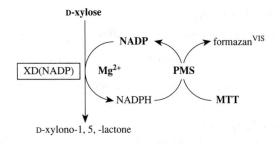

### Staining Solution[1]
A. 1 $M$ Tris–HCl buffer, pH 8.0
   12 m$M$ MgCl$_2$
   0.48 m$M$ NADP
   2 m$M$ MTT
   0.6 m$M$ PMS
   0.2 $M$ D-Xylose
B. 1.8% Agar solution (60°C)

### Procedure
Mix A and B components of the staining solution and pour the mixture over the gel surface. Incubate the gel at 37°C in the dark until dark blue bands appear. Fix stained gel in 50% ethanol.

*Notes:* The enzyme also acts, more slowly, on L-arabinose, D-ribose, D-glucose, D-galactose, L-fucose, D-fucose, 6-deoxy-D-glucose, and 2-deoxy-D-glucose. No activity was detected with ethanol, D-erythrose, D-fructose, glycerol, D-mannose, ribitol, sorbitol, sucrose, xylitol, D-glucose-1-phosphate, D-glucose-6-phosphate, and D-ribose-5-phosphate.

### REFERENCE

1. Newton, M. F., Nash, H. R., Peters, J., and Andrews, S. J., Xylose dehydrogenase-1, a new gene on mouse chromosome 7, *Biochem. Genet.*, 20, 733, 1982.

## 1.1.1.204 — Xanthine Dehydrogenase; XDH

REACTIONS     1. Hypoxanthine + NAD + H$_2$O = xanthine + NADH
                2. Xanthine + NAD + H$_2$O = urate + NADH

ENZYME SOURCE  Green algae, fungi, plants, invertebrates, vertebrates

## METHOD

### Visualization Scheme

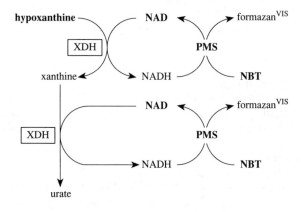

### Staining Solution[1]

| | |
|---|---|
| 0.1 $M$ Tris–HCl buffer, pH 8.0 | 97 ml |
| 1 $M$ Hypoxanthine (dissolved in water by hitting or in minimal volume of 1 $M$ KOH) | 3 ml |
| NAD | 60 mg |
| NBT | 30 mg |
| PMS | 2 mg |

### Procedure
Incubate the gel in staining solution in the dark at 37°C until dark blue bands appear. Wash stained gel in water and fix in 50% ethanol.

*Notes:* Xanthine oxidase (see 1.1.3.22 — XOX) bands can also develop in XDH staining solution. Therefore, an additional gel should be stained for XOX as a control. In invertebrates much of the activity of isozymes developed on gels stained for XDH can be attributed to XOX. Moreover, there is some doubt that XDH exists in vertebrates.[2]

### REFERENCES

1. Shaw, C. R. and Prasad, R., Starch gel electrophoresis of enzymes: a compilation of recipes, *Biochem. Genet.*, 4, 297, 1970.
2. Adams, M., Baverstock, P. R., Watts, C. H. S., and Gutman, G. A., Enzyme markers in inbred rat strains: genetics of new markers and strain profiles, *Biochem. Genet.*, 22, 611, 1984.

## 1.1.1.205 — IMP Dehydrogenase; IMPDH

REACTION     Inosine-5′-phosphate + NAD + H$_2$O = xanthosine-5-phosphate + NADH

ENZYME SOURCE   Bacteria, plants, vertebrates

## METHOD

### Visualization Scheme

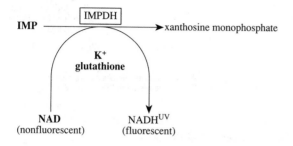

### Staining Solution[1]

165 m$M$ Tris–HCl buffer, pH 8.1
300 m$M$ KCl
6 m$M$ Glutathione (reduced)
6 m$M$ NAD
3 m$M$ Inosine-5′-phosphate

### Procedure

Lay a piece of filter paper saturated with the staining solution on top of the gel and incubate at 37°C in a moist chamber for 30 to 60 min. Remove the filter paper and view the gel under long-wave UV light. Light (fluorescent) bands of IMPDH are visible on the dark (nonfluorescent) background of the gel. Record the zymogram or photograph using a yellow filter.

*Notes:* When a zymogram visible in daylight is required, counterstain the processed gel with MTT/PMS solution to obtain dark blue bands on a light blue background. The post-coupling technique is recommended because of nonspecific reduction of MTT via reduced glutathione. Reduced glutathione is required for activity of bacterial IMPDH. When the enzyme from plant or animal sources is studied, reduced glutathione may be omitted from the staining solution and PMS and MTT added directly to the staining solution to develop IMPDH activity bands visible in daylight by a routine one-step procedure.

### REFERENCE

1. Van Diggelen, O. P. and Shin, S., A rapid fluorescence technique for electrophoretic identification of hypoxanthine phosphoribosyl-transferase allozymes, *Biochem. Genet.*, 12, 375, 1974.

## 1.1.1.X — Choline Dehydrogenase (NAD); CD(NAD)

REACTION (supposed)   Choline + NAD = betaine aldehyde + NADH

ENZYME SOURCE     Plants, vertebrates (?)

## METHOD

### Visualization Scheme

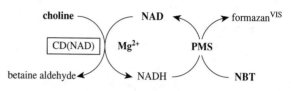

### Staining Solution[1]

| | |
|---|---|
| 0.05 $M$ Tris–HCl buffer, pH 7.5 | 25 ml |
| Choline chloride | 175 mg |
| MgSO$_4$ | 25 mg |
| 10 mg/ml NAD | 1.5 ml |
| 10 mg/ml NBT | 0.5 ml |
| 5 mg/ml PMS | 0.5 ml |

### Procedure

Incubate the gel in staining solution in the dark at 37°C until dark blue bands appear. Wash developed gel in water and fix in 50% ethanol.

*Notes:* This enzyme is not yet included in the enzyme list.[2] It may be that the activity bands developed in the staining solution presented above are caused by choline oxidase (EC 1.1.3.17), which uses oxygen as acceptor. This enzyme contains a tightly bound FAD group that can interchange between the oxidized and reduced states. The reduced flavoprotein can chemically reduce NBT via PMS without the need for NAD. Unlike CD(NAD), choline oxidase produces hydrogen peroxide, which can be detected using the linked–peroxidase reaction (see 1.11.1.7 — PER). Another enzyme, choline dehydrogenase (EC 1.1.99.1), can use PMS as acceptor and, thus, can also be developed in a staining solution for CD(NAD). The bands caused by this enzyme can be identified by the use of the staining solution identical to that presented above but lacking NAD.

### REFERENCES

1. Cheliak, W. M. and Pitel, J. A., Techniques for Starch Gel Electrophoresis of Enzymes from Forest Tree Species, Information Report PI-X-42, Petawawa National Forestry Institute, Canadian Forestry Service, Agriculture Canada, Chalk River, Ont., 1984.
2. Nomenclature Committee of the International Union of Biochemistry, *Enzyme Nomenclature*, Academic Press, Orlando, 1984.

OTHER NAMES    Glucose oxyhydrase

REACTION    β-D-Glucose + $O_2$ = D-glucono-1,5-lactone + $H_2O_2$

ENZYME SOURCE  Fungi, plants, invertebrates, vertebrates

## METHOD 1

### Visualization Scheme

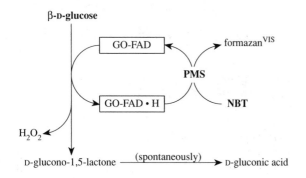

### Staining Solution[1]
    0.05 $M$ Tris–HCl buffer, pH 8.0
    37 m$M$ β-D-Glucose
    0.24 m$M$ NBT
    0.16 m$M$ PMS

### Procedure
Incubate the gel in staining solution in the dark at 37°C until dark blue bands appear. Wash stained gel in water and fix in 50% ethanol.

*Notes:*  An additional gel should be stained in a staining solution lacking glucose as a control. GO activity bands also may develop on glucose dehydrogenase (1.1.1.47 — GD) and hexokinase (2.7.1.1 — HK) zymograms, as well as on the zymograms of other enzymes where exogenous hexokinase and glucose-6-phosphate dehydrogenase are included in the staining solution to catalyze coupled reactions in the presence of MTT (or NBT) and PMS.

## METHOD 2

### Visualization Scheme

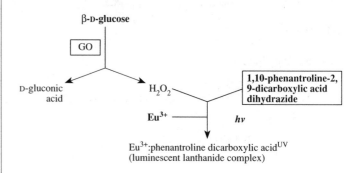

Eu$^{3+}$:phenantroline dicarboxylic acid$^{UV}$
(luminescent lanthanide complex)

### Staining Solution[2] (adapted)
    0.1 $M$ Acetate buffer, pH 6.0
    10 m$M$ β-D-Glucose
    0.01 m$M$ 1,10-Phenantroline-2,9-dicarboxylic acid dihydrazide
    0.02 m$M$ EuCl$_3$

### Procedure
Apply the staining solution to the gel surface using filter paper or 1% agarose overlay. Incubate the gel at 37°C and monitor under UV lamp emitting in the mid-ultraviolet region, 300–340 nm, for fluorescent (luminescent) bands. Record the zymogram or photograph developed gel on Polaroid instant film using a time-resolved photographic camera (e.g., TRP 100 camera produced by Kronem Systems, Inc., Mississauga, Canada) and filters that pass 320- to 340-nm excitation and above 515-nm emission wavelengths.

*Notes:*  The method allows detection of less than $10^{-3}$ U/ml of GO.

The main disadvantage of the method is that 1,10-phenantroline-2,9-dicarboxylic acid dihydrazide is not yet commercially available and should be synthesized under laboratory conditions.

Applications of the staining solution as 1% agarose overlay is preferable because it prevents rapid diffusion of a soluble lanthanide chelate.

## OTHER METHODS

The product hydrogen peroxide can be detected using exogenous peroxidase as a linking enzyme (see 1.11.1.7 — PER).

### REFERENCES
1. Cavener, D. R., Genetics of male-specific glucose oxidase and the identification of other unusual hexose enzymes in *Drosophila melanogaster*, *Biochem. Genet.*, 18, 929, 1980.
2. Evangelista, R. A., Pollak, A., and Templeton, E. F. G., Enzyme-amplified lanthanide luminescence for enzyme detection in bioanalytical assays, *Anal. Biochem.*, 197, 213, 1991.

OTHER NAMES    L-2-Hydroxyacid oxidase (recommended name), hydroxyacid oxidase A, hydroxyacid oxidase B

REACTION    L-2-Hydroxyacid + $O_2$ = 2-oxo acid + $H_2O_2$

ENZYME SOURCE    Bacteria, plants, vertebrates

## METHOD 1

### Visualization Scheme

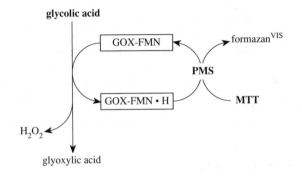

### Staining Solution[1]

A.  0.5 *M* Tris–HCl buffer, pH 7.5                          25 ml
    Glycolic acid                                            50 mg
    5 mg/ml MTT                                              1 ml
    5 mg/ml PMS                                              1 ml
B.  2% Agar solution (60°C)                                  25 ml

### Procedure

Mix A and B components of the staining solution and pour the mixture over the surface of the gel. Incubate the gel in the dark at 37°C until dark blue bands appear. Fix stained gel in 50% ethanol.

*Notes:*   Human GOX also works well with α-hydroxyisocaproic acid as substrate. The rat enzyme also oxidizes phenyllactic and D-lactic (2-hydroxypropionic) acids.[2]

    To decrease nonspecific staining of gel background the use of acid stain buffer (pH 6.5 to 6.8) is recommended.

## METHOD 2

### Visualization Scheme

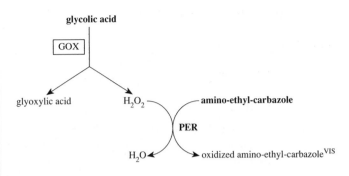

### Staining Solution[3] (modified)

A.  0.5 *M* Tris–HCl buffer, pH 7.4
    8 U/ml Peroxidase (PER)
    2 mg/ml Glycolic (or α-hydroxyisocaproic) acid
    1 mg/ml 3-Amino-9-ethyl-carbazole (dissolved in minimal volume of acetone)
B.  2% Agarose solution (60°C)

### Procedure

Mix A and B components of the staining solution and pour the mixture over the surface of the gel. Incubate the gel at 37°C until reddish-brown bands appear. Fix stained gel in 50% glycerol.

*Notes:*   The resolution and sensitivity of this method are less good than those of MTT/PMS stain used in Method 1.

    *o*-Dianisidine dihydrochloride may be used instead of amino-ethyl-carbazole. It should be remembered, however, that this dye is a possible carcinogen and should be handled with great care.

## GENERAL NOTES

The enzyme exists as two major isoenzymes; the A form preferentially oxidizes short-chain aliphatic hydroxyacids, and was previously listed as glycolate oxidase (EC 1.1.3.1); the B form preferentially oxidizes long-chain and aromatic hydroxyacids. The rat isoenzyme B also acts as L-amino acid oxidase (EC 1.4.3.2).

## REFERENCES

1.  Harris, H. and Hopkinson, D. A., *Handbook of Enzyme Electrophoresis in Human Genetics*, North-Holland, Amsterdam (Loose leaf with supplements in 1977 and 1978), 1976.
2.  Feinstein, R. N. and Lindahl, R., Detection of oxidases on polyacrylamide gels, *Anal. Biochem.*, 56, 353, 1973.
3.  Duley, J. and Holmes, R. S., α-Hydroxyacid oxidase in the mouse: evidence for two genetic loci and a tetrameric subunit structure for the liver isozyme, *Genetics*, 76, 93, 1974.

OTHER NAMES    Hypoxanthine oxidase

REACTION    Hypoxanthine + $H_2O$ + $O_2$ = xanthine + $H_2O_2$

ENZYME SOURCE    Bacteria, vertebrates

## METHOD 1

### Visualization Scheme

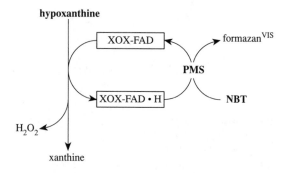

### Staining Solution[1]

| | |
|---|---|
| 0.1 $M$ Phosphate buffer, pH 6.8 | 60 ml |
| 0.01 $M$ Hypoxanthine (dissolved by hitting or in minimal volume of 1 $M$ KOH) | 10 ml |
| 1 mg/ml NBT | 5 ml |
| 0.5 mg/ml PMS | 5 ml |

### Procedure

Incubate the gel in staining solution in the dark at 37°C until dark blue bands appear. Wash developed gel in water and fix in 50% ethanol.

*Notes:*  An additional (control) gel should be stained for aldehyde oxidase (see 1.2.3.1 — AOX), for which activity bands also can be developed by this method.

## METHOD 2

### Visualization Scheme

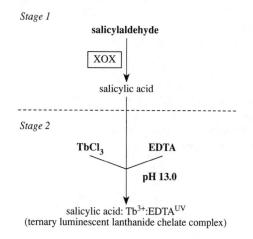

### Staining Solution[2] (adapted)
A.  0.05 $M$ Hepes, pH 7.4
    1 m$M$ Salicylaldehyde
      (dissolved in ethylene glycol dimethyl ether)
B.  0.01 $M$ HCl
    5 m$M$ $TbCl_3$
    5 m$M$ EDTA (tetrasodium salt)
C.  2.5 $M$ Tris, pH 13.0

### Procedure

Apply substrate solution A to the gel surface with filter paper or 1% agarose overlay. Incubate the gel with application at 37°C for 30 min. Remove the first application and apply the next one containing developing solution (one part of solution B, one part of solution C, and three parts of deionized water). Observe luminescent XOX bands under 300- to 400-nm UV light. Photograph developed gel on Polaroid instant film with a TRP 100 time-resolved photographic camera (Kronem Systems, Inc., Mississauga, Canada) using a filter combination providing excitation in the range 320-400 nm and measuring emission above 515 nm with a measurement time delay and gate of 440 µs and 4.1 ms, respectively.

## OTHER METHODS

An immunoblotting procedure (for details see Part II) using monoclonal antibodies specific to bovine XOX[3] can also be used to localize the enzyme protein on electrophoretic gels. This procedure has some disadvantages but may be of great value in special analyses of XOX.

## GENERAL NOTES

The enzyme also oxidizes some other purines and pterins. It has a broad substrate specificity, being able to oxidize a variety of compounds containing aldehyde moieties.

### REFERENCES

1.  Feinstein, R. N. and Lindahl, R., Detection of oxidases on polyacrylamide gels, *Anal. Biochem.*, 56, 353, 1973.
2.  Evangelista, R. A., Pollak, A., and Templeton, E. F. G., Enzyme-amplified lanthanide luminescence for enzyme detection in bioanalytical assays, *Anal. Biochem.*, 197, 213, 1991.
3.  Mather, I. H., Nace, C. S., Johnson, V. G., and Goldsby, R. A., Preparation of monoclonal antibodies to xanthine oxidase and other proteins of bovine milk-fat globule membrane, *Biochem. J.*, 188, 925, 1980.

## 1.1.3.23 — Thiamin Dehydrogenase; TDH

OTHER NAMES    Thiamin oxidase (recommended name)

REACTION      Thiamin + 2O$_2$ = thiaminacetic acid + 2H$_2$O$_2$

ENZYME SOURCE  Bacteria

## METHOD

### Visualization Scheme

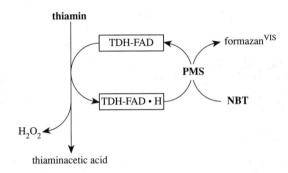

### Staining Solution[1]
    50 m$M$ Sodium phosphate buffer, pH 7.0
    0.015% Thiamin
    0.04% NBT
    0.004% PMS

### Procedure
Incubate the gel in staining solution in the dark at 37°C until dark blue bands appear. Wash stained gel in water and fix in 50% ethanol.

*Notes:* The two-step oxidation of thiamin proceeds without the release of the intermediate aldehyde from the enzyme.

### REFERENCE
1. Neal, R. A., Bacterial metabolism of thiamine. III. Metabolism of thiamine to 3-(2'-methyl-4'-amino-5'-pyrimidylmethyl)-4-methyl-thiazole-5-acetic acid (thiamine acetic acid) by a flavoprotein isolated from a soil microorganism, *J. Biol. Chem.*, 245, 2599, 1970.

## 1.1.99.5 — Glycerol-3-phosphate Dehydrogenase (FAD); G-3-PD(FAD)

REACTION      D-Glycerol-3-phosphate + acceptor = glycerone phosphate + reduced acceptor

ENZYME SOURCE  Invertebrates, vertebrates

## METHOD

### Visualization Scheme

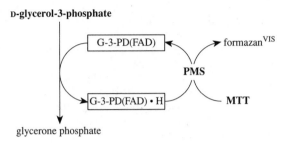

### Staining Solution[1]
    100 m$M$ Sodium phosphate buffer, pH 7.5
    370 m$M$ DL-Glycerol-3-phosphate
    0.4 m$M$ PMS
    0.6 m$M$ MTT

### Procedure
Incubate the gel in staining solution in the dark at 37°C until dark blue bands appear. Wash developed gel in water and fix in 50% ethanol.

*Notes:* The enzyme is a flavoprotein tightly bound to mitochondrial membranes. Preparation of enzyme samples for electrophoresis includes purification of mitochondria, their disruption by sonication, and subsequent dissolving of mitochondrial membranes in 0.125% Triton X-100. Starch gels used for G-3-PD(FAD) electrophoresis contain 0.5% Triton X-100 and 0.3% egg yolk L-α-phosphatidylcholine. Before being added to the heated gel just prior to degassation, phosphatidylcholine is suspended in 10 ml of gel buffer by sonication. Triton X-100 is added after degassation of starch gel.

### REFERENCE
1. Shaw, M.-A., Edwards, Y. H., and Hopkinson, D. A., Human mitochondrial glycerol phosphate dehydrogenase (GPDm) isozymes, *Ann. Hum. Genet.*, 46, 11, 1982.

## 1.2.1.1 — Formaldehyde Dehydrogenase (Glutathione); FDH

REACTION      Formaldehyde + glutathione + NAD = *S*-formylglutathione + NADH

ENZYME SOURCE  Bacteria, fungi, plants, invertebrates, vertebrates

## METHOD

### Visualization Scheme

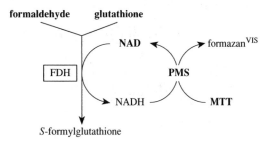

### Staining Solution[1]

| | |
|---|---|
| 0.05 *M* Tris–HCl buffer, pH 8.0 | 100 ml |
| 40% Formaldehyde | 0.08 ml |
| Glutathione (reduced) | 300 mg |
| NAD | 50 mg |
| MTT | 6 mg |
| PMS | 4 mg |

### Procedure

Incubate the gel in staining solution in the dark at 37°C until dark blue bands appear. Wash stained gel in water and fix in 50% ethanol.

*Notes:* The presence of reduced glutathione in the staining solution causes nonspecific reduction of MTT and staining of the gel background. To avoid this problem PMS and MTT may be omitted from the stain and fluorescent bands of FDH activity observed in long-wave UV light.[2]

Unlike FDH (EC 1.2.1.1), the enzyme from *Pseudomonas* (EC 1.2.1.46) does not need reduced glutathione.

### REFERENCES

1. Lush, I. E., Genetic variation of some aldehyde-oxidizing enzymes in the mouse, *Anim. Blood Groups Biochem. Genet.*, 9, 85, 1978.
2. Balakirev, E. S. and Zaykin, D. V., Allozyme variability of formaldehyde dehydrogenase in marine invertebrates, *Genetika (USSR)*, 24, 1504, 1988 (in Russian).

## 1.2.1.2 — Formate Dehydrogenase; FD

REACTION      Formate + NAD = $CO_2$ + NADH

ENZYME SOURCE  Bacteria, fungi

## METHOD

### Visualization Scheme

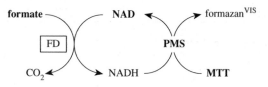

### Staining Solution[1]

| | |
|---|---|
| 0.05 *M* Tris–HCl buffer, pH 8.0 | 50 ml |
| Formic acid (sodium salt) | 200 mg |
| NAD | 30 mg |
| MTT | 10 mg |
| PMS | 2 mg |

### Procedure

Incubate the gel in staining solution in the dark at 37°C until dark blue bands appear. Wash developed gel in water and fix in 50% ethanol.

### REFERENCE

1. Royse, D. J. and May, B., Use of isozyme variation to identify genotypic classes of *Agaricus brunnescens*, *Mycologia*, 74, 93, 1982.

REACTION        Aldehyde + NAD + $H_2O$ = acid + NADH

ENZYME SOURCE   Bacteria, fungi plants, invertebrates, vertebrates

## METHOD

### Visualization Scheme

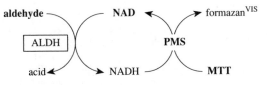

### Staining Solution[1]

| | |
|---|---:|
| 0.05 *M* Tris–HCl buffer, pH 8.5 | 100 ml |
| Salicylaldehyde | 0.15 ml |
| NAD | 50 mg |
| MTT | 12 mg |
| PMS | 4 mg |

### Procedure

Incubate the gel in staining solution in the dark at 37°C until dark blue bands appear. Wash stained gel in water and fix in 50% ethanol.

*Notes:* Possible alternative substrates are acetaldehyde, benzaldehyde, and propionaldehyde. Human ALDH-1 isoenzyme also acts on pyruvaldehyde and furfuraldehyde and is activated by $Mg^{2+}$ and $Ca^{2+}$ ions.[2] The related plant enzyme (see 1.2.1.X — IADH) catalyzes conversion of indol-3-acetaldehyde into indol-3-acetic acid (heteroauxin), which plays an important role in plant organogenesis.[3] Animal ALDH is part of a very complex system of aldehyde-metabolizing enzymes.

A gel stained for ALDH can also exhibit aldehyde oxidase (see 1.2.3.1 — AOX), xanthine oxidase (see 1.1.3.22 — XOX), and alcohol dehydrogenase (see 1.1.1.1 — ADH) activities. The AOX bands can be identified by omitting NAD from the staining solution. The addition of 1 to 2 mg/ml pyrazole to the stain can be used to prevent development of ADH bands.

The addition of NAD to electrophoretic gels or to acetate cellulose soaking buffers often proves beneficial for detection of ALDH activity bands.

### REFERENCES

1. Lush, I. E., Genetic variation of some aldehyde-oxidizing enzymes in the mouse, *Anim. Blood Groups Biochem. Genet.*, 9, 85, 1978.
2. Teng, Y.-S., Human liver aldehyde dehydrogenase in Chinese and Asiatic Indians: gene deletion and its possible implications in alcohol metabolism, *Biochem. Genet.*, 19, 107, 1981.
3. Ballal, S. K. and Harris, J. W., Differential expression of isozymes in relation to organogenesis in two closely related species, *Experientia*, 44, 255, 1988.

## 1.2.1.12 — Glyceraldehyde-3-phosphate Dehydrogenase; GA-3-PD

OTHER NAMES    Triosephosphate dehydrogenase

REACTION    D-Glyceraldehyde-3-phosphate + orthophosphate (or arsenate) + NAD = 3-phospho-D-glyceroyl phosphate (or arsenate) + NADH

ENZYME SOURCE    Bacteria, algae, fungi, plants, invertebrates, vertebrates

## METHOD 1

### Visualization Scheme

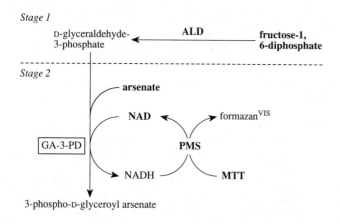

### Staining Solution[1] (modified)

A. 0.1 $M$ Tris–HCl buffer, pH 7.5 — 2 ml
    Fructose-1,6-diphosphate (sodium salt) — 50 mg
    Aldolase (ALD) — 50 units
B. 0.1 $M$ Tris–HCl buffer, pH 7.5 — 18 ml
    NAD — 20 mg
    MTT — 6 mg
    PMS — 2 mg
    Sodium arsenate — 50 mg
C. 2% Agarose solution (60°C) — 20 ml

### Procedure

Incubate mixture A at 37°C for 1 h before use. Mix A and B components of the staining solution and then add agar solution (C). Pour the mixture over the gel surface. Incubate the gel in the dark at 37°C until dark blue bands appear. Fix stained gel together with stained agarose overlay in 50% ethanol.

*Notes:* The addition of NAD to electrophoretic gel or to acetate cellulose soaking buffer often proves beneficial for GA-3-PD detection. The use of 1 to 2 mg/ml pyruvate and pyrazole in the stain is sometimes desirable to prevent or minimize nonspecific development of LDH and ADH activity bands.

The substrate D-glyceraldehyde-3-phosphate can be prepared directly from the diethylacetal barium salt using Dowex 50x4-200R, following the instructions supplied by the manufacturer (Sigma Chemical Company), or from di(cyclohexylammonium) salt using 2 $M$ H₂SO₄.

## METHOD 2

### Visualization Scheme

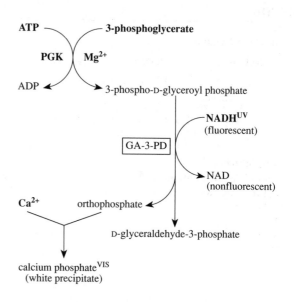

### Staining Solution[2]

100 m$M$ Tris–HCl buffer, pH 8.8
150 m$M$ NADH
1 m$M$ ATP
5 m$M$ 3-Phospho-D-glycerate
1 m$M$ Dithiothreitol
10 µg/ml Phosphoglycerate kinase (PGK)
20 m$M$ Mg²⁺
20 m$M$ Ca²⁺

### Procedure

Before staining, presoak electrophorized gel in 100 m$M$ Tris–HCl buffer (pH 8.8) for 20 to 30 min. Incubate the gel in staining solution at 37°C until bands of white precipitate appear. The stained gel can be stored for several months in 50 m$M$ glycine–KOH buffer (pH 10.0), 5 m$M$ Ca²⁺ either at 5°C or at room temperature in the presence of an antibacterial agent.

*Notes:* This method is developed for PAG. However, it is also applicable to acetate cellulose and starch gels, where GA-3-PD bands can be observed under long-wave UV light as dark (nonfluorescent) bands on a light (fluorescent) background. In this case Ca²⁺ ions should be omitted from the staining solution. It should also be taken into account that the amount of NADH added to the staining solution is critical for development of nonfluorescent bands. If too much NADH is added, the enzyme should not be able to convert enough NADH into NAD for nonfluorescent bands to become visible.

When unclean gels (e.g., starch or acetate cellulose) are used for electrophoresis, the zones of calcium phosphate precipitation can be counterstained with Alizarin Red S.

### REFERENCES

1. Siciliano, M. J. and Shaw, C. R., Separation and visualization of enzymes on gels, in *Chromatographic and Electrophoretic Techniques, Vol. 2, Zone Electrophoresis*, Smith, I., Ed., Heinemann, London, 1976, 185.
2. Nimmo, H.G. and Nimmo, G.A., A general method for the localization of enzymes that produce phosphate, pyrophosphate, or CO₂ after polyacrylamide gel electrophoresis, *Anal. Biochem.*, 121, 17, 1982.

## 1.2.1.13 — Glyceraldehyde-3-phosphate Dehydrogenase (NADP); GA-3-PD(NADP)

OTHER NAMES   Triosephosphate Dehydrogenase (NADP)

REACTION   D-Glyceraldehyde-3-phosphate + orthophosphate (or arsenate) + NADP = 3-phospho-D-glyceroyl phosphate (or arsenate) + NADPH

ENZYME SOURCE  Bacteria, plants

## METHOD

### Visualization Scheme

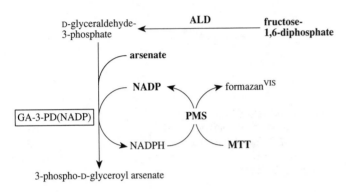

### Staining Solution[1]

| | |
|---|---|
| 0.2 M Tris–HCl buffer, pH 8.0 | 40 ml |
| Fructose-1,6-diphosphate (cyclohexylammonium salt) | 100 mg |
| Aldolase (ALD) | 10 units |
| Sodium arsenate (7H$_2$O) | 50 mg |
| 1.25% MTT | 1 ml |
| 1% PMS | 0.5 ml |
| 1% NADP | 2 ml |

### Procedure

Incubate the gel in staining solution in the dark at 37°C until dark blue bands appear. Wash stained gel in water and fix in 50% ethanol.

*Notes:* The enzyme from some sources can utilize both NADP and NAD as cofactors. However, since the enzyme requires about 100 times more NAD than NADP for equal activity, it is supposed that NADP is the physiological cofactor of GA-3-PD(NADP).

## OTHER METHODS

The reverse reaction can be used to detect GA-3-PD(NADP) activity bands using a staining solution like that given in Method 2 for NAD-dependent GA-3-PD, but containing NADPH in place of NADH (see 1.2.1.12 — GA-3-PD, Method 2).

### REFERENCE

1. Selander, R. K., Caugant, D. A., Ochman, H., Musser, J. M., Gilmour, M. N., and Whittam, T. S., Methods of multilocus enzyme electrophoresis for bacterial population genetics and systematics, *Appl. Environ. Microbiol.*, 51, 873, 1986.

## 1.2.1.16 — Succinate-semialdehyde Dehydrogenase; SSDH

REACTION   Succinate semialdehyde + NAD(P) + H$_2$O = succinate + NAD(P)H

ENZYME SOURCE  Bacteria

## METHOD

### Visualization Scheme

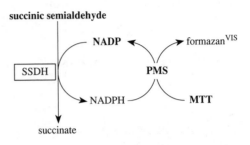

### Staining Solution[1] (adapted)

| | |
|---|---|
| 0.05 M Tris–HCl buffer, pH 8.0 | 80 ml |
| NADP | 15 mg |
| Succinic semialdehyde (Sigma) | 0.1 ml |
| MTT | 10 mg |
| PMS | 1 mg |

### Procedure

Incubate the gel in staining solution in the dark at 37°C until dark blue bands appear. Wash developed gel in water and fix in 50% ethanol.

*Notes:* The reaction catalyzed by SSDH is essentially irreversible.

The enzyme from *Pseudomonas fluorescens* is about eight times more active with NADP than NAD.

### REFERENCE

1. Akers, E. and Aronson, J. N., Detection on polyacrylamide gels of L-glutamic acid decarboxylase activities from *Bacillus thuringiensis*, *Anal. Biochem.*, 39, 535, 1971.

## 1.2.1.X — Indoleacetaldehyde Dehydrogenase; IADH

REACTION         Indole-3-acetaldehyde + NAD + H₂O = indole-3-acetic acid + NADH

$$\text{Indole-3-acetaldehyde} + \text{NAD} + \text{H}_2\text{O} = \text{indole-3-acetic acid} + \text{NADH}$$

ENZYME SOURCE  Plants

## METHOD

### Visualization Scheme

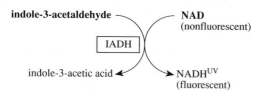

### Staining Solution[1]
0.1 $M$ Tris–HCl buffer, pH 8.8
60 m$M$ Indole-3-acetaldehyde
5 m$M$ NAD
20% Sucrose

### Procedure
Cover gel with staining solution and incubate in a humid chamber at room temperature. View gel under long-wave UV light for fluorescent bands. Record the zymogram or photograph using a yellow filter.

*Notes:*  This is the original method developed for acetate cellulose gel. It can also be applied to PAG and starch gel.

The addition of PMS and MTT (or NBT) to the staining solution will allow development of IADH activity bands visible in daylight. In some cases the addition of PMS and a tetrazolium salt should be made only when fluorescent IADH bands visible under UV light are well developed. This post-coupling technique allows avoidance of the possible inhibitory effect of PMS and/or a tetrazolium salt on IADH activity. When a tetrazolium method is used, sucrose may be omitted from the staining solution.

The enzyme may be identical to aldehyde dehydrogenase (NAD) (see 1.2.1.3 — ALDH).

### REFERENCE
1. Ballal, S. K. and Harris, J. W., Differential expression of isozymes in relation to organogenesis in two closely related species, *Experientia*, 44, 255, 1988.

## 1.2.3.1 — Aldehyde Oxidase; AOX

REACTION         Aldehyde + H₂O + O₂ = acid + O₂·⁻

$$\text{Aldehyde} + \text{H}_2\text{O} + \text{O}_2 = \text{acid} + \text{O}_2^{\cdot -}$$

ENZYME SOURCE  Invertebrates, vertebrates

## METHOD

### Visualization Scheme

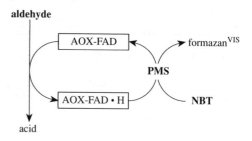

### Staining Solution[1]
| | |
|---|---|
| 0.1 $M$ Phosphate buffer, pH 6.8 | 60 ml |
| 0.01 $M$ 2-Furaldehyde (or benzaldehyde) | 10 ml |
| 1 mg/ml NBT | 5 ml |
| 0.5 mg/ml PMS | 5 ml |

### Procedure
Incubate the gel in staining solution in the dark at 37°C until dark blue bands appear. Wash stained gel in water and fix in 50% ethanol.

*Notes:*  Other substrates can be used such as acetaldehyde, *p*-anisaldehyde, butyraldehyde, 2-ethylbutyraldehyde, heptaldehyde, 2-methylbutyraldehyde, propionaldehyde, and salicylaldehyde.

Gels stained for AOX may also exhibit bands of xanthine oxidase (see 1.1.3.22 — XOX) activity.

In *Drosophila*, the artificial substrate *p*-(dimethylamino)benzaldehyde can be oxidized by both AOX and pyridoxal oxidase (EC 1.2.3.8).[2] To differentiate AOX, XOX, and pyridoxal oxidase bands on *Drosophila* AOX zymograms, the use of different mutants deficient in expression of correspondent structural genes is recommended.[3] In *Drosophila*, the pyridoxal oxidase bands can also be identified using specific antibodies.[4]

### REFERENCES
1. Feinstein, R. N. and Lindahl, R., Detection of oxidases on polyacrylamide gels, *Anal. Biochem.*, 56, 353, 1973.
2. Cypher, J. J., Tedesco, J. L., Courtright, J. B., and Barman, A. K., Tissue-specific and substrate-specific detection of aldehyde and pyridoxal oxidase in larval and imaginal tissues of *Drosophila melanogaster*, *Biochem. Genet.*, 20, 315, 1982.
3. Dickinson, W. J. and Gaughan, S., Aldehyde oxidases of *Drosophila*: contributions of several enzymes to observed activity patterns, *Biochem. Genet.*, 19, 567, 1981.
4. Warner, C. K., Watts, D. T., and Finnerty, V., Molybdenum hydroxylases in *Drosophila*. 1. Preliminary studies of pyridoxal oxidase, *Mol. Gen. Genet.*, 180, 449, 1980.

## 1.2.4.2 — Oxoglutarate Dehydrogenase; OGDH

OTHER NAMES     Oxoglutarate decarboxylase, α-ketoglutaric dehydrogenase

REACTION     2-Oxoglutarate + NAD + CoA = succinyl-CoA + NADH + $CO_2$

ENZYME SOURCE   Bacteria, fungi, plants, invertebrates, vertebrates

## METHOD

### Visualization Scheme

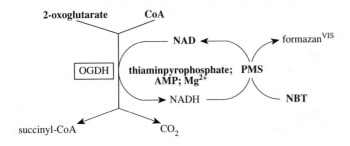

### Staining Solution[1]

    0.1 $M$ Tris–HCl buffer, pH 8.0
    10 m$M$ $MgCl_2$
    1 m$M$ EDTA
    0.1 m$M$ Thiaminpyrophosphate
    5 m$M$ 2-Oxoglutarate
    0.1 m$M$ CoA
    0.5 m$M$ NAD
    0.5 m$M$ AMP
    0.1 mg/ml PMS
    0.3 mg/ml NBT

### Procedure

Incubate the gel in staining solution in the dark at 37°C until dark blue bands appear. Fix stained gel in 50% ethanol.

*Notes:*   OGDH is a component of the multienzyme 2-oxoglutarate dehydrogenase complex.

### REFERENCE

  1. Parker, M. G. and Weitzman, D. J., The purification and regulatory properties of α-oxoglutarate dehydrogenase from *Acinetobacter lwoffi*, *Biochem. J.*, 135, 215, 1973.

## 1.3.1.2 — Dihydrouracil Dehydrogenase (NADP); DHUD

REACTION     5,6-Dihydrouracil + NADP = uracil + NADPH

ENZYME SOURCE   Invertebrates, vertebrates

## METHOD

### Visualization Scheme

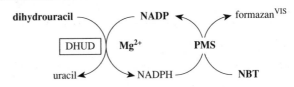

### Staining Solution[1]

  A. 0.25 $M$ Potassium phosphate buffer, pH 7.5
      15 m$M$ Dihydrouracil
      1.5 m$M$ NADP
      15 m$M$ $MgCl_2$
  B. 1 mg/ml NBT               25 ml
      1 mg/ml PMS            2.5 ml
      0.1 $M$ NaCl             10 ml

### Procedure

Mix 15 ml of A with B. Incubate the gel in the mixture in the dark at 37°C until dark blue bands appear. Wash stained gel in water and fix in 50% ethanol.

*Notes:*   The enzyme is inactivated during electrophoresis in tris–barbitone buffer. Dihydrothymine can also be used as substrate.

### REFERENCE

  1. Hallock, R. O. and Yamada, E. W., Visualization of dihydrouracil dehydrogenase (NADP+) activity after disc gel electrophoresis, *Anal. Biochem.*, 56, 84, 1973.

## 1.3.1.14 — Dihydroorotate Dehydrogenase; DHOD

**OTHER NAMES**  Orotate reductase (NADH) (recommended name)

**REACTION**  L-Dihydroorotate + NAD = orotate + NADH

**ENZYME SOURCE**  Bacteria, fungi, protozoa, vertebrates

## METHOD

### Visualization Scheme

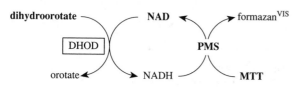

### Staining Solution[1] (adapted)

| | |
|---|---|
| 0.1 $M$ Tris–HCl buffer, pH 8.0 | 50 ml |
| L-Dihydroorotic acid | 50 mg |
| NAD | 30 mg |
| MTT | 10 mg |
| PMS | 1 mg |

### Procedure

Incubate the gel in staining solution in the dark at 37°C until dark blue bands appear. Wash stained gel in water and fix in 50% ethanol.

### REFERENCE

1. Gaal, Ö., Medgyesi, G. A., and Vereczkey, L., *Electrophoresis in the Separation of Biological Macromolecules*, John Wiley & Sons, Chichester, 1980.

## 1.3.1.24 — Biliverdin Reductase; BLVR

**REACTION**  Bilirubin + NAD(P) = biliverdin + NAD(P)H

**ENZYME SOURCE**  Vertebrates

## METHOD

### Visualization Scheme

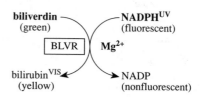

### Staining Solution[1]

| | | |
|---|---|---|
| A. | 0.36 $M$ Tris–HCl buffer, pH 8.0 | 1 ml |
| | Biliverdin | 1 mg |
| B. | 0.36 $M$ Tris–HCl buffer, pH 8.0 | 0.5 ml |
| | NADPH | 2 mg |
| | 1 $M$ MgCl$_2$ | 0.2 ml |

### Procedure

Mix A and B components of the staining solution and apply the mixture dropwise to the gel surface. Incubate the gel at 37°C in a moist chamber until yellow bands against a light green background appear.

*Notes:*  The original method is developed for cellulose acetate gel. However, there are no obvious reasons that can restrict its application to starch gel or PAG.

The enzyme bands can also be observed under UV light (nonfluorescent bands on the fluorescent background of the gel).

### REFERENCE

1. Meera Khan, P., Rijken, H., Wijnen, J. Th., Wijnen, L. M. M., and De Boer, L. E. M., Red cell enzyme variation in the orang utan: electrophoretic characterization of 45 enzyme systems in cellogel, in *The Orang Utan. Its Biology and Conservation*, De Boer, L. E. M., Ed., Dr. W. Junk Publishers, The Hague, 1982, 61.

# 1.3.99.1 — Succinate Dehydrogenase; SUDH

OTHER NAMES    Fumarate reductase, fumaric hydrogenase

REACTION    Succinate + acceptor = fumarate + reduced acceptor

ENZYME SOURCE    Bacteria, fungi, plants, protozoa, invertebrates, vertebrates

## METHOD

### Visualization Scheme

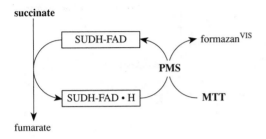

### Staining Solution[1]

A.  200 m$M$ Potassium phosphate buffer, pH 7.5     5 ml
    200 m$M$ Succinic acid (neutralized with NaOH)     2 ml
    10 m$M$ KCN     2 ml
    32.5 mg/ml PMS     0.5 ml
    5 mg/ml MTT     0.5 ml
B.  2% Agar solution (60°C)     9.5 ml

### Procedure

Mix A and B components of the staining solution and pour the mixture over the surface of the gel. Incubate the gel in the dark at 37°C until dark blue bands appear. Fix stained gel in 50% ethanol.

*Notes:*    KCN is added in the staining solution to prevent development of superoxide dismutase (1.15.1.1 — SOD) bands. PMS is used as acceptor.

The enzyme is a flavoprotein bound to mitochondrial membranes. Preparation of enzyme samples for electrophoresis includes purification of mitochondria, their disruption by sonication, and subsequent dissolving of mitochondrial membranes in 0.125% Triton X-100. Starch gels used for SUDH electrophoresis contain 0.5% Triton X-100 and 0.144% phosphatidylethanolamine. Before being added to the heated gel (just prior to degassation) phosphatidylethanolamine is suspended in 10 ml of gel buffer by sonication. Triton X-100 is added after degassation of the starch gel.

### REFERENCE

1.  Shaw, M.-A., Edwards, Y., and Hopkinson, D. A., Human succinate dehydrogenase: biochemical and genetic characterization, *Biochem. Genet.*, 19, 741, 1981.

# 1.3.99.2 — Butyryl-CoA Dehydrogenase; BCD

OTHER NAMES    Butyryl dehydrogenase, unsaturated acyl-CoA reductase

REACTION    Butanoyl-CoA + acceptor = 2-butenoyl-CoA + reduced acceptor

ENZYME SOURCE    Vertebrates

## METHOD

### Visualization Scheme

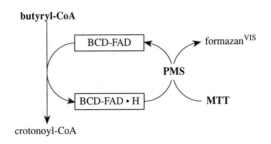

### Staining Solution[1]

A.  0.2 $M$ Tris–HCl buffer, pH 8.0
    0.3 m$M$ Butyryl-CoA
    1.8 m$M$ MTT
    0.6 m$M$ PMS
    0.5 m$M$ KCN
B.  2% Agar solution (60°C)

### Procedure

Mix equal volumes of A and B components of the staining solution. Pour the mixture over the surface of the gel. Incubate the gel in the dark at 37°C until dark blue bands appear. Fix stained gel in 50% ethanol.

*Notes:*    KCN is added in the staining solution to prevent development of superoxide dismutase (1.15.1.1 — SOD) bands. PMS is used as acceptor.

Control stain should be used to reveal nonspecific staining of additional bands in the absence of substrate. Acyl-CoA dehydrogenase (see 1.3.99.3 — ACD) bands also develop on BCD zymograms when butyryl-CoA is used as substrate. These bands also develop when octanoyl-CoA is used as substrate, whereas BCD bands do not.

### REFERENCE

1.  Seeley, T.-L. and Holmes, R. S., Genetics and ontogeny of butyryl CoA dehydrogenase in the mouse and linkage of *Bcd*-1 with *Dao*-1, *Biochem. Genet.*, 19, 333, 1981.

## 1.3.99.3 — Acyl-CoA Dehydrogenase; ACD

**OTHER NAMES** Acyl dehydrogenase, oleoyl-CoA dehydrogenase

**REACTION** Acyl-CoA + acceptor = 2,3-dehydroacyl-CoA + reduced acceptor

**ENZYME SOURCE** Vertebrates

## METHOD

### Visualization Scheme

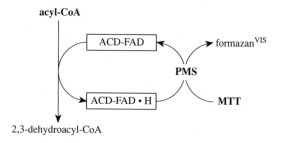

### Staining Solution[1]
A. 0.2 $M$ Tris–HCl buffer, pH 8.0
   0.3 m$M$ Octanoyl-CoA
   1.8 m$M$ MTT
   0.6 m$M$ PMS
   0.5 m$M$ KCN
B. 2% Agar solution (60°C)

### Procedure
Mix equal volumes of A and B components of the staining solution. Pour the mixture over the surface of the gel. Incubate the gel in the dark at 37°C until dark blue bands appear. Fix stained gel in 50% ethanol.

*Notes:* KCN is used to inhibit superoxide dismutase (1.15.1.1 — SOD) activity. PMS is used as acceptor.

Control stain should be used to reveal nonspecific staining of additional bands in the absence of substrate.

Three categories of acyl-CoA dehydrogenases are recognized, which exhibit overlapping substrate specificities: butyryl-CoA dehydrogenase (see 1.3.99.2 — BCD) acts on $C_4$–$C_6$ acyl-CoA; general or acyl-CoA dehydrogenase (ACD) acts on $C_4$–$C_{16}$ acyl-CoA with peak activity towards $C_{10}$ acyl-CoA; and long-chain or oleoyl-CoA dehydrogenase acts on $C_6$–$C_{18}$ acyl-CoA, with peak activity towards $C_{14}$ acyl-CoA.

### REFERENCE
1. Seeley, T.-L. and Holmes, R. S., Genetics and ontogeny of butyryl CoA dehydrogenase in the mouse and linkage of *Bcd*-1 with *Dao*-1, *Biochem. Genet.*, 19, 333, 1981.

## 1.4.1.1 — Alanine Dehydrogenase; ALADH

**REACTION** L-Alanine + $H_2O$ + NAD = pyruvate + $NH_3$ + NADH

**ENZYME SOURCE** Bacteria

## METHOD

### Visualization Scheme

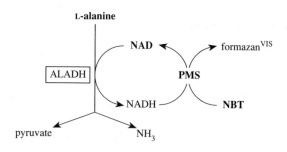

### Staining Solution[1]
| | |
|---|---|
| 0.1 $M$ Phosphate buffer, pH 7.0 | 100 ml |
| D,L-Alanine | 100 mg |
| NAD | 50 mg |
| NBT | 30 mg |
| PMS | 2 mg |

### Procedure
Incubate the gel in staining solution in the dark at 37°C until dark blue bands appear. Wash stained gel in water and fix in 50% ethanol.

*Notes:* Some isozymes of mammal NAD(P)-dependent glutamate dehydrogenase (see 1.4.1.2-4 — GDH) also display ALADH activity.[2]

### REFERENCES
1. Shaw, C. R. and Prasad, R., Starch gel electrophoresis of enzymes: a compilation of recipes, *Biochem. Genet.*, 4, 297, 1970.
2. Lan, N., Frieden, E. H., and Rawitch, A. B., Activity staining for glutamate and alanine dehydrogenases in polyacrilamide gels of varying porosity, *Enzyme*, 24, 416, 1979.

OTHER NAMES    Glutamic dehydrogenase

REACTION    L-Glutamate + $H_2O$ + NAD(P) = 2-oxoglutarate + $NH_3$ + NAD(P)H

ENZYME SOURCE    Bacteria, algae, fungi, plants, protozoa, invertebrates, vertebrates

## METHOD 1

### Visualization Scheme

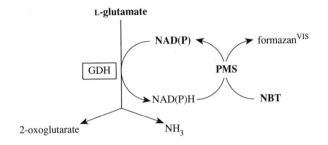

### Staining Solution[1]

| | |
|---|---|
| 0.125 *M* Phosphate buffer, pH 7.0 | 25 ml |
| 1 *M* L-Glutamate | 5 ml |
| NAD | 60 mg |
| NBT | 30 mg |
| PMS | 2 mg |

### Procedure

Incubate the gel in staining solution in the dark at 37°C until dark blue bands appear. Wash stained gel in water and fix in 50% ethanol.

*Notes:*   In higher organisms, GDH is capable of using either NAD or NADP as a cofactor and is activated by ADP. NADP is the cofactor of choice for detection of the enzyme in vertebrates, since its use avoids the problem of artifacts caused by NAD-dependent "nothing dehydrogenase" activities.[2] If NAD is chosen, the inclusion of 1 to 2 mg/ml pyruvate and/or pyrazole in the stain may be desirable to prevent nonspecific development of LDH and/or ADH bands, respectively. The addition of ADP (2 m*M* final concentration) in the stain is usually beneficial.

The GDH reaction is usually displaced towards the production of L-glutamate. To displace the reaction towards production of NAD(P)H and 2-oxoglutarate, the latter should be trapped using such carbonyl-trapping reagents as hydrazyne hydrate or aminooxyacetic acid. When reduced positive fluorescent modification of the method is used, the latter reagent is usually preferable because the use of hydrazyne hydrate can influence the NAD(P)H fluorescence. Therefore, the use of staining buffer (pH 8.6) containing 0.5 *M* glycine and 0.05 *M* aminooxyacetic acid is recommended to enhance the sensitivity of the positive fluorescent method.[3]

## METHOD 2

### Visualization Scheme

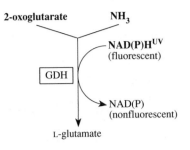

### Staining Solution[4]

| | |
|---|---|
| 0.5 *M* Tris–HCl buffer, pH 7.6 | 10 ml |
| 2-Oxoglutarate | 25 mg |
| NAD(P)H | 10 mg |
| $NH_4Cl$ | 10 mg |

### Procedure

Apply the staining solution to the gel surface on filter-paper overlay and incubate the gel in a moist chamber. After 20 to 30 min of incubation, monitor gel under long-wave UV light for dark (nonfluorescent) bands visible on a light (fluorescent) background. Record the zymogram or photograph using a yellow filter.

*Notes:*   If too much NAD(P)H is added to the staining solution or when GDH activity is too low, the enzyme should not be able to convert enough NAD(P)H into NAD(P) for nonfluorescent bands to become visible.

## GENERAL NOTES

Three types of GDH are recognized, which exhibit different specificities to NAD and NADP as cofactors:

- GDH (EC 1.4.1.2) is specific to NAD and predominates in plants and invertebrates. Plant GDH-NAD is activated by $Ca^{2+}$ ions.
- GDH (EC 1.4.1.4) is specific to NADP. This enzyme was found in some bacteria, fungi, some plants, and in coelenterates. GDH-NADP is not activated by ADP and L-leucine and is not inhibited by GTP.
- GDH (EC 1.4.1.3) capable of using either NAD or NADP is described in some invertebrates and is predominant in vertebrates. It is activated by ADP and L-leucine and inhibited by GTP.

Some GDH isozymes of bovine liver and placental NAD-dependent GDH also display alanine dehydrogenase (see 1.4.1.1 — ALADH) activity.[5] This activity of GDH is stimulated by GTP and inhibited by ADP.

### REFERENCES

1. Shaw, C. R. and Prasad, R., Starch gel electrophoresis of enzymes: a compilation of recipes, *Biochem. Genet.*, 4, 297, 1970.
2. Richardson, B. J., Baverstock, P. R., and Adams, M., *Allozyme Electrophoresis: A Handbook for Animal Systematics and Population Studies*, Academic Press, Sydney, 1986, 182.
3. Pérez-de la Mora, M., Mendez-Franco, J., Salceda, R., and Riesgo-Escovar, J. R., A glutamate dehydrogenase-based method for the assay of L-glutamic acid: formation of pyridine nucleotide fluorescent derivatives, *Anal. Biochem.*, 180, 248, 1989.
4. Harris, H., and Hopkinson, D. A., *Handbook of Enzyme Electrophoresis in Human Genetics*, North-Holland, Amsterdam (Loose leaf with supplements in 1977 and 1978), 1976.
5. Lan, N., Frieden, E. H., and Rawitch, A. B., Activity staining for glutamate and alanine dehydrogenases in polyacrilamide gels of varying porosity, *Enzyme*, 24, 416, 1979.

## 1.4.1.9 — Leucine Dehydrogenase; LEUDH

REACTION      L-Leucine + $H_2O$ + NAD = 4-methyl-2-oxopentanoate + $NH_3$ + NADH

ENZYME SOURCE  Bacteria

## METHOD

### Visualization Scheme

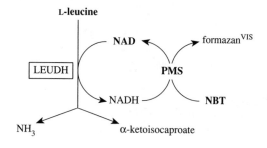

### Staining Solution[1]

| | |
|---|---:|
| 0.1 *M* Phosphate buffer, pH 7.0 | 100 ml |
| L-Leucine | 50 mg |
| NAD | 50 mg |
| NBT | 30 mg |
| PMS | 2 mg |

### Procedure

Incubate the gel in staining solution in the dark at 37°C until dark blue bands appear. Wash stained gel in water and fix in 50% ethanol.

*Notes:*    The enzyme also acts on isoleucine, valine, norvaline, and norleucine.

### REFERENCE

1. Shaw, C. R. and Prasad, R., Starch gel electrophoresis of enzymes: a compilation of recipes, *Biochem. Genet.*, 4, 297, 1970.

## 1.4.1.15 — Lysine Dehydrogenase; LYSDH

REACTION      L-Lysine + NAD = 1,2-didehydropiperidine-2-carboxylate + $NH_3$ + NADH

ENZYME SOURCE  Bacteria

## METHOD

### Visualization Scheme

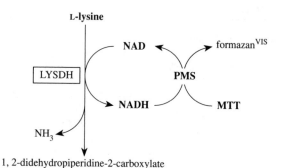

1, 2-didehydropiperidine-2-carboxylate

### Staining Solution[1]

| | |
|---|---:|
| 0.015 *M* Sodium phosphate buffer, pH 7.0 | 50 ml |
| L-Lysine | 5 mg |
| 1.25% MTT | 1 ml |
| 1% PMS | 0.5 ml |
| 1% NAD | 2 ml |

### Procedure

Incubate the gel in staining solution in the dark at 37°C until dark blue bands appear. Wash stained gel in water and fix in 50% ethanol.

### REFERENCE

1. Selander, R. K., Caugant, D. A., Ochman, H., Musser, J. M., Gilmour, M. N., and Whittam, T. S., Methods of multilocus enzyme electrophoresis for bacterial population genetics and systematics, *Appl. Environ. Microbiol.*, 51, 873, 1986.

REACTION (presumed)   L-Aspartate + $H_2O$ + NAD = oxaloacetate + $NH_3$ + NADH

ENZYME SOURCE   Bacteria

## METHOD

### Visualization Scheme

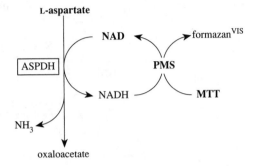

### Staining Solution[1]

| | |
|---|---|
| 0.015 $M$ Sodium phosphate buffer, pH 7.0 | 50 ml |
| L-Aspartate acid (sodium salt) | 50 mg |
| 1.25% MTT | 1 ml |
| 1% PMS | 0.5 ml |
| 1% NAD | 2 ml |

### Procedure

Incubate the gel in staining solution in the dark at 37°C until dark blue bands appear. Wash stained gel in water and fix in 50% ethanol.

*Notes:*  This enzyme is not yet included in the enzyme list.[2] The exact reaction catalyzed by ASPDH is not known. Thus, the proposed product, oxaloacetate, may be misleading. It is not excluded that ASPDH is identical to L-amino acid dehydrogenase (EC 1.4.1.5).

### REFERENCES

1. Selander, R. K., Caugant, D. A., Ochman, H., Musser, J. M., Gilmour, M. N., and Whittam, T. S., Methods of multilocus enzyme electrophoresis for bacterial population genetics and systematics, *Appl. Environ. Microbiol.*, 51, 873, 1986.
2. Nomenclature Committee of the International Union of Biochemistry, *Enzyme Nomenclature*, Academic Press, Orlando, 1984.

OTHER NAMES     Aspartic oxidase

REACTION     D-Aspartate + $H_2O$ + $O_2$ = oxaloacetate + $NH_3$ + $H_2O_2$

ENZYME SOURCE    Vertebrates

## METHOD 1

### Visualization Scheme

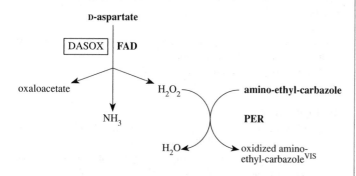

### Staining Solution[1]

| | |
|---|---|
| 0.5 $M$ Tris–HCl buffer, pH 8.0 | 50 ml |
| D-Aspartic acid (monosodium salt) | 200 mg |
| FAD | 8 mg |
| Peroxidase (PER; 100 U/mg) | 5 mg |
| 3-Amino-9-ethyl-carbazole (dissolved in a few drops of acetone) | 25 mg |

### Procedure

Incubate the gel in staining solution at 37°C until red-brown bands appear. Wash stained gel in water and fix in 50% glycerol.

*Notes:* With prolonged staining, weak additional bands due to superoxide dismutase (see 1.15.1.1 — SOD) activity can also develop in tissues such as mammalian liver and kidney. Development of these bands depends on the presence of amino-ethyl-carbazole and FAD in the staining solution but not on the presence of D-aspartate. Presumably, under these conditions of staining, sufficient amounts of superoxide radical are generated to allow the SOD isozymes to catalyze the oxidation of amino-ethyl-carbazole and hence be detected as red-brown bands.

## METHOD 2

### Visualization Scheme

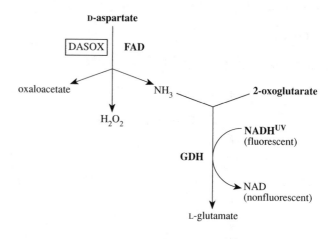

### Staining Solution[2]

| | |
|---|---|
| 0.1 $M$ Tris–HCl buffer, pH 7.6 | 5 ml |
| D-Aspartic acid | 100 mg |
| FAD | 0.1 mg |
| 2-Oxoglutarate | 25 mg |
| NADH | 10 mg |
| Glutamate dehydrogenase (GDH; 500 U/ml) | 0.05 ml |

### Procedure

Apply the staining solution to the gel surface on filter-paper overlay and incubate at 37°C in a moist chamber. After 20 to 30 min of incubation monitor gel under long-wave UV light. Dark (nonfluorescent) bands of DASOX are visible on a light (fluorescent) background. Record the zymogram or photograph using a yellow filter.

*Notes:* When a zymogram that is visible in daylight is required, the processed gel should be counterstained with MTT/PMS solution. This treatment results in the appearance of white bands of DASOX on a blue background of the gel.

## METHOD 3

### Visualization Scheme

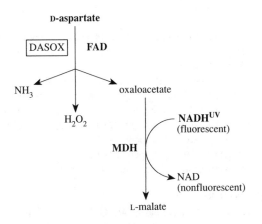

### Staining Solution[1]

| | |
|---|---|
| 0.5 $M$ Tris–HCl buffer, pH 8.0 | 5 ml |
| D-Aspartic acid (monosodium salt) | 20 mg |
| FAD | 1 mg |
| NADH | 10 mg |
| Malate dehydrogenase (MDH) | 100 units |

### Procedure

Apply the staining solution to the gel surface on filter-paper overlay and incubate the gel with application at 37°C in a moist chamber. After 20 to 30 min of incubation monitor gel under long-wave UV light. Dark (nonfluorescent) bands of DASOX are visible on a light (fluorescent) background. Record the zymogram or photograph using a yellow filter.

*Notes:* When a zymogram that is visible in daylight is required, the processed gel should be counterstained with MTT/PMS solution. This treatment results in the appearance of white bands of DASOX on a blue background of the gel.

### GENERAL NOTES

The enzyme is a flavoprotein with FAD as a prosthetic group. It was shown, however, that development of human DASOX isozymes was not dependent significantly on the presence of FAD in the stain.[1] The enzyme–FAD complex perhaps does not dissociate during the course of electrophoresis; therefore, FAD may be omitted from the staining solutions.

The enzyme from human liver and rabbit kidney is specific to D-aspartic acid and does not act on other D-amino acids.

### REFERENCES

1. Barker, R. F. and Hopkinson, D. A., The genetic and biochemical properties of the D-amino acid oxidase in human tissues, *Ann. Hum. Genet.*, 41, 27, 1977.
2. Nelson, R. L., Povey, S., Hopkinson, D. A., and Harris, H., The detection after electrophoresis of enzymes involved in ammonia metabolism using L-glutamate dehydrogenase as a linking enzyme, *Biochem. Genet.*, 15, 1023, 1977.

**OTHER NAMES**     Ophio-amino acid oxidase

**REACTION**     L-amino acid + $H_2O$ + $O_2$ = 2-oxo acid + $NH_3$ + $H_2O_2$

**ENZYME SOURCE**     Bacteria, fungi, vertebrates

## METHOD

### Visualization Scheme

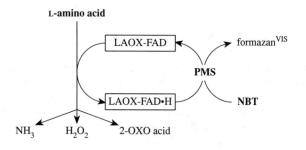

### Staining Solution[1]

| | |
|---|---|
| 65 m$M$ Phosphate buffer, pH 6.8 | 60 ml |
| 10 m$M$ L-Amino acid (see *Notes*) | 10 ml |
| 1 mg/ml NBT | 5 ml |
| 0.5 mg/ml PMS | 5 ml |

### Procedure

Incubate the gel in staining solution in the dark at 37°C until dark blue bands appear. Wash developed gel in water and fix in 50% ethanol.

*Notes:*     The enzyme from *Neurospora*, rat kidney, and snake venom displays the highest rate of reaction when L-amino acids with five or six C atoms are used as substrates. L-Leucine is the substrate more frequently used for LAOX from vertebrates. Good results were also obtained with L-phenylalanine, L-arginine, and L-glutamine as substrates for snake venom LAOX. This enzyme displays trace activity with L-aspartate and L-proline and no histochemically detectable activity with L-glutamate, L-cysteine, and L-serine. The enzyme from liver and kidney also acts on some 2-oxo acids while that from snake venom does not.

## OTHER METHODS

A. The product hydrogen peroxide can be detected using exogenous peroxidase and amino-ethyl-carbazole (e.g., see 1.4.3.3 — DAOX, Method 1).

B. The product ammonia can be detected using exogenous glutamate dehydrogenase in a negative fluorescent stain (e.g., see 1.4.3.3 — DAOX, Method 2).

C. A procedure has been developed for spectrophotometric detection of LAOX on PAG using gel scanning.[2] The method is based on the strong absorbance at 296 nm of aminoethyl cysteine ketimine which originates as a result of oxidation of $S$-aminoethyl-L-cysteine by LAOX. Photocopies of gels stained by this method can be obtained using a special optical device for two-dimensional spectroscopy of electrophoretic gels.[3]

## REFERENCES

1. Feinstein, R. N. and Lindahl, R., Detection of oxidases on polyacrylamide gels, *Anal. Biochem.*, 56, 353, 1973.
2. Ricci, G., Caccuri, A. M., Lo Bello, M., Solinas, S. P., and Nardini, M., Ketimine rings: useful detectors of enzymatic activities in solution and on polyacrylamide gel, *Anal. Biochem.*, 165, 356, 1987.
3. Klebe, R. J., Mancuso, M. G., Brown, C. R., and Teng, L., Two-dimensional spectroscopy of electrophoretic gels, *Biochem. Genet.*, 19, 655, 1981.

REACTION $\qquad$ D-amino acid + H$_2$O + O$_2$ = 2-oxo acid + NH$_3$ + H$_2$O$_2$

ENZYME SOURCE Fungi, vertebrates

## METHOD 1

### Visualization Scheme

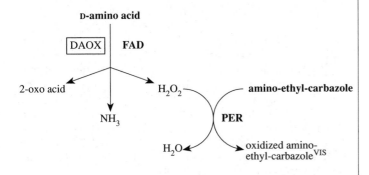

### Staining Solution[1] (modified)
A. 0.018 M Tris–HCl buffer, pH 7.4
  0.0125 M D-Phenylalanine
  0.001 M FAD
B. 3-Amino-9-ethyl-carbazole (dissolved in a few drops of acetone)                        3 mg
  Peroxidase (PER)                        100 units
C. 2% Agar solution (60°C)

### Procedure
Add B components to 12.5 ml of solution A and mix with 12.5 ml of solution C. Pour the mixture over the surface of the gel and incubate at 37°C until brown bands appear. Fix stained gel in 50% glycerol.

*Notes:* With prolonged staining, weak additional bands due to superoxide dismutase (see 1.15.1.1 — SOD) activity can also be developed in tissues such as liver and kidney. Development of these bands depends on the presence of amino-ethyl-carbazole and FAD in the stain but not on the presence of D-amino acid. Presumably, under these conditions of staining, sufficient amounts of superoxide radical are generated to allow the SOD isozymes to catalyze the oxidation of amino-ethyl-carbazole and hence be detected as brown bands.

## METHOD 2

### Visualization Scheme

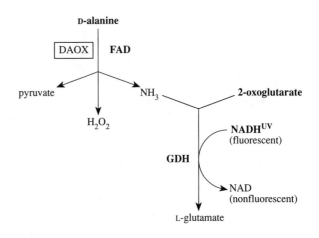

### Staining Solution[2]
| | |
|---|---:|
| 0.1 M Tris–HCl buffer, pH 7.6 | 5 ml |
| D-Alanine | 100 mg |
| FAD | 0.1 mg |
| 2-Oxoglutarate | 25 mg |
| NADH | 10 mg |
| Glutamate dehydrogenase (GDH; 500 U/ml) | 0.05 ml |

### Procedure
Apply the staining solution to the gel surface on a filter-paper overlay and incubate the gel at 37°C in a moist chamber. After 20 to 30 min of incubation monitor gel under long-wave UV light. Dark (nonfluorescent) bands of DAOX are visible on a light (fluorescent) background. Record the zymogram or photograph using a yellow filter.

*Notes:* When a zymogram that is visible in daylight is required, the processed gel should be counterstained with MTT/PMS solution. This treatment results in the appearance of white bands of DAOX on a blue background of the gel.

It should be taken into account when using this method that the amount of NADH added to the staining solution is critical for development of nonfluorescent DAOX bands. If too much NADH is added, the enzyme should not be able to convert enough NADH into NAD for nonfluorescent bands to become visible.

## METHOD 3

### Visualization Scheme

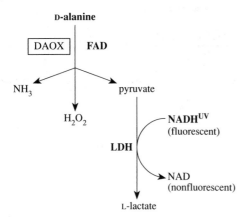

### Staining Solution[3]

A. 0.5 $M$ Tris–HCl buffer, pH 8.0
   30 m$M$ D-Alanine

B. FAD                                                          1 mg
   NADH                                                        10 mg
   Lactate dehydrogenase (LDH)                     50 units

### Procedure

Add B components to 5 ml of solution A and apply the mixture to the gel surface on a filter-paper overlay. Incubate the gel with application at 37°C in a moist chamber for 20 to 30 min and view under long-wave UV light. Dark (nonfluorescent) bands of DAOX are visible on a light (fluorescent) background. Record the zymogram or photograph using a yellow filter.

*Notes:* When a zymogram that is visible in daylight is required, the processed gel should be counterstained with MTT/PMS solution. This treatment results in the appearance of white bands of DAOX on a blue background of the gel.

## GENERAL NOTES

The resolution and sensitivity of the positive stain (Method 1) is better than that obtained with any of the negative fluorescent stains (Methods 2 and 3).

Human DAOX acts on many D-amino acids, except D-aspartic acid, D-cysteine, D-cystine, and D-glutamic acid. The highest activity was revealed with D-phenylalanine, D-leucine, D-alanine, D-isoleucine, D-norleucine, D-proline, and D-tyrosine.

Better staining of DAOX bands can be obtained with higher concentrations of FAD in the staining solution. The staining intensity of DAOX can also be enhanced if FAD (final concentration 0.2 m$M$) is added to the gel and bridge buffers prior to electrophoresis. Under these conditions, however, the enzyme from human liver exhibits a single band of higher activity and greater anodal mobility than either of the two bands seen on the zymogram after electrophoresis in the absence of FAD. This effect of enhanced activity and altered electrophoretic mobility is not observed when homogenates are treated with FAD (final concentration 0.5 m$M$) prior to electrophoresis.[3]

### REFERENCES

1. Duley, J. and Holmes, R. S., α-Hydroxyacid oxidase in the mouse: evidence for two genetic loci and a tetrameric subunit structure for the liver isozyme, *Genetics*, 76, 93, 1974.
2. Nelson, R. L., Povey, S., Hopkinson, D. A., and Harris, H., The detection after electrophoresis of enzymes involved in ammonia metabolism using L-glutamate dehydrogenase as a linking enzyme, *Biochem. Genet.*, 15, 1023, 1977.
3. Barker, R. F. and Hopkinson, D. A., The genetic and biochemical properties of the D-amino acid oxidase in human tissues, *Ann. Hum. Genet.*, 41, 27, 1977.

## 1.4.3.4 — Monoamine Oxidase; MAOX

OTHER NAMES    Amine oxidase (flavin-containing) (recommended name), tyramine oxidase, tyraminase, amine oxidase, adrenaline oxidase

REACTION    $RCH_2NH_2 + H_2O + O_2 = RCHO + NH_3 + H_2O_2$ (Acts on primary amines, and usually also on secondary and tertiary amines with small substituents.)

ENZYME SOURCE   Fungi, plants, invertebrates, vertebrates

## METHOD 1

### Visualization Scheme

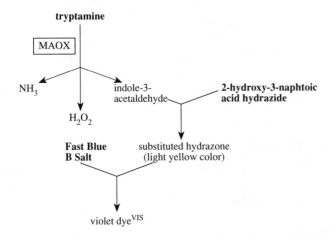

### Staining Solution[1]

| | | |
|---|---|---|
| A. | KH$_2$PO$_4$ | 3.71 g |
| | 0.5 $M$ NaOH | 46.8 ml |
| | H$_2$O | 953 ml |
| B. | 40% H$_2$SO$_4$ | 50 ml |
| | 1 $M$ NaOH | 1 ml |
| | 0.2 $M$ K$_2$HPO$_4$ | 20 ml |
| C. | 2-Hydroxy-3-naphtoic acid hydrazide | 25 mg |
| D. | 0.1 $M$ Tryptamine hydrochloride | 10 ml |
| E. | Fast Blue B salt | 200 mg |
| | Solution A, pH 8.0 | 100 ml |

### Procedure

Dissolve C component in heated solution B (80 to 90°C). Filtrate cooled mixture and add solution D. Incubate the gel in resulting mixture at 37°C until light yellow bands appear. Place gel in solution E for 10 min and then transfer it in 7% acetic acid. Violet bands clearly visible on a blue background appear after about 30 min.

## METHOD 2

### Visualization Scheme

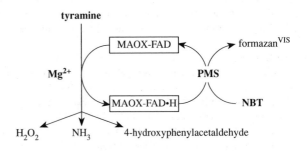

### Staining Solution[2]

| | |
|---|---|
| 0.5 $M$ Phosphate buffer, pH 7.4 | 5 ml |
| 0.2 $M$ Tyramine (or benzylamine, or isoamylamine, or tryptamine) | 2 ml |
| 5 m$M$ MgCl$_2$ | 2 ml |
| 1 mg/ml NBT | 5 ml |
| 1 mg/ml PMS | 0.5 ml |
| 10 m$M$ KCN | 2 ml |

### Procedure

Incubate the gel in staining solution in the dark at 37°C until dark blue bands appear. Wash stained gel in water and fix in 50% ethanol.

*Notes:*   KCN is used to prevent development of superoxide dismutase (see 1.15.1.1 — SOD) bands. It should be remembered, however, that MAOX is also inhibited by cyanide ions.

## OTHER METHODS

A. Two-dimensional spectroscopy of electrophoretic gel (see Part II for details) can be used to visualize MAOX activity bands by purely optical means.[3] In this procedure MAOX is detected due to its formation of H$_2$O$_2$ as a reaction product. With the use of peroxidase as a coupling enzyme and homovanillic acid as a peroxidase substrate, a highly fluorescent product is formed, which is detected fluorimetrically in substrate-containing agarose overlay at an excitation of 313 nm and an emission of 421 nm. A special optical device permits photocopies of the developed agarose overlay to be obtained. This method is not widely used because several simpler procedures for visualization of MAOX activity bands on electrophoretic gels are available.

B. A linked peroxidase reaction also can be used to develop MAOX bands visible in daylight (see, for example, 1.4.3.3 — DAOX, Method 1).

C. A linked glutamate dehydrogenase reaction can be used in a negative fluorescent stain to detect ammonia produced by MAOX (see, for example, 1.4.3.3 — DAOX, Method 2).

D. The immunoblotting procedure (for details see Part II) using monoclonal antibodies specific to human MAOX[4] can also be used for localization of the enzyme protein on electrophoretic gels. This procedure, however, is time consuming and very expensive, thus being unsuitable for routine laboratory use in MAOX electrophoretic studies.

## GENERAL NOTES

The enzyme is a flavoprotein with FAD as the prosthetic group. Flavoprotein complex does not dissociate during electrophoresis because FAD is tightly bound to the enzyme molecule. Therefore, the addition of FAD to MAOX staining solutions is not needed.

## REFERENCES

1. Shaw, C. R. and Prasad, R., Starch gel electrophoresis of enzymes: a compilation of recipes, *Biochem. Genet.*, 4, 297, 1970.
2. Allen, J. M. and Beard, M. E., α-Hydroxy acid oxidase: localization in renal microbodies, *Science*, 149, 1507, 1965.
3. Klebe, R. J., Mancuso, M. G., Brown, C. R., and Teng, L., Two-dimensional spectroscopy of electrophoretic gels, *Biochem. Genet.*, 19, 655, 1981.
4. Denney, R. M., Fritz, R. R., Patel, N. T., and Abell, C. W., Human liver MAO-A and MAO-B separated by immunoaffinity chromatography with MAO-B specific monoclonal antibody, *Science*, 215, 1400, 1982.

OTHER NAMES     Diamine oxidase, diamino oxhydrase, histaminase, amine oxidase (pyridoxal-containing)

REACTION     $RCH_2NH_2 + H_2O + O_2 = RCHO + NH_3 + H_2O_2$ (also see *Notes*)

ENZYME SOURCE     Bacteria, fungi, plants, invertebrates, vertebrates

## METHOD

### Visualization Scheme

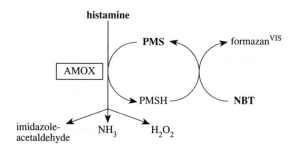

### Staining Solution[1]

| | |
|---|---|
| 65 m$M$ Phosphate buffer, pH 6.8 | 60 ml |
| 10 m$M$ Histamine | 10 ml |
| 1 mg/ml NBT | 5 ml |
| 0.5 mg/ml PMS | 5 ml |

### Procedure

Incubate the gel in staining solution in the dark at 37°C until dark blue bands appear. Wash stained gel in water and fix in 50% ethanol.

*Notes:* The enzyme isolated from a number of sources exhibits low substrate specificity. Primary monoamines, diamines, and histamine are all oxidized by the enzyme.

## OTHER METHODS

A. A coupled peroxidase reaction can be used to detect hydrogen peroxide produced by AMOX (see, for example, 1.4.3.3 — DAOX, Method 1).
B. A coupled glutamate dehydrogenase reaction can be used in a negative fluorescent stain to detect ammonia produced by AMOX (see, for example, 1.4.3.3 — DAOX, Method 2).
C. 2-Hydroxy-3-naphtoic acid hydrazide can be used to detect imidazoleacetaldehyde produced by AMOX. This method is based on the capture of aldehyde by a hydrazide and subsequent coupling of the product with Fast Blue B salt resulting in violet dye (for details see 1.4.3.4 — MAOX, Method 1).

## REFERENCE

1. Feinstein, R. N. and Lindahl, R., Detection of oxidases on polyacrylamide gels, *Anal. Biochem.*, 56, 353, 1973.

## 1.5.1.3 — Dihydrofolate Reductase; DHFR

**OTHER NAMES**  Tetrahydrofolate dehydrogenase, dihydrofolate dehydrogenase

**REACTIONS**
1. 5,6,7,8-Tetrahydrofolate + NADP = 7,8-dihydrofolate + NADPH
2. 7,8-Dihydrofolate + NADP = folate + NADPH

**ENZYME SOURCE**  Bacteria, vertebrates

## METHOD

### Visualization Scheme

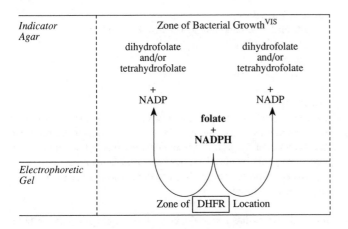

### Indicator agar[1]

1.5% Indicator citrate agar containing 100 ng/ml folate, 400 ng/ml NADPH, and $10^8$ bacteria/ml of *P. cerevisiae* (ATCC 8081) in citrate medium (see Appendix A-2) lacking folinic and folic acids.

### Procedure

Prepare indicator agar and pour it into a sterile plate. After the bacteria-seeded indicator agar solidifies, a slice of electrophoretic starch gel (cut surface down), cellulose acetate strip, or PAG is laid over the agar, avoiding the formation of air bubbles between indicator agar and electrophoretic gels. The bands of bacterial growth become visible in transmitted light after 6 to 12 h of incubation at 37°C.

*Notes:*  As a control for bacterial growth tetrahydrofolate should be spotted at one corner of the indicator agar. The origin and slot locations should be marked on the indicator agar before it is removed.

Bioautographic visualization of DHFR is the only method that is able to detect the enzyme in unconcentrated crude cell extracts.

### REFERENCE

1. Naylor, S. L., Townsend, J. K., and Klebe, R. J., Bioautographic visualization of dihydrofolate reductase in enzyme overproducing BHK mutants, *Biochem. Genet.*, 18, 199, 1980.

## 1.5.1.7 — Saccharopine Dehydrogenase (NAD, L-Lysine-Forming); SD

**OTHER NAMES**  Lysine–2-oxoglutarate reductase

**REACTION**  $N^6$-(L-1,3-Dicarboxypropyl)-L-lysine + NAD + $H_2O$ = L-lysine + 2-oxoglutarate + NADH

**ENZYME SOURCE**  Fungi

## METHOD

### Visualization Scheme

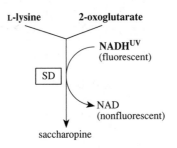

### Staining Solution[1]
0.05 *M* Potassium phosphate buffer, pH 6.8
1 m*M* NADH
10 m*M* 2-Oxoglutarate
10 m*M* L-Lysine

### Procedure

Apply the staining solution to the gel surface with a filter-paper overlay. Incubate the gel at 37°C in a moist chamber. After 20 to 30 min of incubation monitor gel under long-wave UV light. Dark (nonfluorescent) bands of SD are visible on a light (fluorescent) background. Record the zymogram or photograph using a yellow filter.

*Notes:*  If a zymogram that is visible in daylight is required, counterstain the processed gel with MTT/PMS solution. This procedure results in the appearance of white bands of SD on the blue background of the gel.

It should be remembered that if too much NADH is added to the staining solution, the enzyme should not be able to convert enough NADH into NAD for nonfluorescent bands to become visible.

### REFERENCE

1. Nakatani, Y., Motoji, F., and Kazuya, H., Enzymic determination of L-lysine in biological materials, *Anal. Biochem.*, 49, 225, 1972.

OTHER NAMES    D-Octopine synthase

REACTION    $N^2$-(D-1-Carboxyethyl)-L-arginine + NAD + $H_2O$ = L-arginine + pyruvate + NADH

ENZYME SOURCE  Invertebrates

## METHOD 1

### Visualization Scheme

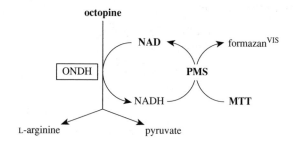

### Staining Solution[1]

80 m$M$ Tris–HCl buffer, pH 9.1
1 m$M$ D(+)-Octopine
0.3 m$M$ NAD
0.49 m$M$ MTT
0.16 m$M$ PMS

### Procedure

Incubate the gel in staining solution in the dark at 37°C until dark blue bands appear. Wash stained gel in water and fix in 50% ethanol.

## METHOD 2

### Visualization Scheme

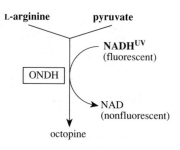

### Staining Solution[1]

100 m$M$ Triethanolamine–HCl buffer, pH 7.0
0.1 m$M$ NADH
2 m$M$ Pyruvate
20 m$M$ L-Arginine

### Procedure

Lay a piece of filter paper saturated with the staining solution on top of the gel, and incubate at 37°C for 10 to 30 min. Remove the filter paper and view the gel under long-wave UV light. Dark (nonfluorescent) bands of ONDH are visible on a light (fluorescent) background of the gel. Record the zymogram or photograph using a yellow filter.

*Notes:* Staining solution may also be applied as 1% agar overlay. When a zymogram that is visible in daylight is required, the processed gel should be counterstained with MTT/PMS solution. This results in the almost immediate appearance of white bands on a blue background.

If the concentration of NADH in the stain is too much, the enzyme should not be able to convert enough NADH into NAD for nonfluorescent ONDH bands to become visible.

In the reverse direction ONDH also acts (but more slowly) on L-ornithine, L-lysine, and L-histidine.

In some invertebrate species LDH bands can also develop on ONDH zymograms obtained by this method. Therefore, an additional gel should be stained for LDH as a control.

### REFERENCE

1. Dando, P. R., Storey, K. B., Hochachka, P. W., and Storey, J. M., Multiple dehydrogenases in marine molluscs: electrophoretic analysis of alanopine dehydrogenase, strombine dehydrogenase, octopine dehydrogenase and lactate dehydrogenase, *Mar. Biol. Lett.*, 2, 249, 1981.

OTHER NAMES    Pyrroline dehydrogenase

REACTION        1-Pyrroline-5-carboxylate + NAD + H$_2$O = L-glutamate + NADH

ENZYME SOURCE  Bacteria, invertebrates

## METHOD

### Visualization Scheme

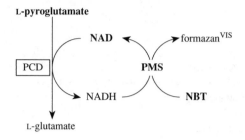

## Staining Solution[1]

| | |
|---|---|
| 0.1 *M* Tris–HCl buffer, pH 8.0 | 100 ml |
| L-Pyroglutamate | 50 mg |
| NAD | 50 mg |
| NBT | 30 mg |
| PMS | 2 mg |

## Procedure

Incubate the gel in staining solution in the dark at 37°C until dark blue bands appear. Wash stained gel in water and fix in 50% ethanol.

## REFERENCE

1. Mulley, J. C. and Latter, B. D. H., Genetic variation and evolutionary relationships within a group of thirteen species of penaeid prawns, *Evolution*, 34, 904, 1980.

REACTION    2,2′-Iminodipropanoate + NAD + $H_2O$ = L-alanine + pyruvate + NADH

ENZYME SOURCE  Invertebrates

## METHOD 1

### Visualization Scheme

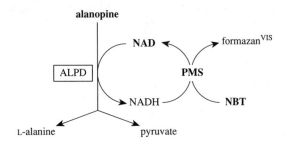

### Staining Solution[1]

| | |
|---|---|
| 50 m$M$ Tris–HCl buffer, pH 8.4 | 24 ml |
| 50 m$M$ Alanopine | 6 ml |
| 10 mg/ml NAD | 6 ml |
| 10 mg/ml NBT | 2 ml |
| 5 mg/ml PMS | 2 ml |

### Procedure

Incubate the gel in staining solution in the dark at 37°C until dark blue bands appear. Wash stained gel in water and fix in 50% ethanol.

*Notes:*  The post-coupling of PMS may prove beneficial.

## METHOD 2

### Visualization Scheme

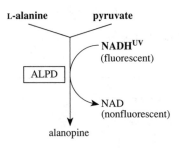

### Staining Solution[2]

100 m$M$ Triethanolamine–HCl buffer, pH 7.0
0.1 m$M$ NADH
2 m$M$ Pyruvate
20 m$M$ L-Alanine

### Procedure

Lay a piece of filter paper saturated with the staining solution on top of the gel, and incubate at 37°C for 10 to 30 min. Remove the filter paper and view the gel under long-wave UV light. Dark (nonfluorescent) bands of ALPD are visible on a light (fluorescent) background of the gel. Record the zymogram or photograph using a yellow filter.

*Notes:*  When a zymogram that is visible in daylight is required, counterstain the processed gel with MTT/PMS solution. This results in the appearance of white bands on a blue background.[3]

In some invertebrate species LDH bands can also develop on ALPD zymograms obtained by this method. Therefore, an additional gel should be stained for LDH as a control.

ALPD from some sources also catalyzes (but more slowly) the reductive imination of glycine and pyruvate to strombine (see, however, 1.5.1.X — STRD).

### GENERAL NOTES

Method 2 is more sensitive than Method 1. The ratio of the maximal ALPD activities in the reverse vs. the forward reactions is about 5:1.[1]

### REFERENCES

1. Plaxton, W. C. and Storey, K. B., Tissue specific isozymes of alanopine dehydrogenase in the channeled whelk *Busycotypus canaliculatum*, *Can. J. Zool.*, 60, 1568, 1982.
2. Dando, P. R., Storey, K. B., Hochachka, P. W., and Storey, J. M., Multiple dehydrogenases in marine molluscs: electrophoretic analysis of alanopine dehydrogenase, strombine dehydrogenase, octopine dehydrogenase and lactate dehydrogenase, *Mar. Biol. Lett.*, 2, 249, 1981.
3. Manchenko, G. P., Nonfluorescent negative stain for alanopine dehydrogenase activity on starch gels, *Anal. Biochem.*, 145, 308, 1985.

## 1.5.1.X — Strombine Dehydrogenase; STRD

REACTION      2-Methyliminodiacetate + NAD + $H_2O$ = glycine + pyruvate + NADH

ENZYME SOURCE  Invertebrates

## METHOD

### Visualization Scheme

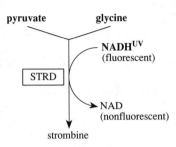

### Staining Solution[1]
100 m$M$ Triethanolamine–HCl buffer, pH 7.0
0.1 m$M$ NADH
2 m$M$ Pyruvate
20 m$M$ Glycine

### Procedure
Apply the staining solution to the gel surface with a filter-paper overlay. Incubate the gel at 37°C in a moist chamber. After 30 min monitor gel under long-wave UV light. Dark (nonfluorescent) bands of STRD are visible on a light (fluorescent) background. Record the zymogram or photograph using a yellow filter.

*Notes:*  When a zymogram that is visible in daylight is required, the processed gel should be counterstained with MTT/PMS solution. This results in the appearance of white bands on a blue background.

In some invertebrate species LDH bands can also develop on STRD zymograms obtained by this Method. Therefore, an additional gel should be stained for LDH as a control.

Alanopine dehydrogenase (see 1.5.1.17 — ALPD) also catalyzes the reductive imination of glycine and pyruvate to strombine. However, it displays high specificity for L-alanine as its substrate and shows very low activity with glycine, whereas STRD shows higher glycine activity than L-alanine activity.[2] To differentiate STRD and ALPD bands, an additional control gel should be stained for ALPD.

### REFERENCES
1. Dando, P. R., Storey, K. B., Hochachka, P. W., and Storey, J. M., Multiple dehydrogenases in marine molluscs: electrophoretic analysis of alanopine dehydrogenase, strombine dehydrogenase, octopine dehydrogenase and lactate dehydrogenase, *Mar. Biol. Lett.*, 2, 249, 1981.
2. Plaxton, W. C. and Storey, K. B., Tissue specific isozymes of alanopine dehydrogenase in the channeled whelk *Busycotypus canaliculatum*, *Can. J. Zool.*, 60, 1568, 1982.

## 1.5.3.1 — Sarcosine Oxidase; SOX

REACTION      Sarcosine + $H_2O$ + $O_2$ = glycine + formaldehyde + $H_2O_2$

ENZYME SOURCE  Bacteria, vertebrates

## METHOD

### Visualization Scheme

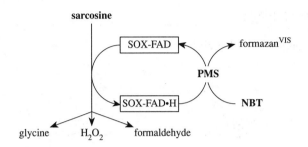

### Staining Solution[1]
| | |
|---|---:|
| 65 m$M$ Phosphate buffer, pH 6.8 | 70 ml |
| 10 m$M$ Sarcosine | 10 ml |
| NBT | 5 mg |
| PMS | 2.5 mg |

### Procedure
Incubate the gel in staining solution in the dark at 37°C until dark blue bands appear. Wash stained gel in water and fix in 50% ethanol.

### REFERENCE
1. Feinstein, R. N. and Lindahl, R., Detection of oxidases on polyacrylamide gels, *Anal. Biochem.*, 56, 353, 1973.

| | |
|---|---|
| OTHER NAMES | Glutathione reductase (NAD(P)H) (recommended name) |
| REACTION | NAD(P)H + GSSG (oxidized glutathione) = NAD(P) + 2GSH (reduced glutathione) |
| ENZYME SOURCE | Bacteria, fungi, plants, invertebrates, vertebrates |

## METHOD 1

### Visualization Scheme

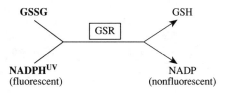

### Staining Solution[1]

A. 0.3 $M$ Tris–HCl buffer, pH 8.0 — 10 ml
   NADPH — 7 mg
   Oxidized glutathione (GSSG) — 30 mg
B. 2% Agar solution (60°C) — 10 ml

### Procedure

Mix A and B components of the staining solution and pour the mixture over the surface of the gel. Incubate the gel at 37°C and view under long-wave UV light. Dark (nonfluorescent) bands of GSR are visible on the light (fluorescent) background of the gel. Record the zymogram or photograph using a yellow filter.

## METHOD 2

### Visualization Scheme

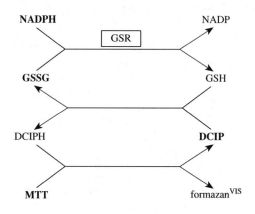

### Staining Solution[2]

0.25 $M$ Tris–HCl buffer, pH 8.4 — 20 ml
Oxidized glutathione (GSSG) — 40 mg
NADPH — 10 mg
2,6-Dichlorophenol indophenol (DCIP) — 0.2 mg
MTT — 10 mg

### Procedure

Incubate the gel in staining solution in the dark at 37°C until purple bands appear on a blue background. When the bands have reached a satisfactory intensity, counterstain gel with 1 $M$ HCl solution to remove a blue background and to allow GSR bands to become more obvious.[3] Wash stained gel in water and fix in 50% ethanol.

*Notes:* The stain also detects NADPH diaphorase [see 1.6.99.1 — DIA(NADPH)]. Its bands can be identified by removing GSSG from the staining solution.

To detect NADH–dependent GSR activity, NADH should be used in the staining solution instead of NADPH. In this case an additional gel should be stained for NADH diaphorase [see 1.8.1.4 — DIA(NADH)] as a control.

## METHOD 3

### Visualization Scheme

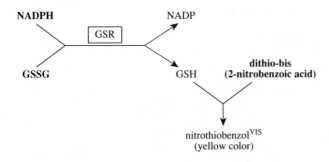

### Staining Solution[4]

    133 m*M* Tris–HCl buffer, pH 8.0
    5.5 m*M* Oxidized glutathione (GSSG)
    0.32 m*M* NADPH
    0.88 m*M* 5,5′-Dithio-bis(2-nitrobenzoic acid)
    33 m*M* EDTA
    1% Agar

### Procedure

Add EDTA and 2-nitrobenzoic acid to half of the tris–HCl buffer and heat to bring the nitrobenzoic acid into solution. When the nitrobenzoic acid is completely dissolved, allow the solution to cool. After the mixture reaches a temperature of 45°C add the NADPH and GSSG. Then add the agar to the remaining half of the tris–HCl buffer and heat to boiling. After the agar solution is cooled to 45°C mix the two solutions and pour the mixture over the surface of the gel. Incubate the gel at 37°C until yellow bands of GSR appear.

*Notes:* Additional nonspecifically stained bands can also develop on GSR zymograms obtained by this method. Thus, it is important to do control staining of an additional gel with a staining solution from which GSSG is absent.

### GENERAL NOTES

Method 2 is usually preferred.

### REFERENCES

1. Nichols, E. A. and Ruddle, F. H., Polymorphism and linkage of glutathione reductase in *Mus musculus*, *Biochem. Genet.*, 13, 323, 1975.
2. Kaplan, J. C. and Beutler, E., Electrophoretic study of glutathione reductase in human erythrocytes and leukocytes, *Nature*, 217, 256, 1968.
3. Richardson, B. J., Baverstock, P. R., and Adams, M., *Allozyme Electrophoresis: A Handbook for Animal Systematics and Population Studies*, Academic Press, Sydney, 1986, 192.
4. Brewer, G. J., *An Introduction to Isozyme Techniques*, Academic Press, New York, 1970, 113.

## 1.6.6.2 — Nitrate Reductase (NAD(P)H); NAR(NAD(P)H)

OTHER NAMES     Assimilatory nitrate reductase

REACTION     NAD(P)H + nitrate = NAD(P) + nitrite + $H_2O$

ENZYME SOURCE   Bacteria, fungi, plants

## METHOD

### Visualization Scheme

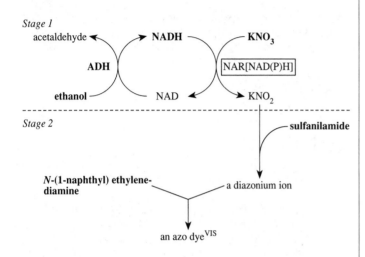

### Staining Solution[1]

A. 0.1 *M* Potassium phosphate buffer, pH 7.5    100 ml
   $KNO_3$    150 mg
   95% Ethanol    2.5 ml
   NADH    30 mg
   Alcohol dehydrogenase (ADH)    100 units
B. 1% Sulfanilamide in 1 *N* HCl    50 ml
   0.01% *N*-(1-Naphthyl)ethylenediamine    50 ml
   dihydrochloride in 0.1 *M* potassium
   phosphate buffer, pH 7.5

### Procedure

Incubate the gel in solution A at 30°C for 30 min. Discard solution A and rinse gel with water. Place the gel in solution B. In a few minutes pink bands develop indicating zones of NAR(NAD(P)H) activity.

*Notes:* Alcohol dehydrogenase and ethanol are used to regenerate NADH. When NADPH is used instead of NADH, NADP-dependent glucose-6-phosphate dehydrogenase (EC 1.1.1.49) and glucose-6-phosphate are recommended for use instead of ADH and ethanol to regenerate NADPH.

### GENERAL NOTES

The activity of NAR(NAD(P)H) from spinach is due to two different proteins: an NAD(P) reductase and a nitrate reductase. The nitrate reductase is inactive with NAD(P)H but serves methyl or benzyl viologen (but not PMS) as electron carriers. The last enzyme may be identical to nitrate reductase (see 1.7.99.4 — NAR).

### REFERENCE

1. Upcroft, J. A. and Done, J., Starch gel electrophoresis of plant NADH–nitrate reductase and nitrite reductase, *J. Exp. Bot.*, 25, 503, 1974.

## 1.6.6.9 — Trimethylamine-*N*-oxide Reductase; TMAOR

REACTION     NADH + trimethylamine-*N*-oxide = NAD + trimethylamine + $H_2O$

ENZYME SOURCE   Bacteria

## METHOD

### Visualization Scheme

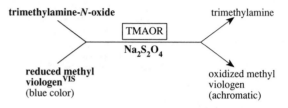

### Staining Solution[1]

A. 100 m*M* Potassium phosphate buffer, pH 6.5    100 ml
   200 m*M* Methyl viologen    1 ml
   50 m*M* Sodium dithionite ($Na_2S_2O_4$)    50 µl
B. 100 m*M* Potassium phosphate buffer, pH 6.5
   2 *M* Trimethylamine-*N*-oxide

### Procedure

Place electrophorized gel in a nitrogen atmosphere in solution A. Then incubate the gel, uniformly colored blue by reduced methyl viologen, in nitrogen atmosphere in solution B. The reduction of the substrate is coupled with the oxidation of reduced methyl viologen, and the resulting achromatic bands on a blue background indicate the areas of TMAOR activity on the gel. Record the zymogram or photograph using a yellow filter.

*Notes:* Methyl viologen is used instead of NADH. Sodium dithionite is used as a powerful reducing agent to reduce methyl viologen, which is of blue color.

Dimethylsulfoxide, tetrahydrothiophene-1-oxide, and pyridine-*N*-oxide can also be used as substrates.

When a permanent negative zymogram is required, the gel should be additionally stained in 2.5% solution of triphenyl tetrazolium chloride (TTC). This counterstaining results in the appearance of white TMAOR bands on a red background. The gel counterstained with TTC can be stored in 50% ethanol for a long time. The procedure of staining gel in a nitrogen atmosphere and counterstaining with TTC is described in detail in the procedure of staining gels for nitrate reductase (see 1.7.99.4 — NAR).

### REFERENCE

1. Silvestro, A., Pommier, J., Pascal, M.-C., and Giordano, G., The inducible trimethylamine *N*-oxide reductase of *Escherichia coli* K12: its localization and inducers, *Biochim. Biophys. Acta*, 999, 208, 1989.

## 1.6.99.1 — NADPH Diaphorase; DIA(NADPH)

OTHER NAMES    NADPH dehydrogenase (recommended name)

REACTION    NADPH + acceptor = NADP + reduced acceptor

ENZYME SOURCE  Bacteria, plants, invertebrates, vertebrates

## METHOD

### Visualization Scheme

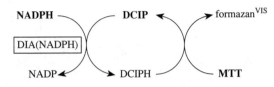

### Staining Solution[1]

| | |
|---|---|
| 0.15 M Tris–HCl buffer, pH 8.2 | 50 ml |
| NADPH | 10 mg |
| 2,6-Dichlorophenol indophenol (DCIP) | 2 mg |
| MTT | 7 mg |

### Procedure

Incubate the gel in staining solution in the dark at 37°C until purple bands appear on a blue background. When the bands have reached a satisfactory intensity, counterstain gel with 1 M HCl solution to remove a blue background and to allow DIA(NADPH) bands to become more obvious.[2] Wash stained gel in water and fix in 50% ethanol.

## OTHER METHODS

Alternative methods of DIA(NADPH) visualization based on defluorescence of NADPH[3] and decoloration of DCIP[4] are also described, but the positive tetrazolium method described above is usually preferred.

## GENERAL NOTES

The term "diaphorase" refers to any enzyme that can catalyze the oxidation of NAD(P)H in the presence of an electron acceptor such as DCIP. A number of enzymes that have specific functions *in vivo* also have general diaphorase activity *in vitro*. This causes well-known difficulties in adequate enzyme classification of diaphorase activity bands on histochemically stained gels. One should beware of homology problems when diaphorase isozymes are used in phylogenetic comparisons [see also 1.6.99.2 — MR and 1.8.1.4 — DIA(NADH)].

### REFERENCES

1. Frischer, H., Nelson, R., Noyes, C., Carson, P. E., Bowman, J. E., Rieckmann, K. H., and Ajmar, F., NAD(P) glycohydrolase deficiency in human erythrocytes and alteration of cytosol NADH–methemoglobin diaphorase by membrane NAD-glycohydrolase activity, *Proc. Natl. Acad. Sci. U.S.A.*, 70, 2406, 1973.
2. Richardson, B. J., Baverstock, P. R., and Adams, M., *Allozyme Electrophoresis: A Handbook for Animal Systematics and Population Studies*, Academic Press, Sydney, 1986, 173.
3. Čepica, S. and Stratil, A., Further studies on sheep polymorphic erythrocyte diaphorase, *Anim. Blood Groups Biochem. Genet.*, 9, 239, 1978.
4. Brewer, G. J., Eaton, J. W., Knutsen, C. S., and Beck, C. C., A starch gel electrophoretic method for the study of diaphorase isozymes and preliminary results with sheep and human erythrocytes, *Biochem. Biophys. Res. Commun.*, 29, 198, 1967.

## 1.6.99.2 — NAD(P)H Dehydrogenase (Quinone); MR

OTHER NAMES    Menadione reductase, phylloquinone reductase, quinone reductase

REACTION    NAD(P)H + acceptor = NAD(P) + reduced acceptor

ENZYME SOURCE  Bacteria, fungi, plants, invertebrates, vertebrates

## METHOD

### Visualization Scheme

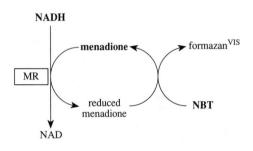

### Staining Solution[1]

| | |
|---|---|
| 0.2 M Tris–HCl buffer, pH 7.0 | 75 ml |
| Menadione | 25 mg |
| NADH | 25 mg |
| NBT | 10 mg |

### Procedure

Incubate the gel in staining solution in the dark at 37°C until dark blue bands appear. Wash stained gel in water and fix in 50% ethanol.

*Notes:*  The enzyme from some sources (e.g., bovine liver) is also active with dichlorophenol indophenol as acceptor. Thus, its bands of activity can also develop on NAD(P)H diaphorase zymograms [see 1.6.99.1 — DIA(NADPH) and 1.8.1.4 — DIA(NADH)].

### REFERENCE

1. Cheliak, W. M. and Pitel, J. A., Techniques for Starch Gel Electrophoresis of Enzymes from Forest Tree Species, Information Report PI-X-42, Petawawa National Forestry Institute, Canadian Forestry Service, Agriculture Canada Chalk River, Ont., 1984.

## 1.7.3.3 — Urate Oxidase; UOX

OTHER NAMES    Uricase

REACTION    Uric acid + $2H_2O$ + $O_2$ = allantoin + $CO_2$ + $H_2O_2$

ENZYME SOURCE  Bacteria, fungi, plants, invertebrates, vertebrates

## METHOD

### Visualization Scheme

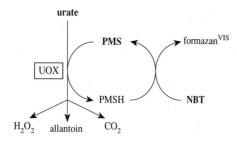

### Staining Solution[1]

| | |
|---|---|
| 0.05 $M$ Phosphate buffer, pH 6.8 | 70 ml |
| 10 m$M$ Urate | 10 ml |
| NBT | 5 mg |
| PMS | 2.5 mg |

### Procedure

Incubate the gel in staining solution in the dark at 37°C until dark blue bands appear. Wash stained gel in water and fix in 50% ethanol.

*Notes:* The enzyme from many sources is more active at alkaline conditions (pH 8.0 to 8.5).

## OTHER METHODS

A. A linked peroxidase reaction can be used to detect the product hydrogen peroxide (see 1.11.1.7 — PER).

B. Calcium ions may be used to detect the product $CO_2$ after electrophoresis of UOX in PAG.[2] Calcium carbonate precipitate forms under alkaline conditions. This results in the appearance of opaque bands visible on transparent PAG (for example, see 4.1.1.1 — PDC). The calcium carbonate method, however, is not as sensitive as the tetrazolium method described above.

## REFERENCES

1. Feinstein, R. N. and Lindahl, R., Detection of oxidases on polyacrylamide gels, *Anal. Biochem.*, 56, 353, 1973.
2. Nimmo, H.G. and Nimmo, G.A., A general method for the localization of enzymes that produce phosphate, pyrophosphate, or $CO_2$ after polyacrylamide gel electrophoresis, *Anal. Biochem.*, 121, 17, 1982.

## 1.7.99.3 — Nitrite Reductase; NIR

REACTION    2 Nitric oxide + $2H_2O$ + acceptor = 2 nitrite + reduced acceptor

ENZYME SOURCE  Bacteria, fungi, plants

## METHOD

### Visualization Scheme

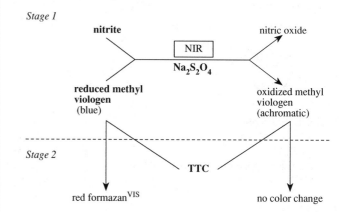

### Staining Solution[1]

| | | |
|---|---|---|
| A. | 50 m$M$ Sodium phosphate buffer, pH 8.0 | 100 ml |
| | $NaNO_2$ | 100 mg |
| B. | 0.1 $M$ $NaHCO_3$ | 3 ml |
| | Sodium hydrosulfite ($Na_2S_2O_4$) | 120 mg |
| C. | 50 m$M$ Sodium phosphate buffer, pH 8.0 | 3 ml |
| | Methyl viologen | 96 mg |
| D. | $H_2O$ | 10 ml |
| | Triphenyl tetrazolium chloride (TTC) | 250 mg |

### Procedure

Prepare solution A and bubble it with nitrogen (or argon) in the staining tray. Immerse the gel in solution A, cover the tray so it is airtight and treat the gel with the gas for 5 min using side ports on the tray. Prepare solutions B and C. Pour C into B and mix thoroughly (the mixture should be blue). Using a syringe inject the mixture into the tray without letting any air in. Incubate the gel until achromatic bands appear on a blue background. Then inject solution D and shake the tray gently to ensure good mixing. Incubate the gel in the dark at 5 to 10°C until the gel background becomes red. Wash negatively stained gel in water and fix in 50% ethanol.

*Notes:* Sodium hydrosulfite is used to reduce methyl viologen, which turns blue in the presence of this reducing agent.

The use of NBT or MTT instead of TTC is not recommended because both give blue formazans upon reduction, thus making it difficult to detect the end point of the last reduction.

Benzyl viologen can be used instead of methyl viologen.

## REFERENCE

1. Vallejos, C. E., Enzyme activity staining, in *Isozymes in Plant Genetics and Breeding*, Part A, Tanskley, S. D. and Orton, T. J., Eds., Elsevier, Amsterdam, 1983, 469.

OTHER NAMES    Respiratory nitrate reductase

REACTION    Nitrite + acceptor = nitrate + reduced acceptor

ENZYME SOURCE  Bacteria, fungi, plants

## METHOD

### Visualization Scheme

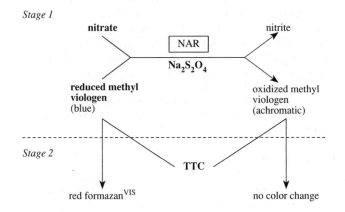

*Stage 1*

*Stage 2*

### Staining Solution[1]

| | | |
|---|---|---|
| A. | 50 m*M* Sodium phosphate buffer, pH 8.0 | 100 ml |
| | KNO$_3$ | 1 g |
| B. | 0.1 *M* NaHCO$_3$ | 3 ml |
| | Sodium hydrosulfite (Na$_2$S$_2$O$_4$) | 120 mg |
| C. | 50 m*M* Sodium phosphate buffer, pH 8.0 | 3 ml |
| | Methyl viologen | 96 mg |
| D. | H$_2$O | 10 ml |
| | Triphenyl tetrazolium chloride (TTC) | 250 mg |

### Procedure

Prepare solution A and bubble it with nitrogen (or argon) in the staining tray. Immerse the gel in solution A, cover the tray so it is airtight and treat the gel with the gas for 5 min using side ports on the tray. Prepare solutions B and C. Pour C into B and mix thoroughly (the mixture should be blue). Using a syringe inject the mixture into the tray without letting any air in. Incubate the gel until achromatic bands appear on a blue background. Then, inject solution D and shake the tray gently to ensure good mixing. Incubate the gel in the dark at 5 to 10°C until the gel background becomes red. Wash negatively stained gel in water and fix in 50% ethanol.

*Notes:*  Sodium hydrosulfite is used to reduce methyl viologen, which turns blue in the presence of this reducing agent.

The use of NBT or MTT instead of TTC is not recommended because both give blue formazans upon reduction, thus making it difficult to detect the end point of the last reduction.

Benzyl viologen can be used instead of methyl viologen.

Nitrate reductase (cytochrome) (EC 1.9.6.1) can also utilize methyl (or benzyl) viologen as electron acceptor and thus be visualized on NAR zymograms.

The activity of nitrate reductase (NAD(P)H) (EC 1.6.6.2) from spinach (and perhaps other plants) is due to two different proteins: an NAD(P) reductase and a nitrate reductase. The nitrate reductase component is inactive with NAD(P)H but serves methyl or benzyl viologen as electron acceptors and thus can also develop on NAR zymograms [see 1.6.6.2 — NAR(NAD(P)H)].

### REFERENCE

1. Vallejos, C. E., Enzyme activity staining, in *Isozymes in Plant Genetics and Breeding*, Part A, Tanskley, S. D. and Orton, T. J., Eds., Elsevier, Amsterdam, 1983, 469.

| | |
|---|---|
| OTHER NAMES | Dihydrolipoamide dehydrogenase (recommended name), lipoamide reductase (NADH), lipoyl dehydrogenase, lipoamide dehydrogenase |
| REACTION | Dihydrolipoamide + NAD = lipoamide + NADH |
| ENZYME SOURCE | Bacteria, fungi, plants, invertebrates, vertebrates |

## METHOD

### Visualization Scheme

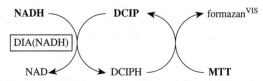

### Staining Solution[1]

| | |
|---|---|
| 0.15 $M$ Tris–HCl buffer, pH 8.2 | 50 ml |
| NADH | 10 mg |
| 2,6-Dichlorophenol indophenol (DCIP) | 2 mg |
| MTT | 7 mg |

### Procedure

Incubate the gel in staining solution in the dark at 37°C until purple bands appear on a blue background. When the bands have reached a satisfactory intensity, treat the gel with 1 $M$ HCl to remove a blue background and to allow DIA(NADH) bands to become more obvious. Wash stained gel in water and fix in 50% ethanol.

## OTHER METHODS

Alternative methods of DIA(NADH) visualization based on defluorescence of NADH[2] and decoloration of DCIP[3] are also available, but the positive tetrazolium method described above is preferable.

## GENERAL NOTES

The name "diaphorase" has been loosely applied to several enzymes that catalyze the oxidation of NAD(P)H in the presence of an electron acceptor such as DCIP. A number of enzymes that have specific functions *in vivo* also have general diaphorase activity *in vitro*. This causes some difficulties in adequate classification of enzymes which display diaphorase activity. For this reason, when DIA(NADH) or DIA(NADPH) isozymes are used as genic markers in phylogenetic studies, the problems of isoenzyme homology can arise [see also 1.6.99.1 — DIA(NADPH) and 1.6.99.2 — MR].

## REFERENCES

1. Frischer, H., Nelson, R., Noyes, C., Carson, P. E., Bowman, J. E., Rieckmann, K. H., and Ajmar, F., NADP glycohydrolase deficiency in human erythrocytes and alteration of cytosol NADH–methemoglobin diaphorase by membrane NAD–glycohydrolase activity, *Proc. Natl. Acad. Sci. U.S.A.*, 70, 2406, 1973.
2. West, C. A., Gomperts, B. D., Huehns, E. R., Kessel, I., and Ashby, J. R., Demonstration of an enzyme variant in a case of congenital methaemoglobinaemia, *Br. Med. J.*, 2, 212, 1967.
3. Brewer, G. J., Eaton, J. W., Knutsen, C. S., and Beck, C. C., A starch gel electrophoretic method for the study of diaphorase isozymes and preliminary results with sheep and human erythrocytes, *Biochem. Biophys. Res. Commun.*, 29, 198, 1967.

## 1.8.3.1 — Sulfite Oxidase; SUOX

REACTION $\quad$ Sulfite + $H_2O$ + $O_2$ = sulfate + $H_2O_2$

ENZYME SOURCE $\quad$ Bacteria, plants, invertebrates, vertebrates

## METHOD

### Visualization Scheme

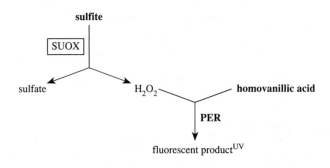

### Staining Solution[1] (modified)
A. 0.1 $M$ Tris–HCl buffer, pH 8.0
    10 m$M$ $Na_2SO_3$
    2 U/ml Peroxidase (PER)
    1 m$M$ Homovanillic acid
B. 2% Agarose solution (60°C)

### Procedure
Mix equal volumes of solutions A and B and pour the mixture over the surface of the gel. Incubate the gel with agarose application at 37°C and observe fluorescent SUOX bands under long-wave UV light. Record the zymogram or photograph using a yellow filter.

*Notes:* Preparation of the enzyme samples for electrophoresis includes partial purification and disruption of mitochondria.

$\quad$ Many chromogenic peroxidase substrates can be used instead of homovanillic acid to develop SUOX activity bands visible in daylight (see 1.11.1.7 — PER).

### REFERENCE
1. Bogaart, A. M. and Bernini, L. F., The molybdoenzyme system of *Drosophila melanogaster*. I. Sulfite oxidase: identification and properties. Expression of the enzyme in maroon-like (mal), low-xanthine dehydrogenase (lxd), and cinnamon (cin) flies, *Biochem. Genet.*, 19, 929, 1981.

## 1.9.3.1 — Cytochrome-*c* Oxidase; CO

OTHER NAMES $\quad$ Cytochrome oxidase, cytochrome $a_3$, cytochrome $aa_3$, indophenolase (misleading name), indophenol oxidase (misleading name)

REACTION $\quad$ 4 Ferrocytochrome $c$ + $O_2$ = 4 ferricytochrome $c$ + $2H_2O$; also catalyzes the Nadi reaction (oxidizing the reaction between α-naphthol and dimethyl-*p*-phenylenediamine)

ENZYME SOURCE $\quad$ Bacteria, plants, vertebrates

## METHOD

### Visualization Scheme

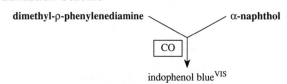

### Staining Solution[1]
| | |
|---|---:|
| 0.1 $M$ Phosphate buffer, pH 7.0 | 100 ml |
| $N,N$-Dimethyl-*p*-phenylenediamine | 100 mg |
| α-Naphthol (predissolved in 0.5 ml acetone) | 150 mg |

### Procedure
Incubate the gel in staining solution in the dark at 37°C until colored bands appear. Wash stained gel in water and fix in 3% acetic acid.

### REFERENCE
1. Brown, A. H. D., Nevo, E., Zohary, D., and Dagan, O., Genetic variation in natural populations of wild barley (*Hordeum spontaneum*), *Genetica*, 49, 97, 1978.

OTHER NAMES Diphenol oxidase, polyphenol oxidase, phenol oxidase, *o*-diphenolase, phenolase, tyrosinase

REACTION 2 Catechol + $O_2$ = 2 1,2-benzoquinone + 2$H_2O$

ENZYME SOURCE Bacteria, fungi, plants, invertebrates, vertebrates

## METHOD 1

### Visualization Scheme

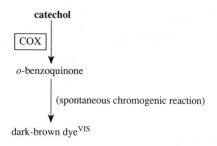

catechol

COX

*o*-benzoquinone

(spontaneous chromogenic reaction)

dark-brown dye[VIS]

### Staining Solution[1]
0.02 *M* Sodium acetate buffer, pH 4.2
0.01 *M* Catechol

### Procedure
Incubate the gel in staining solution at room temperature for about 12 h. The enzyme activity is revealed by the appearance of bands of dark brown catechol melanin, presumably formed as a result of secondary nonenzymatic reactions of the *o*-benzoquinone product of catechol oxidation. Wash stained gel in water and store in 50% glycerol.

## METHOD 2

### Visualization Scheme

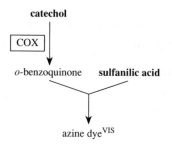

catechol

COX

*o*-benzoquinone    **sulfanilic acid**

azine dye[VIS]

### Staining Solution[2]
| | |
|---|---|
| 0.1 *M* Sodium phosphate buffer, pH 6.8 | 100 ml |
| Catechol | 15 mg |
| Sulfanilic acid | 50 mg |

### Procedure
Incubate the gel in staining solution at 30°C until positively stained bands appear. Wash stained gel in water and store in 50% glycerol.

*Notes:* The azine dye is formed by the condensation of the *o*-quinone and the aromatic amine. Many other coupling amines and diamines can also be used instead of sulfanilic acid.

### GENERAL NOTES

This enzyme represents a group of copper proteins that also act on a variety of substituted catechols, and many of which also catalyze the reactions listed under EC 1.10.3.2 and 1.14.18.1.

Monophenol (tyrosine), diphenols (L-β-3,4-dihydroxyphenylalanine, dopamine, *N*-acetyldopamine, protocatechuic acid, chlorogenic acid, catechin, *m*-cresol), and polyphenol (pyrogallol) also can be used as substrates suitable for visualization of COX activity on electrophoretic gels.

The rate of staining of COX bands on gels is increased by addition to the staining solution of 1 m*M* $Cu^{2+}$.

The phenol oxidases are usually present as inactive proenzymes, which should be activated by incubation of electrophorized gel in solutions containing natural activators extracted from organisms[3] or synthetic activators such as detergents, heavy metals, or alcohols,[4] or proteolytic enzymes such as chymotrypsin.[5] For example, *Drosophila* phenol oxidase is activated by soaking the gel in a 1:1 mixture of propan-2-ol and 0.1 *M* potassium phosphate buffer, pH 6.3, for 2 h at 4°C.[4]

### REFERENCES

1. Pryor, T. and Schwartz, D., The genetic control and biochemical modification of catechol oxidase in maize, *Genetics*, 75, 75, 1973.
2. Sato, M. and Hasegawa, M., The latency of spinach chloroplast phenolase, *Phytochemistry*, 15, 61, 1976.
3. Warner, C. K., Grell, E. H., and Jacobson, K. B., Phenol oxidase activity and the lozenge locus of *Drosophila melanogaster*, *Biochem. Genet.*, 11, 359, 1974.
4. Batterham, P. and MacKechnie, S. W., A phenol oxidase polymorphism in *Drosophila melanogaster*, *Genetica*, 54, 121, 1980.
5. Waite, J. H. and Wilbur, K. M., Phenol oxidase in the periostracum of the marine bivalve *Modiolus demissus* Dillwyn, *J. Exp. Zool.*, 195, 359, 1975.

| OTHER NAMES | Ascorbase |
| --- | --- |

REACTION     2 L-Ascorbate + $O_2$ = 2 dehydroascorbate + $2H_2O$

ENZYME SOURCE  Bacteria, plants

## METHOD 1

### Visualization Scheme

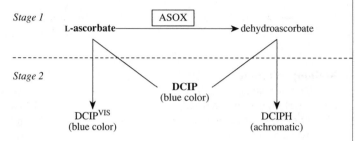

### Staining Solution[1]

A.  0.1 $M$ Tris–HCl buffer, pH 8.0 .............. 100 ml
    Ascorbic acid .............. 20 mg
B.  $H_2O$ .............. 10 ml
    2,6-Dichlorophenol indophenol (DCIP) .............. 2.5 mg

### Procedure

Incubate the gel in solution A at 30°C for 15 min. Discard solution A, blot the surface of the gel to remove excess liquid. Place a piece of filter paper saturated with solution B on top of the gel. Achromatic bands of ASOX activity develop on a blue background of the gel after 5 to 10 min. Bands are ephemeral and the zymogram should be recorded or photographed as soon as possible.

*Notes:*  The application of solution B as 1% agar overlay may prove preferable.

## METHOD 2

### Visualization Scheme

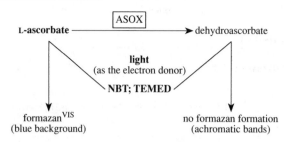

### Staining Solution[2]

A.  0.1 $M$ $H_2O_2$
B.  36 m$M$ Potassium phosphate buffer, pH 7.8
C.  2.45 m$M$ NBT
D.  36 m$M$ Potassium phosphate buffer, pH 7.8
    28 m$M$ $N,N,N',N'$-Tetramethylethylenediamine (TEMED)
    25 μM Ascorbate

### Procedure

After electrophoresis, place PAG (1.5 mm thick) in solution A for 20 min to inhibit superoxide dismutase activity and then wash five times (5 min each) with solution B. Afterwards soak gel in solution C for 30 min and in solution D for a further 30 min in the dark. Finally put gel at a 15 cm distance from a 250-W, HQ1-TS Osram lamp (at a luminous flux of 7.5 ± 0.8 mW cm$^{-2}$ min$^{-1}$ in the interval 400 to 700 nm) and keep the gel temperature at 10°C. After development of the blue color stop the reaction by washing the gel with deionized water. Achromatic ASOX bands are visible on a blue background. The stained gel may be stored in 50% ethanol.

*Notes:*  The method is based on the ability of a mixture of TEMED (or EDTA) and ascorbate (or riboflavin) to give a photoinduced reduction of NBT. The species directly responsible for NBT reduction is thought to be $O_2$. This species is absent in gel areas occupied by active ASOX.

### REFERENCES

1.  Vallejos, C. E., Enzyme activity staining, in *Isozymes in Plant Genetics and Breeding, Part A*, Tanskley, S. D. and Orton, T. J., Eds., Elsevier, Amsterdam, 1983, 469.
2.  Maccarrone, M., Rossi, A., D'Andrea, G., Amicosante, G., and Avigliano, L., Electrophoretic detection of ascorbate oxidase activity by photoreduction of nitroblue tetrazolium, *Anal. Biochem.*, 188, 101, 1990.

REACTION        $H_2O_2 + H_2O_2 = O_2 + 2H_2O$

ENZYME SOURCE   Bacteria, fungi, plants, protozoa, invertebrates, vertebrates

## METHOD 1

### Visualization Scheme

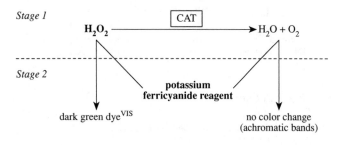

### Staining Solution[1]
A.  3% $H_2O_2$
B.  2% Potassium ferricyanide
C.  2% Ferric chloride

### Procedure
Incubate the gel in solution A for about 15 min. Pour off solution A, rinse gel with water and then immerse it in a 1:1 mixture of solutions B and C. Gently agitate the tray containing the gel for a few minutes. Yellow bands of CAT activity appear on a blue-green background. Wash stained gel in water. Record or photograph zymogram.

*Notes:*   Prepare solutions A, B, and C on the same day as used.

## METHOD 2

### Visualization Scheme

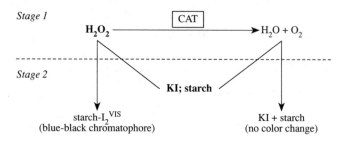

### Staining Solution[2]
A.  60 m$M$ Sodium thiosulfate ($Na_2S_2O_3$)       30 ml
B.  3% $H_2O_2$ (freshly prepared)                   70 ml
C.  90 m$M$ Potassium iodide (KI)                   100 ml
    Acetic acid (glacial)                            0.5 ml

### Procedure
Mix solutions A and B quickly just before use (this is essential). Immerse electrophorized starch gel in the mixture for 30 to 60 s and then place it into solution C. Agitate the staining tray gently. The gel turns a bluish-black color, except at the sites of the CAT activity, which remain achromatic. Record or photograph the zymogram immediately since the bands are ephemeral.

*Notes:*   This method was developed for starch gel but it can also be used with PAG prepared with 0.5% soluble starch.

The method is based on the starch–iodine reaction. Thiosulfate in the staining solution is inactivated by hydrogen peroxide except at the sites of CAT activity, where hydrogen peroxide is destroyed enzymatically. The iodide is oxidized by hydrogen peroxide to iodine, which forms a chromatophore with the starch, and sites of CAT localization remain achromatic. If any iodine diffuses into the achromatic areas, it will be reduced to iodide by thiosulfate, which remains active in these areas.

## METHOD 3

### Visualization Scheme

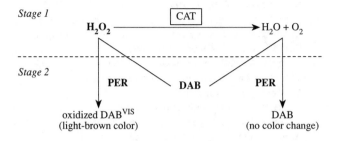

*Stage 1*

*Stage 2*

oxidized DAB$^{VIS}$
(light-brown color)

DAB
(no color change)

### Staining Solution[3]

A.  50 m*M* Potassium phosphate buffer, pH 7.0
    4 mg/ml 3,3′-Diaminobenzidine (DAB)
    10 U/ml Peroxidase (PER)
B.  50 m*M* Potassium phosphate buffer, pH 7.0
    20 m*M* $H_2O_2$

### Procedure

Immerse the gel in solution A and incubate in the dark at room temperature for 45 min to allow peroxidase and DAB to diffuse into the gel matrix. Rinse the gel with water and place in solution B. Hydrogen peroxide is destroyed by CAT prior to the DAB oxidation by peroxidase. As a result, achromatic CAT bands appear on a brown background. Record or photograph zymogram.

*Notes:*   The developed gel may be counterstained with $Cu(NO_3)_2$ solution to obtain a zymogram with achromatic CAT bands on a grey-black background.

DAB is a potential carcinogen. The use of an alternative chromagen (3-amino-9-ethyl-carbazole) is preferable (see 1.11.1.7 — PER).

## OTHER METHODS

A.  The method of simultaneous negative staining of CAT bands and positive staining of peroxidase bands based on modified starch–iodine reaction is also available.[4] This method is applicable to starch gel or PAG prepared with 0.5% soluble starch.
B.  The immunoblotting procedure (for details see Part II) based on the utility of monoclonal antibodies specific to the yeast enzyme[5] can also be used for immunohistochemical visualization of the enzyme protein on electrophoretic gels. This procedure is expensive and unsuitable for routine laboratory use. Monoclonal antibodies, however, may be of great value in special (biochemical, immunochemical, phylogenetic, and genetic) analyses of CAT.

## REFERENCES

1.  Harris, H. and Hopkinson, D. A., *Handbook of Enzyme Electrophoresis in Human Genetics*, North-Holland, Amsterdam (Loose leaf with supplements in 1977 and 1978), 1976.
2.  Thorup, O. A., Strole, W. B., and Leavell, B. S., A method for the localization of catalase on starch gels, *J. Lab. Clin. Med.*, 58, 122, 1961.
3.  Gregory, E. M. and Fridovich, I., Visualization of catalase on acrylamide gels, *Anal. Biochem.*, 58, 57, 1974.
4.  Siciliano, M. J. and Shaw, C. R., Separation and visualization of enzymes on gels, in *Chromatographic and Electrophoretic Techniques, Vol. 2, Zone Electrophoresis*, Smith, I., Ed., Heinemann, London, 1976, 185.
5.  Adolf, G. R., Hartter, E., Ruis, H., and Swetly, P., Monoclonal antibodies to yeast catalase-T, *Biochem. Biophys. Res. Commun.*, 95, 350, 1980.

REACTION         Donor + $H_2O_2$ = oxidized donor + $2H_2O$

ENZYME SOURCE   Bacteria, fungi, plants, invertebrates, verte-
                brates

## METHOD

### Visualization Scheme

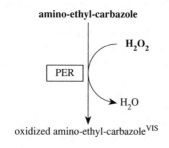

**amino-ethyl-carbazole**

PER

$H_2O_2$

$H_2O$

oxidized amino-ethyl-carbazole[VIS]

### Staining Solution[1]

| | |
|---|---|
| 50 m$M$ Sodium acetate buffer, pH 5.0 | 100 ml |
| 3-Amino-9-ethyl-carbazole (dissolved in a few drops of acetone) | 50 mg |
| 3% $H_2O_2$ (freshly prepared) | 0.75 ml |

### Procedure

Incubate the gel in staining solution in the dark at room temperature or at 4°C until red-brown bands appear. Wash gel in water and
fix in 50% glycerol.

*Notes:*   The use of higher pH of the stain buffer may give faint bands only.[2]
For example, human salivary peroxidase is poorly stained in PAG prepared
in the usual manner with tris–borate buffer, pH 8.6, while good results are
obtained when acidic PAG (polymerized using ferrous sulfate, ascorbic acid,
and hydrogen peroxide) is used.[3]

Many other chromogenic substrates can be used instead of amino-ethyl-
carbazole: *o*-dianisidine dihydrochloride, benzidine dihydrochloride,
diaminobenzidine, tetramethylbenzidine, 3,5-dichloro-2-hydroxybenzene
sulfonate, *o*-tolidine, *p*-phenylenediamine (in couple with catechol),
*p*-hydroxybenzene sulfonate (in couple with 4-aminoantipyrine), *N*-ethyl-*N*-
(3-sulfopropyl)-*m*-anisidine (in couple with 4-aminoantipyrine), guaiacol,
and some others. All of them except guaiacol are carcinogens or possible
carcinogens. Extreme caution should be used when handling these reagents.
Amino-ethyl-carbazole is probably less hazardous, but it also should be
treated with caution.

Eugenol is used as a fluorogenic peroxidase substrate. The product of
the peroxidase reaction, bieugenol, fluoresceces in short-wave UV light.
Using this substrate the bands of PER activity can also be observed in
daylight as areas of bieugenol precipitation.[4] Homovanillic acid is also a very
useful and sensitive fluorogenic substrate for PER (see 1.8.3.1 — SUOX).

Peroxidase conjugated to specific monoclonal antibodies is used as a
coupled enzyme for immunohistochemical visualization of proteins on electrophoretic gels via the immunoblotting technique (for details see Part II).

## REFERENCES

1. Graham, R. C., Lundholm, U., and Karnovsky, M. J., Cytochemi-
cal demonstration of peroxidase activity with 3-amino-9-
ethylcarbazole, *J. Histochem. Cytochem.*, 13, 150, 1964.
2. Vallejos, C. E., Enzyme activity staining, in *Isozymes in Plant
Genetics and Breeding, Part A*, Tanskley, S. D. and Orton, T. J.,
Eds., Elsevier, Amsterdam, 1983, 469.
3. Azen, E. A., Salivary peroxidase (SAPX): genetic modification
and relationship to the proline-rich ($P_r$) and acidic ($P_a$) proteins,
*Biochem. Genet.*, 15, 9, 1977.
4. Liu, E. H., Substrate specificities of plant peroxidase isozymes, in
*Isozymes, Vol. 2, Physiological Function*, Markert, C. L., Ed.,
Academic Press, New York, 1975, 837.

REACTION          2 Glutathione + $H_2O_2$ = oxidized glutathione + $2H_2O$

ENZYME SOURCE  Vertebrates

## METHOD

### Visualization Scheme

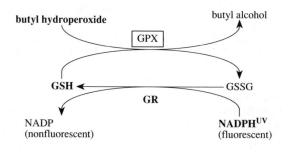

### Staining Solution[1]

| | |
|---|---:|
| 0.1 $M$ Potassium phosphate buffer, pH 7.0 | 10 ml |
| Reduced glutathione (GSH) | 30 mg |
| Glutathione reductase (GR) | 12 units |
| 5.4 m$M$ EDTA (pH 7.0) | 2 ml |
| NADPH | 15 mg |
| $t$-Butyl hydroperoxide (add just before use) | 50 µl |

### Procedure

Apply the staining solution to the gel surface on filter-paper overlay. Incubate the gel at 37°C for 10 to 30 min. Remove filter-paper and view gel under long-wave UV light. Dark (nonfluorescent) bands of GPX are visible on the light (fluorescent) background of the gel. Record the zymogram or photograph using a yellow filter.

*Notes:*  Mammalian erythrocyte GPX displays activity at the pH optimum of 8.8, about 10 times that at pH 7.0.

### REFERENCE

1. Wijnen, L. M. M., Monteba-van Heuvel, M., Pearson, P. L., and Meera Khan, P., Assignment of a gene for glutathione peroxidase (GPX 1) to human chromosome 3, *Cytogenet. Cell Genet.*, 22, 223, 1978.

OTHER NAMES    Lipoxidase, carotene oxidase

REACTION    Linoleate + $O_2$ = 13-hydroperoxy-octadeca-9,11-dienoate

ENZYME SOURCE  Plants

## METHOD 1

### Visualization Scheme

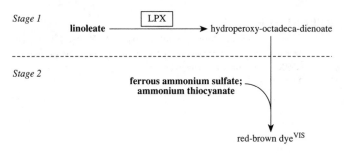

### Staining Solution[1]
  A.  0.2 *M* Phosphate buffer, pH 6.5
      0.25% Tween-20
      7.5 m*M* Linoleic acid
  B.  5% Ferrous ammonium sulfate
      3% HCl
  C.  20% Ammonium thiocyanate

### Procedure
Prepare suspension A by sonication for 5 min at 0°C. Immediately before using, oxygenate the substrate suspension for 20 to 30 min at room temperature. Incubate the gel in suspension A for 20 to 50 min. Rinse gel with distilled water, immerse in solution B for 30 s, and then in solution C also for 30 s. Areas of LPX activity develop as red-brown bands. Rinse stained gel with water. Record the zymogram or photograph because the color development continues upon storage.

*Notes:*  Substantial background staining makes detection of LPX in low-activity samples difficult.

## METHOD 2

### Visualization Scheme

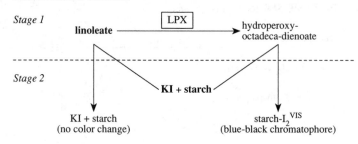

### Staining Solution[2]
  A.  Linoleic acid           500 mg
      $H_2O$                50 ml
      Tween-80          1 drop
  B.  0.05 *M* Tris–HCl buffer, pH 8.3
  C.  15% Acetic acid
  D.  Saturated solution of KI in water

### Procedure
Prepare stock substrate solution A by dispersing 0.5 g of linoleic acid in 25 ml of freshly deionized $H_2O$ with the aid of a drop of Tween-80 and sonication under a stream of nitrogen. Make total volume to 50 ml with water. Store this stock solution at 2 to 5°C in the dark under nitrogen (prepare fresh stock solution weekly). Incubate the gel (see *Notes*) for 30 min at room temperature in freshly prepared 20-fold dilution of the stock substrate solution A in buffer B with agitation of the gel to ensure aeration. During the period of incubation of the gel prepare C+D mixture: 100 ml of solution C purged with nitrogen and then, also under nitrogen, mix with 5 ml of solution D. After 30 min of incubation in substrate solution, rinse the gel and gel tray with water, fill the tray completely with C+D mixture and cover so it is airtight to prevent autooxidation of iodine into iodide and to avoid excessive background staining of the gel. Zones of LPX activity become visible as dark brown to blue bands in about 5 min and reach maximum intensity in 15 to 20 min. Record the zymogram or photograph because the color development continues upon storage.

*Notes:*  The method is applicable to starch gel or PAG containing 0.5% soluble starch. Substantial background staining makes detection of low-activity samples difficult. The high percentage of failure in the stain development with this method is due possibly to a high threshold requirement for hydroperoxide to release iodine in the gel.

## METHOD 3

### Visualization Scheme

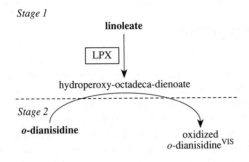

*Stage 1*

**linoleate**

LPX

hydroperoxy-octadeca-dienoate

- - - - - - - - - - - - - - - - - - - - - - -

*Stage 2*

**o-dianisidine**

oxidized
*o*-dianisidine$^{VIS}$

### Staining Solution[3]
A. Linoleic acid           0.62 ml
    H$_2$O                  50 ml
    Triton X-100       2 drops
B. 0.1 *M* Tris–HCl buffer, pH 8.6
C. 0.1 *M* Citrate–phosphate buffer, pH 5.8
D. 0.1% *o*-Dianisidine dihydrochloride

### Procedure
Prepare stock substrate solution A by dispersing linoleic acid in water containing Triton X-100 with a sonifier for 5 min at 0°C. Dilute this solution with water to give a stock solution of 20 m*M* linoleic acid. Then prepare the working substrate solution by dilution of the stock solution to 2 m*M* either with B or C buffers. Immediately before use, oxygenate working substrate solution for 20 to 30 min at room temperature. Rinse the gel with distilled water and place in working substrate solution. Incubate the gel at room temperature for 30 min. Rinse the gel with distilled water and immerse in solution D. Stain gel overnight at room temperature. Red-brown bands appear on the gel with practically no background staining. Wash the dye off and store stained gel in water.

*Notes:* The stained gel may be stored in water at 4°C for as long as 18 months without color deterioration.

Heme proteins also oxidize linoleic acid and produce the hydroperoxide. Lipoxygenase is a far more powerful catalyst than heme proteins. Nevertheless, 1 m*M* sodium cyanide is usually included in the working substrate solution to inhibit any contribution of heme proteins to the formation of hydroperoxide.

When PAG prepared in the usual manner is stained by this method, dark bands usually also appear in the anodal end of the gel due to oxidation of *o*-dianisidine by ammonium persulfate.

### REFERENCES
1. Grossman, S., Pinsky, A., and Goldwetz, Z., A convenient method for lipoxygenase isoenzyme determination, *Anal. Biochem.*, 44, 642, 1971.
2. Hart, G. E. and Langston, P. J., Chromosomal location and evolution of isozyme structural genes in hexaploid wheat, *Heredity*, 39, 263, 1977.
3. De Lumen, B. O. and Kazeniac, S. J., Staining for lipoxygenase activity in electrophoretic gels, *Anal. Biochem.*, 72, 428, 1976.

## 1.15.1.1 — Superoxide Dismutase; SOD

OTHER NAMES      Tetrazolium oxidase, indophenol oxidase (misleading name)

REACTION      $O_2^{\cdot-} + O_2^{\cdot-} + 2H^+ = O_2 + H_2O_2$

ENZYME SOURCE    Bacteria, fungi, plants, protozoa, invertebrates, vertebrates

## METHOD

### Visualization Scheme

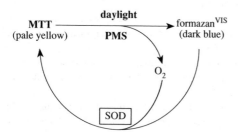

### Staining Solution[1]

| | |
|---|---|
| 50 m$M$ Tris–HCl buffer, pH 8.5 | 80 ml |
| MTT | 10 mg |
| PMS | 6 mg |
| MgCl$_2$·6H$_2$O | 15 mg |

### Procedure

Incubate the gel in staining solution in daylight. The enzyme bands are seen as pale zones on a dark blue background.

*Notes:*   When SOD activity is low, the amount of PMS should be diminished three times.

NBT may be used instead of MTT.

It is often not necessary to stain specifically for SOD, as its bands may appear on any gels stained by means of MTT(NBT)/PMS linked reactions.

## OTHER METHODS

A. Francke and Taggart[2] obtained negative SOD zymograms using a modification of the method developed by Weisiger and Fridovich.[3] The gel was incubated in two changes of 50 m$M$ phosphate buffer (pH 7.8) for a total of 10 min, then in 1 mg/ml NBT solution for 10 min, and finally in 50 m$M$ phosphate buffer (pH 7.8) containing 0.01 mg/ml riboflavin and 3.25 mg/ml $N,N,N',N'$-tetramethylethylenediamine for 10 min at 24°C with gentle agitation. Areas of SOD activity remained clear after exposure of the gel to fluorescent light (see also 1.10.3.3 — ASOX, Method 2).

B. Positively stained bands of SOD can be developed using the method proposed by Misra and Fridovich.[4] According to this method, the gel is incubated in a staining solution containing 10 m$M$ potassium phosphate buffer (pH 7.2), 2 m$M$ o-dianisidine, and 0.1 m$M$ riboflavin at room temperature in the dark for 1 h. Then the gel is rinsed in water and exposed to the light. Brown bands of SOD activity appear after 1 min. Intensity of the bands increases during the next 10 to 15 min of lighting the gel. Presumably, under these conditions of staining, sufficient amounts of superoxide radical are generated to allow the SOD to catalyze the oxidation of o-dianisidine. The use of amino-ethyl-carbasole

instead of o-dianisidine is recommended because o-dianisidine is known to be a carcinogen. The bands of peroxidase can also develop on SOD zymograms obtained by this method, but they only begin to develop when the SOD bands are well stained.

## GENERAL NOTES

Two phylogenetically independent isozymes of SOD are known for eukaryotes. Cytoplasmic isozyme contains both copper and zinc, while mitochondrial isozyme contains manganese. Prokaryotic enzyme contains manganese or iron. Cytoplasmic and mitochondrial isozymes of eukaryotic SOD can be distinguished using the inhibitory effect of 2% SDS on mitochondrial isozyme,[5] or using differences of isozymes in their subunit structure (cytoplasmic SOD is a dimer while mitochondrial SOD is a tetramer).

## REFERENCES

1. Brewer, G. J., Achromatic regions of tetrazolium stained starch gels: inherited electrophoretic variation, *Am. J. Hum. Genet.*, 19, 674, 1967.
2. Francke, U. and Taggart, R. T., Assignment of the gene for cytoplasmic superoxide dismutase (*Sod-1*) to a region of chromosome 16 and of *Hprt* to a region of the X-chromosome in the mouse, *Proc. Natl. Acad. Sci. U.S.A.*, 76, 5230, 1979.
3. Weisiger, R. A. and Fridovich, I., Superoxide dismutase: organelle specificity, *J. Biol. Chem.*, 248, 3582, 1973.
4. Misra, H. P. and Fridovich, I., Superoxide dismutase and peroxidase: a positive activity stain applicable of polyacrylamide gel electropherograms, *Arch. Biochem. Biophys.*, 183, 511, 1977.
5. Geller, B. L. and Winge, D. R., A method for distinguishing Cu-, Zn-, and Mn-containing superoxide dismutases, *Anal. Biochem.*, 128, 86, 1983.

OTHER NAMES     Ferroxidase (recommended name)

REACTION        $4Fe(II) + 4H^+ + O_2 = 4Fe(III) + 2H_2O$

ENZYME SOURCE   Mammals (serum)

## METHOD

### Visualization Scheme

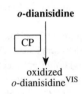

**o-dianisidine**

CP

oxidized
o-dianisidine[VIS]

### Staining Solution[1]

| | |
|---|---|
| 40 m$M$ Acetate buffer, pH 5.5 | 100 ml |
| o-Dianisidine (dissolved in minimal volume of ethanol) | 100 mg |

### Procedure

Incubate the gel in staining solution at 37°C until brown bands appear. Wash gel in water and fix in 50% glycerol.

*Notes:*   o-Dianisidine is used as an electron acceptor in place of oxygen, and $Fe^{2+}$ ions are tightly bound by the enzyme protein molecules.

The method is specific for mammalian serum. When other mammalian tissues or other organisms are used for sample preparation, nonspecific staining of some oxidases can also occur.

The use of o-dianisidine dihydrochloride instead of o-dianisidine free base is preferable in all instances.

The use of p-phenylenediamine instead of o-dianisidine is preferable when electrophoresis is carried out in PAG.

It should be remembered that both o-dianisidine and p-phenylenediamine are strong carcinogens.

### REFERENCE

1. Brewer, G. J., *An Introduction to Isozyme Techniques*, Academic Press, New York, 1970, 133.

Some NAD(P)-dependent dehydrogenases have the interesting property of showing stained bands in the absence of substrate in a staining solution, leading to the term "nothing dehydrogenase" (NDH).

The NDH phenomenon is wide-spread among living organisms, including bacteria, fungi, plants, protozoa, invertebrate and vertebrate animals, and man. Several different causes of this phenomenon are known.

The NDH effect may originate as a result of the binding of endogenous substrates by NAD(P)-dependent dehydrogenase molecules.[1-4]

Another cause of the NDH effect is the contamination of some commercial preparations (e.g., acrylamide, NAD, phosphosugars) with ethanol.[4,5]

In some cases, the NDH effect may be caused by the reducing action of –SH groups present in specific proteins.[6,7] In a strict sense, this cannot be attributed to the NDH phenomenon because free –SH groups are able to reduce a tetrazolium salt in alkaline medium even in the absence of NAD and PMS. Artefact bands also can develop in MTT(NBT)/PMS-containing solutions as the result of direct chemical reaction of PMS in zones of high local pH of electrophoretic gels.[5]

Finally, the detection mechanism used may not be specific for the intended enzyme and can allow the simultaneous development of bands of other enzymes. For example, a gel stained for aldehyde dehydrogenase (see 1.2.1.3 — ALDH) can also exhibit aldehyde oxidase (1.2.3.1 — AOX), xanthine oxidase (1.1.3.22 — XOX), and alcohol dehydrogenase 1.1.1.1 — ADH) activities as well as other stained bands.[8] Lactate dehydrogenase (1.1.1.27 — LDH) and glycerol-3-phosphate dehydrogenase (1.1.1.8 — G-3-PD) bands can develop on triose-phosphate isomerase zymograms (see 5.3.1.1 — TPI, Method 2).

Overlapping substrate specificity of some enzymes can also cause the appearance of additional bands on the zymograms of certain NAD-dependent dehydrogenases. It is shown, for example, that *Drosophila* alcohol dehydrogenase is capable of catalyzing the reaction of lactate oxidation[9] and chicken lactate dehydrogenase is capable of reducing oxaloacetate in the presence of NADH, i.e., to catalyze the reverse reaction of malate dehydrogenase.[10]

Fortunately, many of the stain artifacts listed above usually occur repetitively on gels stained for different enzymes. Thus, it is very important to compare zymograms obtained using similar detection mechanisms to ensure that the same bands are not being scored for supposedly different enzymes.

The observation of data presented in numerous experimental works evidences that nonspecific staining of lactate dehydrogenase and alcohol dehydrogenase in animals (especially in vertebrates), and alcohol dehydrogenase and glutamate dehydrogenase in plants is the most frequent reason for the "nothing dehydrogenase" phenomenon.

**REFERENCES**

1. Ressler, N. and Stitzer, K., Starch-gel investigations of the relationships between dehydrogenase proteins, *Biochim. Biophys. Acta*, 146, 1, 1967.

2. Falkenberg, F., Lehmann, F.-G., and Pfleiderer, G., LDH (lactate dehydrogenase) isozymes as cause of nonspecific tetrazolium salt staining in gel enzymograms. ("Nothing dehydrogenase"), *Clin. Chim. Acta*, 23, 265, 1969.

3. White, H. A., Coulson, C. J., Kemp, C. M., and Rabin, B. R., The presence of lactic acid in purified lactate dehydrogenase, *FEBS Lett.*, 34, 155, 1973.

4. Marshall, J. H., Bridge, P. D., and May, J. W., Source and avoidance of the "nothing dehydrogenase" effect, a spurious band produced during polyacrylamide gel electrophoresis of dehydrogenase enzymes from yeasts, *Anal. Biochem.*, 139, 359, 1984.

5. Wood, T. and Muzariri, C. C., The electrophoresis and detection of transketolase, *Anal. Biochem.*, 118, 221, 1981.

6. Somer, H., "Nothing dehydrogenase" reaction as an artefact in serum isoenzyme analyses, *Clin. Chim. Acta*, 60, 223, 1975.

7. Sri Venugopal, K. S. and Adiga, P. R., Artifactual staining of proteins on polyacrylamide gels by nitro blue tetrazolium chloride and phenazine methosulfate, *Anal. Biochem.*, 101, 215, 1980.

8. Holmes, R. S., Electrophoretic analyses of alcohol dehydrogenase, aldehyde dehydrogenase, aldehyde oxidase, sorbitol dehydrogenase, and xanthine oxidase from mouse tissues, *Comp. Biochem. Physiol.*, 61B, 339, 1978.

9. Onoufriou, A. and Alahiotis, S. N., Enzyme specificity: "pseudopolymorphism" of lactate dehydrogenase in *Drosophila melanogaster*, *Biochem. Genet.*, 19, 277, 1981.

10. Busquets, M., Baro, J., Cortes, A., and Bosal, J., Separation and properties of the two forms of chicken liver (*Gallus domesticus*) cytoplasmic malate dehydrogenase, *Int. J. Biochem.*, 10, 823, 1979.

OTHER NAMES    Catechol-*O*-methyltransferase

REACTION    *S*-Adenosyl-L-methionine + catechol =
*S*-adenosyl-L-homocysteine + guaiacol

ENZYME SOURCE   Vertebrates

## METHOD

### Visualization Scheme

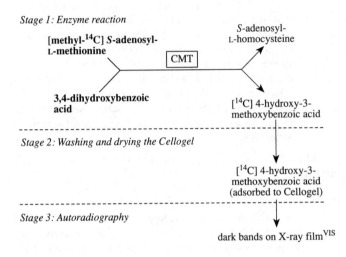

*Stage 1: Enzyme reaction*

[methyl-$^{14}$C] *S*-adenosyl-L-methionine

CMT

*S*-adenosyl-L-homocysteine

3,4-dihydroxybenzoic acid

[$^{14}$C] 4-hydroxy-3-methoxybenzoic acid

*Stage 2: Washing and drying the Cellogel*

[$^{14}$C] 4-hydroxy-3-methoxybenzoic acid
(adsorbed to Cellogel)

*Stage 3: Autoradiography*

dark bands on X-ray film[VIS]

### Reaction Mixture[1]

0.1 *M* Tris–HCl buffer, pH 8.0
1 m*M* MgCl$_2$
0.5 m*M* Dithiothreitol
1 m*M* 3,4-Dihydroxybenzoic acid
0.028 m*M* [methyl-$^{14}$C] *S*-Adenosyl-L-methionine
 (60 mCi/mmol; Amersham)

## Procedure

*Stage 1.* Soak the electrophorized Cellogel strip in the reaction mixture and incubate in a moist chamber at 37°C for 2 h.
*Stage 2.* Wash the strip in 2 l of 0.02 *N* HCl for 4 min and dry in an oven at 60°C for about 2 h.
*Stage 3.* Put dry strip directly in tight contact with a medical X-ray film Kodak-X-OMAT G and expose for 8 d at room temperature or 4°C. Develop exposed X-ray film by a Kodak X-OMAT processor ME-1.

Zones of enzyme activity appear as dark bands on the X-ray film.

*Notes:*   The method is developed for cellulose acetate gel. The soluble molecules of the unreacted [$^{14}$C]*S*-adenosyl-L-methionine can be easily removed from the gel matrix by soaking the gel in water, while the relatively insoluble radioactive product remains adsorbed to the gel at sites of enzyme location.

The addition of adenosine deaminase to the reaction mixture does not improve the final result though this enzyme is known to decrease the inhibitory effect of the product *S*-adenosyl-L-homocysteine on CMT.

The mammalian enzyme acts more rapidly on catecholamines (such as adrenaline or noradrenaline) than on catechols.

## REFERENCE

1. Brahe, C., Crosti, N., Meera Khan, P., and Serra, A., Catechol-*o*-methyltransferase: a method for autoradiographic visualization of isozymes in Cellogel, *Biochem. Genet.*, 22, 125, 1984.

| | |
|---|---|
| OTHER NAMES | DNA-methyltransferase |
| REACTION | S-Adenosyl-L-methionine + DNA = S-adenosyl-L-homocysteine + DNA containing 5-methylcytosine (and 6-methylaminopurine) |
| ENZYME SOURCE | Bacteria, vertebrates |

## METHOD

### Visualization Scheme

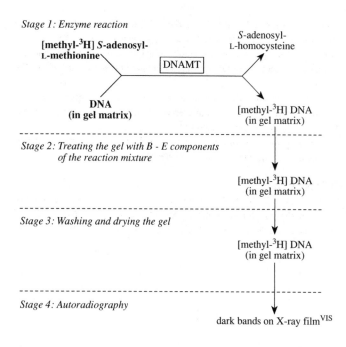

*Stage 1: Enzyme reaction*

*Stage 2: Treating the gel with B - E components of the reaction mixture*

*Stage 3: Washing and drying the gel*

*Stage 4: Autoradiography*

dark bands on X-ray film$^{VIS}$

### Reaction Mixture[1]

A. 25 mM Tris–HCl buffer, pH 7.5
   10 µl/ml [methyl-$^3$H] S-Adenosyl-L-methionine (1 mCi/ml)
   20 mM EDTA
   1 µM S-Adenosyl-L-methionine
B. 1 mg/ml Proteinase K (Boehringer)
   1% Sodium dodecyl sulfate (SDS)
C. 5% Trichloroacetic acid
   1% Sodium pyrophosphate
D. 100% Acetic acid
E. 20% 2,5-Diphenyloxazole (dissolved in 100% acetic acid)

## Procedure

Rinse electrophorized PAG containing 0.1% SDS and 66 mg/ml DNA (mol wt >5·10⁶) with water and then wash twice for 15 min in renaturing solution: 50 mM tris–HCl (pH 7.5), 10 mM EDTA, 10 mM 2-mercaptoethanol. Place the gel in renaturing solution at 0°C and wash with gentle shaking for 12 h. During this period change renaturing solution three times.

*Stage 1.* After renaturing, incubate the gel in solution A at 37°C for 16 h with gentle shaking.

*Stage 2.* Remove the gel from solution A and place in solution B for 2 h at 37°C (this treatment of the gel is carried out for proteolytic inactivation of nucleases). Then place the gel in solution C and wash for 12 h. During the washing change solution C three times. Finally, put the gel in solution D for 30 min and then in solution E also for 30 min.

*Stage 3.* Wash the gel 1 h in warm water, place it on a sheet of Whatman 3 MM chromatographic paper and dry.

*Stage 4.* Put dry gel in tight contact with medical X-ray film and expose for an appropriate period of time. Develop exposed X-ray film.

The enzyme activity zones appear as dark bands on the developed film.

### REFERENCE

1. Hübscher, U., Pedrali-Noy, G., Knust-Kron, B., Doerfler, W., and Spadari, S., DNA methyltransferases: acting minigel analysis and determination with DNA covalently bound to a solid matrix, *Anal. Biochem.*, 150, 442, 1985.

OTHER NAMES   Carbamylaspartotranskinase, aspartate trans-carbamylase

REACTION   Carbamoyl phosphate + L-aspartate = orthophosphate + N-carbamoyl-L-aspartate

ENZYME SOURCE  Bacteria, fungi, plants, vertebrates

## METHOD

### Visualization Scheme

*Stage 1*

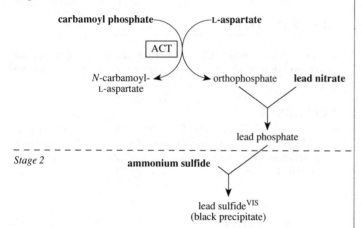

*Stage 2*

### Staining Solution[1]

A.  0.5 $M$ Tris–HCl buffer, pH 7.0     95 ml
    Carbamoyl phosphate (Li$_2$ salt)     50 mg
    L-Aspartic acid (Na salt)     100 mg
    2% Lead nitrate (aqueous solution)     5 ml
B.  1% Ammonium sulfide

### Procedure

Incubate electrophorized gel in freshly prepared filtered solution A for 10 to 20 min at room temperature. Discard solution A, rinse the gel in water and immerse it in solution B, wash the gel again with water. The black zones indicate ACT activity.

## OTHER METHODS

Three other methods for detection of the product orthophosphate may also be used:

A.  A method that involves the formation of white calcium phosphate precipitate (e.g., see 3.1.3.2 — ACP, Method 5). This method is applicable only for clean gels (e.g., PAG).
B.  A method that depends on the generation of blue phosphomolybdic acid (e.g., see 3.6.1.1 — PP, Method 1).
C.  A method that involves the formation of blue formazan as a result of two coupled reactions catalyzed by the auxiliary enzymes purine-nucleoside phosphorylase and xanthine oxidase (e.g., see 3.1.3.1 — ALP, Method 8).

## GENERAL NOTES

The enzymatic method (C) is preferable due to its sensitivity and generation of a nondiffusible formazan as a result of a one-step procedure.

### REFERENCE

1.  Shanley, M. S., Foltermann, K. F., O'Donovan, G. A., and Wild, J. R., Properties of hybrid aspartate transcarbamoylase formed with native subunits from divergent bacteria, *J. Biol. Chem.*, 259, 12672, 1984.

OTHER NAMES    Citrulline phosphorylase, ornithine trans-carbamylase

REACTION    Carbamoyl phosphate + L-ornithine = ortho-phosphate + L-citrulline

ENZYME SOURCE  Bacteria, plants, vertebrates

## METHOD

### Visualization Scheme

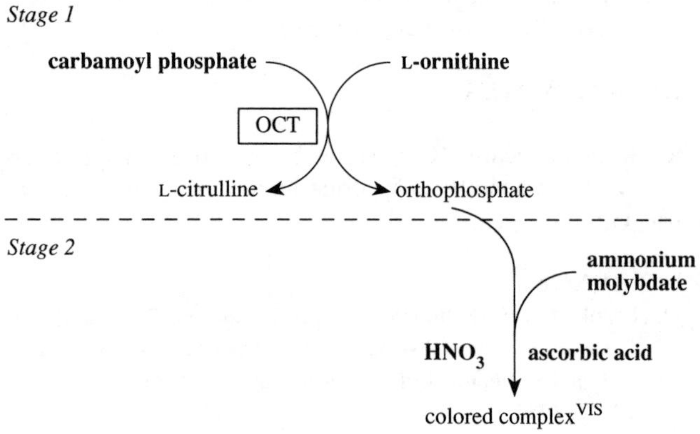

*Stage 1*

carbamoyl phosphate —    L-ornithine

OCT

L-citrulline    orthophosphate

- - - - - - - - - - - - - - - - - - - - - - - - -

*Stage 2*

ammonium molybdate

$HNO_3$   ascorbic acid

colored complex[VIS]

### Staining Solution[1]

A. 0.27 $M$ Triethanolamine buffer, pH 7.5
   5 m$M$ L-Ornithine
   15 m$M$ Carbamoyl phosphate
B. 20 m$M$ Ammonium molybdate
   0.5% Nitric acid
C. 10% Ascorbic acid

### Procedure

Incubate electrophorized gel in solution A at 37°C for 10 min. Rinse gel in distilled water and place in solution B for 5 min. Rinse gel again in water and immerse in solution C. Blue bands of OCT activity appear after a few minutes. Record the zymogram or photograph because the stained bands diffuse rapidly.

## OTHER METHODS

Three other methods for detection of the product orthophosphate may also be used:

A. A method that involves the formation of black lead sulfide (e.g., see 2.1.3.2 — ACT).
B. A method that involves the formation of white calcium phosphate precipitate (e.g., see 3.1.3.2 — ACP, Method 5) visible in clean gels.
C. A method that involves the formation of blue formazan as a result of two coupled reactions catalyzed by auxiliary enzymes purine-nucleoside phosphorylase and xanthine oxidase (e.g., see 3.1.3.1 — ALP, Method 8).

## GENERAL NOTES

The enzymatic method (C) is preferable due to its sensitivity and generation of a nondiffusible formazan as the result of a one-step procedure.

## REFERENCE

1. Farkas, D. H., Skombra, C. J., Anderson., G. R., and Hughes, R. G., Jr., *In situ* staining procedure for the detection of ornithine transcarbamylase activity in polyacrylamide gels, *Anal. Biochem.*, 160, 421, 1987.

OTHER NAMES    Glycolaldehyde-transferase

REACTION    Sedoheptulose 7-phosphate + D-glyceraldehyde 3-phosphate = D-ribose 5-phosphate + D-xylulose 5-phosphate

ENZYME SOURCE    Bacteria, fungi, plants, vertebrates

## METHOD 1

### Visualization Scheme

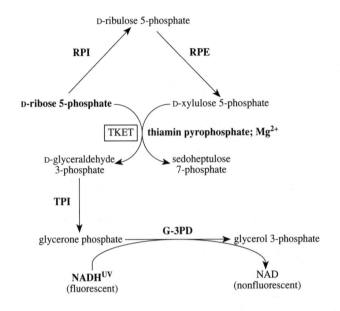

### Staining Solution[1]

| | |
|---|---|
| 0.1 $M$ Glycyl-glycine buffer, pH 7.4 | 10 ml |
| Ribose 5-phosphate (Na$_2$ salt) | 5 mg |
| Thiamin pyrophosphate | 1 mg |
| 1 $M$ MgCl$_2$ | 0.2 ml |
| NADH | 4 mg |
| Ribose-5-phosphate isomerase (RPI) | 50 units |
| Ribulose-phosphate 3-epimerase (RPE) | 5 units |
| Glycerol-3-phosphate dehydrogenase (G-3PD) | 40 µl |
| and triosephosphate isomerase (TPI) | |
| mixture (Sigma) | |

### Procedure

Apply the staining solution to gel on filter-paper overlay. Incubate the gel at 37°C for 1 to 2 h and view under long-wave UV light. Dark (nonfluorescent) bands of TKET activity are visible on a light (fluorescent) background. Record the zymogram or photograph using a yellow filter.

*Notes:* When a zymogram that is visible in daylight is required, counterstain the processed gel with MTT/PMS solution. White bands of TKET appear on a blue background almost immediately. Wash stained gel in water and fix in 50% ethanol.

When D-xylulose 5-phosphate is available it may be included in the staining solution instead of ribose-5-phosphate isomerase and ribulose-phosphate 3-epimerase preparations.

## METHOD 2

### Visualization Scheme

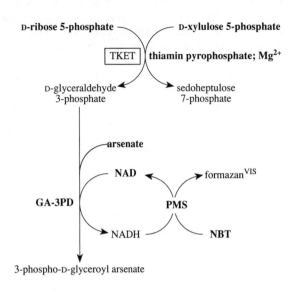

### Staining Solution[2]

A. 100 m$M$ Glycyl–glycine buffer, pH 7.4
     0.4 m$M$ D-Xylulose 5-phosphate
     4 m$M$ D-Ribose 5-phosphate
     0.5 m$M$ NAD
     0.16 m$M$ Sodium arsenate
     0.76 m$M$ EDTA
     5 m$M$ MgCl$_2$
     0.6 m$M$ Thiamin pyrophosphate
     0.4 m$M$ NBT
     0.1 m$M$ PMS
     24 U/ml Glyceraldehyde-3-phosphate dehydrogenase
       (GA-3PD)
B. 1% Agarose solution (60°C)

### Procedure

Mix equal volumes of A and B components of the stain to prepare 0.5% indicator agarose solution. Pour the mixture over the surface of the gel. After agarose solidification incubate the gel with indicator agarose plate at 37°C in the dark until blue bands appear. Fix stained indicator agarose plate in 50% ethanol.

*Notes:* This method was developed for detection of TKET after electrophoresis in 7.5% PAG. However, there are no obvious restrictions for application of the method for starch or acetate cellulose gels. When 7.5% PAG is used for TKET electrophoresis, the use of 9% indicator starch gel in place of 0.5% indicator agarose gel results in faster development of TKET activity bands. In both cases colored bands appear in indicator gels, because the auxiliary glyceraldehyde-3-phosphate dehydrogenase is unable to penetrate the 7.5% PAG, and the staining of an indicator gel is due to TKET diffusion out of 7.5% PAG. The use of 5.5% PAG for TKET electrophoresis does not aid in the detection of TKET activity but markedly impairs the resolution of TKET bands.

To prevent possible nonspecific development of alcohol dehydrogenase activity bands, the phosphosugars, NAD, NBT, and PMS should be prepared alcohol-free by lyophilization.

## GENERAL NOTES

Transketolase/D-glyceraldehyde-3-phosphate dehydrogenase complexes are known to exist in yeasts and mammalian erythrocytes. This information should be taken into account during interpretation of multiple TKET bands detected after electrophoresis of the enzyme preparations obtained from these organisms.

## REFERENCES

1. Anderson, J. E., Teng, Y.-S. and Giblett, E. R., Stains for six enzymes potentially applicable to chromosomal assignment by cell hybridization, *Cytogenet. Cell Genet.*, 14, 465, 1975.
2. Wood, T. and Muzarriri, C. C., The electrophoresis and detection of transketolase, *Anal. Biochem.* 118, 221, 1981.

OTHER NAMES    Dihydroxyacetone transferase, glycerone transferase

REACTION    Sedoheptulose 7-phosphate + D-glyceraldehyde 3-phosphate = D-erythrose 4-phosphate + D-fructose 6-phosphate

ENZYME SOURCE    Fungi, plants, vertebrates

## METHOD 1

### Visualization Scheme

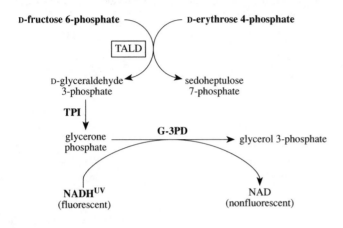

### Staining Solution[1]

| | |
|---|---|
| 40 mM Tris–citrate buffer, pH 7.6 | 5 ml |
| D-Fructose 6-phosphate | 6.6 mg |
| D-Erythrose 4-phosphate | 3.3 mg |
| NADH | 4 mg |
| Glycerol-3-phosphate dehydrogenase (G-3PD) and triosephosphate isomerase (TPI) mixture (Sigma) | 40 µl |

### Procedure

Apply the staining solution to the gel on filter-paper overlay. Incubate the gel with application in a moist chamber at 37°C for 1 to 2 h and view under long-wave UV light. Dark (nonfluorescent) bands of TALD are visible on a light (fluorescent) background. Record the zymogram or photograph using a yellow filter.

*Notes:* When a zymogram that is visible in daylight is required, counterstain the processed gel with MTT/PMS solution. White bands of TALD appear on a blue background almost immediately. Wash negatively stained gel in water and fix in 50% ethanol.

## METHOD 2

### Visualization Scheme

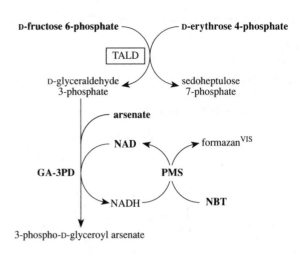

### Staining Solution[2]

A.  100 mM Triethanolamine buffer, pH 7.4
    1 mM EDTA
    0.16 mM Sodium arsenate
    3 mM D-Fructose 6-phosphate
    0.4 mM D-Erythrose 4-phosphate
    0.5 mM NAD
    0.4 mM NBT
    0.1 mM PMS
    16 U/ml Glyceraldehyde-3-phosphate dehydrogenase (GA-3PD)
B.  1% Agarose solution (60°C)

### Procedure

Mix equal volumes of A and B components of the staining solution and pour the mixture over the surface of the gel. Incubate the gel with agarose application at 37°C in the dark until blue bands appear. Fix stained agarose application in 50% ethanol.

*Notes:* When 7.5% PAG is used for electrophoresis, colored bands of TALD activity appear only in agarose plate. This is because the auxiliary glyceraldehyde-3-phosphate dehydrogenase is unable to penetrate the 7.5% PAG, and the staining of agarose plate is due to TALD diffusion out of 7.5% PAG.

To prevent nonspecific development of alcohol dehydrogenase activity bands, the phosphosugars, NAD, NBT and PMS should be prepared alcohol-free by lyophilization.

### REFERENCES

1. Anderson, J. E., Teng, Y.-S., and Giblett, E. R., Stains for six enzymes potentially applicable to chromosomal assignment by cell hybridization, *Cytogenet. Cell Genet.*, 14, 465, 1975.
2. Wood, T. and Muzarriri, C. C., The electrophoresis and detection of transketolase, *Anal. Biochem.*, 118, 221, 1981.

REACTION      Acetyl-CoA + n malonyl-CoA + 2n NADPH = long-chain fatty acid + (n+1) CoA + n $CO_2$ + 2n NADP

ENZYME SOURCE   Bacteria, fungi, invertebrates, vertebrates

## METHOD

### Visualization Scheme

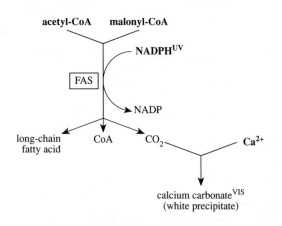

### Staining Solution[1]
100 mM Tris–HCl buffer, pH 7.5
0.1 mM Acetyl-CoA
0.1 mM Malonyl-CoA
0.1 mM NADPH
100 mM $Ca^{2+}$

### Procedure
After completion of electrophoresis in 3.5% PAG soak gel in 0.1 M tris–HCl buffer, pH 7.5, at 37°C for 20 to 30 min and transfer to the staining solution. Incubate the gel at room temperature or 37°C. View PAG against a dark background and, when white bands of calcium carbonate precipitation of sufficient intensity are obtained, remove the gel from staining solution and store in 50 mM glycine–KOH, pH 10, 5 mM $Ca^{2+}$, either at 5°C or at room temperature in the presence of an antibacterial agent.

*Notes:* The yeast and animal enzyme is a multifunctional protein catalyzing the reactions of EC 2.3.1.38, 2.3.1.39, 2.3.1.41, 1.1.1.100, 4.2.1.61, 1.3.1.10 and 3.1.2.14.

Because of its very high molecular weight, FAS is not able to penetrate into 7% PAG. Thus, the use of 3.5% PAG is recommended for FAS electrophoresis.

## OTHER METHODS

A. The product CoA-SH can reduce ferricyanide to ferrocyanide, which further reacts with mercury and yields reddish-brown precipitate (e.g., see 4.1.3.2 — MS).
B. The product CoA-SH can reduce tetrazolium salt via intermediary catalyst dichlorophenol indophenol, resulting in the formation of insoluble formazan (e.g., see 4.1.3.7 — CS).

## REFERENCE
1. Nimmo, H. G. and Nimmo, G. A., A general method for the localization of enzymes that produce phosphate, pyrophosphate, or $CO_2$ after polyacrylamide gel electrophoresis, *Anal. Biochem.*, 121, 17, 1982.

## 2.3.2.2 — Glutamyl Transpeptidase; GTP

**OTHER NAMES**  γ-Glutamyltransferase (recommended name), L-glutamyl transpeptidase, γ-glutamyl transpeptidase

**REACTION**  (5-L-Glutamyl)-peptide + amino acid = peptide + 5-L-glutamyl-amino acid

**ENZYME SOURCE**  Invertebrates, vertebrates

### METHOD

#### Visualization Scheme

*Stage 1*

5-L-glutamyl-2-naphthylamide ⟶ glycyl-glycine

GTP

5-L-glutamyl-glycyl-glycine ⟵ ⟶ 2-naphthylamine

*Stage 2*                         Fast Blue B ⟶

colored dye$^{VIS}$

#### Staining Solution[1]
A. 0.01 *M* Tris–0.05 *M* glycyl-glycine-NaOH buffer, pH 10.0    100 ml
B. 5-L-Glutamyl-2-naphthylamide    100 mg
C. 0.05% Fast Blue B salt in 8% acetic acid

#### Procedure
Add the B component to solution A and dissolve by boiling for 15 min. The final pH of this mixture should be 9.5 at room temperature. Incubate the gel in this mixture at 37°C for 30 min and then place in solution C. Positively stained GTP bands appear after a few minutes.

*Notes:*  The two-step staining procedure is recommended because of the presumed inhibitory effect of Fast Blue B on GTP activity.

#### REFERENCE
1. Patel, S. and O'Gorman, P., Demonstration of serum gamma-glutamyl transpeptidase isoenzymes, using Cellogel electrophoresis, *Clin. Chim. Acta*, 49, 11, 1973.

## 2.3.2.4 — γ-Glutamylcyclotransferase; GCT

**REACTION**  (5-L-Glutamyl)-L-amino acid = 5-oxoproline + L-amino acid

**ENZYME SOURCE**  Plants, vertebrates

### METHOD

#### Visualization Scheme

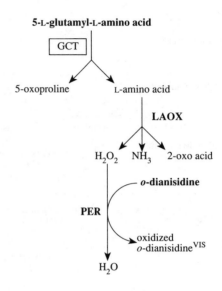

#### Staining Solution[1]
A. 0.05 *M* Tris–HCl buffer, pH 8.0    30 ml
    5-L-Glutamyl-L-methionine (or 5-L-glutamyl-L-glutamine)    17 mg
    L-Amino acid oxidase (LAOX)    6 mg
    *o*-Dianisidine dihydrochloride    6 mg
    Peroxidase (PER)    12 mg
B. 2% Agar solution (60°C)    30 ml

#### Procedure
Mix A and B components of the staining solution and pour the mixture over the surface of the gel. Incubate the gel at room temperature or 37°C until brown bands appear. Fix zymogram in 2 *M* acetic acid and store in 50% glycerol.

*Notes:*  The use of 3-amino-9-ethyl-carbazole instead of *o*-dianisidine is preferable because the latter is a possible carcinogen.

#### REFERENCE
1. Orlowski, M. and Meister, A., γ-Glutamyl cyclotransferase: distribution, isozymic forms, and specificity, *J. Biol. Chem.*, 248, 2836, 1973.

OTHER NAMES   Transamidase, transglutaminase, fibrin stabilizing factor, coagulation factor XIIIa, fibrinoligase

REACTION   Protein glutamine + alkylamine = protein $N^5$-alkylglutamine + $NH_3$

ENZYME SOURCE   Invertebrates, vertebrates

## METHOD

### Visualization Scheme

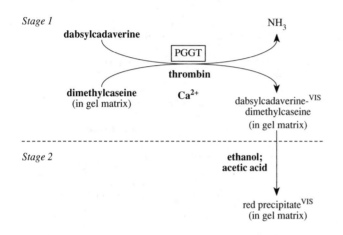

### Staining Solution[1]

A.  0.05 $M$ Tris–HCl buffer, pH 7.5
    0.2 m$M$ Dabsylcadaverine
    20 m$M$ CaCl$_2$
    2 m$M$ Dithiothreitol
    14 U/ml Thrombin
B.  45% Ethanol in 10% acetic acid

### Procedure

Incubate 1% agarose electrophoretic gel containing 0.3% $N,N'$-dimethylcaseine in solution A at 37°C for 60 min and then place gel in solution B for 30 min. The zones of PGGT activity appear as red bands. To intensify positively stained bands, a few drops of diluted HCl can be added to solution B.

## OTHER METHODS

The fluorescent activity staining method for transamidating enzymes is also available. The method is based on the transamidase-catalyzed incorporation of the fluorescent (at 254 nm) monodansylthiacadaverine or dansylcadaverine into casein.[2,3]

## GENERAL NOTES

Transamidases comprise a group of $Ca^{2+}$-dependent thiol enzymes with the specialized function of catalyzing the formation of intermolecular γ-glutamyl-ε-lysine bridges between some native proteins. These enzymes also catalyze the incorporation of low-molecular-weight primary amines into proteins.[2]

It should be emphasized that for each new member of the transamidase family of enzymes one should be prepared to modify conditions of the visualization procedure regarding time of enzyme reaction, pH value and concentration of staining buffers, use of activators, $Ca^{2+}$ ion concentration, and selection of substrates other than caseine or $N,N'$-dimethylcaseine, so as to obtain the best results.[3]

Good results can also be obtained when dimethylcaseine is added to the staining solution, but incorporation of this substrate into the gel matrix is preferable.

Thrombin is used to activate PGGT. Some other transglutaminases are not thrombin-dependent.

### REFERENCES

1.  Lorand, L., Parameswaran, K. N., Velasco, P. T., Hsu, L. K.-H., and Siefring, G. E., New colored and fluorescent amine substrates for activated fibrin stabilizing factor (factor XIIIa) and for transglutaminase, *Anal. Biochem.*, 131, 419, 1983.
2.  Stenberg, P. and Stenflo J., A rapid and specific fluorescent activity staining procedure for transamidating enzymes, *Anal. Biochem.*, 93, 445, 1979.
3.  Lorand, L., Siefring, G. E., Tong, Y. S., Bruner-Lorand, J., and Gray, A. J., Dansylcadaverine specific staining for transamidating enzymes, *Anal. Biochem.*, 93, 453, 1979.

OTHER NAMES   Muscle phosphorylase *a* and *b*, amylophosphorylase, polyphosphorylase. The recommended name is qualified in each instance by adding the name of the natural substrate (e.g., maltodextrin phosphorylase, starch phosphorylase, glycogen phosphorylase).

REACTION   $(1,4\text{-}\alpha\text{-}\text{D-Glucosyl})_n$ + orthophosphate = $(1,4\text{-}\alpha\text{-}\text{D-Glucosyl})_{n-1}$ + $\alpha$-D-glucose 1-phosphate

ENZYME SOURCE   Bacteria, green algae, plants, invertebrates, vertebrates

## METHOD 1

### Visualization Scheme

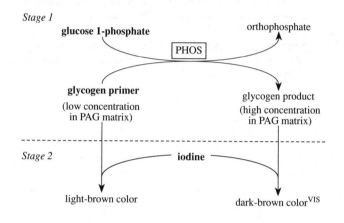

### Staining Solution[1]
A. 0.1 *M* Sodium citrate buffer, pH 5.0
   25 m*M* Glucose 1-phosphate
B. 10 m*M* $I_2$
   14 m*M* KI

### Procedure
Incubate electrophorized PAG (polymerized with 0.1% glycogen primer or 0.1% starch primer) in solution A at room temperature for 5 h and then place in solution B. The gel background is stained light brown (with glycogen primer) or light blue (with starch primer), while PHOS activity bands are stained dark brown or dark blue, respectively, due to increased concentration of glycogen or starch.

*Notes:*   In some cases (e.g., when plant leaf preparations are used as the enzyme source), additional positively stained bands can also develop. These bands also develop when gels are incubated in solution A lacking glucose 1-phosphate and perhaps are caused by action of debranching enzyme (see 3.2.1.41 — DEG), which hydrolyzes the $\alpha$-1,6-branch linkages of the glycogen and the starch (amylopectin form) resulting in a greater capacity of the unit chains to adopt the helical configuration for iodine complex formation.

The colorless bands of amylase activity can also develop on gels stained using this method (see 3.2.1.1 — $\alpha$-AMY, Method 1).

## METHOD 2

### Visualization Scheme

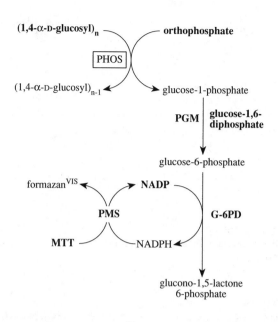

### Staining Solution[2]

| | |
|---|---|
| 0.1 *M* Sodium phosphate buffer, pH 7.0 | 1 ml |
| Glycogen | 10 mg |
| Glucose-6-phosphate dehydrogenase (G-6PD) | 5 units |
| Phosphoglucomutase (PGM) | 5 units |
| Glucose-1,6-diphosphate | trace |
| NADP | 2 mg |
| PMS | 0.1 mg |
| MTT | 0.4 mg |

### Procedure
Apply the staining solution dropwise to the surface of the gel and incubate in the dark at 37°C until dark blue bands appear. Fix stained gel in 50% ethanol.

*Notes:*   The stain is less expensive when NAD-dependent G-6PD (Sigma; G 5760, G 5885) is used.[3]

## METHOD 3

### Visualization Scheme

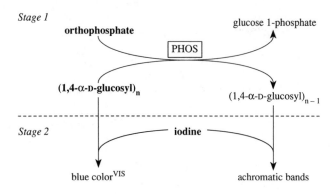

*Stage 1*

orthophosphate → glucose 1-phosphate

PHOS

$(1,4\text{-}\alpha\text{-D-glucosyl})_n$ → $(1,4\text{-}\alpha\text{-D-glucosyl})_{n-1}$

- - - - - - - - - - - - - - - - - - - - - - - - - - - - - - - - - - - - -

*Stage 2* — iodine

blue color$^{VIS}$ — achromatic bands

### Staining Solution[4]

A. 0.1 *M* Sodium phosphate buffer, pH 5.1      100 ml
B. 10 m*M* $I_2$
    14 m*M* KI

### Procedure

Incubate electrophorized starch gel (or PAG containing 0.1 to 0.5% soluble starch or glycogen) in solution A at 37°C for 3 to 5 h. Discard solution A and stain gel with solution B. The presence of achromatic to light brown bands on a blue background of starch gel marks areas of PHOS localization. When starch- or glycogen-containing PAG are used, zones of PHOS activity are indicated by the presence of achromatic or light brown bands on a dark brown background. Record or photograph zymogram.

*Notes:* Achromatic bands of amylase activity can also be developed by this method, so the control staining for amylase could be carried out in parallel (see 3.2.1.1 — α-AMY, Method 1).

## GENERAL NOTES

It is known that the muscle enzyme exists in two forms: phosphorylase *a* (tetramer) and phosphorylase *b* (dimer). AMP activates both forms of the enzyme; in its absence phosphorylase *a* possesses 60 to 70% of the maximum activity and phosphorylase *b* is inactive. Thus, the addition of AMP (about 0.25 mg/ml) to the staining solution is beneficial.

## REFERENCES

1. Gerbrandy, S. J. and Verleur, J. D., Phosphorylase isoenzymes: localization and occurrence in different plant organs in relation to starch metabolism, *Phytochemistry*, 10, 261, 1971.
2. Colgan, D. J., Evidence for the evolutionary significance of developmental variation in an abundant protein of orthopteran muscle, *Genetica*, 67, 81, 1985.
3. Black, W. C., IV and Krafsur, E. S., Electrophoretic analysis of genetic variability in the house fly (*Musca domestica* L.), *Biochem. Genet.*, 23, 193, 1985.
4. Siepmann, R. and Stegemann, H., Enzym-elektrophorese in einschluß-polymerisaten des acrylamids. A. Amylasen, phosphorylasen, *Z. Naturforsch.*, 22, 949, 1967.

OTHER NAMES    Sucrose 6-glucosyltransferase

REACTION    Sucrose + (1,6-$\alpha$-D-glucosyl)$_n$ = D-fructose + (1,6-$\alpha$-D-glucosyl)$_{n+1}$

ENZYME SOURCE    Bacteria, green algae

## METHOD 1

### Visualization Scheme

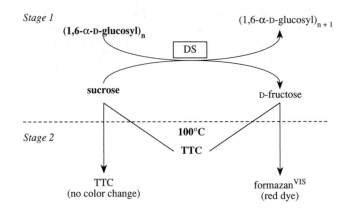

### Staining Solution[1]
A. 0.2 *M* Sodium acetate buffer, pH 5.0     100 ml
    Sucrose     860 mg
    Dextran T10 (Pharmacia)     100 mg
B. 2,3,5-Triphenyltetrazolium chloride (TTC)     100 mg
    1 *N* NaOH     100 ml

### Procedure
Incubate electrophorized PAG in solution A for 30 min and dip into boiling solution B for 1 to 4 min until red-colored bands of DS appear. Too much heating causes the gel background to be stained pink. Immediately after the bands become well visible, wash and fix gel in 7.5% acetic acid.

## METHOD 2

### Visualization Scheme

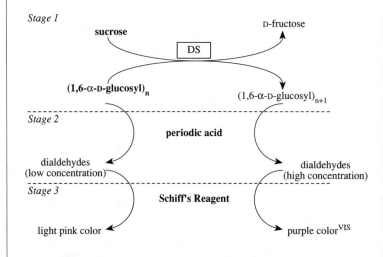

### Staining Solution[1]
A. 0.2 *M* Sodium acetate buffer, pH 5.0     100 ml
    Sucrose     860 mg
    Dextran T10 (Pharmacia)     100 mg
    Merthiolate     10 mg
B. 1% Periodic acid (dissolved in ethanol) in 0.02 *M* sodium acetate
C. Schiff's reagent

### Procedure
Incubate electrophorized PAG in solution A for 15 h at 37°C. Treat the incubated gel with solution B, wash with distilled water, stain with Schiff's reagent, and wash with 7% acetic acid. The zones of DS activity develop as purple bands on a light pink background. Store the stained gel covered with Saran wrap.

*Notes:* When the gel is incubated in solution A containing more dextran primer, the gel background is stained pink more intensely. Therefore, an addition of a minimum amount of a polysaccharide primer is recommended in this method.

## METHOD 3

### Visualization Scheme

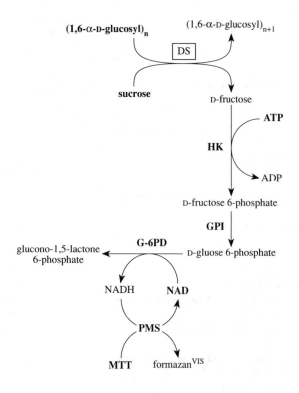

### Staining Solution*

| | | |
|---|---|---|
| A. | 0.005 *M* Sodium acetate buffer, pH 6.5 | 20 ml |
| | Sucrose | 170 mg |
| | Dextran (low molecular weight) | 50 mg |
| | ATP | 30 mg |
| | NAD | 20 mg |
| | MTT | 10 mg |
| | PMS | 1 mg |
| | Hexokinase (HK) | 50 units |
| | Glucose-6-phosphate isomerase (GPI) | 50 units |
| | Glucose-6-phosphate dehydrogenase (G-6PD; NAD-dependent; Sigma) | 50 units |
| B. | 2% Agarose solution (60°C) | 20 ml |

### Procedure

Mix A and B components of the staining solution and pour the mixture over the surface of the gel. Incubate the gel at 37°C in the dark until dark blue bands appear. Fix stained agarose overlay in 50% ethanol.

*Notes:* The main advantage of the method is the one-step staining of DS activity bands. This method is based on the ability of yeast HK to convert D-fructose to fructose-6-phosphate in the presence of ATP.

### REFERENCE

1. Mukasa, H., Shimamura, A., and Tsumori, H., Direct activity stains for glycosidase and glucosyltransferase after isoelectric focusing in horizontal polyacrylamide gel layers, *Anal. Biochem.*, 123, 276, 1982.

---

\* New; recommended for use.

## 2.4.1.7 — Sucrose Phosphorylase; SP

OTHER NAMES     Sucrose glucosyltransferase

REACTION     Sucrose + orthophosphate = D-fructose + α-D-glucose 1-phosphate

ENZYME SOURCE   Bacteria, green algae

## METHOD

### Visualization Scheme

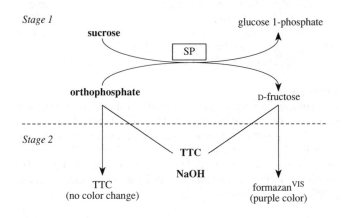

### Staining Solution[1]
A. 3 mM Sodium phosphate buffer, pH 6.9
   200 mM Sucrose
B. 0.1% 2,3,5-Triphenyltetrazolium chloride (TTC)
   1 N NaOH

### Procedure
Wash electrophorized PAG in distilled water thoroughly and incubate in solution A at 30°C for 20 min. Wash gel in distilled water again and place in solution B. Incubate the gel in this solution in the dark at room temperature until purple bands of SP activity appear on the pink background of the gel. Wash stained gel in water and fix in 7.5% acetic acid.

*Notes:* This method is based on the capacity of D-fructose to reduce TTC at room temperature and alkaline conditions resulting in the formation of purple formazan.

### OTHER METHODS

A. The zones of D-fructose production can be visualized using the PMS/MTT system and coupled reactions catalyzed by exogenous hexokinase (with sufficient fructokinase activity), glucose-6-phosphate isomerase, and glucose-6-phosphate dehydrogenase (e.g., see 2.4.1.5 — DS, Method 3).
B. The zones of glucose-1-phosphate production can be visualized using the PMS/MTT system and coupled reactions catalyzed by exogenous phosphoglucomutase and glucose-6-phosphate dehydrogenase (e.g., see 2.4.1.1 — PHOS, Method 2).

### REFERENCE
1. Gabriel, O. and Wang, S.-F., Determination of enzymatic activity in polyacrylamide gels. I. Enzymes catalyzing the conversion of nonreducing substrates to reducing products, *Anal. Biochem.*, 27, 545, 1969.

## 2.4.1.16 — Chitin Synthase; CHS

OTHER NAMES     Chitin–UDP acetylglucosaminyltransferase

REACTION

1. UDP-*N*-acetyl-D-glucosamine + [1,4-(*N*-acetyl-β-D-glucosaminyl)]$_n$ = UDP + [1,4-(*N*-acetyl-β-D-glucosaminyl)]$_{n+1}$

2. Converts UDP-*N*-acetyl-D-glucosamine into UDP and chitin

ENZYME SOURCE   Fungi, invertebrates

## METHOD

### Visualization Scheme

UDP-*N*-acetyl-D-glucosamine

CHS    phosphatidylserine;
*N*-acetylglucosamine

UDP        chitin[VIS]

### Staining Solution[1]
30 mM Tris–HCl buffer, pH 7.5
32 mM *N*-Acetylglucosamine
4 mM Magnesium acetate
0.18 mg/ml Phosphatidylserine
1 mM UDP-*N*-Acetyl-D-glucosamine

### Procedure
Incubate electrophorized PAG in a staining solution at 30°C for 12 h. The zones of CHS activity develop as opaque bands visible in daylight on a clean PAG background.

*Notes:* The enzyme catalyzes the synthesis of chitin directly from UDP-*N*-acetyl-D-glucosamine without the participation of a primer. The synthesis is markedly stimulated by *N*-acetylglucosamine. When the enzyme is solubilized its properties are altered. Thus, the soluble enzyme requires a primer for activity and it is not stimulated by *N*-acetylglucosamine. In the presence of phosphatidylserine the solubilized enzyme catalyzes the synthesis of chitin without the participation of a primer and is stimulated by *N*-acetylglucosamine.

### REFERENCE
1. Kang, M. S., Elango, N., Mattia, E., Au-Young, J., Robbins, P. W., and Cabib, E., Isolation of chitin synthetase from *Saccharomyces cerevisiae*, *J. Biol. Chem.*, 259, 14966, 1984.

OTHER NAMES | UDPgalactose-*N*-acetyl-glucosamine β-D-galactosyltransferase, *N*-acetyl-galactosamine synthase, galactosyltransferase

REACTION | UDPgalactose + *N*-acetyl-D-glucosamine = UDP + *N*-acetyllactosamine

ENZYME SOURCE | Invertebrates, vertebrates

## METHOD 1

### Visualization Scheme

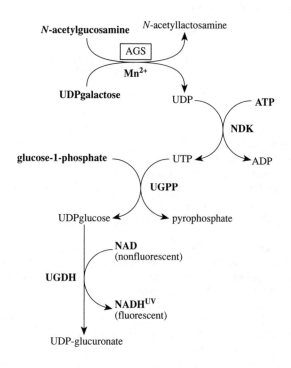

## Staining Solution[1]

A. 0.1 *M* Sodium cacodylate buffer, pH 7.5          0.28 ml
   0.1 *M* MnCl₂                                     0.5 ml
   25 U/ml Uridine-5′-diphosphoglucose               0.02 ml
      pyrophosphorylase (UGPP)
   1000 U/ml Nucleoside-diphosphate                  0.02 ml
      kinase (NDK)
   2 U/ml UDPglucose dehydrogenase (UGDH)            0.02 ml
   200 mg/ml NAD                                     67 µl
   200 mg/ml ATP                                     0.05 ml
   200 mg/ml Glucose 1-phosphate                     0.05 ml
   0.1 *M* UDPgalactose                              0.02 ml
   5 *M* *N*-Acetylglucosamine                       0.02 ml

B. 4% Agarose solution in 0.1 *M* sodium
   cacodylate buffer, pH 7.5 (60°C)

## Procedure

Mix solution A with an equal volume of solution B (temperature of the mixture should be about 40°C) and pour over the surface of the gel. Incubate the gel at room temperature in a moist chamber for 4 to 15 h and view under long-wave UV light. The zones of AGS activity appear as light (fluorescent) bands on a dark (nonfluorescent) background. Record the zymogram or photograph using a yellow filter.

*Notes:* Inclusion of diaphorase and *p*-iodonitrotetrazolium violet in solution A allows one to develop AGS bands visible in daylight. This method, however, is less sensitive than the fluorescent one described above. Diaphorase cannot be replaced by PMS because the latter does not work as an electron acceptor at high Mn²⁺ concentration.

## METHOD 2

### Visualization Scheme

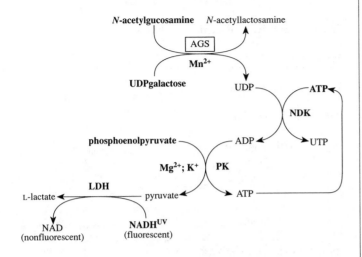

### Staining Solution*

| | |
|---|---:|
| 0.05 *M* Tris–HCl buffer, pH 7.5 | 5 ml |
| NADH | 3 mg |
| ATP | 5 mg |
| Phosphoenolpyruvate | 10 mg |
| Nucleoside-diphosphate kinase (NDK) | 10 units |
| Pyruvate kinase (PK) | 20 units |
| Lactate dehydrogenase (LDH) | 5 units |
| UDP–galactose | 3 mg |
| *N*-Acetylglucosamine | 10 mg |
| MnCl$_2$ | 10 mg |
| MgCl$_2$ | 10 mg |
| KCl | 15 mg |

### Procedure

Apply the staining solution to gel on filter-paper overlay and incubate at 37°C in a moist chamber until dark (nonfluorescent) bands visible in long-wave UV light appear on a light (fluorescent) background. Record the zymogram or photograph using a yellow filter.

*Notes:* Nucleoside-diphosphate kinase and ATP may be omitted from the staining solution because pyruvate kinase works sufficiently well with UDP.

## GENERAL NOTES

The AGS reaction is catalyzed by a component of EC 2.4.1.22, which is identical to EC 2.4.1.38, and by an enzyme from the Golgi apparatus of animal tissues.

### REFERENCE

1.
    Pierce, M., Cummings, R. D., and Roth, S., The localization of galactosyltransferases in polyacrylamide gels by a coupled enzyme assay, *Anal. Biochem.*, 102, 441, 1980.

---

* New; recommended for use.

## 2.4.2.1 — Purine-nucleoside Phosphorylase; PNP

**OTHER NAMES**    Inosine phosphorylase, nucleoside phosphorylase

**REACTION**    Purine nucleoside + orthophosphate = purine + α-D-ribose 1-phosphate

**ENZYME SOURCE**  Bacteria, fungi, invertebrates, vertebrates

## METHOD

### Visualization Scheme

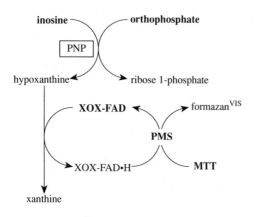

### Staining Solution[1]

A. 0.05 *M* Phosphate buffer, pH 7.5 ......... 25 ml
   Inosine ............................................. 5 mg
   MTT ................................................. 5 mg
   PMS ................................................. 5 mg
   Xanthine oxidase (XOX) .................. 0.4 unit
B. 2% Agar solution (60°C) ................... 25 ml

### Procedure

Mix A and B components of the staining solution and pour the mixture over the surface of the gel. Incubate the gel in the dark at 37°C until dark blue bands appear. Fix stained agarose overlay in 50% ethanol.

*Notes:*   The enzyme from animal species commonly exhibits stain artifacts consisting of one or two diffuse bands in the cathodal half of the gel. These bands do not represent endogenous enzyme and usually also develop on ADA (EC 3.5.4.4) and GDA (EC 3.5.4.3) zymograms.[2]

Specificity of PNP is not completely determined. The enzyme can also catalyze ribosyltransferase reactions of the type catalyzed by nucleoside ribosyltransferase (EC 2.4.2.5).

### REFERENCES
1. Edwards, Y. H., Hopkinson, D. A., and Harris, H., Inherited variants of human nucleoside phosphorylase, *Ann. Hum. Genet.*, 34, 395, 1971.
2. Richardson, B. J., Baverstock, P. R., and Adams, M., *Allozyme Electrophoresis: A Handbook for Animal Systematics and Population Studies*, Academic Press, Sydney, 1986, 204.

## 2.4.2.3 — Uridine Phosphorylase; UP

**OTHER NAMES**    Pyrumidine phosphorylase

**REACTION**    Uridine + orthophosphate = uracil + α-D-ribose 1-phosphate

**ENZYME SOURCE**  Bacteria, vertebrates

## METHOD

### Visualization Scheme

*Stage 1: Enzyme reaction*

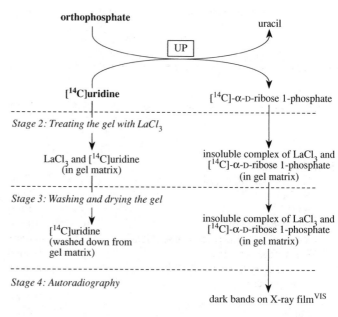

### Reaction mixture[1]

A. 0.2 *M* Potassium phosphate buffer, pH 7.5
   6 μCi [U-¹⁴C]Uridine (specific activity 50 mCi/mmol) labeled on ribose
B. 0.1 *M* Tris–HCl buffer, pH 7.0
   0.1 *M* LaCl₃

### Procedure

*Stage 1.* Incubate electrophorized gel in solution A at 37°C for 2 h.
*Stage 2.* Place gel in solution B and incubate at 4°C for 6 h.
*Stage 3.* Wash gel for 12 h in deionized water. Dry the gel.
*Stage 4.* Expose dry gel in tight contact with X-ray film (Kodak B-54) for 2 to 4 weeks. Develop exposed X-ray film.

Dark bands on developed X-ray film correspond to localization of UP activity in the gel.

### OTHER METHODS

The reaction catalyzed by UP is readily reversible. Thus, in principle, UP activity bands may be detected using histochemical methods of detection of orthophosphate (see 3.6.1.1 — PP), the product of the reverse UP reaction. This approach, however, has not yet been realized. Perhaps this is because D-ribose-1-phosphate, the substrate of the reverse UP reaction, is too expensive.

### REFERENCE
1. Denney, R. M., Nichols, E. A., and Ruddle, F. H., Assignment of a gene for uridine phosphorylase to chromosome 7, *Cytogenet. Cell Genet.*, 22, 195, 1978.

OTHER NAMES    AMP pyrophosphorylase,
transphosphoribosidase

REACTION    AMP + pyrophosphate = adenine + 5-phospho-
α-D-ribose 1-diphosphate

ENZYME SOURCE  Bacteria, plants, invertebrates, vertebrates

## METHOD

### Visualization Scheme

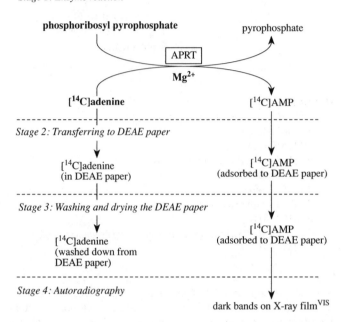

*Stage 1: Enzyme reaction*

phosphoribosyl pyrophosphate → pyrophosphate

APRT, $Mg^{2+}$

[$^{14}$C]adenine    [$^{14}$C]AMP

*Stage 2: Transferring to DEAE paper*

[$^{14}$C]adenine (in DEAE paper)    [$^{14}$C]AMP (adsorbed to DEAE paper)

*Stage 3: Washing and drying the DEAE paper*

[$^{14}$C]adenine (washed down from DEAE paper)    [$^{14}$C]AMP (adsorbed to DEAE paper)

*Stage 4: Autoradiography*

dark bands on X-ray film[VIS]

### Reaction Mixture[1]

| | |
|---|---|
| 55 m*M* Tris–HCl buffer, pH 7.4 | 10 ml |
| [$^{14}$C]Adenine (specific activity 50 µCi/µmol; 50 µCi/ml) labeled on ribose | 0.3 ml |
| 0.2 *M* MgCl$_2$ | 2 ml |
| 10 m*M* Phosphoribosyl pyrophosphate | 1 ml |

### Procedure[2]

*Stages 1, 2.* Apply a sheet of Whatman DE 81 (DEAE cellulose) paper to the surface of the electrophorized gel and pipette on the reaction mixture. Wrap the gel/DEAE paper combination in "Saran Wrap" and incubate at 37°C for 1 h.

*Stage 3.* Remove the DEAE paper and wash on a Bucher funnel with 15 l of distilled water to remove the unreacted [$^{14}$C]adenine leaving [$^{14}$C]AMP adsorbed to the DEAE paper at the sites of the enzyme reaction. Dry the DEAE paper.

*Stage 4.* Apply DEAE paper to a sheet of X-ray film (Blue Brand, Kodak). Place the X-ray film/DEAE paper combination between two glass plates and wrap in a dark bag. Develop the X-ray film exposed for 4 d with Kodak D 19 developer (Kodak Safelight 6B may be used).

Dark bands on developed X-ray film correspond to localization of APRT activity on the gel.

*Notes:* Precipitation of [$^{14}$C]AMP with LaCl$_3$ directly in the gel matrix also may be used in visualization of APRT by the autoradiographic procedure.[3]

## OTHER METHODS

A. A bioautographic method of visualization of APRT activity on electrophoretic gels was developed by Naylor and Klebe.[4] The principle of this method is the use of a microbial reagent to locate the enzyme after gel electrophoresis. Electrophorized gel is placed on indicator agar seeded with mutant (pur A⁻) *E. coli*, which requires the product (adenine) of APRT reaction. Bacteria proliferate to form visible bands at the sites of the enzymatic reaction. This method, however, is not appropriate for routine laboratory use and is recommended for visualization of enzymes that are difficult or impossible to detect with standard histochemical or other methods.

B. A general method for the localization of enzymes that produce pyrophosphate is available.[5] The method is based on insolubility of white calcium pyrophosphate precipitate forming as a result of interaction between $Ca^{2+}$ ions included in the reaction mixture and pyrophosphate molecules produced by an enzyme reaction. This method can also be applied to APRT electrophorized in clean gels (e.g., PAG or agarose gel). The zones of calcium pyrophosphate precipitation can be subsequently counterstained with Alizarin Red S. This procedure would be of advantage for starch or acetate cellulose gels.

### REFERENCES
1. Mowbray, S., Watson, B., and Harris, H., A search for electrophoretic variants of human adenine phosphoribosyl transferase, *Ann. Hum. Genet.*, 36, 153, 1972.
2. Harris, H. and Hopkinson, D. A., *Handbook of Enzyme Electrophoresis in Human Genetics*, North-Holland, Amsterdam (Loose leaf with supplements in 1977 and 1978), 1976.
3. Tischfield, J. A., Bernhard, H. P., and Ruddle, F. H., A new electrophoretic–autoradiographic method for visual detection of phosphotransferases, *Anal. Biochem.*, 53, 545, 1973.
4. Naylor, S. L. and Klebe, R. J., Bioautography: a general method for the visualization of isozymes, *Biochem. Genet.*, 15, 1193, 1977.
5. Nimmo, H. G. and Nimmo, G. A., A general method for the localization of enzymes that produce phosphate, pyrophosphate, or CO$_2$ after polyacrylamide gel electrophoresis, *Anal. Biochem.*, 121, 17, 1982.

OTHER NAMES    Hypoxanthine–guanine phosphoribosyltransferase, IMP pyrophosphorylase, transphosphoribosidase, guanine phosphoribosyltransferase

REACTIONS    1. IMP + pyrophosphate = hypoxanthine + 5-phospho-α-D-ribose 1-diphosphate
2. GMP + pyrophosphate = guanine + 5-phospho-α-D-ribose 1-diphosphate

ENZYME SOURCE    Bacteria, fungi, plants, invertebrates, vertebrates

## METHOD 1

### Visualization Scheme

*Stage 1: Enzyme reaction*

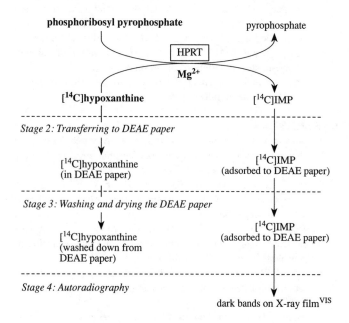

**phosphoribosyl pyrophosphate**                    pyrophosphate

HPRT

$Mg^{2+}$

[$^{14}$C]hypoxanthine                    [$^{14}$C]IMP

- - - - - - - - - - - - - - - - - - - - - - - - - - - - - - - - -

*Stage 2: Transferring to DEAE paper*

[$^{14}$C]hypoxanthine (in DEAE paper)          [$^{14}$C]IMP (adsorbed to DEAE paper)

- - - - - - - - - - - - - - - - - - - - - - - - - - - - - - - - -

*Stage 3: Washing and drying the DEAE paper*

[$^{14}$C]hypoxanthine (washed down from DEAE paper)          [$^{14}$C]IMP (adsorbed to DEAE paper)

- - - - - - - - - - - - - - - - - - - - - - - - - - - - - - - - -

*Stage 4: Autoradiography*

dark bands on X-ray film[VIS]

### Reaction Mixture[1]

| | |
|---|---|
| 55 m$M$ Tris–HCl buffer, pH 7.4 | 10 ml |
| [$^{14}$C]Hypoxanthine (specific activity 50 μCi/μmol; 50 μCi/ml) | 0.3 ml |
| 0.2 $M$ MgCl$_2$ | 2 ml |
| 10 m$M$ Phosphoribosyl pyrophosphate | 1 ml |

### Procedure

The procedure of HPRT detection by this method is similar to that described for APRT (see 2.4.2.7 — APRT).

*Notes:*    [$^{14}$C]Hypoxanthine may be replaced by [$^{14}$C]guanine in the reaction mixture.[2]

Precipitation of [$^{14}$C]IMP with LaCl$_3$ directly in the gel matrix also may be used in visualization of HPRT by an autoradiographic procedure.[3]

## METHOD 2

### Visualization Scheme

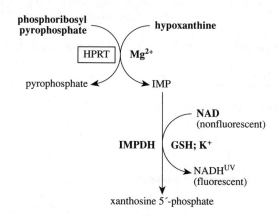

**phosphoribosyl pyrophosphate**                    **hypoxanthine**

HPRT    $Mg^{2+}$

pyrophosphate                    IMP

**NAD** (nonfluorescent)

IMPDH    GSH; K$^+$

NADH$^{UV}$ (fluorescent)

xanthosine 5′-phosphate

### Staining Solution[4]

165 m$M$ Tris–HCl buffer, pH 8.1
15 m$M$ MgSO$_4$
300 m$M$ KCl
6 m$M$ Reduced glutathione (GSH)
3 m$M$ Allopurinol
3 m$M$ Hypoxanthine
2 m$M$ Phosphoribosyl pyrophosphate
6 m$M$ NAD
0.3 U/ml IMP dehydrogenase from *Aerobacter aerogenes* (IMPDH)

### Procedure

Pour staining solution onto a clean glass plate (0.1 ml/10 cm$^2$ of gel to be stained). Place electrophorized acetate cellulose sheet on the top of a glass plate with the porous side down (or starch gel with the cut surface down). Allow the staining solution to absorb completely into the gel matrix. Cover gel with a thin plastic sheet to stop evaporation and incubate for 1 to 2 h at 37°C. View gel under long-wave UV light for fluorescent bands. Record the zymogram or photograph using a yellow filter.

*Notes:*    On prolonged incubation with staining solution, minor fluorescent bands in addition to the major HPRT bands can also appear. These bands also develop in a staining solution from which phosphoribosyl pyrophosphate and Mg$^{2+}$ are lost. The appearance of some of these minor bands could be due to endogenous xanthine dehydrogenase and/or xanthine oxidase. Allopurinol is incorporated in a staining solution to inhibit these activities. Other minor bands can also sometimes develop in certain extracts used for electrophoresis. These bands can be eliminated completely by heating the extracts for 2 min at 70°C. This pretreatment does not decrease the HPRT activity.[5]

The linking enzyme IMPDH is not commercially available, however, it can be relatively easily obtained from a guanine-requiring mutant of *Aerobacter aerogenes*.[6]

## METHOD 3

### Visualization Scheme

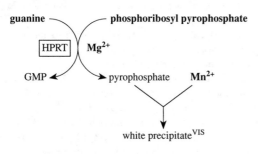

### Staining Solution[7]

50 m$M$ Tris–HCl buffer, pH 7.4
0.15 m$M$ Guanine
1 m$M$ Monothioglycerol
1 m$M$ MgCl$_2$
1 m$M$ MnCl$_2$
0.45 m$M$ Phosphoribosyl pyrophosphate

### Procedure

Wash electrophorized PAG in 0.2 $M$ tris–HCl buffer, pH 7.4, for 15 min. Incubate the gel in staining solution at 37°C for about 45 to 60 min. The manganese pyrophosphate bands are visible due to light scattering. They are not apparent when the processed gel is placed directly on a dark background, but they are very distinct when the gel is held a few inches from a dark background and lighted indirectly. Submerge the stained gel in a solution of 0.01 $M$ MnCl$_2$ in 0.02 $M$ succinate, pH 6.0, for 30 to 60 min and store in 0.02 $M$ succinate, pH 6.0.

*Notes:* The dense white band, which presumably arises from precipitation of anions that run at the dye front, usually develops near the anodal end of the PAG.

The use of Ca$^{2+}$ instead of Mn$^{2+}$ ions in the staining solution is preferable because the white calcium pyrophosphate precipitate is clearly visible on a dark background.[8] The use of Ca$^{2+}$ ions is also preferable because the zones of calcium pyrophosphate precipitation can be subsequently stained with Alizarin Red S. This procedure is of advantage for unclean gels (e.g., starch or acetate cellulose gels).

## METHOD 4

### Visualization Scheme

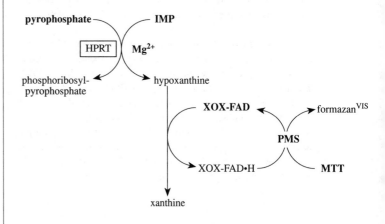

### Staining Solution[9]

| | |
|---|---|
| 55 m$M$ Tris–HCl buffer, pH 7.4, containing | 8 ml |
| 8.3 m$M$ MgSO$_4$ | |
| IMP (disodium salt) | 50 mg |
| Xanthine oxidase (XOX) | 0.1 unit |
| 22.5 mg/ml Na$_4$P$_2$O$_7$·10H$_2$O | 1 ml |
| 2 mg/ml MTT | 1 ml |
| 0.4 mg/ml PMS | 1 ml |

### Procedure

Pour staining solution over the surface of the gel, or apply it dropwise, and incubate the gel in the dark at 37°C until dark blue bands appear. Fix stained gel in 50% ethanol.

## REFERENCES

1. Watson, B., Gormley, I. P., Gardiner, S. E., Evans, H. J., and Harris, H., Reappearance of murine hypoxanthine guanine phosphoribosyl transferase activity in mouse A9 cells after attempted hybridization with human cell lines, *Exp. Cell Res.*, 75, 401, 1972.
2. Der Kaloustian, V. M., Byrne, R., Young, W, J., and Childs, B., An electrophoretic method for detecting hypoxanthine guanine phosphoribosyl transferase variants, *Biochem. Genet.*, 3, 299, 1963.
3. Tischfield, J. A., Bernhard, H. P., and Ruddle, F. H., A new electrophoretic-autoradiographic method for visual detection of phosphotransferases, *Anal. Biochem.*, 53, 545, 1973.
4. Van Diggelen, O. P. and Shin, S., A rapid fluorescent technique for electrophoretic identification of hypoxanthine phosphoribosyl transferase allozymes, *Biochem. Genet.*, 12, 375, 1974.
5. Van Diggelen, O. P., personal communication, 1977.
6. Hampton, A. and Nomura, A., Inosine 5′-phosphate dehydrogenase: site of inhibition by guanosine 5′-phosphate and of inactivation by 6-chloro and 6-mercapto purine ribonucleoside 5′-phosphates, *Biochemistry*, 3, 679, 1967.
7. Vasquez, B. and Bieber, A. L., Direct visualization of IMP-GMP: pyrophosphate phosphoribosyl transferase in polyacrylamide gels, *Anal. Biochem.*, 84, 504, 1978.
8. Chang, G.-G., Deng, R.-Y., and Pan, F., Direct localization and quantitation of aminoacyl-tRNA synthetase activity in polyacrylamide gel, *Anal. Biochem.*, 149, 474, 1985.
9. Van Someren, H., Van Henegouwen, H. B., Los, W., Wurzer-Figurelli, E., Doppert, B., Vervloet, M., and Meera Khan, P., Enzyme electrophoresis on cellulose acetate gel. II. Zymogram patterns in man–chinese hamster somatic cell hybrids, *Humangenetik*, 25, 189, 1974.

OTHER NAMES    Poly(ADP-ribose) polymerase, poly(ADP) polymerase, poly(adenosine diphosphate ribose) polymerase, ADP-ribosyltransferase (polymerizing)

REACTION    NAD + (ADP-D-ribosyl)$_n$ = nicotinamide + (ADP-D-ribosyl)$_{n+1}$

ENZYME SOURCE    Fungi, plants, invertebrates, vertebrates

## METHOD

### Visualization Scheme

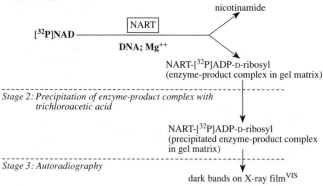

*Stage 1: Enzyme Reaction*

*Stage 2: Precipitation of enzyme-product complex with trichloroacetic acid*

*Stage 3: Autoradiography*

### Reaction Mixture[1]

0.1 $M$ Tris–HCl buffer, pH 8.0
10 m$M$ MgCl$_2$
1 m$M$ Dithiothreitol
1 m$M$ NAD
10 µCi/ml [Adenin-2,8-$^{32}$P]NAD

## Procedure

The method is developed for PAG containing 1% SDS and 100 µg/ml calf thymus DNA activated by pancreatic deoxyribonuclease.

After completion of electrophoresis wash SDS–PAG in 1 l of renaturing buffer (5 m$M$ tris–HCl, pH 8.0; 3 m$M$ 2-mercaptoethanol) for 4 h with two changes at room temperature. Then wash gel in 100 ml of renaturing buffer containing 6 $M$ guanidine hydrochloride for 2 h with two changes at room temperature. Place gel again in 1 l of renaturing buffer and wash at 2°C for 16 to 18 h with several changes. After this, preincubate the gel in 50 ml of 100 m$M$ tris–HCl buffer, pH 8.0; 10 m$M$ MgCl$_2$; 1 m$M$ dithiotreitol for 1 h. The processed gel is renatured and ready for NART detection by autoradiography.

*Stage 1.* Incubate renatured gel in 10 ml of reaction mixture at 37°C for 8 to 12 h.

*Stage 2.* Wash incubated gel five times in 1 l of cold 5% (w/v) trichloroacetic acid. Dry the gel.

*Stage 3.* Autoradiograph dry gel with X-ray film (Kodak AR). Dark bands on developed X-ray film correspond to localization of NART activity on the gel.

## GENERAL NOTES

The NART is a eukaryotic enzyme that transfers the ADP-ribose moiety of the NAD molecule to unclear proteins and extends the reaction by terminal addition to produce an ADP-ribose homopolymer of different lengths (20 to 30 units). The polymer is synthesized in the presence of DNA and is transferred to a variety of acceptor proteins, including NART itself.

The enzyme is activated when cells are subjected to the action of DNA-damaging agents, but the exact role of NART in DNA reparation is not known.

## REFERENCE

1. Scovassi, A. I., Stefanini, M., and Bertazzoni, U., Catalytic activities of human poly(ADP-ribose) polymerase from normal and mutagenized cells detected after sodium dodecyl sulfate–polyacrylamide gel electrophoresis, *Anal. Biochem.*, 259, 10973, 1984.

OTHER NAMES   Glutathione *S*-alkyltransferase, glutathione *S*-aryltransferase, glutathione *S*-transferase, *S*-(hydroxyalkyl)-glutathione lyase, glutathione *S*-aralkyltransferase

REACTION   RX + glutathione-SH = HX + glutathione-*S-R*

ENZYME SOURCE   Bacteria, fungi, plants, invertebrates, vertebrates

## METHOD 1

### Visualization Scheme

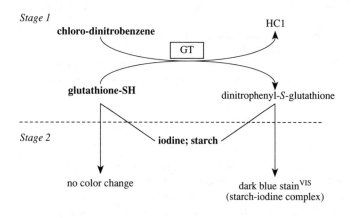

### Staining Solution[1]

A. 0.1 *M* Sodium phosphate buffer, pH 6.5     20 ml
   1-Chloro-2,4-dinitrobenzene (dissolved in   8 mg
     0.8 ml ethanol)
   Reduced glutathione               14 mg
B. 1.0% $I_2$ in 1.0% KI            0.9 ml
   $H_2O$                        30 ml
C. 2% Agar solution (60°C)        30 ml

### Procedure

Saturate a filter paper with solution A and place it on the cut surface of electrophorized starch gel or PAG containing 0.04% (w/v) of soluble starch. Take care to avoid the formation of air bubbles between paper overlay and gel. Incubate overlayed gel at 37°C for 40 min. Remove the paper sheet. Mix solutions B and C and apply the mixture to the gel surface. Intense blue color appears immediately in areas where reduced glutathione has been conjugated to 1-chloro-2,4-dinitrobenzene by the action of GT. Record or photograph the zymogram.

## METHOD 2

### Visualization Scheme

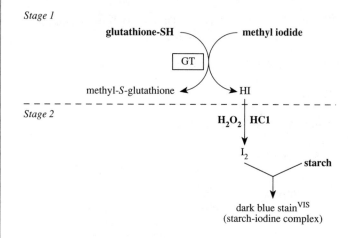

### Staining Solution[2]

A. 0.1 *M* Potassium phosphate buffer, pH 7.0
   7 m*M* Methyl iodide
   6 m*M* Reduced glutathione
B. 0.3 *M* HCl
   0.3% $H_2O_2$

### Procedure

Preincubate electrophorized PAG containing 0.04% (w/v) soluble starch in two changes of 0.1 *M* potassium phosphate buffer, pH 7.0, for 10 min at room temperature with gentle agitation. Then place gel in solution A and incubate at 37°C for periods of from 6 to 20 min with periodic agitation. At the end of the incubation period transfer gel to solution B. Keep the gel under observation until blue bands indicating the local formation of iodine are observed. The bands appear abruptly following a lag period, the length of which depends on the amount of GT catalytic activity present. When the bands are well developed record or photograph the zymogram quickly. After full development, the bands retain their definition for 2 to 3 h and then fade.

*Notes:*   2 m*M* 1,3-Dinitro-4-iodobenzene (IDNB) can be used as substrate instead of methyl iodide. To increase the solubility of IDNB, 0.33 vol of glycerol should be added to 0.1 *M* potassium phosphate buffer, pH 7.0, containing 1.67 m*M* reduced glutathione.

## METHOD 3

### Visualization Scheme

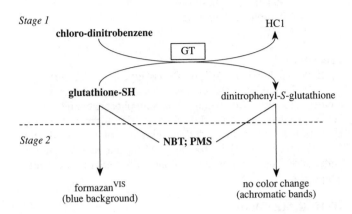

*Stage 1*

chloro-dinitrobenzene

HCl

GT

glutathione-SH

dinitrophenyl-*S*-glutathione

*Stage 2*

NBT; PMS

formazan<sup>VIS</sup>
(blue background)

no color change
(achromatic bands)

### Staining Solution[3]

A. 0.1 *M* Potassium phosphate buffer, pH 6.5
   4.5 m*M* Reduced glutathione
   1 m*M* 1-Chloro-2,4-dinitrobenzene
   1 m*M* NBT

B. 0.1 *M* Tris–HCl buffer, pH 9.6
   3 m*M* PMS

### Procedure

Incubate electrophorized PAG in solution A at 37°C for 10 min under gentle agitation. Wash gel with water and incubate in solution B at room temperature. Blue insoluble formazan appears on the gel surface in about 3 to 5 min, except in the GT areas. Wash negatively stained gel with water and place in 1 *M* NaCl. Under these conditions the achromatic bands remain clearly visible for almost 1 month.

*Notes:* Artifactual achromatic bands, perhaps due to superoxide dismutase (see 1.15.1.1 — SOD), can be observed on gels stained using this method. These artifactual bands do not impair the method since they can be easily identified by comparing the test gel with a control gel incubated with all reagents except chloro-dinitrobenzene.

### REFERENCES

1. Board, P. G., A method for the localization of glutathione *S*-transferase isozymes after starch gel electrophoresis, *Anal. Biochem.*, 105, 147, 1980.
2. Clark, A. G., A direct method for the visualization of glutathione *S*-transferase activity in polyacrylamide gels, *Anal. Biochem.*, 123, 147, 1982.
3. Ricci, G., Bello, M. L., Caccuri, A. M., Galiazzo, F., and Federici, G., Detection of glutathione transferase activity on polyacrylamide gels, *Anal. Biochem.*, 143, 226, 1984.

OTHER NAMES    3-Phosphoshikimate 1-carboxyvinyltransferase (recommended name)

REACTION    Phosphoenolpyruvate + shikimate-5-phosphate = orthophosphate + 3-enol-pyruvoylshikimate-5-phosphate

ENZYME SOURCE   Bacteria, fungi

## METHOD

### Visualization Scheme

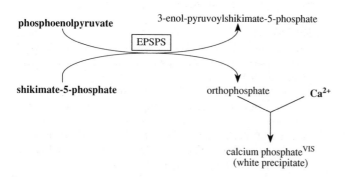

## Staining Solution[1]

50 m$M$ Glycine–KOH buffer, pH 10.0
1 m$M$ Shikimate-5-phosphate
2 m$M$ Phosphoenolpyruvate
10 m$M$ $Ca^{2+}$

## Procedure

Soak electrophorized PAG in 50 m$M$ glycine–KOH buffer, pH 10.0, for 20 to 30 min and incubate in a staining solution at room temperature until white bands of calcium phosphate precipitation become visible against a dark background. Photograph stained gel by reflected light against a dark background. Store stained gel in 50 m$M$ glycine–KOH buffer, pH 10.0, containing 5 m$M$ $Ca^{2+}$ either at 5°C or in the presence of an antibacterial agent at room temperature.

## OTHER METHODS

The product orthophosphate may be detected using some other histochemical Methods (e.g., see 3.6.1.1 — PP).

## REFERENCE

1. Nimmo, H. G. and Nimmo, G. A., A general method for the localization of enzymes that produce phosphate, pyrophosphate, or $CO_2$ after polyacrylamide gel electrophoresis, *Anal. Biochem.*, 121, 17, 1982.

OTHER NAMES    Aspartate aminotransferase (recommended name), glutamic–aspartic transaminase, transaminase A

REACTION    L-Aspartate + 2-oxoglutarate = oxaloacetate + L-glutamate

ENZYME SOURCE    Bacteria, fungi, plants, protozoa, invertebrates, vertebrates

## METHOD 1

### Visualization Scheme

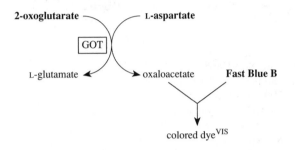

### Staining Solution[1] (modified)

| | |
|---|---:|
| 0.05 $M$ Tris–HCl buffer, pH 7.5 | 100 ml |
| L-Aspartic acid (monosodium salt) | 400 mg |
| 2-Oxoglutaric acid (disodium salt) | 180 mg |
| Fast Blue B salt | 150 mg |

### Procedure

Incubate the gel in staining solution in the dark at 37°C until dark brown bands appear. Wash gel in water and fix in 50% glycerol or in water solution of reduced glutathione.

*Notes:* Some authors recommend including cofactor pyridoxal 5-phosphate in the staining solution. Usually, there is no need to do this because native GOT molecules contain sufficient amounts of tightly bound pyridoxal 5-phosphate molecules.

Fast Violet B, Fast Blue BB, and Fast Garnet GBC may be used instead of Fast Blue B.

Where enzyme activity is low, greater sensitivity of the Method may be obtained using a post-coupling technique. When using this technique, apply all necessary ingredients except a diazo dye to the gel in the normal manner. Incubate the gel for a period of time (depending upon the expected activity of the enzyme) and then add a diazo dye dissolved in a minimal volume of staining buffer.

## METHOD 2

### Visualization Scheme

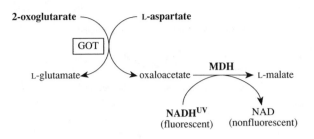

### Staining Solution[2] (modified)

| | |
|---|---:|
| A. 0.1 $M$ Sodium phosphate buffer, pH 7.5 | 25 ml |
| L-Aspartic acid (monosodium salt) | 200 mg |
| 2-Oxoglutaric acid (disodium salt) | 90 mg |
| Malate dehydrogenase (MDH) | 60 units |
| NADH | 7 mg |
| B. 1.5% Agar solution (60°C) | 25 ml |

### Procedure

Mix A and B components of the staining solution and pour the mixture over the surface of the gel. Incubate the gel at 37°C for 20 to 60 min and monitor under long-wave UV light. The zones of GOT activity appear as dark (nonfluorescent) bands on a light (fluorescent) background. Record the zymogram or photograph using a yellow filter.

*Notes:* When a zymogram that is visible in daylight is required, counterstain the processed gel with MTT/PMS solution. Achromatic bands of GOT appear almost immediately.

## METHOD 3

### Visualization Scheme

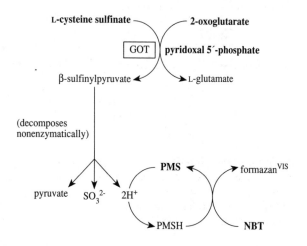

### Staining Solution[3]

500 µM Tris–HCl buffer, pH 8.5
250 µM L-Cysteine sulfinate
25 µM 2-Oxoglutarate
0.5 µM Pyridoxal 5′-phosphate
0.4 mg/ml NBT
0.1 mg/ml PMS

### Procedure

Incubate the gel in staining solution in the dark at 37°C until dark blue bands appear. Wash gel in water and fix in 3% acetic acid or 50% ethanol.

*Notes:* This method is based on the cysteine sulfinate transamination activity of GOT. The method is highly sensitive. It is capable of detecting 0.3 milliunits per band of GOT activity. It is difficult to detect such a low level of activity on the gel by any of the other methods except Method 4 (see below).

## METHOD 4

### Visualization Scheme

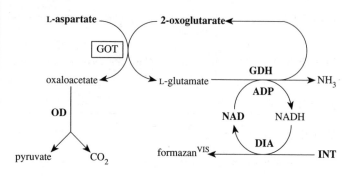

### Staining Solution[4]

A.  180 mM Tris–HCl buffer, pH 8.1
    20 mM L-Aspartate
    10 mM 2-Oxoglutarate
    4 mM ADP
B.  80 mM NAD
C.  30 mM Iodonitrotetrazolium Violet (INT)
D.  100 mM Tris–HCl buffer, pH 7.5
    9.8 U/ml Diaphorase (DIA)
E.  1200 U/ml Glutamate dehydrogenase (GDH) in 50% glycerol
F.  125 U/ml Oxaloacetate decarboxylase (OD) in 100 mM Tris–HCl buffer, pH 7.5
G.  2% Agarose solution (45°C) in 100 mM tris–HCl buffer, pH 7.5

### Procedure

Mix 5 ml of solution A with 1 ml each of solutions B through F and incubate in the dark at 37°C for 15 min. Add this mixture to 10 ml of solution G and pour the mixture over the surface of the gel. Incubate the gel in the dark at 37°C until pink bands appear. Fix gel in 5% acetic acid.

*Notes:* This method is suitable for quantitative detection of GOT isoenzymes. Product inhibition of GOT isozymes (especially mitochondrial isozyme) by oxaloacetate is prevented by oxaloacetate decarboxylase, which is included in the stain. GOT activity as low as 30 µU per band can be quantitated by incubating the gel overnight at room temperature in the dark. Pyruvate kinase (EC 2.7.1.40) has been reported to have decarboxylase activity and perhaps can be used instead of oxaloacetate decarboxylase to remove the excess of oxaloacetate.

This method is the most expensive in comparison with the other three described above.

### REFERENCES

1.  Decker, L. E. and Rau, E. M., Multiple forms of glutamic–oxalacetic transaminase in tissues, *Proc. Soc. Exp. Biol. Med.*, 112, 144, 1963.
2.  Boyd, J. W., The extraction and purification of two isoenzymes of L-aspartate:2-oxoglutarate aminotransferase, *Biochim. Biophys. Acta*, 113, 302, 1966.
3.  Yagi, T., Kagamiyama, H., and Nozaki, M., A sensitive method for the detection of aspartate:2-oxoglutarate aminotransferase activity on polyacrylamide gels, *Anal. Biochem.*, 110, 146, 1981.
4.  Nealon, D. A. and Rej, R., Quantitation of aspartate aminotransferase isoenzymes after electrophoretic separation, *Anal. Biochem.*, 161, 64, 1987.

OTHER NAMES    Alanine aminotransferase (recommended name), glutamic–alanine transaminase, alanine transaminase

REACTION    L-Alanine + 2-oxoglutarate = pyruvate + L-glutamate

ENZYME SOURCE    Bacteria, fungi, plants, protozoa, invertebrates, vertebrates

## METHOD 1

### Visualization Scheme

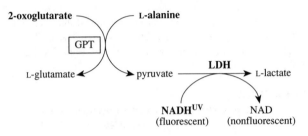

### Staining Solution[1]

| | |
|---|---|
| 0.1 *M* Tris–HCl buffer, pH 7.6 | 10 ml |
| L-α-Alanine | 178 mg |
| 2-Oxoglutaric acid | 13 mg |
| NADH | 7 mg |
| Lactate dehydrogenase (LDH) | 8 units |

### Procedure

Apply the staining solution to gel on filter-paper overlay and, after incubation at 37°C for 30 to 60 min, view gel under long-wave UV light. Dark (nonfluorescent) bands of GPT activity are visible on a light (fluorescent) background. Photograph developed gel through a yellow filter. Nonfluorescent GPT bands may be made visible in daylight (achromatic bands on a blue background) after treating the processed gel with MTT/PMS solution.

*Notes:*    When LDH suspension in $(NH_4)_2SO_4$ is used, glutamate dehydrogenase activity bands can also develop on a GPT zymogram obtained by this method. Thus, the use of $NH_3$-free preparations of LDH is recommended in this method.

## METHOD 2

### Visualization Scheme

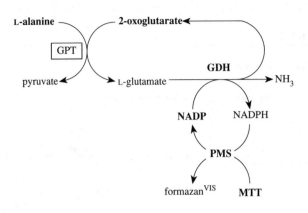

### Staining Solution[2]

| | | |
|---|---|---|
| A. | 0.2 *M* Tris–HCl buffer, pH 8.0 | 10 ml |
| | 400 mg/ml L-Alanine | 5 ml |
| | 40 mg/ml 2-Oxoglutarate | 2.5 ml |
| | 10 mg/ml NADP | 0.5 ml |
| | Glutamate dehydrogenase (GDH) | 90 units |
| | 10 mg/ml MTT | 0.5 ml |
| | 2.5 mg/ml PMS | 0.5 ml |
| | 65 mg/ml KCN | 0.5 ml |
| B. | 0.15% Agar solution (60°C) | 10 ml |

### Procedure

Mix A and B components of the staining solution, pour the mixture over the surface of the gel and allow to solidify. Incubate the gel in the dark at 37°C until dark blue bands appear. Fix stained gel in 50% ethanol.

*Notes:*    The linking enzyme, glutamate dehydrogenase (EC 1.4.1.3), also works well with NAD as cofactor. The use of NAD instead of NADP is preferable because NAD is several times cheaper than NADP.

ADP may be included in the staining solution to stimulate the coupled reaction catalyzed by GDH (e.g., see 2.6.1.1 — GOT, Method 4).

### REFERENCES

1. Chen, S.-H. and Giblett, E. R., Polymorphism of soluble glutamic–pyruvic transaminase: a new genetic marker in man, *Science*, 173, 148, 1971.
2. Eicher, E. M. and Womack, J. E., Chromosomal location of soluble glutamic–pyruvic transaminase-1 (*Gpt-1*) in the mouse, *Biochem. Genet.*, 15, 1, 1977.

REACTION           L-Tyrosine + 2-oxoglutarate =
                   4-hydroxyphenylpyruvate + L-glutamate

ENZYME SOURCE  Bacteria, protozoa, invertebrates, vertebrates

## METHOD

### Visualization Scheme

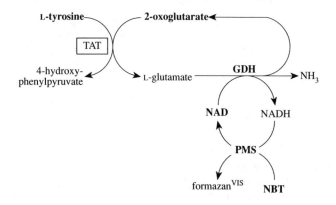

### Staining Solution[1]

| | |
|---|---:|
| 0.1 *M* Sodium phosphate buffer, pH 7.0 | 50 ml |
| NBT | 30 mg |
| PMS | 2 mg |
| NAD | 50 mg |
| 10 mg/ml 2-Oxoglutaric acid (neutralized) | 10 ml |
| L-Tyrosine | 100 mg |
| Glutamate dehydrogenase (GDH) | 16 units |
| $H_2O$ | 30 ml |

### Procedure

Incubate the gel in staining solution in the dark at 37°C until dark blue bands appear. Wash gel in water and fix in 50% ethanol.

*Notes:*   ADP may be added to the staining solution to stimulate a coupled reaction catalyzed by GDH (e.g., see 2.6.1.1 — GOT, Method 4).

The mitochondrial isozyme of TAT may be identical to EC 2.6.1.1 (GOT).

### REFERENCE

1. Shaw, C. R. and Prasad, R., Starch gel electrophoresis of enzymes: a compilation of recipes, *Biochem. Genet.*, 4, 297, 1970.

OTHER NAMES     L-Ornithine aminotransferase

REACTION     L-Ornithine + 2-oxo acid = L-glutamate 5-semialdehyde + L-amino acid

ENZYME SOURCE   Fungi, vertebrates

## METHOD 1

### Visualization Scheme

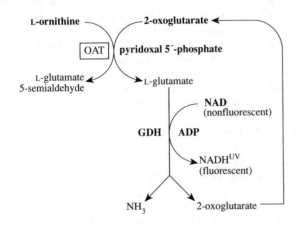

### Staining Solution[1] (adapted)

A. 100 mM Tris–HCl buffer, pH 8.0
   0.1 mM Pyridoxal 5′-phosphate
   0.1 mM ADP
   2 mM NAD
   2 mM 2-Oxoglutarate
   10 mM L-Ornithine
   20 U/ml Glutamate dehydrogenase (GDH)
B. 2% Agarose solution (60°C)

### Procedure

Mix equal volumes of A and B components of the staining solution and pour the mixture over the surface of the gel. Incubate the gel at 37°C for 30 min and view under long-wave UV light. Light (fluorescent) bands of OAT are visible on a dark (nonfluorescent) background of the gel. Record the zymogram or photograph using a yellow filter.

*Notes:* MTT and PMS may be added to the staining solution to obtain OAT zymograms visible in daylight.

## METHOD 2

### Visualization Scheme

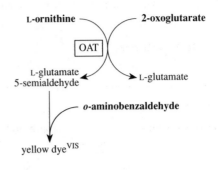

### Staining Solution[2]

A. 0.1 M Potassium phosphate buffer, pH 8.15
   50 mM L-Ornithine
   25 mM 2-Oxoglutarate
   0.1% o-Aminobenzaldehyde
B. 3% Agar solution (60°C)

### Procedure

Mix 19 ml of solution A with 5 ml of solution B and pour the mixture over the surface of the gel. Incubate the gel at 30°C until yellow bands appear. Record the zymogram or photograph by contact printing on a photographic paper placed under the stained agar overlay with a photographic enlarger lamp as a light source.

## GENERAL NOTES

OAT is a mitochondrial enzyme. To prepare a mitochondrial extract for electrophoresis, the mitochondrial fraction should be isolated and suspended in an appropriate buffer at a concentration of 30% with respect to the original tissue weight. After sonication the mitochondrial suspension should be centrifuged at 100,000 g for 1 h. The supernatant may be used for electrophoresis.

## REFERENCES

1. Akabayashi, A. and Kato, T., One-step and two-step fluorometric assay methods for general aminotransferases using glutamate dehydrogenase, *Anal. Biochem.*, 182, 129, 1989.
2. Yanagi, S., Tsutsumi, T., Saheki, S., Saheki, K., and Yamamoto, N., Novel and sensitive activity stains on polyacrylamide gel of serine and threonine dehydratase and ornithine aminotransferase, *Enzyme*, 28, 400, 1982.

OTHER NAMES    Glutaminase II, glutamine transaminase, glutamine–oxoacid transaminase

REACTION    L-Glutamine + pyruvate = 2-oxoglutaramate + L-alanine

ENZYME SOURCE  Vertebrates

## METHOD

### Visualization Scheme

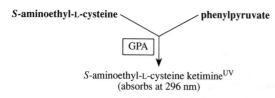

S-aminoethyl-L-cysteine ketimine$^{UV}$
(absorbs at 296 nm)

### Reaction Mixture[1]
0.1 M Pyrophosphate buffer, pH 8.5
20 mM S-2-Aminoethyl-L-cysteine
0.4 mM Phenylpyruvate

### Procedure
Incubate electrophorized PAG in reaction mixture at 20°C for 30 min. Wash gel with water and scan at 296 nm using a scanning spectrophotometer. Sharp peaks on the photometric scan correspond to GPA bands on PAG.

*Notes:*   The method is based on the ability of GPA to act on S-aminoethyl-L-cysteine (as well as on L-cystathionine, L-methionine, and other sulfur compounds) in the presence of a number of keto acids, including phenylpyruvate.

The use of borate-containing buffers should be avoided because of the strong absorbance of phenylpyruvate enol-borate complex at 300 nm.

Using an optical instrument constructed for two-dimensional spectroscopy of electrophoretic gels[2] and interference filter with peak transmission wavelength near 296 nm a photocopy of the GPA zymogram can be made.

## OTHER METHODS

A. Zymograms of GPA visible in daylight can be obtained using auxiliary alanine dehydrogenase (see 1.4.1.1 — ALADH) to detect the product L-alanine. The recommended staining solution should include L-glutamine, pyruvate, NAD, alanine dehydrogenase, MTT (or NBT), PMS, and pyrophosphate buffer, pH 8.5.

B. An auxiliary enzyme, alanopine dehydrogenase (see 1.5.1.17 — ALPD), can also be used to detect the product L-alanine. Staining solution recommended for the trial should include L-glutamine, pyruvate, NADH, and ALPD. Dark GPA bands will be visible in long-wave UV light on the fluorescent background of the gel. This method, however, has two obvious disadvantages: (1) the ALPD preparations are not yet commercially available and (2) the control staining of an additional gel for lactate dehydrogenase is necessary. Nevertheless, when ALPD preparations are available, this method will be more appropriate for routine laboratory use than the spectrophotometric method described above.

## REFERENCES
1. Ricci, G., Caccuri, A. M., Bello, M. L., Solinas, S. P., and Nardini, M., Ketimine rings: useful detectors of enzymatic activities in solution and on polyacrylamide gel, *Anal. Biochem.*, 165, 356, 1987.
2. Klebe, R. J., Mancuso, M. G., Brown, C. R., and Teng, L., Two-dimensional spectroscopy of electrophoretic gels, *Biochem. Genet.*, 19, 655, 1981.

OTHER NAMES     γ-Aminobutyric acid transaminase, β-Alanine–oxoglutarate aminotransferase

REACTION     4-Aminobutyrate + 2-oxoglutarate = succinate semialdehyde + L-glutamate

ENZYME SOURCE  Bacteria, vertebrates

## METHOD 1

### Visualization Scheme

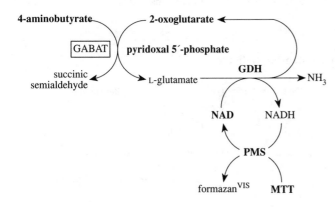

### Staining Solution[1]

A. 0.5 $M$ Tris–HCl buffer, pH 7.5     25 ml
    4-Aminobutyric acid     250 mg
    NAD     20 mg
    Glutamate dehydrogenase (GDH)     50 units
    0.1 $M$ 2-Oxoglutaric acid (neutralized)     0.4 ml
    5 mg/ml MTT     1 ml
    5 mg/ml PMS     1 ml
B. 1.5% Agar solution (60°C)     25 ml

### Procedure

Mix A and B components of the staining solution and pour the mixture over the surface of the gel. Incubate the gel in the dark at 37°C until dark blue bands appear. Fix stained gel in 50% ethanol.

*Notes:* When the enzyme from mammalian tissues is detected, β-alanine may be used instead of 4-aminobutyric acid. The cofactor pyridoxal 5′-phosphate is recommended to be included in starch gel after degassing (final concentration 3 m$M$) and to cathode buffer compartment (final concentration 0.4 m$M$). A small amount of pyruvate may be added to the staining solution to inhibit lactate dehydrogenase activity.

## METHOD 2

### Visualization Scheme

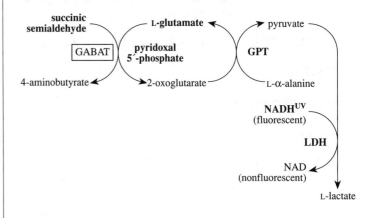

### Staining Solution[1]

    0.5 $M$ Tris–HCl buffer, pH 7.5     10 ml
    Succinic semialdehyde     0.1 ml
    L-Glutamic acid     20 mg
    D,L-α-Alanine     100 mg
    Glutamic–pyruvic transaminase (GPT)     80 units
    Lactate dehydrogenase (LDH)     150 units
    NADH     20 mg

### Procedure

Soak a piece of filter paper in a staining solution and apply to the gel surface. Wrap gel in Saran wrap and incubate at 37°C for 30 to 60 min. View gel under long-wave UV light. Dark (nonfluorescent) bands of GABAT activity are visible on a light (fluorescent) background. Record the zymogram or photograph using a yellow filter.

*Notes:* When a zymogram that is visible in daylight is required, counterstain the processed gel with MTT/PMS solution. Achromatic bands of GABAT activity appear on a blue background almost immediately.

    The cofactor pyridoxal 5′-phosphate is recommended to be added to starch gel after degassing (final concentration 3 m$M$) and to cathodal buffer (final concentration 0.4 m$M$).

### REFERENCE

1. Jeremiah, S. and Povey, S., The biochemical genetics of human γ-aminobutyric acid transaminase, *Ann. Hum. Genet.*, 45, 231, 1981.

## 2.6.1.42 — Branched-Chain Amino Acid Aminotransferase; BCT

OTHER NAMES    Transaminase B

REACTION    L-Leucine + 2-oxoglutarate = 2-oxoisocaproate + L-glutamate

ENZYME SOURCE    Bacteria, plants, invertebrates, vertebrates

## METHOD

### Visualization Scheme

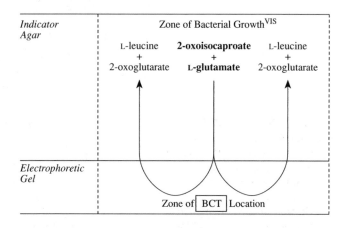

### Indicator Agar[1]

1.5% indicator agar containing 100 µg/ml 2-oxoisocaproate, 100 µg/ml pyridoxal 5′-phosphate, and $10^8$ bacteria/ml of *P. cerevisiae* ATCC 8081 in citrate medium (for details see Appendix A-2) containing L-glutamate and lacking L-leucine.

### Procedure

Prepare indicator agar and pour it onto a sterile plate of appropriate size. After the bacteria-seeded indicator agar solidifies, a slice of electrophoretic starch gel (cut surface down), cellulose acetate strip, or PAG is laid over the agar in order to expose the indicator agar to the enzyme (BCT) entrapped in the electrophoretic gel. The gel is applied to the indicator agar avoiding the formation of air bubbles. L-Leucine should be spotted at one corner of the indicator agar as a control of bacterial proliferation. The bands of bacterial growth become visible in transmitted light after 6 to 12 h of incubation at 37°C. The origin and slot locations should be marked on the indicator agar before the electrophoretic gel is removed.

### REFERENCE

1. Naylor, S. L. and Klebe, R. J., Bioautography: a general method for the visualization of isozymes, *Biochem. Genet.*, 15, 1193, 1977.

## 2.6.1.64 — Glutamine Transaminase K; GTK

OTHER NAMES    Glutamine–phenylpyruvate aminotransferase (recommended name), glutamine transaminase from kidney

REACTION    Broad specificity. The enzyme is active with glutamine, methionine, phenylalanine, tyrosine, cystine, and the corresponding α-keto acids. It may be regarded as a fully reversible glutamine (methionine) aromatic amino acid aminotransferase.

ENZYME SOURCE    Vertebrates (mammals)

## METHOD

### Visualization Scheme

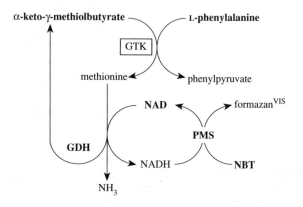

### Staining Solution[1]

0.1 *M* Potassium phosphate buffer, pH 7.2
0.02 *M* L-Phenylalanine
0.005 *M* α-Keto-γ-methiolbutyrate
0.032 *M* NAD
0.1 m*M* PMS
1 m*M* NBT
12 U/ml Glutamate dehydrogenase from bovine liver (GDH)

### Procedure

Wash electrophorized PAG twice with distilled water and incubate in a staining solution in the dark at 37°C until dark blue bands appear. Fix stained gel in 50% ethanol.

*Notes:*    This method is based on the ability of an auxiliary enzyme, glutamate dehydrogenase (EC 1.4.1.3), to exhibit catalytic activity towards methionine.

The cytosolic enzyme from rat kidney was shown to be identical with cytosolic cysteine conjugate β-lyase (see 4.4.1.13 — CCL) from the same source.[2]

### REFERENCES

1. Abraham, D. G. and Cooper, A. J. L., Glutamine transaminase K and cysteine S-conjugate β-lyase activity stains, *Anal. Biochem.*, 197, 421, 1991.
2. Cooper, A. J. L. and Anders, M. W., Glutamine transaminase K and cysteine conjugate β-lyase, *Ann. NY Acad. Sci.*, 585, 118, 1990.

| OTHER NAMES | Glucokinase |
|---|---|
| REACTION | ATP + D-hexose = ADP + D-hexose 6-phosphate |
| ENZYME SOURCE | Bacteria, green algae, fungi, plants, protozoa, invertebrates, vertebrates |

## METHOD

### Visualization Scheme

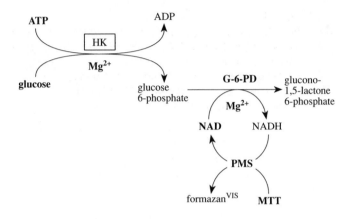

### Staining Solution[1] (modified)

A. 0.1 $M$ Tris–HCl buffer, pH 7.8 .......... 25 ml
   D-Glucose .......... 50 mg
   ATP (disodium salt) .......... 30 mg
   NAD .......... 15 mg
   MTT .......... 5 mg
   PMS .......... 1 mg
   MgCl$_2$·6H$_2$O .......... 10 mg
   Glucose-6-phosphate dehydrogenase (G-6-PD; NAD-dependent; Sigma G5760 or G5885) .......... 20 units
B. 2% Agarose solution (60°C) .......... 25 ml

## Procedure

Mix A and B components of the staining solution and pour the mixture over the surface of the gel. Incubate the gel in the dark at 37°C until dark blue bands appear. Fix stained gel in 50% ethanol.

*Notes:* D-Mannose, D-fructose, and D-glucosamine also can act as acceptors; ITP can act as a donor.

The enzyme from microorganisms and some invertebrates is known as glucokinase (EC 2.7.1.2). It is highly specific for glucose. The HK isozyme from mammalian liver also has sometimes been called glucokinase. Final glucose concentrations of 1 m$M$ and 100 m$M$ are usually used to identify hexokinase and glucokinase isozymes, respectively.[2,3]

When NADP-dependent G-6-PD is used as a linking enzyme, NADP should be substituted for NAD in the staining solution. However, the use of NAD-dependent G-6-PD results in a cost saving because NAD is several times cheaper than NADP.

When high concentrations of glucose are used in the staining solution, the bands of glucose oxidase (see 1.1.3.4 — GO) and glucose dehydrogenase (see 1.1.1.47 — GD) can sometimes also be developed on hexokinase zymograms.

## REFERENCES

1. Eaton, G. M., Brewer, G. J., and Tashian, R. E., Hexokinase isozyme patterns of human erythrocytes and leukocytes, *Nature*, 212, 944, 1966.
2. Harris, H. and Hopkinson, D. A., *Handbook of Enzyme Electrophoresis in Human Genetics*, North-Holland, Amsterdam (Loose leaf with supplements in 1977 and 1978), 1976.
3. Richardson, B. J., Baverstock, P. R., and Adams, M., *Allozyme Electrophoresis: A Handbook for Animal Systematics and Population Studies*, Academic Press, Sydney, 1986, 198.

REACTION          ATP + D-fructose = ADP + D-fructose 6-phosphate

ENZYME SOURCE   Plants, invertebrates

## METHOD

### Visualization Scheme

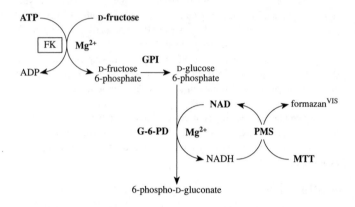

### Staining Solution[1] (modified)

A. 0.1 $M$ Tris–HCl buffer, pH 7.8     25 ml
    D-Fructose     100 mg
    ATP     50 mg
    NAD     20 mg
    MTT     7 mg
    PMS     1 mg
    $MgCl_2 \cdot 6H_2O$     10 mg
    Glucose-6-phosphate isomerase (GPI)     20 units
    Glucose-6-phosphate dehydrogenase (G-6-PD;     20 units
      NAD-dependent; Sigma G5760 or G5885)
B. 2% Agarose solution (60°C)     25 ml

## Procedure

Mix A and B components of the staining solution and pour the mixture over the surface of the gel. Incubate the gel in the dark at 37°C until dark blue bands appear. Fix stained gel in 50% ethanol.

*Notes:* In mushrooms and invertebrates this enzyme is perhaps identical to hexokinase (2.7.1.1 — HK). Identical allozymic patterns were observed on FK and HK zymograms in mushrooms, nemerteans, sea urchins, sea stars, and insects.[2] Some FK isozymes, however, are specific for fructose and are not active with glucose. Such a fructose-specific isozyme was found, for example, in the nemertean *Tetrastemma nigrifrons*.[3]

## REFERENCES

1. Jelnes, J. E., Identification of hexokinases and localization of a fructokinase and tetrazolium oxidase locus in *Drosophila melanogaster, Hereditas*, 67, 291, 1971.
2. Manchenko, G. P., The use of allozyme patterns in genetic identification of enzymes, *Isozyme Bull.*, 23, 102, 1990.
3. Manchenko, G. P., unpublished data, 1990.

REACTION      ATP + D-galactose = ADP + α-D-galactose 1-phosphate

ENZYME SOURCE   Bacteria, fungi, protozoa, vertebrates

## METHOD 1

### Visualization Scheme

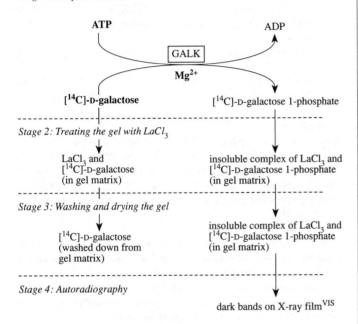

*Stage 1: Enzyme reaction*

*Stage 2: Treating the gel with LaCl₃*

*Stage 3: Washing and drying the gel*

*Stage 4: Autoradiography*

### Reaction Mixture[1]

A.   0.2 *M* Tris–HCl buffer, pH 7.2
     3.61 m*M* ATP
     7.84 m*M* MgCl₂
B.   [¹⁴C] = D-Galactose (specific activity 45 to 50 mCi/mmol)
C.   0.1 *M* Tris–HCl buffer, pH 7.0
     0.1 *M* LaCl₃

### Procedure

*Stage 1.*   Add 50 µl of B to 15 ml of A. Incubate the gel in resultant mixture at 37°C for 1 to 2 h.

*Stage 2.*   After incubation place gel in solution C and expose at 4°C for 6 h.

*Stage 3.*   Wash gel for 3 h in distilled water. Dry the gel.

*Stage 4.*   Autoradiograph dry gel with X-ray film (Kodak Blue Brand BB-54) for 1 to 2 weeks. Develop exposed X-ray film.

Dark bands on developed X-ray film correspond to localization of GALK activity in the gel.

## METHOD 2

### Visualization Scheme

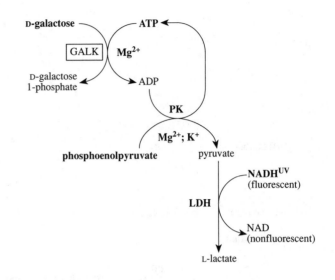

### Staining Solution*

| | |
|---|---:|
| 0.1 *M* Tris–HCl buffer, pH 7.5 | 5 ml |
| ATP | 10 mg |
| D-Galactose | 15 mg |
| KCl | 1.5 mg |
| MgCl₂·6H₂O | 2 mg |
| NADH | 3.5 mg |
| Pyruvate kinase (PK) | 40 units |
| Lactate dehydrogenase (LDH) | 30 units |
| Phosphoenolpyruvate | 10 mg |

### Procedure

Apply the staining solution to the gel surface on filter-paper overlay. Incubate the gel at 37°C for 30 to 60 min and view under long-wave UV light. Dark (nonfluorescent) bands of GALK are visible on a light (fluorescent) background. Record the zymogram or photograph using a yellow filter.

*Notes:*   When a final zymogram that is visible in daylight is required, counterstain the processed gel with MTT/PMS solution. Achromatic bands of GALK activity appear on a blue background. Wash negatively stained gel in water and fix in 50% ethanol.

Two additional gels should be stained for phosphoenolpyruvate phosphatase (see 3.1.3.18 — PGP, Method 2) and ATPase (see 3.6.1.3 — ATPASE) activities, which can also be developed by this method.

---

\*   New; recommended for use.

## METHOD 3

### Visualization Scheme

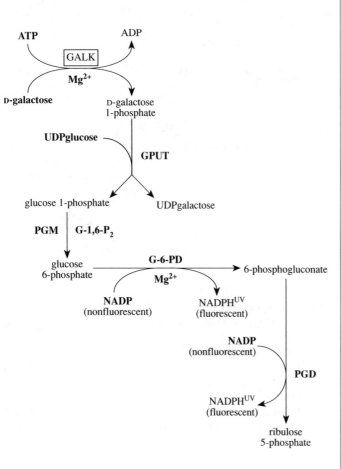

### Staining Solution[2]

A.  1 *M* Tris–HCl buffer, pH 8.0                                          1.5 ml
     7.2 mg/ml D-Galactose                                                0.1 ml
     182 mg/ml ATP (disodium salt)                                        0.2 ml
     8 mg/ml UDPglucose (disodium salt)                                   0.75 ml
     1.4 mg/ml Glucose-1,6-diphosphate (G-1,6-P$_2$;                       75 µl
     tetracyclohexylammonium salt, 4H$_2$O)
     8 mg/ml MgCl$_2$·6H$_2$O                                             0.75 ml
     16 mg/ml NADP (disodium salt)                                        0.75 ml
     20 U/mg Galactose-1-phosphate uridyl                                 0.2 mg
     transferase (GPUT)
     2000 U/ml Phosphoglucomutase (PGM)                                   30 µl
     700 U/ml Glucose-6-phosphate dehydrogenase                           60 µl
     (G-6-PD)
     120 U/ml Phosphogluconate dehydrogenase                              30 µl
     (PGD)
     10 µl/ml 2-Mercaptoethanol                                           0.75 ml
B.  1% Agar solution (60°C)                                               5 ml

### Procedure

Mix A and B components of the staining solution and pour the mixture over the surface of the gel. Incubate the gel at 37°C for 30 to 60 min and monitor under long-wave UV light. Light (fluorescent) bands of GALK activity appear on a dark (nonfluorescent) background of the gel. Record the zymogram or photograph using a yellow filter.

*Notes:*  Phosphogluconate dehydrogenase is included in the staining solution to obtain additional reduction of NADP to NADPH and so enhance the sensitivity of the method.

When preparations with high activity of GALK are used for electrophoresis, phosphogluconate dehydrogenase may be omitted from the staining solution. This will allow the use of NAD-dependent glucose-6-phosphate dehydrogenase (Sigma; G 5760 or 5885) instead of the NADP-dependent form of the enzyme and NAD instead of NADP.

### REFERENCES

1.  Nichols, E. A., Elsevier, S. M., and Ruddle, F. H., A new electrophoretic technique for mouse, human and chinese hamster galactokinase, *Cytogenet. Cell Genet.*, 13, 275, 1974.
2.  Harris, H. and Hopkinson, D. A., *Handbook of Enzyme Electrophoresis in Human Genetics*, North-Holland, Amsterdam (Loose leaf with supplements in 1977 and 1978), 1976.

REACTION      ATP + D-mannose = ADP + D-mannose 6-phosphate

ENZYME SOURCE   Bacteria, invertebrates

## METHOD

### Visualization Scheme

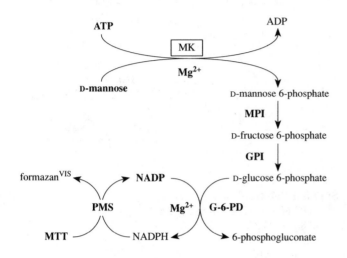

### Staining Solution[1]

A. 60 m$M$ Tris–HCl buffer, pH 8.0    25 ml
   D-Mannose    100 mg
   ATP    25 mg
   NADP    2.5 mg
   MTT    2.5 mg
   PMS    1.25 mg
   Glucose-6-phosphate dehydrogenase (G-6-PD)    0.7 unit
   Glucose-6-phosphate isomerase (GPI)    7 units
   Mannose-6-phosphate isomerase (MPI)    0.4 unit
B. 2% Agarose solution containing    25 ml
   25 m$M$ MgCl$_2$ (60°C)

### Procedure

Mix A and B components of the staining solution and pour the mixture over the surface of the gel. Incubate the gel in the dark at 37°C until dark blue bands appear. Fix stained gel in 50% ethanol.

*Notes:* In *Drosophila melanogaster* MK is identical to one of the three isozymes revealed on a hexokinase (2.7.1.1 — HK) zymogram.[1]

## OTHER METHODS

Coupled reactions catalyzed by exogenous pyruvate kinase and lactate dehydrogenase can be used to detect the production of ADP by MK (e.g., see 2.7.1.6 — GALK, Method 2). Two additional gels should be stained for phosphoenolpyruvate phosphatase (see 3.1.3.18 — PGP, Method 2) and ATPase (see 3.6.1.3 — ATPASE), for which activity bands can also be developed by this method.

### REFERENCE

1. Jelnes, J. E., Identification of hexokinases and localization of a fructokinase and tetrazolium oxidase locus in *Drosophila melanogaster*, *Hereditas*, 67, 291, 1971.

| | |
|---|---|
| OTHER NAMES | Phosphofructokinase, phosphofructokinase 1 |
| REACTION | ATP + D-fructose-6-phosphate = ADP + D-fructose-1,6-bisphosphate |
| ENZYME SOURCE | Bacteria, fungi, plants, protozoa, invertebrates, vertebrates |

## METHOD 1

### Visualization Scheme

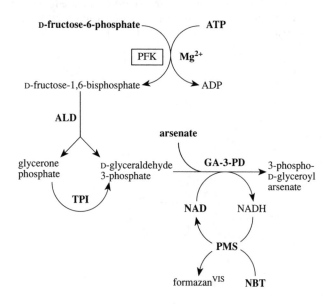

### Staining Solution[1] (modified)

| | | |
|---|---|---|
| A. | 100 m$M$ Tris–HCl buffer, pH 8.3 | 5 ml |
| | NBT | 4 mg |
| | PMS | 0.24 mg |
| | NAD | 8.6 mg |
| | MgCl$_2$ (anhydrous) | 3.8 mg |
| | ATP | 6.25 mg |
| | D-Fructose-6-phosphate (sodium salt) | 3.5 mg |
| | EDTA | 7.5 mg |
| | Triose-phosphate isomerase (TPI) | 250 units |
| | Aldolase (ALD) | 18 units |
| | Glyceraldehyde-3-phosphate dehydrogenase (GA-3-PD) | 20 units |
| | Sodium arsenate | 13 mg |
| B. | 1% Agarose solution (60°C) | 5 ml |

### Procedure

Mix A and B components of the staining solution and pour the mixture over the surface of the gel. Incubate the gel in the dark at 37°C until dark blue bands appear. Fix stained gel in 50% ethanol.

## METHOD 2

### Visualization Scheme

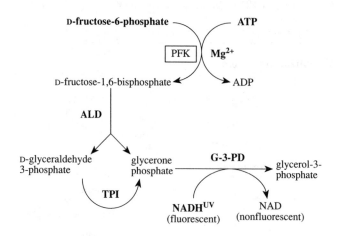

### Staining Solution[2]

0.07 $M$ Tris–HCl buffer, pH 8.1
2.8 m$M$ MgCl$_2$
1.1 m$M$ NADH
1.8 m$M$ ATP
2.2 m$M$ D-Fructose-6-phosphate
1.5 U/ml Glycerol-3-phosphate dehydrogenase (G-3-PD)
2 U/ml Aldolase (ALD)
111 U/ml Triose-phosphate isomerase (TPI)

### Procedure

Apply the staining solution to the gel surface on filter-paper overlay. Incubate the gel at 37°C and monitor under long-wave UV light. Dark (nonfluorescent) bands of PFK activity are visible on a light (fluorescent) background. Record the zymogram or photograph using a yellow filter.

*Notes:* When a zymogram that is visible in daylight is required, counterstain the processed gel with MTT/PMS solution. Achromatic bands of PFK activity become readily visible on a blue background of the gel.

## METHOD 3

### Visualization Scheme

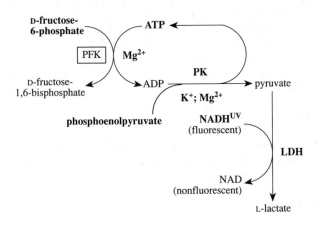

### Staining Solution*

| | |
|---|---|
| 0.1 $M$ Tris–HCl buffer, pH 8.3 | 5 ml |
| ATP (disodium salt) | 10 mg |
| D-Fructose-6-phosphate | 8 mg |
| Phosphoenolpyruvate | 7 mg |
| NADH | 3 mg |
| MgCl$_2$·6H$_2$O | 8 mg |
| KCl | 12 mg |
| Pyruvate kinase (PK) | 18 units |
| Lactate dehydrogenase (LDH) | 25 units |

### Procedure

Apply the staining solution to the gel surface on filter-paper overlay. Incubate the gel at 37°C and monitor under long-wave UV light. Dark (nonfluorescent) bands of PFK activity are visible on a light (fluorescent) background. Record the zymogram or photograph using a yellow filter. When a zymogram that is visible in daylight is required, counterstain the processed gel with MTT/PMS solution to obtain white bands of PFK activity on a blue background of the gel.

*Notes:* Stain a control gel in a staining solution lacking ATP, fructose-6-phosphate, and pyruvate kinase to identify possible bands of phosphoenolpyruvate phosphatase activity (see 3.1.3.18 — PGP, Method 2). An additional gel also should be stained for ATPase (see 3.6.1.3 — ATPASE), for which bands also can be developed by this method.

### OTHER METHODS

The immunoblotting procedure (for details see Part II) can be used for visualization of PFK on electrophoretic gels using monoclonal antibodies against the human enzyme.[3]

### REFERENCES

1. Niessner, H. and Beutler, E., Starch gel electrophoresis of phosphofructokinase in red cells, *Biochem. Med.*, 9, 73, 1974.
2. Anderson, J. E. and Giblett, E. R., Intraspecific red cell enzyme variation in the pigtailed macaque (Macaca nemestrina), *Biochem. Genet.*, 13, 189, 1975.
3. Vora, S., Wims, L. A., Durham, S., and Morrison, S. I., Production and characterization of monoclonal antibodies to the subunits of human phosphofructokinase: new tools for the immunochemical and genetic analyses of isozymes, *Blood*, 58, 823, 1981.

* New; recommended for use.

REACTION          ATP + adenosine = ADP + AMP

ENZYME SOURCE  Fungi, protozoa, invertebrates, vertebrates

## METHOD

### Visualization Scheme

*Stage 1: Enzyme reaction*

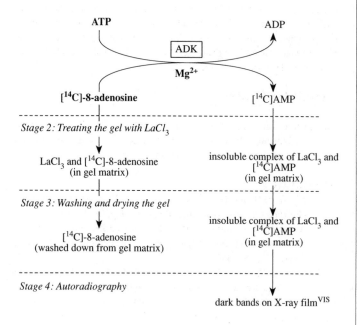

*Stage 2: Treating the gel with LaCl₃*

*Stage 3: Washing and drying the gel*

*Stage 4: Autoradiography*

### Reaction Mixture[1]

A.  20 m$M$ Potassium phosphate buffer, pH 6.2          20 ml
    ATP (disodium salt)                                                    4 mg
    MgCl$_2$ (anhydrous)                                                 1 mg
    [$^{14}$C]-8-Adenosine (40 to 60 µCi/mmol)                   5 µCi
B.  0.1 $M$ Tris–HCl buffer, pH 7.0
    0.1 $M$ LaCl$_3$

### Procedure

*Stage 1.* Incubate the gel in solution A at 37°C for 1 h.
*Stage 2.* Place gel in solution B and incubate at 4°C for 6 h.
*Stage 3.* Wash gel for 3 h with distilled water and dry.
*Stage 4.* Autoradiograph dry gel with X-ray film for 2 weeks. Dark bands on developed X-ray film correspond to localization of ADK activity in the gel.

*Notes:*  The addition of dithiothreitol (about 0.2 mg/ml) to the electrophoretic starch gel is recommended during the last 30 s of gel cooking.

## OTHER METHODS

Areas of ADK localization and production of ADP can also be detected in long-wave UV light (dark bands on a fluorescent background) using linked reactions catalyzed by two auxiliary enzymes, pyruvate kinase and lactate dehydrogenase, in the presence of phosphoenolpyruvate and NADH. This method, however, requires a control staining of two additional gels for phosphoenolpyruvate phosphatase (see 3.1.3.18 — PGP, Method 2) and ATP-ase (see 3.6.1.3 — ATPASE).

## GENERAL NOTES

The reaction catalyzed by ADK is essentially irreversible. Thus, the backward ADK reaction may not be used to develop some other practical methods for ADK detection.

## REFERENCE

1. Klobutcher, L., Nichols, E., Kucherlapati, R., and Ruddle, F. H., Assignment of the gene for human adenosine kinase to chromosome 10 using a somatic cell hybrid clone panel, *Cytogenet. Cell Genet.*, 16, 171, 1976.

REACTION        ATP + thymidine = ADP + thymidine 5′-phosphate

ENZYME SOURCE  Bacteria, plants, invertebrates, vertebrates

## METHOD

### Visualization Scheme

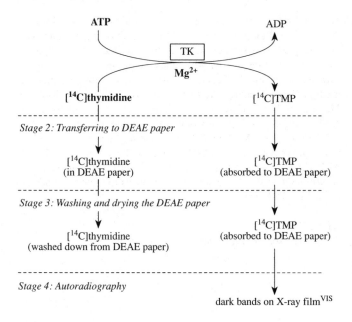

*Stage 1: Enzyme reaction*

*Stage 2: Transferring to DEAE paper*

*Stage 3: Washing and drying the DEAE paper*

*Stage 4: Autoradiography*

dark bands on X-ray film[VIS]

### Reaction Mixture[1]

0.01 *M* Tris–HCl buffer, pH 8.0
57 μ*M* [$^{14}$C]-Thymidine (26.9 to 29.6 mCi/mmol)
5 m*M* ATP
5 m*M* MgCl$_2$

### Procedure

*Stages 1, 2.* Apply a sheet of Whatman DE 81 (DEAE cellulose) paper to the surface of the electrophorized gel and pipette on the reaction mixture. Wrap the gel-DEAE paper combination in Saran Wrap and incubate at 37°C for 1.5 h.

*Stage 3.* Remove the DEAE paper and wash with 15 l of distilled water on a Buchner funnel to remove the unreacted [$^{14}$C]-thymidine, leaving [$^{14}$C]-TMP absorbed to the DEAE paper at the sites of the enzyme reaction. Dry the DEAE paper.

*Stage 4.* Apply DEAE paper to a sheet of X-ray film (Blue Brand, Kodak). Place the X-ray film-DEAE paper combination between two glass plates wrapped in a dark bag. Develop the X-ray film exposed for 2 to 4 weeks with Kodak D 19 developer.

Dark bands on the developed X-ray film correspond to localization of TK activity on the gel.

*Notes:*    The phosphorylated products of thymidine, iododeoxycytidine, and iododeoxyuridine are much more negatively charged than the substrates and bind firmly to DEAE paper. Thus, the paper binds labeled reaction products but not labeled substrates.

Using $^{125}$iododeoxycytidine or $^{125}$iododeoxyuridine as substrates, TK can also be visualized after electrophoresis, transferring to ion-exchange DEAE paper and subsequent autoradiography.[2]

The Herpes virus and mammalian TK differ in substrate specificity. Halogenated deoxyuridine is efficiently phosphorylated by both mammalian and viral TK, whereas only viral TK efficiently utilizes halogenated deoxycytidine.

## OTHER METHODS

Gel areas occupied by TK (areas of ADA production) can be detected using two auxiliary enzymes, pyruvate kinase and lactate dehydrogenase, as dark bands visible in long-wave UV light on a fluorescent background of the gel. This method, however, requires a control staining of two additional gels for phosphoenolpyruvate phosphatase (see 3.1.3.18 — PGP, Method 2) and ATPase (see 3.6.1.3 — ATPASE), whose activity bands also can be developed by this method.

### REFERENCES

1. Migeon, B. R., Smith, S. W., and Leddy, C. L., The nature of thymidine kinase in the human–mouse hybrid cell, *Biochem. Genet.*, 3, 583, 1969.
2. Van Den Berg, K. J., Direct assay of thymidine kinase bound to ion-exchange paper for dot spotting and enzyme blotting analysis, *Anal. Biochem.*, 155, 149, 1986.

OTHER NAMES    Triose kinase

REACTION    ATP + D-glyceraldehyde = ADP + D-glyceraldehyde 3-phosphate

ENZYME SOURCE    Vertebrates

## METHOD

### Visualization Scheme

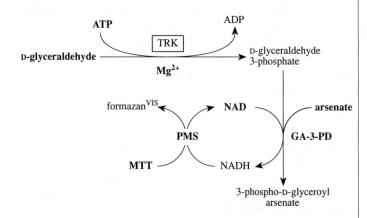

### Staining Solution[1]

A. 0.2 $M$ Tris–HCl buffer, pH 8.0                          15 ml
     D,L-Glyceraldehyde                              20 mg
   ATP                                                      15 mg
   1.0 $M$ MgCl$_2$                                          0.3 ml
   Sodium arsenate                                          50 mg
   0.5% NAD                                                 0.5 ml
   0.5% MTT                                                 0.5 ml
   0.5% PMS                                                 0.5 ml
   Glyceraldehyde-3-phosphate dehydrogenase            12 units
     (GA-3-PD)
B. 2% Agar solution (60°C)                                  10 ml

### Procedure

Mix A and B components of the staining solution and pour the mixture over the surface of the gel. Incubate the gel in the dark at 37°C until dark blue bands appear. Fix stained gel in 50% ethanol.

*Notes:*   In some species nonspecific staining of NAD-dependent dehydrogenases (e.g., aldehyde dehydrogenase) and/or aldehyde oxidase can occur with this method. Thus, interpretation of TRK zymograms should be made with caution.

### OTHER METHODS

To avoid the problem of nonspecific stainings described above, the negative fluorescent method of detection of the product ADP may be used. This method involves two auxiliary enzymes, pyruvate kinase and lactate dehydrogenase (e.g., see 2.7.1.11 — PFK, Method 3). It should be taken into account, however, that this method also can detect aldehyde reductase (see 1.1.1.1 — ADH, Method 2) bands (due to the presence of glyceraldehyde and NADH in the stain), phosphoenolpyruvate phosphatase (see 3.1.3.18 — PGP, Method 2) bands (due to the presence of phosphoenolpyruvate and NADH) and ATPase (see 3.6.1.3 — ATPASE) bands (due to the presence of ATP). Thus, at least three additional gels should be stained as controls to identify bands not caused by TRK activity.

### REFERENCE

1. Aebersold, P. B., personal communication, 1991.

REACTION    ATP + glycerol = ADP + glycerol-3-phos-
            phate

ENZYME SOURCE  Bacteria, fungi, protozoa, invertebrates, verte-
               brates

## METHOD 1

### Visualization Scheme

*Stage 1: Enzyme reaction*

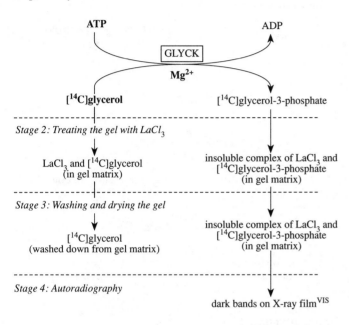

*Stage 2: Treating the gel with LaCl₃*

*Stage 3: Washing and drying the gel*

*Stage 4: Autoradiography*

### Reaction Mixture[1]

A.  49.5 m$M$ Tris–384 m$M$ glycine buffer, pH 8.4
    50 m$M$ ATP
    50 m$M$ MgCl$_2$
    7.4 μ$M$ [$^{14}$C]Glycerol (specific activity 134 mCi/mmol)
B.  0.1 $M$ Tris–HCl buffer, pH 7.0
    0.1 $M$ LaCl$_3$

### Procedure

*Stage 1.*  Incubate the gel in solution A at 37°C for 30 to 45 min.
*Stage 2.*  Rinse gel in water, place it in solution B, and incubate at 4°C for 6 h.
*Stage 3.*  Wash gel in deionized water for 12 h and dry.
*Stage 4.*  Autoradiograph dry gel with X-ray film for 2 to 6 d. Develop exposed X-ray film.

Dark bands on X-ray film correspond to localization of GLYCK activity in the gel.

## METHOD 2

### Visualization Scheme

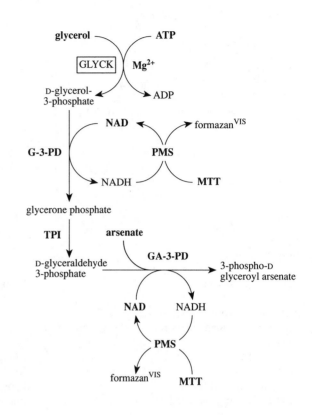

### Staining Solution*

| A. | | |
|---|---|---|
| 0.1 $M$ Tris–HCl buffer, pH 8.5 | | 25 ml |
| Glycerol | | 0.3 ml |
| ATP (disodium salt) | | 20 mg |
| MgCl$_2$·6H$_2$O | | 5 mg |
| NAD | | 25 mg |
| MTT | | 7 mg |
| PMS | | 1 mg |
| Sodium arsenate | | 50 mg |
| Glycerol-3-phosphate dehydrogenase (G-3-PD) | | 90 units |
| Triose-phosphate isomerase (TPI) | | 1000 units |
| Glyceraldehyde-3-phosphate dehydrogenase (GA-3-PD) | | 90 units |
| B. | 2% Agarose solution (60°C) | 15 ml |

### Procedure

Mix A and B components of the staining solution and pour the mixture over the surface of the gel. Incubate the gel in the dark at 37°C until dark blue bands appear. Fix stained gel in 50% ethanol.

*Notes:*  Auxiliary enzymes, triosephosphate isomerase and glyceraldehyde-3-phosphate dehydrogenase, are included to double the NAD into NADH conversion and formation of blue formazan. When preparations with high activity of GLYCK are used for electrophoresis, these enzymes and arsenate may be omitted from the staining solution.

---

*   New; recommended for use.

## METHOD 3

### Visualization Scheme

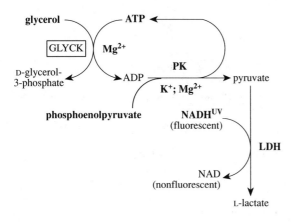

### Staining Solution*

| | |
|---|---|
| 0.05 $M$ Tris–HCl buffer, pH 8.5 | 10 ml |
| ATP (disodium salt) | 10 mg |
| Glycerol | 0.2 ml |
| Phosphoenolpyruvate | 8 mg |
|   (tricyclohexylammonium salt) | |
| NADH | 4 mg |
| MgCl$_2$·6H$_2$O | 8 mg |
| KCl | 20 mg |
| Pyruvate kinase (PK) | 60 units |
| Lactate dehydrogenase (LDH) | 50 units |

### Procedure

Apply the staining solution to gel on filter-paper overlay. Incubate the gel at 37°C and monitor under long-wave UV light. Dark (nonfluorescent) bands of GLYCK activity are visible on a light (fluorescent) background. Record the zymogram or photograph using a yellow filter.

*Notes:* Stain two additional gels as controls for phosphoenolpyruvate phosphatase (see 3.1.3.18 — PGP, Method 2) and ATPase (see 3.6.1.3 — ATPASE), which also can develop on GLYCK zymograms obtained by this method.

### REFERENCE

1. Tischfield, J. A., Bernhard, H. P., and Ruddle, F. H., A new electrophoretic–autoradiographic method for visual detection of phosphotransferases, *Anal. Biochem.*, 53, 545, 1973.

---

OTHER NAMES     Pyridoxal kinase (recommended name)

REACTION
1. Pyridoxine + ATP = pyridoxine-5-phosphate + ADP

2. Pyridoxal + ATP = pyridoxal-5-phosphate + ADP

ENZYME SOURCE  Bacteria, fungi, vertebrates

## METHOD

### Visualization Scheme

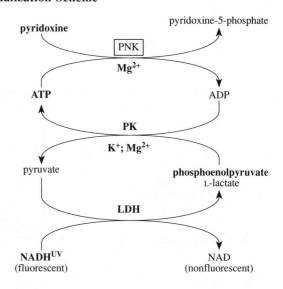

### Staining Solution[1]

0.1 $M$ Tris–HCl buffer, pH 8.0
0.2 m$M$ Pyridoxine
0.5 m$M$ ATP
0.2 m$M$ NADH
5 m$M$ Phosphoenolpyruvate
0.1 $M$ KCl
0.01 $M$ MgCl$_2$
7.8 U/ml Lactate dehydrogenase (LDH)
10.2 U/ml Pyruvate kinase (PK)

### Procedure

Apply the staining solution to the gel surface on filter-paper overlay. Incubate the gel at 37°C and monitor under long-wave UV light. Dark (nonfluorescent) bands of PNK are visible on a light (fluorescent) background. Record the zymogram or photograph using a yellow filter.

*Notes:* Faint additional bands of activity may also appear due to other kinases or phosphatases that catalyze the ATP into ADP conversion or formation of pyruvate from phosphoenolpyruvate. It is necessary, therefore, to carry out control stains on additional gels. Composition of a control stain for phosphoenolpyruvate phosphatase is given in 3.1.3.18 — PGP (Method 2) and for ATPase in 3.6.1.3 — ATPASE.

### REFERENCE

1. Chern, C. J. and Beutler, E., Biochemical and electrophoretic studies of erythrocyte pyridoxine kinase in White and Black Americans, *Am. J. Hum. Genet.*, 28, 9, 1976.

---

* New; recommended for use.

OTHER NAMES      Phosphorylase *b* kinase kinase, glycogen synthase *a* kinase, hydroxylalkyl-protein kinase, serine (threonine) protein kinase

REACTION      ATP + protein = ADP + a phosphoprotein

ENZYME SOURCE      Fungi, plants, protozoa, invertebrates, vertebrates

## METHOD

### Visualization Scheme

*Stage 1: Enzyme reaction*

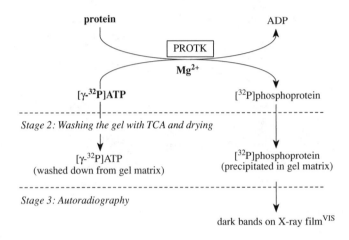

*Stage 2: Washing the gel with TCA and drying*

*Stage 3: Autoradiography*

### Reaction Mixture[1]

A. 10 m$M$ Tris–HCl buffer, pH 6.75
   10 m$M$ MgCl$_2$
   0.1 m$M$ 2-Mercaptoethanol
   0.1 m$M$ EDTA
   0.2 m$M$ Ethylene glycol-bis(β-aminoethyl ether) *N,N,N′,N′*-tetraacetic acid
B. [γ-$^{32}$P]ATP (specific activity 20 to 40 Ci/mmol; 1 mCi/ml)
C. 5 mg/ml Casein, or histone, in solution A containing 0.4 $M$ NaCl
D. 5 mg/ml Protamine sulfate, or phosvitin, in solution A containing 0.2 $M$ NaCl
E. 0.1 g/ml Trichloroacetic acid (TCA)
   5 m$M$ Sodium pyrophosphate
   5 m$M$ NaH$_2$PO$_4$

### Procedure

*Stage 1.* Mix 150 µl of solution A with 15 µl of B and apply onto the "running" acetate cellulose strip (5.7 × 5.7 cm) with a fine brush. Prepare "substrate" acetate cellulose by incubation of another strip in solution C or D depending on specificity of investigated PROTK. Press together the "substrate" and "running" strips between two glass slides for 30 min.

*Stage 2.* Fix the "running" strip in solution E. After extensive washing in this solution (five baths of 300 ml changed each 30 min) dry the strip.

*Stage 3.* Autoradiograph dry "running" strip at room temperature with "no screen" film for 6 to 16 h. Develop exposed X-ray film.

Dark bands on the film correspond to localization of PROTK activity on "running" acetate cellulose gel.

*Notes:* 3′,5′-cAMP should be added to solution A (0.01 m$M$ final concentration) when PROTK stimulated by cAMP is studied.

The method is highly sensitive. Bands corresponding to PROTK activity of 0.25 pmol of phosphate transferred per minute at 30°C are easily detected after an overnight exposure. The method using acetate cellulose gel seems to be at least 50-fold more sensitive than methods using routine PAG.

## OTHER METHODS

A. cAMP-dependent PROTK may be visualized on SDS–containing PAG by autoradiography using a method based on photoactivated covalent binding of radiolabeled 8-azido cAMP with the regulatory subunit of PROTK in sample preparations before electrophoresis.[2]
B. The method of detection of calmodulin-dependent PROTK in substrate-containing SDS–PAG is also available.[3] This method includes five steps:
   · The renaturation of electrophorized SDS–PAG
   · The incubation of renatured PAG in a buffered solution containing [γ-$^{32}$P]ATP and calmodulin
   · The extensive washing of the gel in 5% TCA containing 1% sodium pyrophosphate
   · The drying of the gel and
   · The autoradiography of dry PAG with X-ray film
C. Bands of PROTK can be detected using an ADP-detecting system consisting of two auxiliary enzymes (pyruvate kinase and lactate dehydrogenase) and observed in long-wave UV light (for example see 2.7.1.30 — GLYCK, Method 3). This method also detects phosphoenolpyruvate phosphatase (see 3.1.3.18 — PGP, Method 2) and ATPase (see 3.6.1.3 — ATPASE) activity bands. Thus, when using this method, two additional gels should be stained as controls to identify bands caused by phosphatase activities.

## GENERAL NOTES

There is evidence that PROTK from a particular source preferentially attacks the phosphoprotein from the same source.

## REFERENCES

1. Phan-Dinh-Tuy, F., Weber, A., Henry, J., Cottreau, D., and Kahn, A., Cellulose acetate electrophoresis of protein kinases: detection of the active forms using various substrates, *Anal. Biochem.*, 127, 73, 1982.
2. Sato, M., Hiragun, A., and Mitsui, H., Differentiation-associated increase of cAMP-dependent type II protein kinase in murine preadipose cell line (ST 13), *Biochim. Biophys. Acta*, 844, 296, 1985.
3. Kameshita, I. and Fujisawa, H., A sensitive method for detection of calmodulin-dependent protein kinase II activity in sodium dodecyl sulfate–polyacrylamide gel, *Anal. Biochem.*, 183, 139, 1989.

OTHER NAMES   Phosphoenolpyruvate kinase, phosphoenol transphosphorylase

REACTION   ATP + pyruvate = ADP + phosphoenolpyruvate

ENZYME SOURCE   Bacteria, green algae, fungi, plants, protozoa, invertebrates, vertebrates

## METHOD 1

### Visualization Scheme

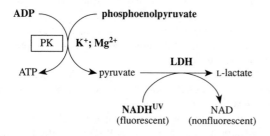

### Staining Solution[1] (modified)

| | |
|---|---|
| 0.2 $M$ Tris–HCl buffer, pH 8.0 | 10 ml |
| Phosphoenolpyruvate (monopotassium salt) | 15 mg |
| ADP (disodium salt) | 25 mg |
| NADH | 7 mg |
| MgCl$_2$·6H$_2$O | 30 mg |
| KCl | 40 mg |
| Lactate dehydrogenase (LDH) | 50 units |

### Procedure

Apply the staining solution to the gel surface on filter-paper overlay. Incubate the gel at 37°C for 30 to 60 min and monitor under long-wave UV light. Dark (nonfluorescent) bands visible on a light (fluorescent) background correspond to localization of PK activity. Record the zymogram or photograph using a yellow filter.

*Notes:* In some organisms additional bands caused by phosphoenolpyruvate phosphatase (see 3.1.3.18 — PGP, Method 2) can also be developed on PK zymograms obtained by this method. Thus, the control staining of an additional gel in staining solution lacking ADP is required.

## METHOD 2

### Visualization Scheme

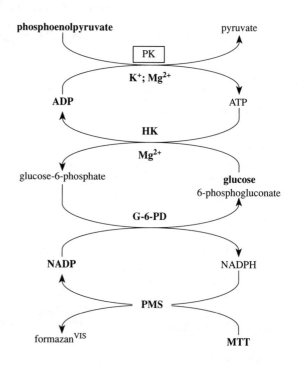

### Staining Solution[2]

A. 0.1 $M$ Tris–HCl buffer, pH 8.0
   0.1 $M$ KCl
   10 m$M$ MgCl$_2$
   5 m$M$ Phosphoenolpyruvate
   3 m$M$ ADP
   10 m$M$ Glucose

| B. | | |
|---|---|---|
| | NADP | 10 mg |
| | MTT | 10 mg |
| | PMS | 1 mg |
| | Hexokinase (HK) | 16 units |
| | Glucose-6-phosphate dehydrogenase (G-6-PD) | 12 units |

C. 1% Agarose solution (60°C)

### Procedure

Add reagents B to 10 ml of solution A and then add 10 ml of solution C. Pour the resulting mixture over the surface of the gel and incubate in the dark at 37°C until dark blue bands appear. Fix stained gel in 50% ethanol.

*Notes:* Additional bands caused by adenylate kinase activity can also develop on PK zymograms obtained by this method. Thus, an adenylate kinase control gel should also be available for comparison (see 2.7.4.3 — AK). The use of AMP (2 mg/ml final concentration) in the PK stain may inhibit AK activity.

   NAD-dependent G-6-PD is available (Sigma G 5760 or G 5885). When this form of the enzyme is used, NAD should be substituted for NADP in the staining solution. This substitution will result in a cost saving because NAD is several times cheaper than NADP.

## METHOD 3

### Visualization Scheme

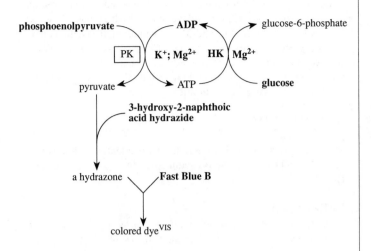

### Staining Solution[3]

| | |
|---|---|
| 50 m$M$ Tris–HCl buffer, pH 7.5 | 100 ml |
| 1 $M$ MgCl$_2$·6H$_2$O | 1 ml |
| 5 $M$ KCl | 3 ml |
| Phosphoenolpyruvate (trisodium salt; 5H$_2$O) | 50 mg |
| ADP (sodium salt) | 20 mg |
| Glucose | 180 mg |
| 3-Hydroxy-2-naphthoic acid hydrazide | 50 mg |
| Fast Blue B salt | 50 mg |
| Hexokinase (HK) | 30 units |

### Procedure

Incubate the gel in staining solution in the dark at 36°C until colored bands appear. Rinse stained gel in water and fix in 50% glycerol.

*Notes:* In this method, the carbonyl group of pyruvate condenses with the hydrazine group of 3-hydroxy-2-naphthoic acid hydrazide. Hydrazone molecules so formed are cross-linked with each other by the addition of a tetrazonium salt. The coupling reaction is directed by the 2-hydroxy group.

The role of glucose and HK is the regeneration of ADP.

## OTHER METHODS

An immunoblotting procedure (for details see Part II) using monoclonal antibodies specific to rabbit PK[4] can also be used for immunohistochemical localization of the enzyme protein on electrophoretic gels. This procedure, however, is not as suitable for routine laboratory use as methods described above.

### GENERAL NOTES

The enzyme from some mammalian species is activated by fructose-1,6-diphosphate (2 mg/ml final concentration).

### REFERENCES

1. Shaw, C. R. and Prasad, R., Starch gel electrophoresis of enzymes: a compilation of recipes, *Biochem. Genet.*, 4, 297, 1970.
2. Chern, C. J. and Croce, C. M., Confirmation of the synteny of the human genes for mannose phosphate isomerase and pyruvate kinase and their assignment to chromosome 15, *Cytogenet. Cell Genet.*, 15, 299, 1975.
3. Vallejos, C. E., Enzyme activity staining, in *Isozymes in Plant Genetics and Breeding, Part A*, Tanskley, S. D. and Orton, T. J., Eds., Elsevier, Amsterdam, 1983, 469.
4. Hance, A. J., Lee, J., and Feitelson, M., The M1 and M2 isozymes of pyruvate kinase are the products of the same gene, *Biochem. Biophys. Res. Commun.*, 106, 492, 1982.

REACTION    Nucleoside triphosphate + deoxycytidine = nucleoside diphosphate + dCMP

ENZYME SOURCE   Vertebrates

## METHOD

### Visualization Scheme

*Stage 1: Enzyme reaction*

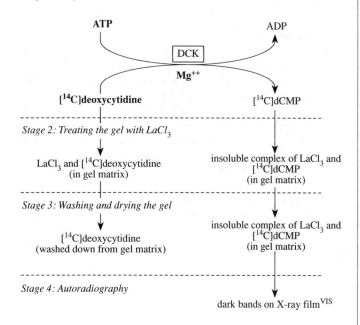

*Stage 2: Treating the gel with LaCl₃*

*Stage 3: Washing and drying the gel*

*Stage 4: Autoradiography*

### Reaction Mixture[1]

A. 20 m$M$ Potassium phosphate buffer, pH 6.2    20 ml
   ATP (disodium salt)    4 mg
   MgCl$_2$ (anhydrous)    1 mg
   [$^{14}$C]Deoxycytidine    5 μCi
B. 0.1 $M$ Tris–HCl buffer, pH 7.0
   0.1 $M$ LaCl$_3$

### Procedure

*Stage 1.* Incubate the gel in solution A at 37°C for 1 h.
*Stage 2.* Remove solution A and incubate the gel in solution B at 4°C for 6 h.
*Stage 3.* Wash gel for 3 h with distilled water. Dry the gel.
*Stage 4.* Autoradiograph dry gel with X-ray film for 2 weeks.

Dark bands on developed X-ray film correspond to localization of DCK activity on the gel.

## OTHER METHODS

The areas of ADP production can be detected as dark bands visible in long-wave UV light using reactions catalyzed by two auxiliary enzymes, pyruvate kinase and lactate dehydrogenase (e.g., see 2.7.1.30 — GLYCK, Method 3). This method also detects phosphoenolpyruvate phosphatase and ATPase activity bands. Thus, a control staining of two additional gels for phosphoenolpyruvate phosphatase (see 3.1.3.18 — PGP, Method 2) and ATPase (see 3.6.1.3 — ATPASE) is desirable.

## GENERAL NOTES

The enzyme may be identical to deoxyadenosine kinase (see 2.7.1.76 — DAK) and deoxyguanosine kinase (see 2.7.1.113 — DGK).

## REFERENCE

1. Osborne, W. R. A. and Scott, C. R., Nucleoside kinases in B and T lymphoblastoid cells, *Isozyme Bull.*, 18, 68, 1985.

REACTION          ATP + deoxyadenosine = ADP + dAMP

ENZYME SOURCE  Vertebrates

## METHOD

### Visualization Scheme

*Stage 1: Enzyme reaction*

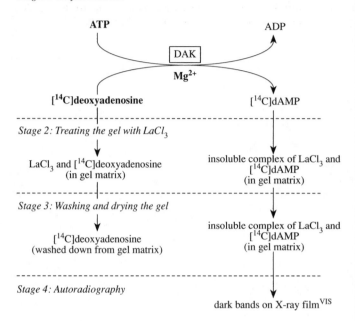

*Stage 2: Treating the gel with LaCl₃*

*Stage 3: Washing and drying the gel*

*Stage 4: Autoradiography*

### Reaction Mixture[1]

A.  20 m$M$ Potassium phosphate buffer, pH 6.2          20 ml
    ATP (disodium salt)                                    4 mg
    MgCl₂ (anhydrous)                                      1 mg
    [¹⁴C]Deoxyadenosine                                    5 µCi
B.  0.1 $M$ Tris–HCl buffer, pH 7.0
    0.1 $M$ LaCl₃

### Procedure

*Stage 1*.  Incubate the gel in solution A at 37°C for 1 h.
*Stage 2*.  Remove solution A and incubate the gel in solution B at 4°C for 6 h.
*Stage 3*.  Wash gel for 3 h with distilled water. Dry the gel.
*Stage 4*.  Autoradiograph dry gel with X-ray film for 2 weeks.

Dark bands on developed X-ray film correspond to localization of DAK activity in the gel.

## OTHER METHODS

Bands of DAK activity can be detected in long-wave UV light (dark bands on a fluorescent background) using the ADP-detecting system of two auxiliary enzymes, pyruvate kinase and lactate dehydrogenase (for example, see 2.7.1.30 — GLYCK, Method 3). This method, however, requires two additional gels to be stained for phosphoenolpyruvate phosphatase (see 3.1.3.18 — PGP, Method 2) and ATPase (see 3.6.1.3 — ATPASE), for which activity bands also can develop on DAK zymograms obtained by this method.

## GENERAL NOTES

This enzyme may be identical to deoxycytidine kinase (see 2.7.1.74 — DCK) and deoxyguanosine kinase (see 2.7.1.113 — DGK).

## REFERENCE

1.  Osborne, W. R. A. and Scott, C. R., Nucleoside kinases in B and T lymphoblastoid cells, *Isozyme Bull.*, 18, 68, 1985.

OTHER NAMES   6-Phosphofructokinase (pyrophosphate), pyrophosphate-dependent phosphofructokinase

REACTION   Pyrophosphate + D-fructose-6-phosphate = orthophosphate + D-fructose-1,6-bisphosphate

ENZYME SOURCE  Bacteria, plants

## METHOD

### Visualization Scheme

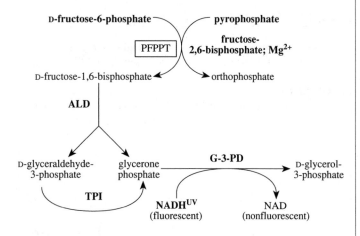

### Staining Solution[1] (adapted)

A. 50 mM HEPES (N-2-Hydroxyethylpiperazine-N′-2-ethanesulfonate) buffer, pH 8.0
0.5 mM EDTA
4 mM Mg(CH$_3$COO)$_2$
1 mM NADH
10 mM D-Fructose-6-phosphate
2 mM Pyrophosphate
0.2 U/ml Aldolase (ALD)
0.2 U/ml Triose-phosphate isomerase (TPI)
0.2 U/ml Glycerol-3-phosphate dehydrogenase (G-3-PD)
100 nM D-Fructose-2,6-bisphosphate
B. 1.4% Agar solution (60°C)

### Procedure

Mix equal volumes of A and B components of the staining solution and pour the mixture over the surface of the gel. Incubate the gel at 37°C and monitor under long-wave UV light. Dark (nonfluorescent) bands on a light (fluorescent) background indicate the sites of localization of PFPPT activity in the gel. Record the zymogram or photograph using a yellow filter.

*Notes:*  Plant enzyme requires fructose-2,6-biphosphate for its activity. Bacterial enzyme is not activated by this cofactor.

Fructose-2,6-bisphosphate may be replaced by 6-phosphofructo-2-kinase (EC 2.7.1.105) and ATP. This substitution, however, causes additional development of 6-phosphofructokinase (see 2.7.1.11 — PFK) activity bands on PFPPT zymograms.

## OTHER METHODS

When a zymogram of PFPPT that is visible in daylight is required, G-3-PD and NADH in the staining solution given above should be replaced by glyceraldehyde-3-phosphate dehydrogenase, arsenate, NAD, PMS, and MTT (for example, see 4.1.2.13 — ALD, Method 1).

## REFERENCE

1. Kora-Miura, Y., Fujii, S., Matsuda, M., Sato, Y., Kaku, K., and Kaneko, T., Electrophoretic determination of fructose 6-phosphate, 2-kinase, *Anal. Biochem.*, 170, 372, 1988.

| | |
|---|---|
| OTHER NAMES | Neomycin–kanamycin phosphotransferase, neomycin phosphotransferase |
| REACTION | ATP + kanamycin = ADP + kanamycin 3′-phosphate |
| ENZYME SOURCE | Bacteria |

## METHOD

### Visualization Scheme

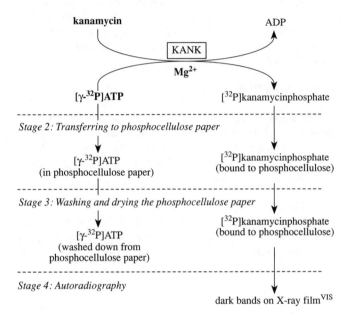

*Stage 1: Enzyme reaction*

*Stage 2: Transferring to phosphocellulose paper*

*Stage 3: Washing and drying the phosphocellulose paper*

*Stage 4: Autoradiography*

### Reaction Mixture[1]

20 m$M$ Tris–HCl buffer, pH 7.3
13 m$M$ MgCl$_2$
100 m$M$ NH$_4$Cl
0.5 m$M$ Dithiothreitol
62.5 µg/ml Kanamycin
1.25 m$M$ ATP
10-20 µCi/ml [γ-$^{32}$P]ATP

### Procedure

*Stage 1*. Soak electrophorized gel in reaction mixture at 4°C for 15 min in a plastic box to permit the reactants to diffuse into the gel. Then place the container in a 37°C incubator for 30 min to enable the reaction to occur.

*Stage 2*. Remove the reaction mixture and rinse the gel once with distilled water. Transfer the reaction products from the gel to prewetted Whatman P-81 phosphocellulose paper by capillary blotting overnight using distilled water as a transfer solution.

*Stage 3*. Wash the P-81 paper in 70°C distilled water twice and three times at room temperature and then dry.

*Stage 4*. Apply dry Whatman P-81 paper to a sheet of X-ray film and expose for 6 d.

Dark bands on developed X-ray film correspond to localization of KANK activity on the gel.

### REFERENCE

1. Fregien, N. and Davidson, N., Quantitative *in situ* gel electrophoretic assay for neomycin phosphotransferase activity in mammalian cell lysates, *Anal. Biochem.*, 148, 101, 1985.

OTHER NAMES     Phosphofructokinase 2

REACTION     ATP + D-fructose-6-phosphate = ADP + D-fructose-2,6-bisphosphate

ENZYME SOURCE  Vertebrates

## METHOD

**Visualization Scheme**

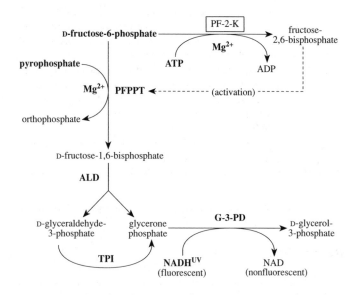

**Staining Solution[1]**

A. 50 mM HEPES (N-2-Hydroxyethylpiperazine-N'-2-ethanesulfonate) buffer, pH 8.0
   0.5 mM EDTA
   4 mM Mg(CH₃COO)₂
   1 mM NADH
   10 mM ATP
   10 mM D-Fructose-6-phosphate
   2 mM Pyrophosphate
   0.2 U/ml Aldolase (ALD)
   0.2 U/ml Triose-phosphate isomerase (TPI)
   0.2 U/ml Glycerol-3-phosphate dehydrogenase (G-3-PD)
   0.1 U/ml Pyrophosphate-fructose-6-phosphate 1-phosphotransferase (PFPPT)

B. 1.4% Agar solution (60°C)

**Procedure**

Mix equal volumes of A and B components of the staining solution and pour the mixture over the surface of the gel. Incubate the gel at 37°C and monitor under long-wave UV light. Dark (nonfluorescent) bands on a light (fluorescent) background indicate the sites of localization of PF-2-K activity in the gel. Record the zymogram or photograph using a yellow filter.

*Notes:* 6-Phosphofructokinase (EC 2.7.1.11) activity bands can also develop on PF-2-K zymograms obtained by this method. However, PF-2-K bands do not develop when pyrophosphate is excluded from the staining solution. This difference may be used to differentiate activity bands of these two enzymes.

   The visualization of PF-2-K activity on electrophoretic gels is based on the production of fructose-2,6-bisphosphate, coupled to the activation of auxiliary potato enzyme pyrophosphate–fructose-6-phosphate 1-phosphotransferase (see 2.7.1.90 — PFPPT). The product of PFPPT reaction (fructose-1,6-bisphosphate) is then detected using three auxiliary enzymes: ALD, TPI, and G-3-PD.

## OTHER METHODS

When a zymogram of PF-2-K that is visible in daylight is required, G-3-PD and NADH in the staining solution given above should be replaced by glyceraldehyde-3-phosphate dehydrogenase, arsenate, NAD, PMS, and MTT (e.g., see 4.1.2.13 — ALD, METHOD 1).

## REFERENCE

1. Kora-Miura, Y., Fujii, S., Matsuda, M., Sato, Y., Kaku, K., and Kaneko, T., Electrophoretic determination of fructose 6-phosphate, 2-kinase, *Anal. Biochem.*, 170, 372, 1988.

OTHER NAMES  Tyrosylprotein kinase, protein kinase (tyrosine), hydroxyaryl-protein kinase

REACTION  ATP + protein tyrosine = ADP + protein tyrosine phosphate

ENZYME SOURCE  Fungi, plants, invertebrates, vertebrates

## METHOD

### Visualization Scheme

*Stage 1: Enzyme reaction*

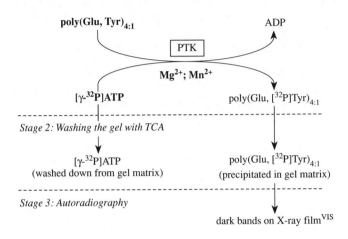

*Stage 2: Washing the gel with TCA*

*Stage 3: Autoradiography*

### Reaction Mixture[1]

A.  20 mM HEPES (*N*-[2-Hydroxyethyl]piperazine-*N'*-[2-ethanesulfonate]) buffer, pH 7.4
    5 mg/ml Poly(Glu, Tyr)$_{4:1}$
    33 µCi/ml [γ-$^{32}$P]ATP
    50 µM ATP
    10 mM MgCl$_2$
    10 mM MnCl$_2$
B.  5% Trichloroacetic acid (TCA)
    10 mM Sodium pyrophosphate

## Procedure

*Stage 1.*  Soak electrophorized PAG (containing 10% glycerol, 0.1% Triton X-100) twice for 15 min in 20 mM HEPES buffer, pH 7.4, at 4°C. Remove the buffer and overlay gel with solution A (35 µl/cm$^2$). Incubate the gel at 37°C for 30 min and then rinse gel once with water.

*Stage 2.*  Wash gel several times (usually five 10-min washes) at room temperature on a shaker with solution B.

*Stage 3.*  Dry gel and autoradiograph with Kodak X-Omat XK-1 film.

Dark bands on developed X-ray film correspond to localization of PTK activity on the gel.

*Notes:*  PTK acts on specific tyrosine-containing proteins associated with membrane vesicles. Nucleotides other than ATP may also act as phosphate donors.

If protein-tyrosine phosphatase (EC 3.1.3.48), which may be present in preparations under analysis, comigrates with some PTK isozymes, it can decrease the intensity of development of these isozymes on autoradiographs. To inhibit this phosphatase activity, sodium vanadate (0.1 mM final concentration) should be included in solution A of the reaction mixture.

## REFERENCE

1.  Glazer, R. I., Yu, G., and Knode, M. C., Analysis of tyrosine kinase activity in cell extracts using nondenaturing polyacrylamide gel electrophoresis, *Anal. Biochem.*, 164, 214, 1987.

REACTION        ATP + deoxyguanosine = ADP + dGMP

ENZYME SOURCE  Vertebrates

## METHOD

### Visualization Scheme

*Stage 1: Enzyme reaction*

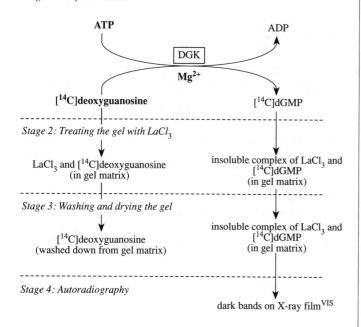

*Stage 2: Treating the gel with LaCl$_3$*

*Stage 3: Washing and drying the gel*

*Stage 4: Autoradiography*

### Reaction Mixture[1]

A.  20 m$M$ Potassium phosphate buffer, pH 6.2          20 ml
    ATP (disodium salt)                                4 mg
    MgCl$_2$ (anhydrous)                               1 mg
    [$^{14}$C]Deoxyguanosine                           5 μCi
B.  0.1 $M$ Tris–HCl buffer, pH 7.0
    0.1 $M$ LaCl$_3$

### Procedure

*Stage 1.*  Incubate the gel in solution A at 37°C for 1 h.
*Stage 2.*  Remove solution A and incubate the gel in solution B at 4°C for 6 h.
*Stage 3.*  Wash gel for 3 h with distilled water. Dry the gel.
*Stage 4.*  Autoradiograph dry gel with X-ray film for 2 weeks.

Dark bands on developed X-ray film correspond to localization of DGK activity on the gel.

## OTHER METHODS

Areas of ADP production can be detected in UV light as dark bands on the fluorescent background of the gel using two auxiliary enzymes, pyruvate kinase and lactate dehydrogenase (for example, see 2.7.1.30 — GLYCK, Method 3). When using this method, stain two additional gels for phosphoenolpyruvate phosphatase (see 3.1.3.18 — PGP, Method 2) and ATPase (see 3.6.1.3 — ATPASE), for which bands can also develop on DGK zymograms obtained by this method.

## GENERAL NOTES

The enzyme may be identical to deoxyadenosine kinase (see 2.7.1.76 — DAK) and deoxycytidine kinase (see 2.7.1.74 — DCK).

Deoxyinosine can also act as an acceptor.

## REFERENCE

1.  Osborne, W. R. A. and Scott, C. R., Nucleoside kinases in B and T lymphoblastoid cells, *Isozyme Bull.*, 18, 68, 1985.

OTHER NAMES    3-Phosphoglycerate kinase, 3-phosphoglyceric phosphokinase

REACTION    ATP + 3-phospho-D-glycerate = ADP + 3-phospho-D-glyceroyl phosphate

ENZYME SOURCE    Bacteria, fungi, plants, protozoa, invertebrates, vertebrates

## METHOD

### Visualization Scheme

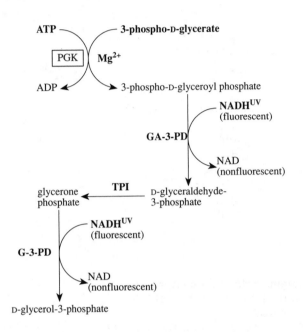

### Staining Solution[1] (modified)

| | |
|---|---:|
| 0.3 $M$ Tris–HCl buffer, pH 8.0 | 5 ml |
| 3-Phosphoglycerate (disodium salt) | 20 mg |
| ATP (disodium salt; $3H_2O$) | 30 mg |
| $MgCl_2·6H_2O$ | 35 mg |
| Glyceraldehyde-3-phosphate dehydrogenase (GA-3-PD) | 40 units |
| NADH | 10 mg |
| Triose-phosphate isomerase (TPI) | 100 units |
| Glycerol-3-phosphate dehydrogenase (G-3-PD) | 10 units |

### Procedure

Apply the staining solution to the gel surface on filter-paper overlay. Incubate the gel at 37°C and monitor under long-wave UV light. Dark (nonfluorescent) bands visible on a light (fluorescent) background indicate the sites of PGK localization. Record the zymogram or photograph using a yellow filter.

*Notes:* Negatively stained bands of PGK visible in daylight can be developed by treating the processed gel with MTT/PMS solution.

Auxiliary enzymes TPI and G-3-PD are used to intensify the process of NADH into NAD conversion. These enzymes may be omitted from the staining solution when preparations with high PGK activity are analyzed.

### OTHER METHODS

A. The reverse PGK reaction can be used to detect ATP production via two linked reactions catalyzed by two auxiliary enzymes, hexokinase and glucose-6-phosphate dehydrogenase (e.g., see 2.7.3.2 — CK, Method 2). However, this method is not specific since the adenylate kinase (AK) activity bands are stained together with PGK bands. Thus, an additional gel should be stained for AK as a control (see 2.7.4.3 — AK, Method 1).

B. Using the forward PGK reaction, the product ADP can be detected via two linked reactions catalyzed by auxiliary enzymes, pyruvate kinase and lactate dehydrogenase (for example, see 2.7.1.11 — PFK, Method 3). This method reveals areas of PGK localization as dark (nonfluorescent) bands visible in long-wave UV light on the light (fluorescent) background of the gel. When using this method, two additional gels should be stained as controls to identify possible bands caused by phosphoenolpyruvate phosphatase (see 3.1.3.18 — PGP, Method 2) and ATPase (see 3.6.1.3 — ATPASE).

### REFERENCE

1. Beutler, E., Electrophoresis of phosphoglycerate kinase, *Biochem. Genet.*, 3, 189, 1969.

REACTION     ATP + creatine = ADP + phosphocreatine

ENZYME SOURCE  Vertebrates

## METHOD 1

### Visualization Scheme

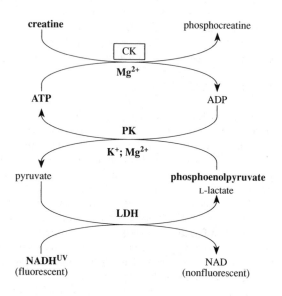

### Staining Solution[1]

| | |
|---|---|
| 0.5 *M* Tris–HCl buffer, pH 8.0 | 10 ml |
| Creatine | 30 mg |
| ATP (disodium salt; 3H$_2$O) | 20 mg |
| Magnesium acetate (4H$_2$O) | 40 mg |
| Potassium acetate | 40 mg |
| Phosphoenolpyruvate (potassium salt) | 15 mg |
| NADH | 10 mg |
| Pyruvate kinase (PK) | 2 units |
| Lactate dehydrogenase (LDH) | 130 units |

### Procedure

Apply the staining solution to the gel surface on filter-paper overlay. Incubate the gel at 37°C and monitor under long-wave UV light. Dark (nonfluorescent) bands visible on a light (fluorescent) background indicate the sites of CK localization. Record the zymogram or photograph using a yellow filter.

*Notes:*  When a zymogram that is visible in daylight is required, the processed gel should be counterstained with MTT/PMS solution, resulting in the appearance of achromatic bands on a blue background of the gel.

In some cases, additional bands of phosphatase activity can also be developed by this method. This is due to the ability of phosphatases from some sources to hydrolyze the phosphoenolpyruvate.[1,2] To identify these bands an additional gel should be stained with staining solution lacking ATP, PK, and creatine (for details see 3.1.3.18 — PGP, Method 2).

## METHOD 2

### Visualization Scheme

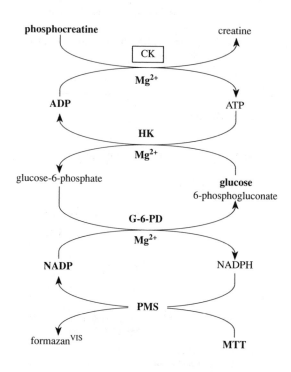

### Staining Solution[3] (modified)

| | |
|---|---|
| A.  0.1 *M* Tris–HCl buffer, pH 8.0 | 20 ml |
| NADP | 10 mg |
| Phosphocreatine (disodium salt; 6H$_2$O) | 25 mg |
| ADP (disodium salt) | 25 mg |
| Glucose | 60 mg |
| MgCl$_2$·6H$_2$O | 60 mg |
| Glucose-6-phosphate dehydrogenase (G-6-PD) | 20 units |
| Hexokinase (HK) | 20 units |
| MTT | 7 mg |
| PMS | 1 mg |
| B.  1.5% Agarose solution (60°C) | 20 ml |

### Procedure

Mix A and B components of the staining solution and pour the mixture over the surface of the gel. Incubate the gel in the dark until dark blue bands appear. Fix stained gel in 50% ethanol.

*Notes:*  Bands of adenylate kinase (see 2.7.4.3 — AK) activity can also be developed with this method. Therefore, an additional gel should be stained for AK as a control. The addition of AMP (2 mg/ml final concentration) to the CK staining solution may be used to inhibit AK activity.

Preparations of NAD-dependent G-6-PD are now commercially available (Sigma G 5760 or G 5885). When this form of G-6-PD is used, NAD should be substituted for NADP in the staining solution. This substitution will result in a cost saving because NAD is about five times less expensive than NADP.

## GENERAL NOTES

Method 1 is more sensitive than Method 2, but the latter is more convenient for routine laboratory use.

## OTHER METHODS

An immunoblotting procedure (for details see Part II) based on the utility of monoclonal antibodies specific to the hen enzyme[4] can also be used for visualization of the enzyme protein on electrophoretic gels. This procedure is not recommended for routine laboratory use; however, it may be of great value in special analyses of the enzyme.

## REFERENCES

1. Harris, H. and Hopkinson, D. A., *Handbook of Enzyme Electrophoresis in Human Genetics*, North-Holland, Amsterdam (Loose leaf with supplements in 1977 and 1978), 1976.
2. Manchenko, G. P., Allozymic variation and substrate specificity of phosphatase from sipunculid *Phascolosoma japonicum*, *Isozyme Bull.*, 21, 168, 1988.
3. Shaw, C. R. and Prasad, R., Starch gel electrophoresis of enzymes: a compilation of recipes, *Biochem. Genet.*, 4, 297, 1970.
4. Morris, G. E. and Head, L. P., A monoclonal antibody against the skeletal muscle enzyme creatine kinase, *FEBS Lett.*, 145, 163, 1982.

REACTION         ATP + L-arginine = ADP + phospho-L-arginine

ENZYME SOURCE   Invertebrates

## METHOD 1

### Visualization Scheme

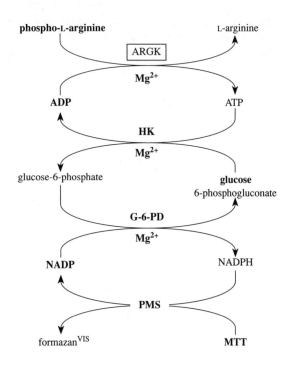

### Staining Solution[1] (modified)

| | |
|---|---:|
| A. 0.1 *M* Tris–HCl buffer, pH 8.0 | 20 ml |
| Phospho-L-arginine | 20 mg |
| ADP | 30 mg |
| Glucose | 80 mg |
| MgCl$_2$·6H$_2$O | 8 mg |
| NADP | 20 mg |
| PMS | 1 mg |
| MTT | 8 mg |
| Hexokinase (HK) | 45 units |
| Glucose-6-phosphate dehydrogenase (G-6-PD) | 100 units |
| B. 1.5% Agarose solution (60°C) | 20 ml |

### Procedure

Mix A and B components of the staining solution and pour the mixture over the surface of the gel. Incubate the gel in the dark at 37°C until dark blue bands appear. Fix stained gel in 50% ethanol.

*Notes:*  Bands of adenylate kinase (see 2.7.4.3 — AK) activity can also be developed with this method. Therefore, an additional gel should be stained for AK as a control. The addition of AMP (2 mg/ml final concentration) to the staining solution may be used to inhibit AK activity.

NAD-dependent G-6-PD is now commercially available (Sigma G 5760 or G 5885). When this form of the linking enzyme is used, NAD should be substituted for NADP in the staining solution. This replacement will result in a cost saving because NAD is about five times less expensive than NADP.

## METHOD 2

### Visualization Scheme

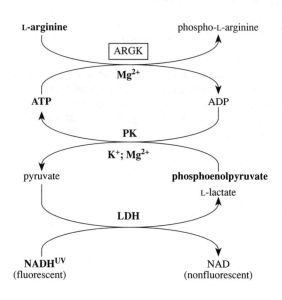

### Staining Solution[2] (modified)

| | |
|---|---:|
| A. 0.1 *M* Tris–HCl buffer, pH 8.0 | 20 ml |
| L-Arginine | 20 mg |
| ATP | 30 mg |
| MgCl$_2$·6H$_2$O | 25 mg |
| KCl | 20 mg |
| Phosphoenolpyruvate (tricyclohexylammonium salt) | 30 mg |
| NADH | 15 mg |
| Pyruvate kinase (PK) | 90 units |
| Lactate dehydrogenase (LDH) | 150 units |
| B. 1.5% Agarose solution (60°C) | 20 ml |

### Procedure

Mix A and B components of the staining solution and pour the mixture over the surface of the gel. Incubate the gel at 37°C and monitor under long-wave UV light. Dark (nonfluorescent) bands visible on a light (fluorescent) background correspond to localization of the enzyme on the gel. Record the zymogram or photograph using a yellow filter.

*Notes:*  When a zymogram that is visible in daylight is required, counterstain the processed gel with MTT/PMS solution to reveal achromatic ARGK bands on a blue background of the gel.

Alkaline phosphatase (ALP; EC 3.1.3.1) and phosphoglycolate phosphatase (PGP; EC 3.1.3.18) activity bands can also be developed by this method. This is due to the ability of ALP and PGP from some animal species to hydrolyze the phosphoenolpyruvate.[3] To identify these bands, an additional gel should be stained in the staining solution lacking ATP, PK, and L-arginine (see also 3.1.3.18 — PGP, Method 2).

## METHOD 3

### Visualization Scheme

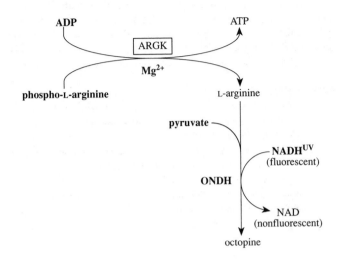

### Staining Solution*

| | |
|---|---|
| 0.1 $M$ Tris–HCl buffer, pH 8.0 | 10 ml |
| ADP | 15 mg |
| Phospho-L-arginine | 10 mg |
| MgCl$_2$·6H$_2$O | 5 mg |
| Pyruvic acid (sodium salt) | 10 mg |
| NADH | 7 mg |
| Octopine dehydrogenase (ONDH) | 20 units |

### Procedure

Apply the staining solution to the gel surface on filter-paper overlay. Incubate the gel in a moist chamber at 37°C for 30 min and monitor under long-wave UV light. Dark (nonfluorescent) bands visible on a light (fluorescent) background indicate the sites of ARGK localization. Record the zymogram or photograph using a yellow filter.

*Notes:* When a zymogram that is visible in daylight is required, counterstain the processed gel with MTT/PMS solution to obtain achromatic ARGK bands on a blue gel background.

Lactate dehydrogenase bands can also be developed by this method. Therefore, an additional gel should be stained for LDH activity as a control. In many invertebrate taxons, however, LDH activity is very low or not detectable at all.

## METHOD 4

### Visualization Scheme

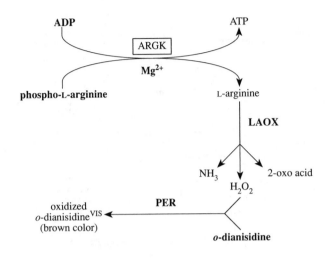

### Staining Solution*

| | | |
|---|---|---|
| A. | 0.1 $M$ Tris–HCl buffer, pH 8.0 | 20 ml |
| | Phospho-L-arginine | 20 mg |
| | ADP | 30 mg |
| | Snake venom L-amino acid oxidase (LAOX) | 1 unit |
| | Peroxidase (PER) | 200 units |
| | MgCl$_2$·6H$_2$O | 16 mg |
| | *o*-Dianisidine (dihydrochloride) | 10 mg |
| B. | 2% Agarose solution (60°C) | 20 ml |

### Procedure

Mix A and B components of the staining solution and pour the mixture over the surface of the gel. Incubate the gel at 37°C until colored bands of good intensity appear. Fix stained gel and agarose overlay in 50% glycerol.

*Notes:* *o*-Dianisidine dihydrochloride is a potential carcinogen. 3-Amino-9-ethyl-carbazole is recommended for use in place of *o*-dianisidine. The use of *o*-dianisidine, however, gives better results.

---

\* New, recommended for use.

\* New; recommended for use.

## METHOD 5

### Visualization Scheme

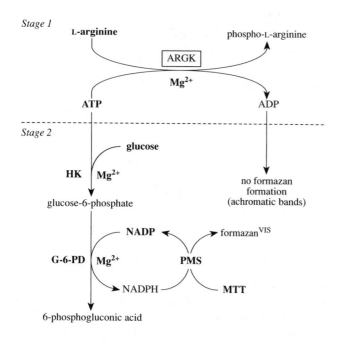

Stage 1
L-arginine → phospho-L-arginine
ARGK
Mg²⁺
ATP → ADP

Stage 2
glucose
HK Mg²⁺
glucose-6-phosphate
no formazan formation (achromatic bands)
NADP → formazan^VIS
G-6-PD Mg²⁺ PMS
NADPH ← MTT
6-phosphogluconic acid

### Staining Solution*

A. 0.05 *M* Tris–HCl buffer, pH 8.0    20 ml
    L-arginine    20 mg
    ATP    30 mg
    MgCl$_2$·6H$_2$O    10 mg
B. 0.05 *M* Tris–HCl buffer, pH 8.0    20 ml
    Hexokinase (HK)    45 units
    Glucose-6-phosphate dehydrogenase (G-6-PD)    100 units
    NADP    15 mg
    Glucose    80 mg
    MgCl$_2$·6H$_2$O    16 mg
    MTT    8 mg
    PMS    1 mg
C. 1.5% Agarose solution (50°C)

### Procedure

Mix solution A with 20 ml of solution C and pour the mixture over the surface of the gel. Incubate the gel at 37°C for 30 to 60 min. Remove first agarose overlay. Mix solution B with 20 ml of solution C and pour the mixture over the surface of the preincubated gel. Incubate the gel covered with second agarose overlay in the dark at 37°C until white bands appear on a blue background. Fix the stained agarose plate in 50% ethanol and dry on a filter paper.

### REFERENCES

1. Fisher, S. E. and Whitt, G. S., Evolution of isozyme loci and their differential tissue expression: creatine kinase as a model system, *J. Mol. Evol.*, 12, 25, 1978.
2. Bulnheim, H.-P. and Scholl, A., Genetic variation between geographic populations of the amphipods *Gammarus zaddachi* and *G. salinus*, *Mar. Biol.*, 64, 105, 1981.
3. Manchenko, G. P., Allozymic variation and substrate specificity of phosphatase from sipunculid *Phascolosoma japonicum*, *Isozyme Bull.*, 21, 168, 1988.

* New; recommended for use.

OTHER NAMES    Myokinase

REACTION    ATP + AMP = ADP + ADP

ENZYME SOURCE    Bacteria, green algae, fungi, plants, protozoa, invertebrates, vertebrates

## METHOD 1

### Visualization Scheme

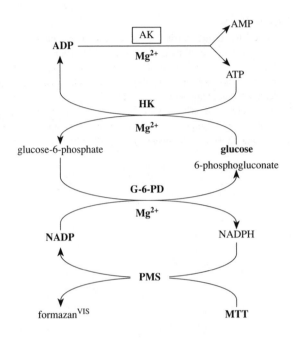

### Staining Solution[1]

A. 0.2 $M$ Tris–HCl buffer, pH 8.0 — 25 ml
   1 $M$ MgCl$_2$ — 1 ml
   ADP (disodium salt) — 25 mg
   Glucose — 180 mg
   NADP — 15 mg
   PMS — 2 mg
   MTT — 10 mg
   Hexokinase (HK) — 25 units
   Glucose-6-phosphate dehydrogenase (G-6-PD) — 15 units
B. 1.5% Agar solution (60°C) — 25 ml

### Procedure

Mix A and B components of the staining solution and pour the mixture over the surface of the gel. Incubate the gel in the dark at 37°C until dark blue bands appear. Fix stained gel or agar overlay in 50% ethanol.

*Notes:* When a preparation of NAD-dependent G-6-PD is included in the staining solution, NAD should be substituted for NADP. The use of NAD-dependent G-6-PD (Sigma G 5760 or G 5885) in a stain results in a cost saving because NAD is about five times less expensive than NADP. Furthermore, such a substitution eliminates the problem of enhancement of some AK bands owing to the activity of comigrating endogenous phosphogluconate dehydrogenase (see 1.1.1.44 — PGD), which bands can develop by Method 1 due to the production of 6-phosphogluconate by the linking enzyme, glucose-6-phosphate dehydrogenase, and the presence of NADP in the stain.

## METHOD 2

### Visualization Scheme

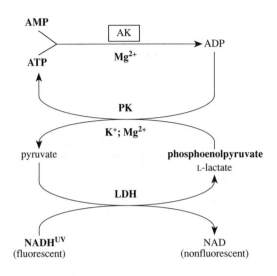

### Staining Solution[2]

A. 0.5 $M$ Tris–HCl buffer, pH 8.0 — 10 ml
   AMP (disodium salt; 6H$_2$O) — 25 mg
   ATP (disodium salt; 3H$_2$O) — 25 mg
   Phosphoenolpyruvate (potassium salt) — 25 mg
   NADH (disodium salt) — 10 mg
   KCl — 150 mg
   0.2 $M$ MgCl$_2$ — 2 ml
   Pyruvate kinase (PK; 400 U/ml) — 0.1 ml
   Lactate dehydrogenase (LDH; 2750 U/ml) — 0.1 ml
B. 2% Agar solution (60°C) — 12 ml

### Procedure

Mix A and B components of the staining solution and pour the mixture over the surface of the gel. Incubate the gel at 37°C and monitor under long-wave UV light. Dark (nonfluorescent) bands of AK activity are visible on a light (fluorescent) background of the gel. Record the zymogram or photograph using a yellow filter.

*Notes:* When preparations containing a phosphoenolpyruvate phosphatase activity are used for electrophoresis, additional bands can be observed on AK zymograms obtained by this method. These bands also develop in a staining solution lacking AMP, ATP, and PK (see 3.1.3.18 — PGP, Method 2), whereas AK bands do not.

## METHOD 3

### Visualization Scheme

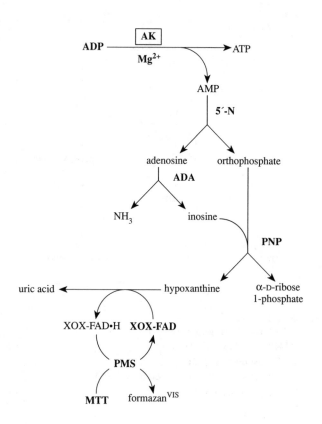

### Staining Solution[3]

| | |
|---|---:|
| A. 0.2 $M$ Tris–HCl buffer, pH 8.0 | 1 ml |
| ADP | 10 mg |
| MgCl$_2$ | 10 mg |
| PMS | 2 mg |
| MTT | 8 mg |
| 5′-Nucleotidase (5′-N) | 12 units |
| Adenosine deaminase (ADA) | 25 units |
| Purine-nucleoside phosphorylase (PNP) | 6 units |
| Xanthine oxidase (XOX) | 2 units |
| B. 1% Agar solution (60°C) | 5 ml |

### Procedure

Mix A and B components of the staining solution and pour the mixture over the surface of the gel. Incubate the gel in the dark at 37°C until dark blue bands appear. Fix stained gel in 50% ethanol.

*Notes:* This method is less practical than the other two described above; however, it demonstrates a general approach for visualizing enzymes releasing AMP.

## GENERAL NOTES

In the forward reaction catalyzed by mammalian AK, AMP cannot be replaced by UMP, GMP, or CMP, using ATP as the second substrate. However, ATP can be replaced by UTP, ITP, CTP, or GTP, using AMP as the other substrate. The enzyme from rabbit muscle is inactive towards IDP, GDP, and UDP in the backward reaction while CDP is a substrate as well as ADP. The enzyme from baker's yeast is specific for ADP as the nucleotide diphosphate. However, GTP or ITP can replace ATP and GMP can replace AMP but CTP, UTP, CDP, and UDP are inactive.

### REFERENCES

1. Fildes, R. A. and Harris, H., Genetically determined variation of adenylate kinase in man, *Nature*, 209, 261, 1966.
2. Harris, H. and Hopkinson, D. A., *Handbook of Enzyme Electrophoresis in Human Genetics*, North-Holland, Amsterdam (Loose leaf with supplements in 1977 and 1978), 1976.
3. Friedrich, C. A., Chakravarti, S., and Ferrell, R. E., A general method for visualizing enzymes releasing adenosine or adenosine-5′-monophosphate, *Biochem. Genet.*, 22, 389, 1984.

OTHER NAMES    Nucleoside monophosphate kinase, uridine monophosphate kinase

REACTION    ATP + nucleoside monophosphate = ADP + nucleoside diphosphate

ENZYME SOURCE  Bacteria, fungi, vertebrates

## METHOD

### Visualization Scheme

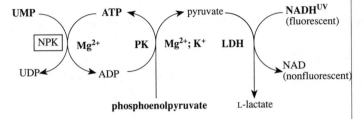

### Staining Solution[1]

    0.1 $M$ Tris–HCl buffer, pH 7.8
    4.4 m$M$ UMP
    3.6 m$M$ ATP
    2.1 m$M$ Phosphoenolpyruvate
    1 m$M$ NADH
    25 m$M$ MgCl$_2$
    100 m$M$ K$_2$SO$_4$
    20 U/ml Pyruvate kinase (PK)
    50 U/ml Lactate dehydrogenase (LDH)

### Procedure

Soak filter paper in the staining solution and apply to the gel surface. Incubate the gel at 37°C and monitor under long-wave UV light. Dark (nonfluorescent) bands of NPK activity are visible on the light (fluorescent) background of the gel. Record the zymogram or photograph using a yellow filter.

*Notes:* When preparations containing a phosphoenolpyruvate phosphatase activity are electrophorized, additional bands can develop on NPK zymograms obtained by this method. These bands also develop in a staining solution lacking UMP, ATP, and PK (see 3.1.3.18 — PGP, Method 2), whereas NPK bands do not.

## OTHER METHODS

The product of the reverse NPK reaction, ATP, can be detected using two linked reactions catalyzed by auxiliary enzymes, hexokinase and glucose-6-phosphate dehydrogenase. This method, however, also develops adenylate kinase activity bands (see 2.7.4.3 — AK, Method 1).

## GENERAL NOTES

Many nucleoside monophosphates can act as acceptors; other nucleoside triphosphates can act as donors.

## REFERENCE

1.  Giblett, E. R., Anderson, J. E., Chen, S.-H., Teng, Y.-S., and Cohen, F., Uridine monophosphate kinase: a new genetic polymorphism with possible clinical implications, *Am. J. Hum. Genet.*, 26, 627, 1974.

OTHER NAMES    Uridine-diphosphate kinase

REACTION    ATP + nucleoside diphosphate = ADP + nucleoside triphosphate

ENZYME SOURCE  Bacteria, fungi, plants, vertebrates

## METHOD 1

### Visualization Scheme

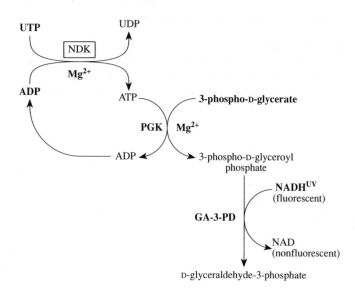

### Staining Solution[1]

| | |
|---|---|
| 0.1 $M$ Tris–HCl buffer, pH 7.8 | 10 ml |
| UTP | 15 mg |
| ADP | 4.9 mg |
| 3-Phospho-D-glycerate (disodium salt) | 8.6 mg |
| 0.2 $M$ KCl; 50 m$M$ MgSO$_4$ | 0.2 ml |
| NADH | 8 mg |
| Phosphoglycerate kinase (PGK) | 60 units |
| Glyceraldehyde-3-phosphate dehydrogenase (GA-3-PD) | 40 units |

### Procedure

Apply filter paper soaked in the staining solution to the surface of the gel. Incubate the gel at 37°C in a moist chamber for 1 to 2 h and monitor under long-wave UV light. Dark (nonfluorescent) bands of NDK activity are visible on the light (fluorescent) background of the gel. Record the zymogram or photograph using a yellow filter.

*Notes:*  Adenylate kinase bands can also develop on NDK zymograms obtained by this method. Therefore, an additional gel should be stained for AK activity (see 2.7.4.3 — AK) as a control.

Additional auxiliary enzymes, triose-phosphate isomerase and glycerol-3-phosphate dehydrogenase, may be included in the staining solution to intensify the process of NADH into NAD conversion (for example see 2.7.2.3 — PGK).

## METHOD 2

### Visualization Scheme

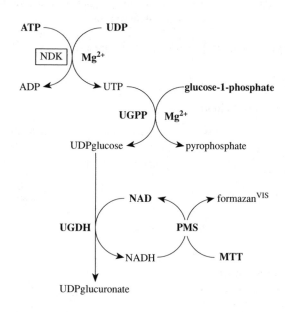

### Staining Solution[2] (adapted)

| | |
|---|---|
| A.  0.2 $M$ Tris–HCl buffer, pH 8.0 | 6 ml |
| 0.1 $M$ MgCl$_2$ | 2 ml |
| 200 mg/ml ATP | 0.5 ml |
| 200 mg/ml UDP | 0.5 ml |
| 200 mg/ml Glucose-1-phosphate | 0.5 ml |
| 200 mg/ml NAD | 0.2 ml |
| 25 U/ml UTPglucose-1-phosphate uridylyltransferase (UGPP) | 0.5 ml |
| 2 U/ml UDPglucose dehydrogenase (UGDH) | 0.2 ml |
| 10 mg/ml PMS | 0.1 ml |
| 50 mg/ml MTT | 0.1 ml |
| B.  2% Agarose solution (60°C) | 10 ml |

### Procedure

Mix A and B components of the staining solution and pour the mixture over the surface of the gel. Incubate the gel in the dark at 37°C until dark blue bands appear. Fix stained gel in 50% ethanol.

*Notes:*  UDPglucose dehydrogenase preparation used in the staining solution should be free of NDK activity.

## GENERAL NOTES

The enzyme is nonspecific with respect to its substrates. For example, the enzyme from human erythrocytes reacts with di- and triphosphate nucleotides containing either ribose or deoxyribose and any of the naturally occurring purine or pyrimidine bases. The enzyme does not catalyze an adenylate kinase type of reaction (see 2.7.4.3 — AK).

## REFERENCES

1. Anderson, J. E., Teng, Y.-S. and Giblett, E. R., Stains for six enzymes potentially applicable to chromosomal assignment by cell hybridization, *Cytogenet. Cell Genet.*, 14, 465, 1975.
2. Pierce, M., Cummings, R. D., and Roth, S., The localization of galactosyltransferases in polyacrylamide gels by a coupled enzyme assay, *Anal. Biochem.*, 102, 441, 1980.

## 2.7.4.8 — Guanylate Kinase; GUK

OTHER NAMES    Deoxyguanylate kinase

REACTION    ATP + GMP = ADP + GDP

ENZYME SOURCE  Fungi, invertebrates, vertebrates

## METHOD 1

### Visualization Scheme

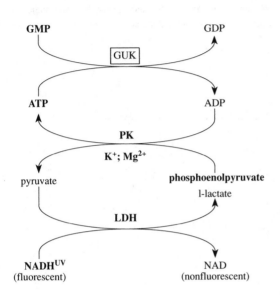

### Staining Solution[1]

A. 0.2 $M$ Tris–HCl buffer, pH 7.9
   1.5 m$M$ ATP
   6 m$M$ GMP
   4 m$M$ Phosphoenolpyruvate
   0.6 m$M$ NADH
   20 m$M$ MgSO$_4$
   100 m$M$ KCl
   1 m$M$ CaCl$_2$
   2 U/ml Pyruvate kinase (PK)
   18 U/ml Lactate dehydrogenase (LDH)
B. 1% Agar solution (60°C)

### Procedure

Mix equal volumes of A and B solutions and pour the mixture over the surface of the gel. Incubate the gel at 37°C and monitor under long-wave UV light. Dark (nonfluorescent) bands of GUK activity are visible on a light (fluorescent) background of the gel. Record the zymogram or photograph using a yellow filter.

*Notes:* When a zymogram that is visible in daylight is required, counterstain the processed gel with MTT/PMS solution. This will result in the appearance of achromatic GUK bands on a blue background of the gel.

When preparations containing a phosphoenolpyruvate phosphatase activity are electrophorized, additional bands can be observed on GUK zymograms obtained by this method. These bands also develop in a staining solution lacking ATP, GMP, and PK (see 3.1.3.18 — PGP, Method 2), whereas GUK bands do not.

## METHOD 2

### Visualization Scheme

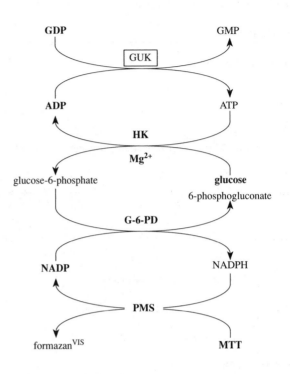

### Staining Solution[1]

A. 0.2 $M$ Tris–HCl buffer, pH 7.9
   1 m$M$ ADP
   4 m$M$ GDP
   20 m$M$ Glucose
   0.8 m$M$ NADP
   0.08% MTT
   0.04% PMS
   20 m$M$ MgSO$_4$
   100 m$M$ KCl
   0.2 U/ml Glucose-6-phosphate dehydrogenase (G-6-PD)
   0.4 U/ml Hexokinase (HK)
B. 1% Agar solution (60°C)

### Procedure

Mix equal volumes of A and B solutions and pour the mixture over the surface of the gel. Incubate the gel in the dark at 37°C until dark blue bands appear. Fix stained gel in 50% ethanol.

*Notes:* Adenylate kinase (AK) bands can also develop on GUK zymograms obtained by this method. Therefore, an additional gel should be stained for AK activity (see 2.7.4.3 — AK, Method 1) as a control.

### REFERENCE

1. Moon, E. and Christiansen, R. O., Guanylate kynase in man: multiple molecular forms, *Hum. Hered.*, 22, 18, 1972.

REACTION    AMP + nucleoside triphosphate = ADP + nucleoside diphosphate

ENZYME SOURCE  Vertebrates

## METHOD

### Visualization Scheme

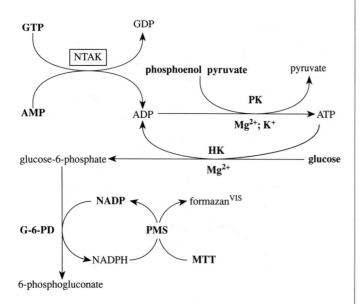

### Staining Solution[1]

| | |
|---|---|
| A. 0.3 $M$ Tris–HCl buffer, pH 8.0 | 10 ml |
| AMP (disodium salt; $6H_2O$) | 25 mg |
| GTP | 15 mg |
| Phosphoenolpyruvate (potassium salt) | 20 mg |
| KCl | 150 mg |
| $MgCl_2 \cdot 6H_2O$ | 40 mg |
| NADP (disodium salt) | 5 mg |
| Glucose | 40 mg |
| Glucose-6-phosphate dehydrogenase (G-6-PD; 140 U/ml) | 25 µl |
| Hexokinase (HK; 280 U/ml) | 25 µl |
| Pyruvate kinase (PK; 400 U/ml) | 50 µl |
| MTT | 5 mg |
| PMS | 0.5 mg |
| B. 1.5% Agar solution (60°C) | 10 ml |

### Procedure

Mix A and B solutions and pour the mixture over the surface of the gel. Incubate the gel in the dark at 37°C until dark blue bands appear. Fix stained gel in 50% ethanol.

*Notes:*  This staining system also detects adenylate kinase activity bands, but NTAK activity is not detected by the ordinary adenylate kinase stains (see 2.7.4.3 — AK, Methods 1 to 3). These differences can be used to differentiate AK and NTAK bands.

It is possible to replace GTP with ITP in the staining solution. However, this will cause significant staining of gel background because of the reaction of auxiliary HK with ITP and glucose and the subsequent reaction of auxiliary G-6-PD with glucose-6-phosphate and NADP in the presence of PMS and MTT.

## OTHER METHODS

NTAK activity can also be detected by negative fluorescent stain using pyruvate kinase and lactate dehydrogenase as linking enzymes. To prepare the necessary staining solution, substitute GTP for ATP in the negative fluorescent stain for adenylate kinase (see 2.7.4.3 — AK, Method 2).

### REFERENCE
1. Wilson, D. E., Povey, S., and Harris, H., Adenylate kinases in man: evidence for a third locus, *Ann. Hum. Genet.*, 39, 305, 1976.

OTHER NAMES    5-Phosphoribosyl-1-pyrophosphate synthetase

REACTION    ATP + D-ribose-5-phosphate = AMP +
5-phospho-$\alpha$-D-ribose 1-diphosphate

ENZYME SOURCE  Bacteria, vertebrates

## METHOD 1

### Visualization Scheme

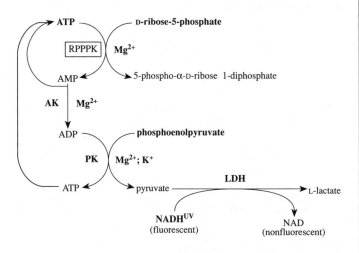

### Staining Solution[1]

| | |
|---|---|
| 0.1 $M$ Tris–HCl buffer, pH 7.8 | 5 ml |
| D-ribose-5-phosphate (disodium salt) | 12.4 mg |
| ATP | 15 mg |
| Phosphoenolpyruvate | 4.5 mg |
| NADH | 3.5 mg |
| 2 $M$ KCl; 0.5 $M$ MgSO$_4$ | 0.25 ml |
| Adenylate kinase (AK; Sigma) | 50 µl |
| Pyruvate kinase (PK; Sigma) | 50 µl |
| Lactate dehydrogenase (LDH; Sigma) | 100 µl |

### Procedure

Soak filter paper in the staining solution and apply to the surface of the gel. Incubate the gel at 37°C for 2 to 3 h in a moist chamber and monitor under long-wave UV light. Dark (nonfluorescent) bands of RPPPK are visible on a light (fluorescent) background of the gel. Record the zymogram or photograph using a yellow filter.

*Notes:*  When preparations containing a phosphoenolpyruvate phosphatase activity are electrophorized, additional bands can be observed on RPPPK zymograms obtained by this method. These bands also develop in a staining solution lacking ATP, D-ribose-5-phosphate, AK, and PK (see 3.1.3.18 — PGP, Method 2), whereas RPPPK activity bands do not.

## METHOD 2

### Visualization Scheme

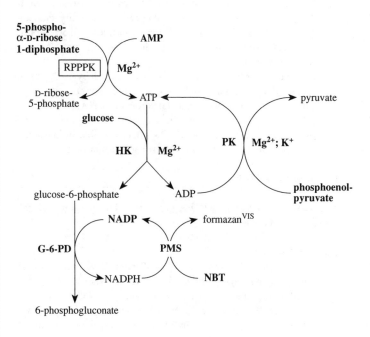

### Staining Solution[2]

75 m$M$ Potassium phosphate buffer, pH 7.4
1 m$M$ 5-Phospho-$\alpha$-D-ribose 1-diphosphate
0.5 m$M$ AMP
1 m$M$ Phosphoenolpyruvate
1 m$M$ D-Glucose
0.4 m$M$ NADP
10 m$M$ MgCl$_2$
0.075 mg/ml PMS
0.75 mg/ml NBT
10 U/ml Pyruvate kinase (PK)
1 U/ml Glucose-6-phosphate dehydrogenase (G-6-PD)
2.25 U/ml Hexokinase (HK)
10% Glycerol

### Procedure

Saturate the glass-supported Whatman 3MM chromatographic paper with staining solution and apply the gel directly to the chromatographic paper. Cover gel with a second glass plate and wrap in aluminum foil to avoid nonspecific light-induced production of blue formazan. Incubate the gel at 37°C until dark blue bands appear. Fix stained gel in 50% ethanol.

*Notes:*  The addition of 3% Nonidet to a homogenization buffer and to electrode and gel buffers is recommended.

Pyruvate kinase and phosphoenolpyruvate are included in the stain to remove ADP which inhibits RPPPK.

Intensely stained nonspecific bands which are not dependent on the 5-phospho-$\alpha$-D-ribose 1-diphosphate also develop on RPPPK zymograms obtained using this method after electrophoresis of human tissue preparations. The nature of these bands is unknown.

## 2.7.6.1 — Ribose-phosphate Pyrophosphokinase; RPPPK (continued)

### OTHER METHODS

A. The product of the forward RPPPK reaction, AMP, can be detected using four reactions catalyzed by auxiliary enzymes 5′-nucleotidase, adenosine deaminase, purine nucleoside phosphorylase, and xanthine oxidase (for example, see 2.7.4.3 — AK, Method 3).

B. Method 2 described above may be modified by inclusion of lactate dehydrogenase and NADH in the staining solution in place of glucose-6-phosphate dehydrogenase, NADP, PMS, and NBT. This modification will result in the development of dark (nonfluorescent) bands of RPPPK activity visible in long-wave UV light on the light (fluorescent) background of the gel.

### GENERAL NOTES

The forward reaction of RPPPK is favored. The enzyme is highly specific for its substrates.

### REFERENCES

1. Anderson, J. E., Teng, Y.-S. and Giblett, E. R., Stains for six enzymes potentially applicable to chromosomal assignment by cell hybridization, *Cytogenet. Cell Genet.*, 14, 465, 1975.
2. Lebo, R. V. and Martin, D. W., Electrophoretic heterogeneity of 5-phosphoribosyl-1-pyrophosphate synthetase within and among humans, *Biochem. Genet.*, 16, 905, 1978.

## 2.7.7.4 — Sulfate Adenylyltransferase; SAT

OTHER NAMES     ATP–sulfurylase, sulfurylase

REACTION     ATP + sulfate (or molybdate) = pyrophosphate + adenylylsulfate (or adenylylmolybdate)

ENZYME SOURCE   Bacteria, fungi, plants

### METHOD

**Visualization Scheme**

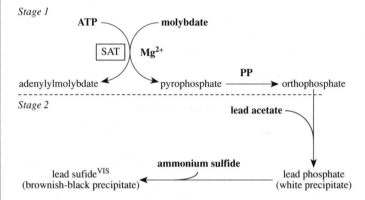

### Staining Solution[1] (modified)
A. 0.1 $M$ Tris–HCl buffer, pH 8.0     20 ml
    ATP     40 mg
    $Na_2MoO_4$     80 mg
    $MgCl_2 \cdot 6H_2O$     30 mg
    Inorganic pyrophosphatase from yeast (PP)     25 units
B. 2% Agarose solution (60°C)     20 ml
C. 0.2% $Pb(CH_3COO)_2$ in 1% $CH_3COOH$
D. 5% Ammonium sulfide

### Procedure
Mix A and B solutions and pour the mixture over the surface of the gel. Incubate the gel at 37°C for 30 to 40 min. Remove agarose overlay and immerse gel in solution C for 10 to 15 min. Discard solution C, rinse gel in water and treat with solution D. A brownish-black precipitate of lead sulfide is generated in areas of SAT localization.

### OTHER METHODS

An enzymatic method for detection of orthophosphate generated by auxiliary inorganic pyrophosphatase is available.[2] This method involves two additional linked reactions catalyzed by auxiliary enzymes purine nucleoside phosphorylase and xanthine oxidase, coupled with the PMS/MTT system (for example, see 3.1.3.1 — ALP, Method 8). The enzymatic method may be preferable due to its sensitivity and generation of a nondiffusable formazan as the result of a one-step procedure.

### REFERENCES

1. Skiring, G. W., Trudinger, P. A., and Shaw, W. H., Electrophoretic characterization of ATP:sulfate adenylyltransferase (ATP–sulfurylase) with use of polyacrylamide gels, *Anal. Biochem.*, 48, 259, 1972.
2. Klebe, R. J., Schloss, S., Mock, L., and Link, C. R., Visualization of isozymes which generate inorganic phosphate, *Biochem. Genet.*, 19, 921, 1981.

| OTHER NAMES | RNA nucleotidyltransferase (DNA-directed), RNA polymerase |
|---|---|
| REACTION | n Nucleoside triphosphate = n pyrophosphate + RNA$_n$ (DNA template is needed) |
| ENZYME SOURCE | Bacteria, fungi, plants, invertebrates, vertebrates |

## METHOD

### Visualization Scheme

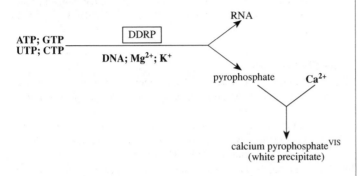

### Staining Solution[1]

10 mM Tris–HCl buffer, pH 8.0
12 mM Mg$^{2+}$
0.1 mM EDTA
1 mM Dithiothreitol
0.2 M KCl
20 mM Ca$^{2+}$
0.8 mM ATP
0.8 mM CTP
0.8 mM GTP
0.8 mM UTP

### Procedure

Soak electrophorized PAG containing 1.6 mg/ml calf thymus DNA in 100 mM tris–HCl buffer, pH 8.0, for 20 to 30 min and incubate in the staining solution at 37°C until white bands of calcium pyrophosphate precipitation appear. These bands are well visible when the gel is viewed against a dark background. When an activity stain of sufficient intensity is obtained, remove gel from the staining solution and store in 50 mM glycine–KOH buffer, pH 10.0, containing 5 mM Ca$^{2+}$ either at 5°C or at room temperature in the presence of an antibacterial agent.

*Notes:* The method is applicable for clean gels (PAG or agarose). When more opaque gels are used (e.g., acetate cellulose or starch gel), precipitated calcium pyrophosphate should be counterstained with Alizarin Red S.

## OTHER METHODS

A. The product pyrophosphate can be detected enzymatically using three coupled reactions sequentially catalyzed by auxiliary enzymes bacterial pyrophosphate–fructose-6-phosphate 1-phosphotransferase, aldolase, and glycerol-3-phosphate dehydrogenase. The activity bands of DDRP developed by this method are visible in long-wave UV light as dark areas on a light (fluorescent) gel background. The substitution of glyceraldehyde-3-phosphate dehydrogenase for glycerol-3-phosphate dehydrogenase and NAD, arsenate, PMS and MTT for NADH results in the development of DDRP activity bands visible in daylight. The use of an additional auxiliary enzyme, triosephosphate isomerase, accelerates reactions occurring in fluorogenic and chromogenic methods and enhances developing bands (for details see 2.7.1.90 — PFPPT). Another enzymatic method for detection of pyrophosphate is available. It involves three auxiliary enzymes (the inorganic pyrophosphatase, the purine-nucleoside phosphorylase and the xanthine oxidase) coupled with a PMS/MTT system (for example, see 2.7.7.4 — SAT, Other Methods).

B. The enzyme can also be detected by autoradiography using a staining solution similar to that described above but lacking Ca$^{2+}$ and containing [$^{14}$C]ATP (1 µCi/ml final concentration) in addition to nonlabeled ATP.[2]

C. An immunoblotting procedure (for details see Part II) based on the utility of monoclonal antibodies specific to the *Drosophila* and bovine enzyme[3-5] can also be used for immunohistochemical visualization of the enzyme protein on electrophoretic gels. This procedure is unsuitable for routine laboratory use in large-scale population genetic studies, but it may be of great value in special (e.g., biochemical, immunochemical, phylogenetic, genetic, etc.) analyses of DDRP.

## REFERENCES

1. Nimmo, H. G. and Nimmo, G. A., A general method for the localization of enzymes that produce phosphate, pyrophosphate, or CO$_2$ after polyacrylamide gel electrophoresis, *Anal. Biochem.*, 121, 17, 1982.

2. Uriel, J. and Lavialle, C., Autoradiographic method for characterization of DNA and RNA polymerases after gel electrophoresis, *Anal. Biochem.*, 42, 509, 1971.

3. Bona, M., Scheer, U., and Bautz, E. K., Antibodies to RNA polymerase-II(B) inhibit transcription in lampbrush chromosomes after microinjection into living amphibian oocytes, *J. Mol. Biol.*, 151, 81, 1981.

4. Christmann, J. L. and Dahmus, M. E., Monoclonal antibody specific for calf thymus RNA polymerases-IIO and polymerase-IIA, *J. Biol. Chem.*, 256, 1798, 1981.

5. Kramer, A. and Bautz, E. K., Immunological relatedness of subunits of RNA polymerase-II from insects and mammals, *Eur. J. Biochem.*, 117, 449, 1981.

OTHER NAMES     DNA nucleotidyltransferase (DNA-directed), DNA polymerase

REACTION     n Deoxynucleoside triphosphate = n pyrophosphate + DNA$_n$ (DNA template is needed)

ENZYME SOURCE     Bacteria, fungi, plants, invertebrates, vertebrates

## METHOD

### Visualization Scheme

*Stage 1: Enzyme reaction*

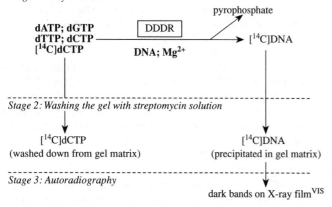

*Stage 2: Washing the gel with streptomycin solution*

[$^{14}$C]dCTP                     [$^{14}$C]DNA
(washed down from gel matrix)        (precipitated in gel matrix)

*Stage 3: Autoradiography*

dark bands on X-ray film$^{VIS}$

### Reaction Mixture[1]

A.   140 m*M* Tris–HCl buffer, pH 7.4
     6 m*M* MgCl$_2$
     2 m*M* 2-Mercaptoethanol
     0.06 m*M* dATP
     0.06 m*M* dGTP
     0.06 m*M* dTTP
     0.06 m*M* dCTP
     0.4 µCi/ml [$^{14}$C]dCTP
     400 µg/ml Calf thymus DNA
B.   2.4% Agar solution (42°C)
C.   2% Streptomycin (water solution)

### Procedure

*Stage 1.*   Mix A and B components of the reaction mixture and pour the mixture over the surface of electrophorized 6% PAG containing 0.8% agarose to form a 1 mm thick reactive agar plate. Incubate the PAG/reactive plate combination at 37°C for 2 h.

*Stage 2.*   Take off the reactive plate and wash it two times for 1 to 2 h in solution C. Dry the reactive plate on a sheet of filter paper.

*Stage 3.*   Autoradiograph dry reactive plate with X-ray film (Kodak, Kodirex film) for 1 to 2 weeks at room temperature.

Dark bands on developed X-ray film correspond to localization of DDDP activity on the gel.

*Notes:*   DNA template (calf thymus DNA activated by DNase I, or poly[d(A-T)]) may be included directly into running 10% PAG containing 0.1% SDS.[2]

## OTHER METHODS

A. The product pyrophosphate can be detected in clean gels (PAG or agarose) using the calcium-pyrophosphate precipitation method.[3] The white bands of the precipitated calcium pyrophosphate are clearly visible when viewed against a dark background and can be photographed or scanned (e.g., see 2.7.7.6 — DDRP).

B. Pyrophosphate can be detected enzymatically using three coupled reactions catalyzed by the auxiliary enzymes inorganic pyrophosphatase, purine-nucleoside phosphorylase, and xanthine oxidase (see 3.6.1.1 — PP, Method 2). Another enzymatic method for detection of pyrophosphate is available. Two variants of this method exist which allow observation of DDDP bands in long-wave UV light or daylight (see 2.7.7.6 — DDRP; Other Methods, A).

## REFERENCES

1. Uriel, J. and Lavialle, C., Autoradiographic method for characterization of DNA and RNA polymerases after gel electrophoresis, *Anal. Biochem.*, 42, 509, 1971.
2. Karawya, E., Swack, J. A., and Wilson, S. H., Improved conditions for activity gel analysis of DNA polymerase catalytic polypeptides, *Anal. Biochem.*, 135, 318, 1983.
3. Nimmo, H. G. and Nimmo, G. A., A general method for the localization of enzymes that produce phosphate, pyrophosphate, or CO$_2$ after polyacrylamide gel electrophoresis, *Anal. Biochem.*, 121, 17, 1982.

OTHER NAMES    Polynucleotide phosphorylase, polyribonucleotide phosphorylase

REACTION    $RNA_{n+1}$ + orthophosphate = $RNA_n$ + nucleoside diphosphate

ENZYME SOURCE    Bacteria, fungi, plants, invertebrates, vertebrates

## METHOD

### Visualization Scheme

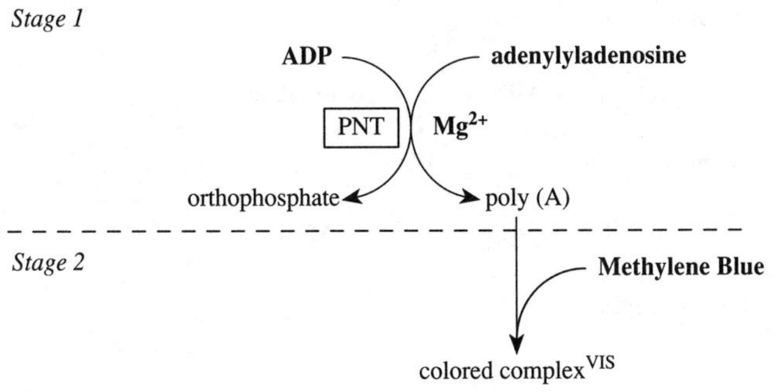

*Stage 1*

*Stage 2*

### Staining Solution[1]
A. 75 m$M$ Tris–HCl buffer, pH 9.0
   20 m$M$ ADP
   5 m$M$ $MgCl_2$
   0.2 m$M$ EDTA
   0.2 mg/ml Adenylyladenosine (ApA)
B. 0.2% Methylene Blue
   0.4 $M$ Sodium acetate buffer, pH 4.7

### Procedure
Incubate electrophorized gel at 37°C for 2 to 48 h in solution A. Rinse gel with a solution of 7% acetic acid and transfer to solution B for 18 h. Destain the stained gel by diffusion with distilled water. Dark blue bands indicate the areas of PNT activity.

*Notes:* A 1% (w/v) solution of Acridine Orange or 1.03% (w/v) solution of lanthanum chloride in 25% acetic acid can also be used to visualize the areas of poly(A) deposition on the gel. Gels stained with Acridine Orange should be destained electrophoretically with 7.5% acetic acid.

## OTHER METHODS

A. The bands of PNT activity can be visualized by autoradiography using labeled substrate [$^{14}$C]ADP (1 µCi/ml final concentration) in a reaction mixture similar to solution A of the staining solution given above.[2] After an appropriate period of gel incubation in the reaction mixture, the poly(A) formed is precipitated in a gel matrix with streptomycin. The washed and dried gel is then autoradiographed with X-ray film.
B. Different methods of detection of orthophosphate can also be used for localization of PNT activity on electrophoretic gels (for details see 3.1.3.1 — ALP; Methods 5, 6, 7, and 8 and 3.1.3.2 — ACP; Methods 4 and 5).

## GENERAL NOTES

ADP, IDP, GDP, UDP, and CDP can act as donors.

## REFERENCES
1. Killick, K. A., Polyribonucleotide phosphorylase from *Dictyostelium discoideum*, *Exp. Mycol.*, 4, 181, 1980.
2. Uriel, J. and Lavialle, C., Autoradiographic method for characterization of DNA and RNA polymerases after gel electrophoresis, *Anal. Biochem.*, 42, 509, 1971.

OTHER NAMES    UDPglucose pyrophosphorylase; glucose-1-phosphate uridylyltransferase

REACTION    UTP + α-D-glucose-1-phosphate = pyrophosphate + UDPglucose

ENZYME SOURCE    Bacteria, fungi, plants, invertebrates, vertebrates

## METHOD 1

### Visualization Scheme

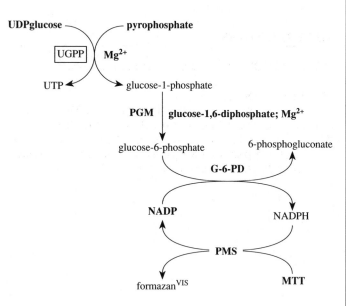

### Staining Solution[1]

| | |
|---|---|
| 0.36 $M$ Tris–HCl buffer, pH 8.0 | 0.8 ml |
| 0.1 $M$ MgCl$_2$ | 0.2 ml |
| UDPglucose (disodium salt) | 6 mg |
| 22.5 mg/ml Pyrophosphate (disodium salt; 10H$_2$O) | 0.2 ml |
| 0.175 mg/ml Glucose-1,6-diphosphate (tetracyclohexylammonium salt; 4H$_2$O) | 0.2 ml |
| 4 mg/ml NADP (disodium salt) | 0.2 ml |
| 0.054 $M$ EDTA (pH 7.0) | 0.2 ml |
| 140 U/ml Glucose-6-phosphate dehydrogenase (G-6-PD) | 5 µl |
| 400 U/ml Phosphoglucomutase (PGM) | 5 µl |
| 2 mg/ml MTT | 0.2 ml |
| 0.4 mg/ml PMS | 0.2 ml |

### Procedure

Apply the staining solution dropwise to the gel surface. Incubate the gel in the dark at 37°C until dark blue bands appear. Fix stained gel in 50% ethanol.

## METHOD 2

### Visualization Scheme

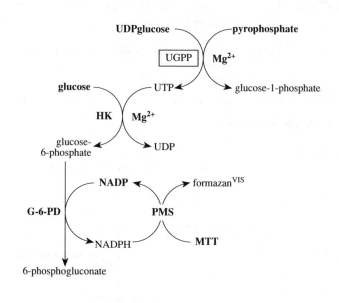

### Staining Solution*

| | |
|---|---|
| A. 0.4 $M$ Tris–HCl buffer, pH 8.0 | 20 ml |
|    UDPglucose (disodium salt) | 50 mg |
|    Pyrophosphate (disodium salt; 10H$_2$O) | 40 mg |
|    MgCl$_2$·6H$_2$O | 10 mg |
|    Glucose | 80 mg |
|    Hexokinase from Bakers yeast (HK) | 40 units |
|    Glucose-6-phosphate dehydrogenase (G-6-PD) | 20 units |
|    NADP | 10 mg |
|    MTT | 6 mg |
|    PMS | 1 mg |
| B. 2% Agarose solution (50°C) | 20 ml |

### Procedure

Mix A and B solutions and pour the mixture over the surface of the gel. Incubate the gel in the dark at 37°C until dark blue bands appear. Fix stained gel in 50% ethanol.

*Notes:* The method is based on the ability of yeast hexokinase to utilize UTP instead of ATP in its forward reaction. The hexokinase reaction rate with UTP is much lower than with ATP but is quite enough to produce essential quantities of glucose-6-phosphate, which is then detected using auxiliary NADP-dependent glucose-6-phosphate dehydrogenase coupled with the PMS/MTT system.

---

\* New; recommended for use.

## METHOD 3

### Visualization Scheme

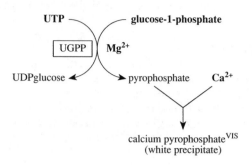

### Staining Solution[2]

50 m$M$ Glycine–KOH buffer, pH 9.0
0.5 m$M$ Glucose-1-phosphate
8 m$M$ Mg$^{2+}$
2 m$M$ UTP
2 m$M$ Ca$^{2+}$

### Procedure

Following electrophoresis, soak PAG in 50 m$M$ glycine–KOH buffer, pH 9.0, for 20 to 30 min and incubate in the staining solution at room temperature until white bands of calcium pyrophosphate precipitation appear. These bands are well visible when the gel is viewed against a dark background. When an activity stain of sufficient intensity is obtained, remove the gel from the staining solution and store in 50 m$M$ glycine–KOH buffer, pH 10.0, containing 5 m$M$ Ca$^{2+}$, either at 5°C or at room temperature in the presence of an antibacterial agent.

*Notes:* The method is developed for clean gels (PAG or agarose). When more opaque gels are used (e.g., acetate cellulose or starch gel), precipitated calcium pyrophosphate can be subsequently counterstained with Alizarin Red S.

## OTHER METHODS

The product of the reverse UGPP reaction, UDPglucose, can be detected using a linked reaction catalyzed by the auxiliary enzyme NAD-dependent UDPglucose dehydrogenase in couple with the PMS/MTT system (see 1.1.1.22 — UGDH).

### REFERENCES

1. Van Someren, H., Van Henegouwen, H. B., Los, W., Wurzer-Figurelli, E., Doppert, B., Vervloet, M., and Meera Khan, P., Enzyme electrophoresis on cellulose acetate gel. II. Zymogram patterns in man–chinese hamster somatic cell hybrids, *Humangenetik*, 25, 189, 1974.
2. Nimmo, H. G. and Nimmo, G. A., A general method for the localization of enzymes that produce phosphate, pyrophosphate, or CO$_2$ after polyacrylamide gel electrophoresis, *Anal. Biochem.*, 121, 17, 1982.

OTHER NAMES  UDPglucose–hexose-1-phosphate uridylyltransferase (recommended name), hexose-1-phosphate uridylyltransferase, uridyl transferase

REACTION  UDPglucose + α-D-galactose-1-phosphate = α-D-glucose-1-phosphate + UDP–galactose

ENZYME SOURCE  Bacteria, fungi, plants, protozoa, vertebrates

## METHOD

### Visualization Scheme

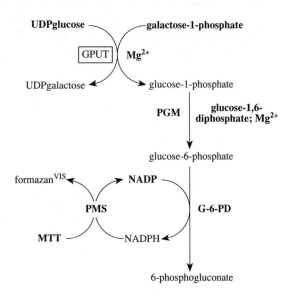

### Staining Solution[1]

A. 0.3 $M$ Tris–acetate buffer, pH 7.8 — 10 ml
   Galactose-1-phosphate (dipotassium salt; $5H_2O$) — 20 mg
   UDPglucose (disodium salt) — 15 mg
   NADP (disodium salt) — 10 mg
   Glucose-1,6-diphosphate — 0.2 mg
   0.2 $M$ $MgCl_2$ — 1 ml
   500 U/ml Phosphoglucomutase (PGM) — 20 μl
   345 U/ml Glucose-6-phosphate dehydrogenase (G-6-PD) — 20 μl
   2 mg/ml MTT — 1 ml
   1 mg/ml PMS — 1 ml
B. 2% Agarose solution (50°C) — 15 ml

### Procedure

Mix A and B components of the staining solution and pour the mixture over the surface of the gel. Incubate the gel in the dark at 37°C until dark blue bands appear. Fix stained gel in 50% ethanol.

*Notes:*  NAD-dependent glucose-6-phosphate dehydrogenase (Sigma G 5760 or G 5885) and NAD may be used instead of NADP-dependent glucose-6-phosphate dehydrogenase and NADP in the staining solution. This substitution will result in a cost saving because NAD is about five times less expensive than NADP.

When NADP is used, 6-phosphogluconate dehydrogenase may be included in the staining solution to enhance NADP into NADPH conversion and thus to increase the sensitivity of the method.[2]

## OTHER METHODS

A product of the backward GPUT reaction, UDPglucose, can be detected using the auxiliary enzyme UDPglucose dehydrogenase (see 1.1.1.22 — UGDH).

## REFERENCES

1. Sparkes, M. C., Crist, M., and Sparkes, R. S., Improved technique for electrophoresis of human galactose-1-P uridyl transferase (EC 2.7.7.12), *Hum. Genet.*, 40, 93, 1977.
2. Harris, H. and Hopkinson, D. A., *Handbook of Enzyme Electrophoresis in Human Genetics*, North-Holland, Amsterdam (Loose leaf with supplements in 1977 and 1978), 1976.

## 2.7.7.48 — RNA-Directed RNA Polymerase; RNAP

**OTHER NAMES**    RNA nucleotidyltransferase (RNA-directed), RNA-directed RNA replicase

**REACTION**    n Nucleoside triphosphate = n pyrophosphate + $RNA_n$

**ENZYME SOURCE**  Plants, vertebrates

## METHOD

### Visualization Scheme

*Stage 1*

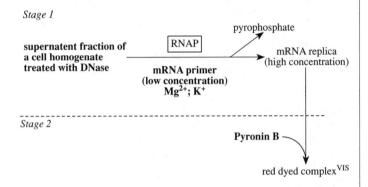

*Stage 2*

### Staining Solution[1]

A. Supernatant fraction of a cell homogenate treated with DNase (see *Notes*)

B. 0.1 *M* Tris–maleate buffer, pH 8.0
   50 m*M* KCl
   10 m*M* Mg(CH$_3$COO)$_2$
   6 m*M* 2-Mercaptoethanol

C. 0.9% NaCl

D. 1% Pyronin B
   7.5% Acetic acid

### Procedure

Following electrophoresis, incubate PAG containing mRNA primer (see *Notes* below) for 5 min at 0°C in A + B mixture (1 part of A + 9 parts of B) and then at 37°C for 5 min. Rinse incubated gel thoroughly in solution C and place in solution D for 5 min. Wash stained gel in 7.5% acetic acid. Red bands indicate RNAP activity areas on the gel.

*Notes:* To prepare mammalian preparations containing RNAP activity, peripheral leukocytes should be grown in a medium containing 1 to 10 µg/ml of antigenic mRNA. Immunocompetitive leukocytes are then homogenized and a supernatant fraction obtained after centrifugation at 24000 rpm is used for electrophoresis.

    Immunocompetitive leukocytes contain mRNA for synthesis of antibody to antigenic mRNA. The antibody mRNA incorporated into PAG during the process of gel polymerization is used as a primer in the reaction catalyzed by RNAP.

    The supernatant fraction of a cell homogenate treated with DNase (component A of the staining solution) is used as a source of nucleoside triphosphates needed for RNA synthesis.

### REFERENCE

1. Neuhoff, V., Schill, W.-B., and Jacherts, D., Nachweis einer RNA-abhängigen RNA-replicase aus immunologisch kompetenten zellen durch mikro-disk-elektrophorese, *Hoppe-Seyler's Z. Physiol. Chem.*, 351, 157, 1970.

## 2.8.1.1 — Thiosulfate Sulfurtransferase; TST

**OTHER NAMES**    Thiosulfate cyanide transsulfurase, thiosulfate thiotransferase, rhodanese

**REACTION**    Thiosulfate + cyanide = sulfite + thiocyanate

**ENZYME SOURCE**  Vertebrates

## METHOD 1

### Visualization Scheme

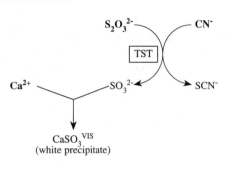

### Staining Solution[1]

0.333 *M* Tris–acetate buffer, pH 8.5
0.1 *M* KCN
0.1 *M* Na$_2$S$_2$O$_3$
0.3 *M* CaCl$_2$

### Procedure

Incubate electrophorized PAG in the staining solution at 37°C until white opaque bands appear. These bands are well visible against a dark background.

*Notes:* Only freshly prepared staining solution should be used.

## METHOD 2

### Visualization Scheme

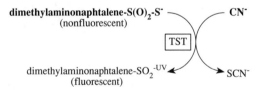

### Staining Solution[2]

A. 0.25 *M* Tris–acetate buffer, pH 8.2
   50 m*M* 5-Dimethylamino-1-naphthalene thiosulfonate

B. 0.25 *M* KCN

### Procedure

Following electrophoresis, coat the top of the gel with solution A (0.7 ml per 8 × 10.5 cm of gel; because of background fluorescence, minimizing the volume of solution A is desirable). Spread solution evenly with a glass rod, and allow to penetrate for 10 min. Then treat the gel with solution B (0.3 ml per 8 × 10.5 cm of gel). After 1 to 2 min view gel under long-wave UV light. Areas of TST activity are indicated by fluorescent bands (emission maximum of 500 to 510 nm; excitation at 325 nm). Record the zymogram or photograph using a yellow filter.

## 2.8.1.1 — Thiosulfate Sulfurtransferase; TST (continued)

*Notes:*    The synthesis of a fluorogenic substrate, 5-dimethylamino-1-naphthalene thiosulfonate anion, is carried out by stirring dansyl chloride in 10 vol of an aqueous solution containing one analytical equivalent of $Na_2S$ at 65°C for 2 to 3 h. The reaction mixture is then dried under reduced pressure in an atmosphere of nitrogen, and the crude product is extracted from the residue with hot ethanol. After crystallization at –20°C and recrystallization from ethanol, the thiosulfonate is contaminated with only trace amounts of the corresponding sulfinate and/or sulfonate and is suitable for use in the method described above.

### REFERENCES

1. Guilbault, G. G., Kuan, S. S., and Cochran, R., Procedure for rapid and sensitive detection of rhodanese separated by polyacrylamide gel electrophoresis, *Anal. Biochem.*, 43, 42, 1971.
2. Aird, B. A., Lane, J., and Westley, J., Methods for *in situ* visualization and assay of sulfurtransferases, *Anal. Biochem.*, 164, 554, 1987.

## 2.8.1.3 — Thiosulfate–thiol Sulfurtransferase; TTST

OTHER NAMES    Glutathione-dependent thiosulfate reductase, sulfane reductase, thiosulfate reductase

REACTION    Thiosulfate + 2 glutathione = sulfite + oxidized glutathione + sulfide

ENZYME SOURCE    Fungi

### METHOD

#### Visualization Scheme

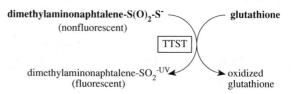

#### Staining Solution[1]
A. 0.25 *M* Tris–acetate buffer, pH 8.2
   50 m*M* 5-Dimethylamino-1-naphthalene thiosulfonate
B. 80 m*M* Glutathione, reduced (pH 9.0)

#### Procedure
Coat the top of the gel with solution A (0.7 ml per 8 × 10.5 cm of gel). Spread solution evenly with a glass rod and allow to penetrate for 10 min. Then treat the gel with solution B (0.3 ml per 8 × 10.5 cm of gel). After 1 to 2 min view gel under long-wave UV light. Areas of TTST activity are indicated by fluorescent bands (emission maximum of 500 to 510 nm; excitation at 325 nm). Record the zymogram or photograph using a yellow filter.

*Notes:*    The fluorogenic substrate is not yet commercially available but is available by a simple one-step synthesis from dansyl chloride (see 2.8.1.1 — TST, *Notes*).

### REFERENCE

1. Aird, B. A., Lane, J., and Westley, J., Methods for *in situ* visualization and assay of sulfurtransferases, *Anal. Biochem.*, 164, 554, 1987.

OTHER NAMES    Nonspecific esterases

REACTION    Hydrolyze ester bonds of various carboxylic esters; wide substrate specificity

ENZYME SOURCE    Bacteria, fungi, plants, protozoa, invertebrates, vertebrates

## METHOD 1

### Visualization Scheme

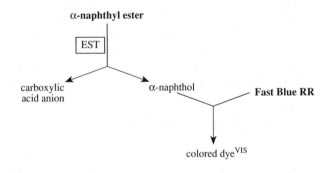

### Staining Solution[1] (modified)

| | |
|---|---|
| 0.05 $M$ Phosphate buffer, pH 7.2 | 100 ml |
| α-Naphthyl acetate (dissolved in 1 ml of acetone) | 10 mg |
| Fast Blue RR | 50 mg |

### Procedure

Incubate the gel in staining solution in the dark at 37°C until dark grey or black bands appear. Wash stained gel with water and fix in 3% acetic acid.

*Notes:* Esters of α-naphthols with acetate, propionate, and butyrate are the most commonly used artificial substrates for nonspecific esterases. Certain esterase isozymes have specificity for β-naphthyl acetate, which gives a reddish dye with Fast Blue RR salt. Thus, both α- and β-naphthyls may be included in the staining solution in some cases. Other dye couplers, such as Fast Blue BB, Fast Garnet GBC, and Fast Red TR, can also be used instead of Fast Blue RR. To reduce nonspecific background staining of the gel, 2 to 5 ml of 4% formaldehyde should be added to the staining solution.

## METHOD 2

### Visualization Scheme

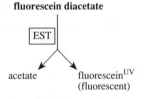

### Staining Solution[2]

| | |
|---|---|
| 50 m$M$ Sodium acetate buffer, pH 5.2 | 10 ml |
| 4-Methylumbelliferyl acetate (dissolved in a few drops of acetone) | 4 mg |

### Procedure

Apply the staining solution to the gel surface on filter-paper overlay. Incubate the gel at room temperature and view under long-wave UV light. Fluorescent bands of EST activity usually appear after a few minutes. Record the zymogram or photograph using a yellow filter.

*Notes:* 4-Methylumbelliferyl butyrate and propionate also may be used as fluorogenic esterase substrates.

## METHOD 3

### Visualization Scheme

fluorescein diacetate

EST

acetate    fluorescein[UV]
(fluorescent)

### Staining Solution[3]

| | |
|---|---|
| 0.1 $M$ Phosphate buffer, pH 6.5 | 100 ml |
| Fluorescein diacetate (dissolved in a few drops of acetone) | 10 mg |

### Procedure

Incubate the gel in staining solution at 37°C for 30 min and inspect under long-wave UV light for yellow fluorescent bands. When the bands are well developed, record the zymogram or photograph using a yellow filter.

## METHOD 4

### Visualization Scheme

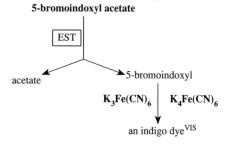

**5-bromoindoxyl acetate**

EST

acetate ← → 5-bromoindoxyl

$K_3Fe(CN)_6$ | $K_4Fe(CN)_6$

an indigo dye[VIS]

### Staining Solution[4]

| | |
|---|---|
| 0.15 $M$ Sodium phosphate buffer, pH 6.5 | 90 ml |
| 1% 5-Bromoindoxyl acetate in dimethyl sulfoxide | 4 ml |
| 10 m$M$ $K_4Fe(CN)_6 \cdot 3H_2O$ | 5 ml |
| 10 m$M$ $K_3Fe(CN)_6$ | 5 ml |

### Procedure

Incubate the gel in staining solution until colored bands appear. Wash gel with water and fix in 3% acetic acid.

*Notes:* Potassium ferricyanide is used to accelerate oxidation of bromoindoxyl to insoluble indigo dye. Potassium ferrocyanide is added to prevent further oxidation of the dye.

The chromogenic substrate 5-bromo-4-chloro-3-indolyl acetate in couple with NBT (or MTT) can also be used to visualize EST activity resulting in the formation of both the dehydroindigo and the formazan (e.g., see 3.1.3.1 — ALP, Method 2).

### GENERAL NOTES

All the methods described above can also detect carbonic anhydrase activity bands (see 4.2.1.1 — CA). Mammalian CA is inhibited by 1 m$M$ acetazolamide. This specific inhibitor is used to identify CA bands on EST zymograms.

The esterases are a complex of enzymes capable of hydrolyzing ester bonds. Nonspecific esterases detected using artificial substrates include five different enzymes. There are carboxylesterase or ali-esterase (EC 3.1.1.1), arylesterase or A(aromatic) esterase (EC 3.1.1.2), acetylesterase (EST 3.1.1.6), acetylcholinesterase or true cholinesterase (EC 3.1.1.7), and cholinesterase or pseudocholinesterase (EC 3.1.1.8). Different artificial substrates and inhibitors can be used to identify and differentiate these esterases on the zymograms.[5-9] The validity of such an approach to esterase differentiation is, however, questionable.[10]

Two esterases can be identified using specific staining procedures. These are acetylcholinesterase (see 3.1.1.7 — ACHE) and cholinesterase (see 3.1.1.8 — CHE).

### REFERENCES

1. Hunter, R. L. and Markert, C. L., Histochemical demonstration of enzymes separated by zone electrophoresis in starch gels, *Science*, 125, 1294, 1957.
2. Bargagna, M., Domenici, R., and Morali, A., Red cell esterase D polymorphism in the population of Tuscany, *Humangenetik*, 29, 251, 1975.
3. Hopkinson, D. A., Coppock, J. S., Mühlemann, M. F., and Edwards, Y. H., The detection and differentiation of the products of the human carbonic anhydrase loci $CA_I$ and $CA_{II}$, using fluorogenic substrates, *Ann. Hum. Genet.*, 38, 155, 1974.
4. Bender, K., Nagel, M., and Gunther, E., *Est*-6, a further polymorphic esterase in the rat, *Biochem. Genet.*, 20, 221, 1982.
5. Augustinson, K.-B., Electrophoretic separation and classification of blood plasma esterase, *Nature*, 181, 1786, 1958.
6. Holmes, R. S. and Masters, C. J., The developmental multiplicity and isoenzyme status of cavian esterases, *Biochim. Biophys. Acta*, 132, 379, 1967.
7. Holmes, R. S. and Masters, C. J., A comparative study of the multiplicity of mammalian esterases, *Biochim. Biophys. Acta*, 151, 147, 1968.
8. Holmes, R. S., Masters, C. J., and Webb, E. C., A comparative study of vertebrate esterase multiplicity, *Comp. Biochem. Physiol.*, 26, 837, 1968.
9. Tashian, R. E., The esterases and carbonic anhydrases in human erythrocytes, in *Biochemical Methods in Red Cell Genetics*, Yunis, J. J., Ed., Academic Press, New York, 1969, 307.
10. Choudhury, S. R., The nature of nonspecific esterase: a subunit concept, *J. Histochem. Cytochem.*, 20, 507, 1972.

## 3.1.1.3 — Triacylglycerol Lipase; TAGL

OTHER NAMES    Lipase, triglyceride lipase, tributyrase

REACTION    Triacylglycerol + $H_2O$ = diacylglycerol + fatty acid anion

ENZYME SOURCE  Bacteria, fungi, plants, invertebrates, vertebrates

### METHOD

### Visualization Scheme

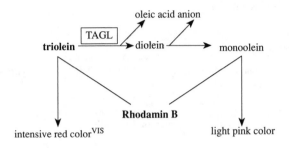

### Staining Solution[1]
A. 2% Agar solution (60°C) in 0.1 $M$     20 ml
    succinate buffer, pH 6.0
B. Rhodamin B                      4 mg
   Triolein                      0.5 g

### Procedure
Add B components to solution A and mix at 60 to 65°C for 1 min using high-speed homogenizer to prepare emulsion. Form a 50-μm reactive agar plate between two glass plates heated to 40°C. Use lower glass plate covered by silanized 100-μm polyester film and upper glass plate covered by 100-μm polyester film treated with alkali.

Apply electrophorized gel gently to the reactive agar plate formed and incubate at 40°C until light pink bands (fluorescent at 366 nm) appear on an intensive red gel background.

### OTHER METHODS

Fluorogenic substrates 4-methylumbelliferil oleate and monodecanoyl fluorescein can also be used to visualize TAGL activity bands on electrophoretic gels.[2]

### REFERENCES
1. Höfelmann, M., Kittsteiner-Eberle, R., and Schreier, P., Ultrathin-layer agar gels: a novel print technique for ultrathin-layer isoelectric focusing of enzymes, *Anal. Biochem.*, 128, 217, 1983.
2. Cortner, J. A. and Swoboda, E., "Wolman's" disease: prenatal diagnosis; electrophoretic identification of the missing lysosomal acid lipase, *Am. J. Hum. Genet.*, 26, 23A, 1974.

## 3.1.1.7 — Acetylcholinesterase; ACHE

OTHER NAMES    True cholinesterase, cholinesterase I, cholinesterase

REACTION    Acetylcholine + $H_2O$ = choline + acetate

ENZYME SOURCE  Vertebrates

### METHOD 1

### Visualization Scheme

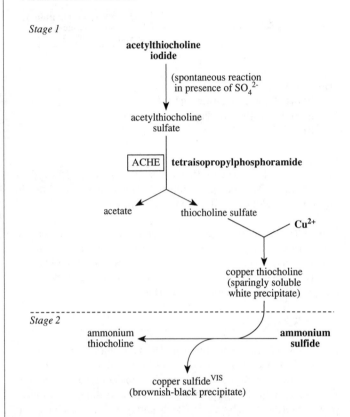

### Staining Solution[1]
A. 2.4 $M$ $Na_2SO_4$ (see Procedure)
   6.9 m$M$ Acetylthiocholine iodide
   6 m$M$ $CuSO_4$
   22 m$M$ Glycine
   75 m$M$ Maleic acid
   150 m$M$ NaOH
   25 m$M$ $MgCl_2$
   0.01 m$M$ Tetraisopropylphosphoramide (dissolved in 95% ethanol)
B. 40% $Na_2SO_4$
C. 10 m$M$ $(NH_4)_2S$

### Procedure
To prepare solution A, dissolve the $Na_2SO_4$ first, because the solution must be heated to effect solution. When $Na_2SO_4$ solution cools, add the other components. The pH of solution A should be 6.0.

Incubate electrophorized gel in solution A at 37°C for 2 h. Rinse gel in solution B and place in solution C. Brown bands that appear quite rapidly denote ACHE activity.

*Notes:*  Tetraisopropylphosphoramide is used to inhibit cholinesterase (see 3.1.1.8 — CHE) which also can hydrolyze acetylthiocholine sulfate.

## METHOD 2

### Visualization Scheme

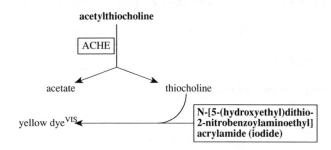

### Staining Solution[2]

50 m$M$ Phosphate buffer, pH 7.4
10 m$M$ Acetylthiocholine
10 µM EDTA

### Procedure

Incubate electrophorized PAG prepared using $N$-[5-(hydroxyethyl)dithio-2-nitrobenzoylaminoethyl] acrylamide (iodide) in the staining solution until yellow bands appear.

*Notes:* To prevent development of cholinesterase (see 3.1.1.8 — CHE) activity bands, electrophorized PAG should be initially preincubated in phosphate buffer, pH 7.4, containing 0.01 m$M$ tetraisopropylphosphoramide.

The method is based on the reduction of disulfide bonds of chromogenic group (dithio-2-nitrobenzene) by thiocholine.

## OTHER METHODS

An immunoblotting procedure (for details see Part II) based on the utility of monoclonal antibodies specific to human ACHE[3] can also be used for immunohistochemical visualization of the enzyme protein on electrophoretic gels. This procedure is not appropriate for routine laboratory use but may be of great value in special analyses of ACHE (e.g., biochemical, immunochemical, phylogenetic, genetic, etc.).

## REFERENCES

1. Brewer, G. J., *An Introduction to Isozyme Techniques*, Academic Press, New York, 1970, 122.
2. Harris, R. B. and Wilson, I. B., Polyacrylamide gels which contain a novel mixed disulfide compound can be used to detect enzymes that catalyze thiol-producing reactions, *Anal. Biochem.*, 134, 126, 1983.
3. Fambrough, D. M., Engel, A. G., and Rosenberry, T. L., Acetylcholinesterase of human erythrocytes and neuromuscular junctions: homologies revealed by monoclonal antibodies, *Proc. Natl. Acad. Sci. U.S.A.*, 79, 1078, 1982.

| OTHER NAMES | Pseudocholinesterase, butyrylcholine esterase, nonspecific cholinesterase, choline esterase II (unspecific), benzoylcholinesterase |
|---|---|
| REACTION | Acetylcholine + H$_2$O = choline + carboxylic acid anion |
| ENZYME SOURCE | Vertebrates |

## METHOD

### Visualization Scheme

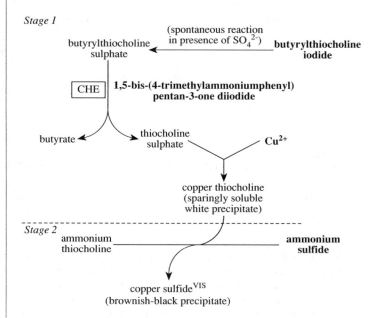

### Staining Solution[1]

A. 2.4 $M$ Na$_2$SO$_4$ (see Procedure)
   6.9 m$M$ Butyrylthiocholine iodide
   6 m$M$ CuSO$_4$
   22 m$M$ Glycine
   75 m$M$ Maleic acid
   150 m$M$ NaOH
   25 m$M$ MgCl$_2$
   0.01 m$M$ 1,5-Bis-(4-trimethylammoniumphenyl) pentan-3-one diiodide
B. 40% Na$_2$SO$_4$
C. 10 m$M$ (NH$_4$)$_2$S

### Procedure

To prepare solution A, dissolve the Na$_2$SO$_4$ first, because the solution must be heated to effect solution. When the Na$_2$SO$_4$ solution cools, add the other components. The pH of solution A should be 6.0.

Incubate electrophorized gel in solution A at 37°C for 2 h. Rinse gel in solution B and place in solution C. Brown bands which appear quite rapidly denote CHE activity.

*Notes:* 1,5-Bis-(4-trimethylammoniumphenyl) pentan-3-one diiodide inhibits acethylcholinesterase (see 3.1.1.7 — ACHE), which also can hydrolyze butyrylthiocholine sulfate. Trimethyl(*p*-aminophenyl)-ammonium chloride can also be used for this purpose.

## OTHER METHODS

PAG prepared using *N*-[5-(hydroxyethyl)dithio-2-nitrobenzoyla-minoethyl] acrylamide (iodide) can also be used to visualize CHE activity bands (for example, see 3.1.1.7 — ACHE, Method 2).

## REFERENCE

1. Brewer, G. J., *An Introduction to Isozyme Techniques*, Academic Press, New York, 1970, 122.

OTHER NAMES    Pectin demethoxylase, pectin methoxylase, pectin methylesterase

REACTION    Pectin + n $H_2O$ = n methanol + pectate

ENZYME SOURCE  Bacteria, fungi, plants

## METHOD

### Visualization Scheme

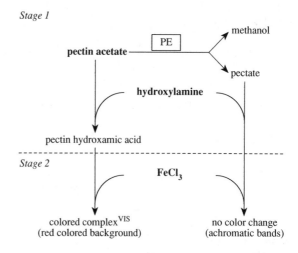

### Staining Solution[1]
A. 2% Agar, 1% pectin solution (60°C) in 0.3 *M* acetate buffer, pH 4.5
B. 14% Hydroxylamine chloride in 60% ethanol
C. 14% NaOH in 60% ethanol
D. 25% HCl
E. 95% Ethanol
F. 2.5% $FeCl_3$ in 60% ethanol containing 0.1 *N* HCl

### Procedure
Using solution A, form a 50-µm reactive agar–pectin plate between two glass plates heated to 40°C. Use lower glass plate covered by silanized 100–µm polyester film and an upper glass plate covered by 100–µm polyester film treated with alkali. Apply electrophorized gel to the reactive agar–pectin plate and incubate the gel/reactive agar–pectin plate combination at 40°C for 20 s. Remove the gel and put the reactive plate in a 1:1 mixture of B and C solutions for 30 s. Then treat the reactive plate for 30 s in a 1:2 mixture of D and E solutions. Finally, place the reactive plate in solution F for 30 s. Achromatic bands of PE activity appear on the reddish-brown background of the gel. Fix the stained agar plate in 50% ethanol and dry on filter paper.

### REFERENCE
1. Höfelmann, M., Kittsteiner-Eberle, R., and Schreier, P., Ultrathin-layer agar gels: a novel print technique for ultrathin-layer isoelectric focusing of enzymes, *Anal. Biochem.*, 128, 217, 1983.

## 3.1.2.1 — Acetyl-CoA Hydrolase; ACoAH

OTHER NAMES      Acetyl-CoA deacylase, acetyl-CoA acylase

REACTION        Acetyl-CoA + $H_2O$ = CoA + acetate

ENZYME SOURCE  Plants, vertebrates

## METHOD

### Visualization Scheme

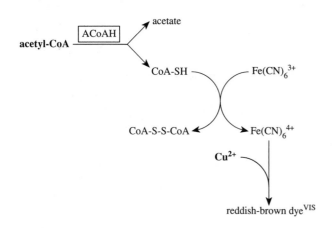

### Staining Solution[1]

| | |
|---|---:|
| 30 m$M$ Phosphate buffer, pH 7.6 | 7.5 ml |
| 100 m$M$ Sodium phosphotartrate | 2.5 ml |
| 50 m$M$ Cupric sulfate | 2.5 ml |
| 15 m$M$ Potassium ferricyanide | 12.5 ml |
| 25 m$M$ Magnesium chloride | 25 ml |
| 10 m$M$ Acetyl-CoA | 2.5 ml |

### Procedure

Incubate the gel in staining solution at 37°C until reddish-brown bands appear.

## OTHER METHODS

A. PAG prepared using $N$-[5-(hydroxyethyl)dithio-2-nitro-benzoylaminoethyl] acrylamide (iodide) can be used to visualize ACoAH activity bands. The method is based on the reduction of disulfide bonds of the chromogenic group (dithio-2-nitrobenzene) by thiol reagents, including CoA-SH produced by ACoAH (e.g., see 3.1.1.7 — ACHE, Method 2).

B. The product CoA-SH can be detected using the redox indicator 2,6-dichlorophenol indophenol in couple with the tetrazolium system (e.g., see 1.6.4.2 — GSR, Method 2).

C. The free thiol group of CoA-SH can also be detected using 5,5′-dithiobis(2-nitrobenzoic acid) (e.g., see 1.6.4.2 — GSR, Method 3).

## REFERENCE

1. Volk, M. J., Trelease, R. N., and Reeves, H. C., Determination of malate synthase activity in polyacrylamide gels, *Anal. Biochem.,* 58, 315, 1974.

## 3.1.2.6 — Hydroxyacylglutathione Hydrolase; HAGH

OTHER NAMES      Glyoxalase II

REACTION        $S$-(2-Hydroxyacyl)glutathione + $H_2O$ = glutathione + 2-hydroxyacid anion

ENZYME SOURCE  Vertebrates

## METHOD 1

### Visualization Scheme

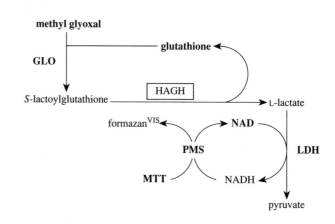

### Staining Solution[1]

| | | |
|---|---|---:|
| A. | 0.1 $M$ Tris–HCl buffer, pH 8.0 | 12.5 ml |
| | Methyl glyoxal | 50 µl |
| | Glyoxalase I (GLO; 200 U/ml) | 25 µl |
| | Lactate dehydrogenase (LDH; 2750 U/ml) | 10 µl |
| | NAD | 40 mg |
| | Glutathione (reduced form) | 40 mg |
| | MTT | 4 mg |
| | PMS | 2 mg |
| B. | 2% Agar solution (60°C) | 12.5 ml |

### Procedure

Mix A and B components of the staining solution and pour the mixture over the gel surface. Incubate the gel in the dark at 37°C until dark blue bands appear. Fix stained gel in 50% ethanol.

## 3.1.2.6 — Hydroxyacylglutathione Hydrolase; HAGH (continued)

### METHOD 2

#### Visualization Scheme

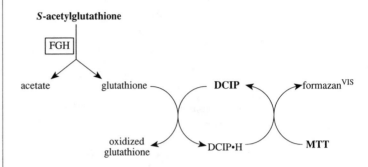

S-lactoylglutathione

HAGH

L-lactate      glutathione      DCIP ← formazan[VIS]

oxidized glutathione ← DCIP·H      MTT

#### Staining Solution[2]
A. 0.2 *M* Tris–HCl buffer, pH 8.0                28.2 ml
   2,6-Dichlorophenol indophenol (DCIP)            6 mg
   MTT                                            24 mg
   50 m*M* S-Lactoylglutathione                   1.8 ml
B. 1.8% Agar solution (50°C)                      30 ml

#### Procedure
Mix A and B components of the staining solution and pour the mixture over the gel surface. Incubate the gel in the dark at 37°C until dark blue bands appear. Fix stained gel in 50% ethanol.

### GENERAL NOTES

Human red cell enzyme is able to catalyze the hydrolysis of S-formylglutathione and gives with this substrate 46% of the rate with S-lactoylglutathione (see also 3.1.2.12 — FGH; Method 1, *Notes*).

### REFERENCES

1. Charlesworth, D., Starch gel electrophoresis of 4 enzymes from human red blood cells: glyceraldehyde-3-phosphate dehydrogenase, fructo-aldolase, glyoxalase II and sorbitol dehydrogenase, *Ann. Hum. Genet.*, 35, 477, 1972.
2. Uotila, L., Polymorphism of red cell S-formylglutathione hydrolase in a Finnish population, *Hum. Hered.*, 34, 273, 1984.

## 3.1.2.12 — S-Formylglutathione Hydrolase; FGH

REACTION    S-Formylglutathione + H₂O = glutathione + formate; also hydrolyzes S-acetylglutathione, more slowly

ENZYME SOURCE  Vertebrates

### METHOD 1

#### Visualization Scheme

S-acetylglutathione

FGH

acetate      glutathione      DCIP ← formazan[VIS]

oxidized glutathione ← DCIP·H      MTT

#### Staining Solution[1]
A. 0.2 *M* Tris–HCl buffer, pH 8.0                28.2 ml
   2,6-Dichlorophenol indophenol (DCIP)            6 mg
   MTT                                            24 mg
   50 m*M* S-Acetylglutathione                    1.8 ml
B. 1.8% Agar solution (50°C)                      30 ml

#### Procedure
Mix A and B components of the staining solution and pour the mixture over the gel surface. Incubate the gel in the dark at 37°C until dark blue bands appear. Fix stained gel in 50% ethanol.

*Notes:*  The use of S-formylglutathione instead of S-acetylglutathione is preferable because it is a much more effective substrate of FGH than is S-acetylglutathione (relative rates 100 and 0.5, respectively). However, S-formylglutathione of sufficient purity was not obtained by the author during development of this method. When using this substrate in the staining solution instead of S-acetylglutathione, the interpretation of FGH electrophoretic patterns should be made with caution because hydroxyacylglutathione hydrolase (see 3.1.2.6 — HAGH, General Notes) also is able to catalyze the hydrolysis of S-formylglutathione (with this substrate human red cell HAGH gives 46% of the rate with S-lactoylglutathione). Thus, when S-formylglutathione is used as substrate in this method, a control staining for HAGH activity should be made for comparison.

## METHOD 2

### Visualization Scheme

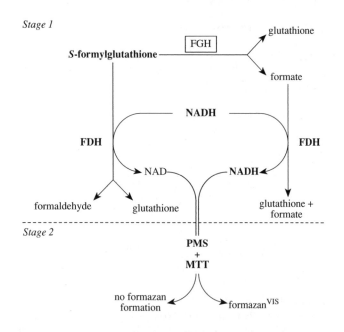

*Stage 1*

*Stage 2*

### Staining Solution[1]
A. 0.1 *M* Sodium phosphate buffer, pH 6.0
   1 m*M* *S*-Formylglutathione
   0.4 m*M* NADH
   0.01 U/ml Formaldehyde dehydrogenase (FDH)
B. 0.1 *M* Sodium phosphate buffer, pH 7.5
   0.03 mg/ml PMS
   0.3 mg/ml NBT

### Procedure
Incubate the gel in solution A at 23°C for 30 min and then transfer to solution B. Incubate the gel in solution B in the dark at 23°C until dark blue bands appear (30 to 60 min). Rinse stained gel with water and fix in 50% ethanol.

*Notes:*  Formaldehyde dehydrogenase is used to catalyze in its reverse reaction the oxidation of NADH to NAD in the presence of *S*-formylglutathione. At the location of FGH activity, however, *S*-formylglutathione is hydrolyzed, preventing there the oxidation of NADH, which is then visualized via the PMS/MTT system.

## GENERAL NOTES

*S*-Formylglutathione is a much more effective substrate of FGH than is *S*-acetylglutathione. However, Method 1 works well even with *S*-acetylglutathione. Using this method it is possible to detect a much lower amount of FGH than with Method 2. The use of Method 2 is recommended only to confirm that the staining results obtained with Method 1 are not affected by using *S*-acetylglutathione instead of *S*-formylglutathione.

Preparations of *S*-acetylglutathione and *S*-formylglutathione are not yet commercially available but can be synthesized and purified under laboratory conditions.[2-4]

### REFERENCES
1. Uotila, L., Polymorphism of red cell *S*-formylglutathione hydrolase in a Finnish population, *Hum. Hered.*, 34, 273, 1984.
2. Uotila, L., Preparation and assay of glutathione thiol esters: survey of human liver glutathione thiol esterases, *Biochemistry*, 12, 3938, 1973.
3. Uotila, L., Thioesters of glutathione, *Meth. Enzymol.*, 77, 424, 1981.
4. Board, P. G. and Coggan, M., Genetic heterogeneity of *S*-formylglutathione hydrolase, *Ann. Hum. Genet.*, 50, 35, 1986.

OTHER NAMES    Alkaline phosphomonoesterase, phosphomo-
               noesterase, glycerophosphatase

REACTION       Orthophosphoric monoester + $H_2O$ = alcohol
               + orthophosphate

ENZYME SOURCE  Bacteria, fungi, green algae, plants, protozoa,
               invertebrates, vertebrates

## METHOD 1

### Visualization Scheme

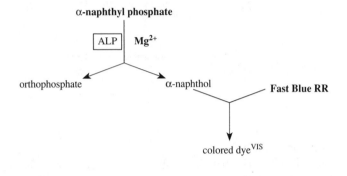

### Staining Solution[1]

| | |
|---|---|
| 60 m$M$ Borate buffer, pH 9.7 | 100 ml |
| α-Naphthyl phosphate | 50 mg |
| Fast Blue RR | 50 mg |
| 10 m$M$ MgCl$_2$ | 1 ml |

### Procedure

Incubate the gel in staining solution in the dark at 37°C until dark grey bands appear. Wash stained gel with water and fix in 50% ethanol.

*Notes:* Other substrates (e.g., α-naphthyl acid phosphate and β-naphthyl phosphate) and other dye couplers (e.g., Fast Blue B) can also be used.

Using this method, nonspecifically stained light-yellow bands of albumin, haptoglobin, and ceruloplasmin can also be developed on ALP zymograms after electrophoresis of blood serum preparations.

## METHOD 2

### Visualization Scheme

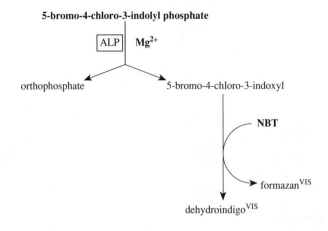

### Staining Solution[2]

| | |
|---|---|
| 0.1 $M$ Tris–HCl buffer, pH 9.0 | 95 ml |
| 2 m$M$ MgCl$_2$ | 5 ml |
| 1% 5-Bromo-4-chloro-3-indolyl phosphate ($p$-toluidine salt, dissolved in dimethylformamide) | 5 ml |
| NBT | |
| | 10 mg |

### Procedure

Incubate the gel in staining solution in the dark at 37°C until dark blue bands appear. Wash stained gel with water and fix in 3% acetic acid.

*Notes:* The hydroxyl group of the product 5-bromo-4-chloro-3-indoxyl tautomerizes, forming a ketone, and under alkaline conditions, dimerization occurs, forming a dehydroindigo. In the process of dimerizing, it releases hydrogen ions which reduce nitro blue tetrazolium to blue formazan. This one-step staining procedure gives distinct bands. Thus, the bands migrating close together can easily be distinguished from each other. The reaction causing formazan formation can be quantitated by reflective densitometry and appears to be a log linear relation over a wide concentration range of ALP.[3]

## METHOD 3

### Visualization Scheme

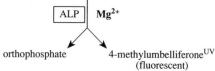

### Staining Solution[4]

A. 0.1 $M$ Borate buffer, pH 9.7     10 ml
    4-Methylumbelliferyl phosphate     1 mg
    $MgSO_4$     50 mg
B. 2% Agar solution (55°C)     20 ml

### Procedure

Mix A and B components of the staining solution and pour the mixture over the gel surface. Incubate the gel at 37°C and monitor under long-wave UV light. Fluorescent bands indicate localization of ALP activity in the gel. Record the zymogram or photograph using a yellow filter.

## METHOD 4

### Visualization Scheme

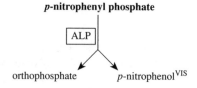

### Staining Solution[5]

A. 0.89 $M$ Diethanolamine     20 ml
    $p$-Nitrophenyl phosphate     4 mg
B. 2% Agarose solution (50°C)     20 ml

### Procedure

Mix A and B components of the staining solution and pour the mixture over the gel surface. Incubate the gel at 37°C until yellow bands appear. Photograph the zymogram using a 436.8-nm interference filter.

## METHOD 5

### Visualization Scheme

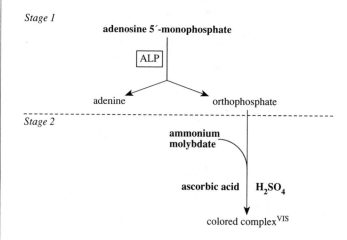

### Staining Solution[5]

A. 0.1 $M$ Tris–HCl buffer, pH 8.0     20 ml
    AMP (sodium salt)     140 mg
B. 2% Agarose solution (60°C)
C. 1.25% Ammonium molybdate
    1 $M$ $H_2SO_4$
    10% Ascorbic acid

### Procedure

Mix equal volumes of A and B solutions and pour the mixture over the gel surface. Incubate the gel at 37°C for 30 min. Remove first agarose overlay and cover the gel surface with a mixture consisting of equal volumes of B and C solutions. Blue bands appear almost immediately at sites of ALP activity. The bands are ephemeral, thus the zymogram should be recorded or photographed immediately.

## METHOD 6

### Visualization Scheme

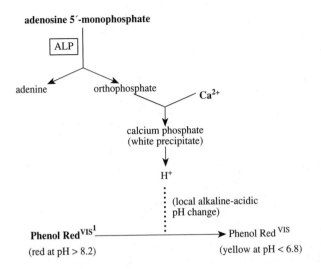

### Staining Solution[5]

A.  1% Phenol Red                     0.25 ml
    AMP (sodium salt)              35 mg
    0.15 $M$ NaCl                   4.1 ml
    1.0 $M$ $CaCl_2$                 1 ml
B.  2% Agarose solution (50°C)      5 ml

### Procedure

Wash electrophorized acetate cellulose gel with water for 2 min to remove gel buffer. Prepare solution A. Prior to the addition of $CaCl_2$ all other components of solution A should be adjusted to pH 8.0. Mix solutions A and B and pour the mixture over the porous side of the acetate cellulose gel. Incubate the gel at 37°C until yellow bands of ALP appear on a red background. Photograph the zymogram using a 570-nm interference filter.

*Notes:* Since changes in the absorption spectrum of Phenol Red occur between pH 6.8 and 8.2, theoretically a change as small as $10^{-7}$ $M$ hydrogen ion could be detected by this method.[6]

A white precipitate of calcium phosphate is visible against a dark background when a transparent gel (e.g., PAG) is used for electrophoresis.[7]

## METHOD 7

### Visualization Scheme

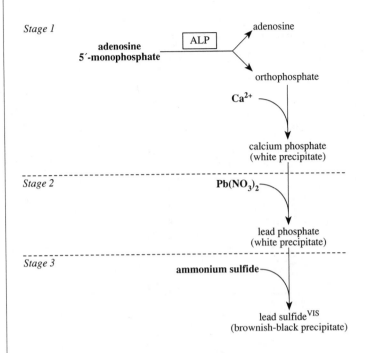

### Staining Solution[5]

A.  90 m$M$ Tris–2 m$M$ EDTA–50 m$M$ boric acid, pH 8.6    16 ml
    1 $M$ $CaCl_2$                              2 ml
    AMP (sodium salt)                     140 mg
    1.5 $M$ NaCl                        1.6 ml
B.  2% Agarose solution (50°C)         20 ml
C.  0.1 $M$ Tris–HCl buffer, pH 7.0
    3 m$M$ $Pb(NO_3)_2$
D.  5% Ammonium sulfide

### Procedure

Mix A and B components of the staining solution and pour the mixture over the gel surface. Incubate the gel at 37°C for 30 to 60 min. Remove agarose overlay and wash gel with water for 15 min. Place gel in solution C for 30 min and then in solution D. Brownish-black bands indicate the sites of ALP activity localization on the gel. Photograph the zymogram using a 436.8-nm interference filter.

## METHOD 8

### Visualization Scheme

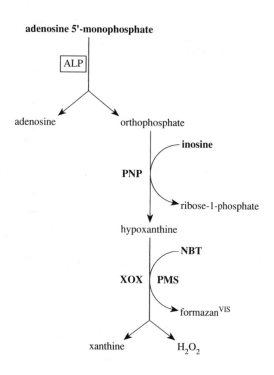

### Staining Solution[5]

A. 0.1 M Tris–HCl buffer, pH 8.0 — 6 ml
0.1 M EDTA — 0.5 ml
10 mg/ml NBT — 1 ml
2 mg/ml PMS — 0.1 ml
0.1 M Inosine — 1.6 ml
AMP (sodium salt) — 140 mg
0.75 U/ml Xanthine oxidase (XOX) — 8 ml
1.67 U/ml Purine-nucleoside phosphorylase (PNP) — 0.2 ml
H$_2$O — 12 ml
B. 2% Agarose solution in 0.1 M Tris–HCl — 20 ml
buffer, pH 8.0 (50°C)

### Procedure

Mix A and B components of the staining solution and pour the mixture over the gel surface. Incubate the gel in the dark at 37°C until dark blue bands appear. Fix stained gel in 50% ethanol.

*Notes:* Alternative enzymatic methods for detection of orthophosphate are available which are based on coupled reactions involving either the glyceraldehyde 3-phosphate dehydrogenase[8] or the phosphorylase *a*[9] reactions. Both methods involve three enzymatic steps and are more complicated than the method presented above. Moreover, the coupled reactions of these alternative enzymatic methods are readily reversible and certain of the substrates used are unstable.

## METHOD 9

### Visualization Scheme

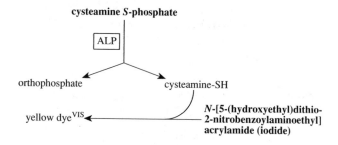

### Staining Solution[10]

0.5 M Tris–HCl buffer, pH 8.0
5 mM Cysteamine *S*-phosphate

### Procedure

Incubate electrophorized PAG prepared using *N*-[5-(hydroxyethyl)-dithio-2-nitrobenzoylaminoethyl] acrylamide (iodide) in the staining solution at 37°C until yellow bands appear.

## METHOD 10

### Visualization Scheme

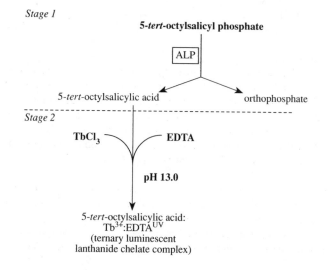

### Staining Solution[11]

A. 0.1 M Tris–HCl buffer, pH 9.0
0.1 M NaCl
1 mM MgCl$_2$
1 mM 5-*tert*-Octylsalicyl phosphate
B. 0.01 M HCl
5 mM TbCl$_3$
5 mM EDTA (tetrasodium salt)
C. 2.5 M Tris, pH 13.0

## Procedure

Transfer proteins from electrophorized gel on Nitran nylon membrane (0.45-μm pore size; Schleicher and Schull) using routine blotting procedure. Incubate the membrane for 2 h in substrate solution A and blot with blotting paper on the non–protein-containing surface. Cover the membrane with developing solution (one part of solution B, one part of solution C, and three parts of deionized water) and observe luminiscent ALP bands under 300 to 400-nm UV light or photograph on Polaroid instant film with a TRP 100 time-resolved photographic camera (Kronem Systems, Inc., Mississauga, Canada) using filters that pass 320 to 400-nm excitation and more than 515-nm emission wavelengths, a 440-μs time delay, and a 4.1-ms measurement gate.

*Notes:* This method may be applied directly to electrophoretic gel without transferring proteins on the nylon membrane. In this situation the substrate and developing solutions should be applied as 1% agar or as filter-paper overlays. The time of incubation of the gel with a substrate-containing overlay should be diminished with the purpose of reducing undesirable diffusion of the product 5-*tert*-octylsalicylic acid. The main disadvantage of non–membrane-based detection of ALP by this method is that the detection should be carried out in a two-step procedure. This is because optimal formation of a luminescent lanthanide chelate complex occurs at pH 12.5, which is too high even for ALP.

The membrane-based method was used to detect biotinylated DNA in dot–blot and Southern blot assays using streptavidin–ALP conjugate. High sensitivity that is comparable with radioisotopic detection was obtained with this method during quantitative assays.

Another substrate, 5-fluorosalicyl phosphate, may be used in non–membrane-based detection of ALP via formation of a ternary luminescent lanthanide chelate complex (5-fluorosalicylic acid:$Tb^{3+}$:EDTA).[12]

## GENERAL NOTES

The enzyme from some sources requires manganese ions for activity.[13]

Alkaline phosphatase zymograms should be compared to those of acid phosphatase (see 3.1.3.2 — ACP) because some taxa possess phosphatases capable of exhibiting activity under both acidic and alkaline conditions.[14]

All methods based on detection of liberated orthophosphate can only be used when electrophoresis is carried out in a phosphate-free buffer system.

ALP from some sources can hydrolyze phosphoenolpyruvate and cause the appearance of additional bands on the zymograms of some enzymes where pyruvate kinase and lactate dehydrogenase are used as linking enzymes to detect the product ADP (e.g., see 3.1.4.17 — CNPE, Method 1).

## REFERENCES

1. Boyer, S. H., Alkaline phosphatase in human sera and placentae, *Science*, 134, 1002, 1961.
2. Dingjan, P. G., Postma, T., and Stroes, J. A. P., Quantitative differentiation of human-serum alkaline phosphatase isoenzymes with polyacrylamide disc gel electrophoresis, *Z. Klin. Chem. Klin. Biochem.*, 11(4), 167, 1973.
3. Blake, M. S., Johnston, K. H., Russell-Jones, G. J., and Gotschlich, E. C., A rapid, sensitive method for detection of alkaline phosphatase-conjugated anti-antibody in western blots, *Anal. Biochem.*, 136, 175, 1984.
4. Benham, F. J., Cottell, P. C., Franks, L. M., and Wilson, P. D., Alkaline phosphatase activity in human bladder tumor cell lines, *J. Histochem. Cytochem.*, 25, 266, 1977.
5. Klebe, R. J., Schloss, S., Mock, L., and Link, G. R., Visualization of isozymes which generate inorganic phosphate, *Biochem. Genet.*, 19, 921, 1981.
6. Klebe, R. J., Mancuso, M. G., Brown, C. R., and Teng, L., Two-dimensional spectroscopy of electrophoretic gels, *Biochem. Genet.*, 19, 655, 1981.
7. Nimmo, H. G. and Nimmo, G. A., A general method for the localization of enzymes that produce phosphate, pyrophosphate, or $CO_2$ after polyacrylamide gel electrophoresis, *Anal. Biochem.*, 121, 17, 1982.
8. Cornell, N. W., Leadbetter, M. G., and Veech, R. L., Modifications in the enzymatic assay for inorganic phosphate, *Anal. Biochem.*, 95, 524, 1979.
9. Lowry, O. H., Schulz, D. W., and Passonneau, J. V., Effects of adenylic acid on the kinetics of muscle phosphorylase a, *J. Biol. Chem.*, 239, 1947, 1964.
10. Harris, R. B. and Wilson, I. B., Polyacrylamide gels which contain a novel mixed disulfide compound can be used to detect enzymes that catalyze thiol-producing reactions, *Anal. Biochem.*, 134, 126, 1983.
11. Templeton, E. F. G., Wong, H. E., Evangelista, R. A., Granger, T., and Pollak, A., Time-resolved fluorescence detection of enzyme-amplified lanthanide luminescence for nucleic acid hybridization assays, *Clin. Chem.*, 37, 1506, 1991.
12. Evangelista, R. A., Pollak, A., and Templeton, E. F. G., Enzyme-amplified lanthanide luminescence for enzyme detection in bioanalytical assays, *Anal. Biochem.*, 197, 213, 1991.
13. Wilcox, F. H., Hirschhorn, L., Taylor, B. A., Womack, J. E., and Roderick, T. H., Genetic variation in alkaline phosphatase of the house mouse (*Mus musculus*) with emphasis on a manganese-requiring isozyme, *Biochem. Genet.*, 17, 1093, 1979.
14. Richardson, B. J., Baverstock, P. R., and Adams, M., *Allozyme Electrophoresis: A Handbook for Animal Systematics and Population Studies*, Academic Press, Sydney, 1986, 170.

OTHER NAMES    Acid phosphomonoesterase, phosphomo-noesterase, glycerophosphatase

REACTION    Orthophosphoric monoester + $H_2O$ = alcohol + orthophosphate

ENZYME SOURCE    Bacteria, fungi, green algae, plants, protozoa, invertebrates, vertebrates

## METHOD 1

### Visualization Scheme

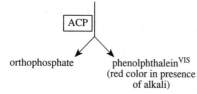

**phenolphtalein monophosphate**

orthophosphate    phenolphthalein[VIS]
(red color in presence
of alkali)

### Staining Solution[1]
A.  0.1 *M* Citrate buffer, pH 5.5     25 ml
    Phenolphthalein monophosphate (disodium salt)     50 mg
B.  $NH_4OH$ (concentrated solution)     5 ml

### Procedure
Pour solution A on top of filter paper; overlay the gel and incubate at 37°C for 1.5 to 2 h. Remove filter paper and cover the gel with solution B. Red bands indicating localization of ACP activity on the gel appear after 1 to 2 min. Record or photograph zymogram.

*Notes:* A method with phenolphthalein diphosphate as chromogenic substrate is also available,[2] but it is less sensitive than that described above. The method with phenolphthalein monophosphate has a sensitivity comparable to the sensitivity of the method that uses 4-methylumbelliferyl phosphate (see Method 2 below).

## METHOD 2

### Visualization Scheme

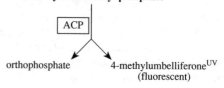

**4-methylumbelliferyl phosphate**

orthophosphate    4-methylumbelliferone[UV]
(fluorescent)

### Staining Solution[1]
    0.1 *M* Citrate buffer, pH 5.5     25 ml
    4-Methylumbelliferyl phosphate     5 mg

### Procedure
Apply the staining solution to the gel surface on a filter-paper overlay and incubate the gel at 37°C for 15 to 30 min. Light (fluorescent) bands of ACP are visible under long-wave UV light. Record the zymogram or photograph using a yellow filter.

*Notes:* Zones of ACP which are very weak after prolonged incubation may be seen more clearly if the gel surface is made alkaline with ammonia to increase the level of fluorescence.[3]

## METHOD 3

### Visualization Scheme

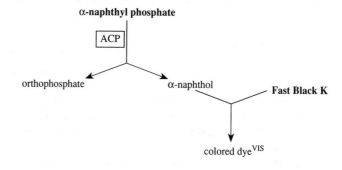

**α-naphthyl phosphate**

orthophosphate    α-naphthol    **Fast Black K**

colored dye[VIS]

### Staining Solution[4]
    50 m*M* Acetate buffer, pH 5.0     100 ml
    α-Naphthyl phosphate (disodium salt)     100 mg
    Fast Black K salt     100 mg

### Procedure
Incubate the gel in staining solution in the dark at 37°C until colored bands appear. Wash stained gel in water and fix in 7% acetic acid.

*Notes:* Where the enzyme activity is weak, greater sensitivity may be obtained using a post-coupling technique. In this situation, all ingredients of the staining solution except Fast Black K (the possible inhibitor) are applied to the gel. The gel is incubated for a period of time (depending upon the expected activity of the enzyme) and Fast Black K is then applied to the gel.

    β-Naphthyl phosphate may be used as substrate instead of α-naphthyl phosphate. Other dye couplers (e.g., Fast Blue B, Fast Blue BB, and Fast Garnet GBC) also may be used instead of Fast Black K.

## METHOD 4

### Visualization Scheme

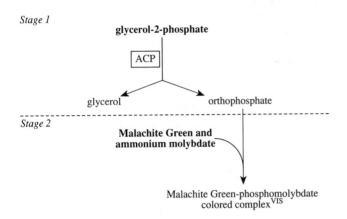

*Stage 1*

**glycerol-2-phosphate**

ACP

glycerol          orthophosphate

*Stage 2*

**Malachite Green and
ammonium molybdate**

Malachite Green-phosphomolybdate
colored complex[VIS]

### Staining Solution[5]

A. 100 m*M* Acetate buffer, pH 5.0
   5 m*M* Glycerol-2-phosphate

B. 4.2% Ammonium molybdate in 4 *N* HCl     30 ml
   0.045% Malachite Green (oxalate salt)     90 ml
   2% Sterox (a detergent diluent)     2.4 ml

C. Solution B     60 ml
   H₂O     40 ml

### Procedure

Preincubate electrophorized gel in 100 m*M* acetate buffer, pH 5.0 for 30 min. Then incubate the gel in solution A (100 ml of solution A for 20 ml of gel volume) for 30 min at 37°C. Following incubation rinse gel quickly with water (usually 2 × 100 ml) to remove substrate and excess orthophosphate from the surface of the gel and place gel in solution C (see *Notes*). Color development is usually complete in 10 to 20 min. Rinse stained gel with several changes of water and store in 5% acetic acid, 20% ethanol.

*Notes:* Prepare stock solution B as follows: mix 30 ml of ammonium molybdate solution and 90 ml of Malachite Green solution for 20 min at room temperature. Then pass resulting mixture through a Whatman No. 5 filter and add 2.4 ml of sterox solution. This stock solution may be prepared in advance and stored at 4°C, at which it is stable for about a week. Solution C is prepared using stock solution B and water immediately prior to use. Malachite Green hydrochloride can be used instead of Malachite Green oxalate salt.

This method is ideal for use in the assay of detergent-solubilized membrane-associated phosphatase activities. The staining procedure is easy to perform, results in a stabler colored product in comparison with the routine acid molybdate method, and is free from interference by detergents. The Malachite Green technique may be used to detect orthophosphate at pH 5.0 to 8.5.

The method can easily determine orthophosphate in a range of 0.5 to 10 nmol. However, it has two restrictions: (1) the use of citrate buffers prevents color development, and (2) the method can only be used with phosphate-free buffer systems.

## METHOD 5

### Visualization Scheme

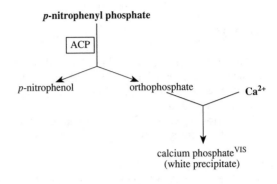

***p*-nitrophenyl phosphate**

ACP

*p*-nitrophenol          orthophosphate          Ca²⁺

calcium phosphate[VIS]
(white precipitate)

### Staining Solution[6]

0.1 *M* Acetate buffer, pH 5.0
0.6 m*M p*-Nitrophenyl phosphate
0.2 *M* Ca²⁺

### Procedure

Soak electrophorized PAG in 0.1 *M* acetate buffer, pH 5.0, for 20 to 30 min and incubate in the staining solution at 37°C. View the gel against a dark background and, when white bands of calcium phosphate precipitation of sufficient intensity are obtained, remove the gel from staining solution and store in 50 m*M* glycine–KOH, pH 10.0, 5 m*M* Ca²⁺, either at 5°C or at room temperature in the presence of an antibacterial agent.

*Notes:* The method can only be used when electrophoresis is carried out in a phosphate-free buffer system.

The precipitated calcium phosphate may be converted to brownish-black lead sulfide (e.g., see 3.1.3.1 — ALP, Method 7) or subsequently stained with Alizarin Red S. The lead conversion stain and Alizarin Red S stain do not increase the sensitivity of the staining method for photographs or for scanning, although they would be of advantage for opaque gel systems such as starch or acetate cellulose.

## 3.1.3.2 — Acid Phosphatase; ACP (continued)

### OTHER METHODS

Some other methods developed for alkaline phosphatase (see 3.1.3.1 — ALP) may be adapted for acid phosphatase.

### GENERAL NOTES

Acid phosphatase zymograms should be compared to those of alkaline phosphatase (see 3.1.3.1 — ALP) because some taxa possess phosphatases capable of exhibiting activity under both acidic and alkaline conditions.[7]

The enzyme from some sources requires magnesium or manganese ions or EDTA for activity.

### REFERENCES

1. Sparkes, M. C., Crist, M. L., and Sparkes, R. S., High sensitivity of phenolphthalein monophosphate in detecting acid phosphatase isoenzymes, *Anal. Biochem.*, 64, 316, 1975.
2. Hopkinson, D. A., Spencer, N., and Harris, H., Red cell acid phosphatase variants: a new human polymorphism, *Nature*, 199, 969, 1963.
3. Harris, H. and Hopkinson, D. A., *Handbook of Enzyme Electrophoresis in Human Genetics*, North-Holland, Amsterdam (Loose leaf with supplements in 1977 and 1978), 1976.
4. Shaw, C. R. and Prasad, R., Starch gel electrophoresis of enzymes: a compilation of recipes, *Biochem. Genet.*, 4, 297, 1970.
5. Zlotnick, G. W. and Gottlieb, M., A sensitive staining technique for the detection of phosphohydrolase activities after polyacrylamide gel electrophoresis, *Anal. Biochem.*, 153, 121, 1986.
6. Nimmo, H. G. and Nimmo, G. A., A general method for the localization of enzymes that produce phosphate, pyrophosphate, or $CO_2$ after polyacrylamide gel electrophoresis, *Anal. Biochem.*, 121, 17, 1982.
7. Richardson, B. J., Baverstock, P. R., and Adams, M., *Allozyme Electrophoresis: A Handbook for Animal Systematics and Population Studies*, Academic Press, Sydney, 1986, 162.

## 3.1.3.3. — Phosphoserine Phosphatase; PSP

REACTION      L(or D)-*o*-Phosphoserine + $H_2O$ = L(or D)-serine + orthophosphate

ENZYME SOURCE   Bacteria, fungi, vertebrates

### METHOD

#### Visualization Scheme

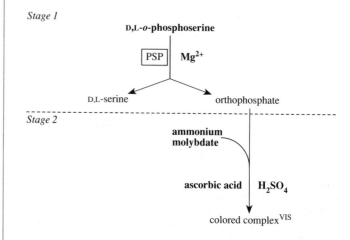

#### Staining Solution[1]

A. 0.1 *M* Tris–HCl buffer, pH 7.5      25 ml
    L-*o*-Phosphoserine      50 mg
    0.2 *M* $MgCl_2$      2 ml
B. 2% Agar solution (55°C)
C. 2.5% Ammonium molybdate in 4 *N* $H_2SO_4$      25 ml
    Ascorbic acid      1.25 g

#### Procedure

Mix solution A with 25 ml of solution B and pour the mixture over the gel surface. Incubate the gel at 37°C for 1 to 4 h. Remove the agar overlay. Mix solution C with 25 ml of solution B and cover preincubated gel with resulting mixture. Dark blue bands due to the presence of orthophosphate appear at the sites of PSP activity. The bands are ephemeral, thus the zymogram should be recorded or photographed immediately.

*Notes:* The best resolution of PSP allozymes is achieved when 2-mercaptoethanol is incorporated in the gel. The method can only be used when electrophoresis is carried out in a phosphate-free buffer systems.

### OTHER METHODS

Some alternative methods of detecting the product orthophosphate also may be used (see 3.1.3.1 — ALP, Methods 6 to 8 and 3.1.3.2 — ACP, Methods 4 and 5).

### REFERENCE

1. Moro-Furlani, A. M., Turner, V. S., and Hopkinson, D. A., Genetical and biochemical studies on human phosphoserine phosphatase, *Ann. Hum. Genet.*, 43, 323, 1980.

REACTION        5'-Ribonucleotide + $H_2O$ = ribonucleoside + orthophosphate

ENZYME SOURCE   Bacteria, fungi, plants, protozoa, invertebrates, vertebrates

## METHOD 1

### Visualization Scheme

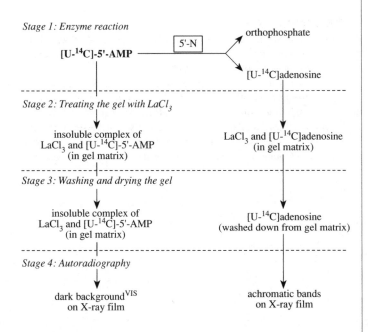

*Stage 1: Enzyme reaction*

$[U\text{-}^{14}C]\text{-}5'\text{-}AMP$ —— 5'-N —— orthophosphate / $[U\text{-}^{14}C]$adenosine

*Stage 2: Treating the gel with $LaCl_3$*

insoluble complex of $LaCl_3$ and $[U\text{-}^{14}C]\text{-}5'\text{-}AMP$ (in gel matrix)

$LaCl_3$ and $[U\text{-}^{14}C]$adenosine (in gel matrix)

*Stage 3: Washing and drying the gel*

insoluble complex of $LaCl_3$ and $[U\text{-}^{14}C]\text{-}5'\text{-}AMP$ (in gel matrix)

$[U\text{-}^{14}C]$adenosine (washed down from gel matrix)

*Stage 4: Autoradiography*

dark background$^{VIS}$ on X-ray film

achromatic bands on X-ray film

### Reaction Mixture[1]
A. 56 m$M$ Sodium phosphate buffer, pH 6.8
   1 µCi/ml $[U\text{-}^{14}C]\text{-}5'\text{-}AMP$
B. 0.1 $M$ Tris–HCl buffer, pH 7.0
   0.1 $M$ $LaCl_3$

### Procedure

*Stage 1.* Incubate electrophorized gel in solution A at 37°C for 1 h.
*Stage 2.* Place gel in solution B and incubate at 4°C for 6 h.
*Stage 3.* Wash gel for 12 h in deionized water. Dry the gel.
*Stage 4.* Autoradiograph dry gel with X-ray film (Kodak PR/R54) for 48 h. Develop exposed X-ray film.

White bands on a dark background of the developed X-ray film correspond to localization of 5'-N activity in the gel.

## METHOD 2

### Visualization Scheme

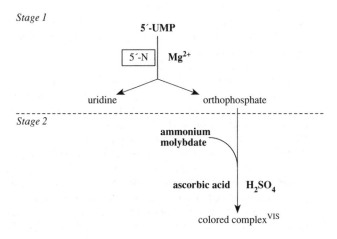

*Stage 1*

**5′-UMP**

5′-N   $Mg^{2+}$

uridine           orthophosphate

*Stage 2*

**ammonium molybdate**

**ascorbic acid**   $H_2SO_4$

colored complex$^{VIS}$

### Staining Solution[2]
A. 0.1 $M$ Tris–HCl buffer, pH 7.8          10 ml
   5'-UMP                           20 mg
   Glutathione (reduced form)      5 mg
   0.5 $M$ $MgSO_4$                 2 ml
B. 2% Agar solution (60°C)
C. 2.5% Ammonium molybdate in 4$N$ $H_2SO_4$   10 ml
   Ascorbic acid                      1 g

### Procedure
Mix solution A with an equal volume of solution B and pour the mixture over the gel surface. Incubate the gel at 37°C for 1 to 2 h. Remove agar overlay containing substrate. Mix solution C with an equal volume of solution B and pour the mixture over the gel surface. Dark blue bands appear at the sites of 5'-N activity. The bands are ephemeral, thus the zymogram should be recorded or photographed immediately.

*Notes:*   The method can only be used when electrophoresis is carried out in a phosphate-free buffer system.

## OTHER METHODS

A. Several alternative methods of detecting the product orthophosphate are also available (see 3.1.3.1 — ALP, Methods 6 to 8 and 3.1.3.2 — ACP, Methods 4 and 5).

B. An immunoblotting procedure (for details see Part II) based on the utility of monoclonal antibodies specific to the rat enzyme[3] can be used for immunohistohemical visualization of the enzyme protein on electrophoretic gels.

C. Positive zymograms of 5′-N can be obtained using IMP as substrate and two linking enzymes, purine-nucleoside phosphorylase and xanthine oxidase, coupled with the PMS/MTT (for example, see 3.5.4.6 — AMPDA, Method 2).

D. Dark (nonfluorescent) bands of 5′-N visible in UV light on a light (fluorescent) background can be developed using AMP as substrate and two coupled reactions catalyzed by auxiliary adenosine deaminase (3.5.4.4 — ADA, forward reaction) and glutamate dehydrogenase (1.4.1.2-4 — GDH, backward reaction). In this method 5′-N bands become visible due to NADH to NAD conversion. Negative zymograms of 5′-N visible in daylight may be then obtained by treating the fluorozymogram with the PMS/MTT mixture.

## GENERAL NOTES

0.75% Amphoteric detergent (zwittergent-314) is recommended to be included in the enzyme-containing preparations and electrophoretic gels. In the absence of the detergent the enzyme activity is very low.

Alkaline phosphatase (see 3.1.3.1 — ALP) can also act on some 5′ribonucleotides (e.g., 5′-AMP). Thus, an additional gel should be stained for ALP activity for comparison using substrates other than 5′-ribonucleotides.

## REFERENCES

1. Tucker-Pian, C., Bakay, B., and Nyhan, W. L., 5′-Nucleotidase: solubilization, radiochemical analysis, and electrophoresis, *Biochem. Genet.*, 17, 995, 1979.

2. Anderson, J. E., Teng, Y.-S., and Giblett, E. R., Stains for six enzymes potentially applicable to chromosomal assignment by cell hybridization, *Cytogenet. Cell Genet.*, 14, 465, 1975.

3. Bailyes, E. M., Newby, A. C., Siddle, K., and Luzio, J. P., Solubilization and purification of rat liver 5′-nucleotidase by use of zwitterionic detergent and monoclonal antibody immunoadsorbent, *Biochem. J.*, 203, 245, 1982.

REACTION  3′-Ribonucleotide + H₂O = ribonucleoside + orthophosphate

ENZYME SOURCE  Plants, protozoa

## METHOD

### Visualization Scheme

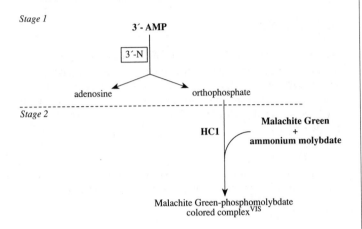

Stage 1

3′- AMP

3′-N

adenosine    orthophosphate

Stage 2

HCl

Malachite Green
+
ammonium molybdate

Malachite Green-phosphomolybdate
colored complex$^{VIS}$

### Staining Solution[1]

A. 100 m$M$ Tris–HCl buffer, pH 8.5
   2.5 m$M$ 3′-AMP
   0.05% CHAPSO (Sigma; a nondenaturing zwitterionic detergent)

| | |
|---|---|
| B. 4.2% Ammonium molybdate in 4 $N$ HCl | 30 ml |
| 0.045% Malachite Green (oxalate salt) | 90 ml |
| 2% Sterox (a detergent diluent) | 2.4 ml |
| C. Solution B | 60 ml |
| H₂O | 40 ml |

### Procedure

Incubate the gel in solution A (100 ml of solution A for 20 ml of gel volume) for 30 min at 37°C. Following incubation rinse gel quickly with water (usually 2 × 100 ml) to remove substrate and excess orthophosphate from the surface of the gel and place gel in solution C (see *Notes*). Color development is complete in 20 to 30 min. Rinse stained gel with several changes of water and store in 5% acetic acid, 20% ethanol.

*Notes:*  Prepare stock solution B as follows: mix 30 ml of ammonium molybdate solution and 90 ml of Malachite Green solution for 20 min at room temperature. Then pass resulting mixture through a Whatman No. 5 filter and add 2.4 ml of sterox solution. This stock solution may be prepared in advance and stored at 4°C, at which it is stable for about a week. Solution C is prepared using stock solution B and water immediately prior to use. Malachite Green hydrochloride can be used instead of Malachite Green oxalate salt.

The method is ideal for use in the assay of detergent-solubilized membrane-associated 3′-N activity.

The staining procedure results in a stabler colored product in comparison with the routine acid molybdate method.

The method can only be used with phosphate-free buffer systems. The use of citrate buffers prevents color development.

## OTHER METHODS

A. Several alternative methods of detecting the product orthophosphate are also available (see 3.1.3.1 — ALP, Methods 6 to 8 and 3.1.3.2 — ACP; Method 5).
B. Both products, adenosine and orthophosphate, can be detected using linked enzymatic reactions catalyzed by auxiliary enzymes adenosine deaminase, purine-nucleoside phosphorylase, and xanthine oxidase (e.g., see 3.5.4.4 — ADA, Method 1).
C. The product adenosine can be detected using two linked reactions catalyzed by auxiliary enzymes adenosine deaminase and glutamate dehydrogenase (see 3.5.4.4 — ADA, Method 2).

## REFERENCE

1. Zlotnick, G. W. and Gottlieb, M., A sensitive staining technique for the detection of phosphohydrolase activities after polyacrylamide gel electrophoresis, *Anal. Biochem.*, 153, 121, 1986.

REACTION    D-Glucose-6-phosphate + $H_2O$ = D-glucose + orthophosphate

ENZYME SOURCE  Invertebrates, vertebrates

## METHOD

### Visualization Scheme

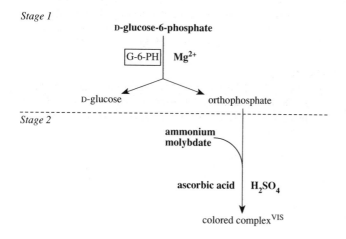

*Stage 1*

D-glucose-6-phosphate

G-6-PH    $Mg^{2+}$

D-glucose        orthophosphate

*Stage 2*

ammonium
molybdate

ascorbic acid    $H_2SO_4$

colored complex[VIS]

### Staining Solution[1]

A.  0.1 *M* Tris–HCl buffer, pH 7.8           25 ml
    20 m*M* D-Glucose-6-phosphate            25 ml
    0.2 *M* $MgCl_2$                           2.5 ml
B.  2% Agar solution (60°C)
C.  2.5% Ammonium molybdate in 4 *N* $H_2SO_4$   50 ml
    Ascorbic acid                              5 g

### Procedure

Mix solution A with an equal volume of solution B and pour the mixture over the gel surface. Incubate the gel at 37°C for 30 min. Remove first agar overlay. Mix solution C with an equal volume of solution B and pour the mixture over the gel surface. Dark blue bands of G-6-PH activity appear almost immediately. The bands are ephemeral, thus the zymogram should be recorded or photographed immediately.

*Notes:*  The method can only be used with phosphate-free electrophoretic and staining buffers.

The $MgCl_2$ may be omitted from the staining solution because the enzyme does not require any divalent ions for activity.

## OTHER METHODS

A.  Several alternative methods of detecting the product orthophosphate are also available (see 3.1.3.1 — ALP, Methods 6 to 8 and 3.1.3.2 — ACP, Methods 4 and 5).
B.  The product glucose may be detected enzymatically using the linking enzyme glucose oxidase in couple with the MTT/PMS system or using two linking enzymes, glucose oxidase and peroxidase (see 1.1.3.4 — GO, Method 1 and Other Methods).

## GENERAL NOTES

The enzyme also catalyzes potent transphosphorylations from carbamoyl phosphate, hexose phosphates, pyrophosphate, phosphoenolpyruvate, and nucleoside di- and triphosphates, to D-glucose, D-mannose, 3-methyl-D-glucose, and 2-deoxy-D-glucose. It may be identical to EC 3.1.3.1, EC 3.6.1.1, EC 3.9.1.1, EC 2.7.1.62, and EC 2.7.1.79.

## REFERENCE

1. Fisher, R. A., Turner, B. M., Dorkin, H. L., and Harris, H., Studies on human erythrocyte inorganic pyrophosphatase, *Ann. Hum. Genet.*, 37, 341, 1974.

OTHER NAMES    Hexosediphosphatase, fructose-1,6-diphosphatase

REACTION    D-Fructose-1,6-bisphosphate + $H_2O$ = D-fructose-6-phosphate + orthophosphate

ENZYME SOURCE    Bacteria, fungi, plants, invertebrates, vertebrates

## METHOD 1

### Visualization Scheme

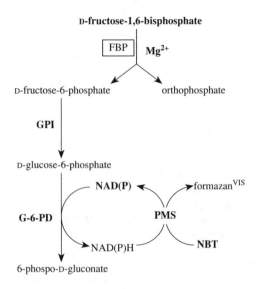

### Staining Solution[1]

| | | |
|---|---|---|
| A. | 0.1 *M* Tris–HCl buffer, pH 7.5 | 25 ml |
| | NADP | 8 mg |
| | $MgSO_4 \cdot 7H_2O$ | 50 mg |
| | 2-Mercaptoethanol | 1 µl |
| | PMS | 1 mg |
| | NBT | 10 mg |
| | D-Fructose-1,6-bisphosphate (sodium salt) | 10 mg |
| | Glucose-6-phosphate isomerase (GPI) | 20 units |
| | Glucose-6-phosphate dehydrogenase (G-6-PD) | 20 units |
| B. | 2% Agar solution (60°C) | 25 ml |

### Procedure

Mix A and B components of the staining solution and pour the mixture over the gel surface. Incubate the gel in the dark at 37°C until dark blue bands appear. Fix stained gel in 50% ethanol.

*Notes:* An NAD-dependent form of the auxiliary enzyme G-6-PD is available (Sigma, G 5760 and G 5885). If NAD-dependent G-6-PD is used, NAD should be substituted for NADP in the staining solution. This substitution is beneficial because NAD is about five times less expensive than NADP.

## METHOD 2

### Visualization Scheme

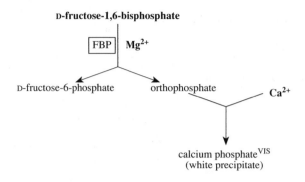

### Staining Solution[2]

50 m*M* Glycine–KOH buffer, pH 10.0
10 m*M* $Mg^{2+}$
10 m*M* $Ca^{2+}$
10 m*M* KCl
5 m*M* D-Fructose-1,6-bisphosphate

### Procedure

Soak electrophorized PAG in 50 m*M* glycine–KOH buffer, pH 10.0, at 37°C for 20 to 30 min and incubate in the staining solution at 37°C. View the gel against a dark background and, when white bands of calcium phosphate precipitation of sufficient intensity are obtained, remove the gel from the staining solution and store in 50 m*M* glycine–KOH, pH 10.0, 5 m*M* $Ca^{2+}$, either at 5°C or at room temperature in the presence of an antibacterial agent.

*Notes:* The method may be used only when electrophoresis is carried out in a phosphate-free buffer system.

The precipitated calcium phosphate may be converted to brownish-black lead sulfide (e.g., see 3.1.3.1 — ALP, Method 7) or subsequently stained with Alizarin Red S. These counterstains would be of advantage for opaque gel systems such as starch or acetate cellulose.

## OTHER METHODS

Some other methods of detecting the product orthophosphate are also available (see 3.1.3.1 — ALP, Methods 5 to 8 and 3.1.3.2 — ACP, Method 4).

### REFERENCES

1. Shaw, C. R. and Prasad, R., Starch gel electrophoresis of enzymes: a compilation of recipes, *Biochem. Genet.*, 4, 297, 1970.
2. Nimmo, H. G. and Nimmo, G. A., A general method for the localization of enzymes that produce phosphate, pyrophosphate, or $CO_2$ after polyacrylamide gel electrophoresis, *Anal. Biochem.*, 121, 17, 1982.

REACTION    2,3-Bisphospho-D-glycerate + H$_2$O = 3-phospho-D-glycerate + orthophosphate (see also General Notes)

ENZYME SOURCE  Fungi, vertebrates

## METHOD 1

### Visualization Scheme

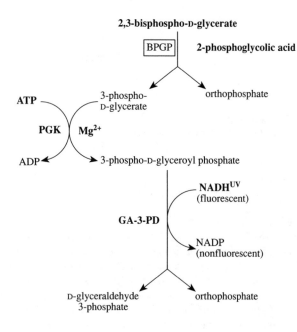

### Staining Solution[1]

50 m*M* Triethanolamine–HCl buffer, pH 7.5
2 m*M* 2,3-Bisphospho-D-glycerate
3 m*M* ATP
1 m*M* MgCl$_2$
1 m*M* 2-Phosphoglycolic acid
0.25 m*M* NADH
1.6 U/ml Glyceraldehyde-3-phosphate dehydrogenase (GA-3-PD)
1.6 U/ml Phosphoglycerate kinase (PGK)

### Procedure

Apply the staining solution to the gel surface on a filter-paper overlay and incubate the gel at 37°C. Inspect gel under long-wave UV light for dark (nonfluorescent) bands. Record the zymogram or photograph using a yellow filter.

*Notes:*  When a zymogram that is visible in daylight is required, counterstain the processed gel with the PMS/MTT solution. Achromatic bands of BPGP appear on a blue background of the gel almost immediately.

## METHOD 2

### Visualization Scheme

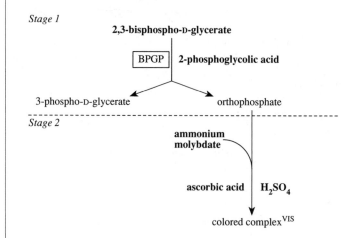

### Staining Solution[2]

A. 0.2 *M* Histidine–HCl buffer, pH 6.5
   1 m*M* 2,3-Bisphospho-D-glycerate
   0.12 m*M* 2-Phosphoglycolate
B. 1.5% Agar solution (55°C)
C. 2% Agar solution (55°C)
D. 1.25% Ammonium molybdate in 1 *M* H$_2$SO$_4$ containing 0.15 *M* ascorbic acid

### Procedure

Mix equal volumes of A and B solutions, pour the mixture over the gel surface and incubate at 37°C for 2 h. Remove the first agar overlay, mix equal volumes of solutions C and D and pour the mixture over the gel surface. Dark blue bands appear within 20 min.

*Notes:*  It should be taken into account that phosphoglycolate phosphatase (see 3.1.3.18 — PGP) activity bands can also be developed by this method. Thus, control staining of an additional gel for PGP should be made. This problem can be avoided if a low concentration of 2-phosphoglycolic acid is used in the staining solution.

## OTHER METHODS

Several other methods may be used to detect the product ortho-phosphate (see 3.1.3.1 — ALP, Methods 6 to 8 and 3.1.3.2 — ACP, Methods 4 and 5). All these methods may be used only when electrophoresis is carried out in a phosphate-free buffer system.

## GENERAL NOTES

Comparative electrophoretic studies show that BPGP, phospho-glycerate mutase (see 5.4.2.1 — PGLM), and bisphosphoglycerate mutase (see 5.4.2.2 — BPGM) activities, at least in mammalian red cells, are determined by a single protein.[3] 2-Phosphoglycolate is used in both methods to activate the enzyme.

## REFERENCES

1. Rosa, R., Gaillardon, J., and Rosa, J., Characterization of 2,3-diphosphoglycerate phosphatase activity: electrophoretic study, *Biochim. Biophys. Acta*, 293, 285, 1973.
2. Scott, E. M. and Wright, R. C., An alternate method for demonstration of bisphosphoglyceromutase (DPGM) on starch gels, *Am. J. Hum. Genet.*, 34, 1013, 1982.
3. Rosa, R., Audit, I., and Rosa, J., Evidence for three enzymatic activities in one electrophoretic band of 3-phosphoglycerate mutase from red cells, *Biochemie*, 57, 1059, 1975.

REACTION      2-Phosphoglycolate + H$_2$O = glycolate + orthophosphate

ENZYME SOURCE   Plants, invertebrates, vertebrates

## METHOD 1

### Visualization Scheme

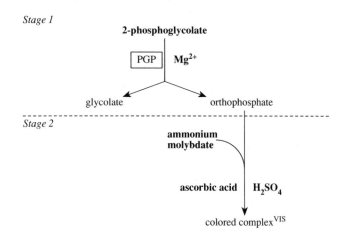

*Stage 1*

*Stage 2*

### Staining Solution[1]

A.   0.1 *M* Tris–HCl buffer, pH 7.5       25 ml
     2-Phosphoglycolic acid       50 mg
     MgSO$_4$·7H$_2$O       10 mg
B.   2% Agar solution (60°C)
C.   2.5% Ammonium molybdate in 4*N* H$_2$SO$_4$    25 ml
     Ascorbic acid       1.25 g

### Procedure

Mix solution A with an equal volume of solution B and pour the mixture over the gel surface. Incubate the gel at 37°C for 1 to 2 h. Remove the agar overlay. Mix solution C with an equal volume of solution B and pour the mixture over the gel surface. Dark blue bands of PGP activity appear after a few minutes. Record the zymogram or photograph because the stain is ephemeral.

*Notes:*   The method may be used only when electrophoresis is carried out in a phosphate-free buffer system.

## METHOD 2

### Visualization Scheme

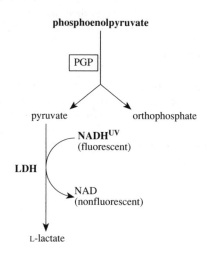

### Staining Solution[1]

   0.1 *M* Tris–HCl buffer, pH 7.5       5 ml
   Phosphoenolpyruvate (potassium salt)       25 mg
   NADH (disodium salt)       10 mg
   2750 U/ml Lactate dehydrogenase (LDH)       50 µl

### Procedure

Apply the staining solution to the gel surface on filter-paper overlay and monitor gel under long-wave UV light. The PGP activity is seen as dark (nonfluorescent) bands on a light (fluorescent) background. When the bands are well developed, record the zymogram or photograph using a yellow filter.

*Notes:*   This method is based on phosphoenolpyruvate phosphatase activity of PGP from some sources (e.g., from human red cells).

## OTHER METHODS

Several alternative methods of detection of the product orthophosphate are also available (see 3.1.3.1 — ALP, Methods 6 to 8 and 3.1.3.2 — ACP, Methods 4 and 5). All these methods may be used only when electrophoresis is carried out in a phosphate-free buffer system.

## GENERAL NOTES

PGP and alkaline phosphatase activities towards phosphoenolpyruvate can cause the development of additional bands on the zymograms of some other enzymes for which linked reactions catalyzed by pyruvate kinase and lactate dehydrogenase are used (for example, see 2.7.1.40 — PK, Method 1 and 2.7.3.3 — ARGK, Method 2).

## REFERENCE

1.   Barker, R. F. and Hopkinson, D. A., Genetic polymorphism of human phosphoglycolate phosphatase (PGP), *Ann. Hum. Genet.*, 42, 143, 1978.

OTHER NAMES    5′-Exonuclease

REACTION    Hydrolytically removes 5′-nucleotides succes-sively from the 3′-hydroxy termini of 3′-hy-droxy-terminated oligonucleotides

ENZYME SOURCE    Bacteria, plants, protozoa, invertebrates, ver-tebrates

## METHOD 1

### Visualization Scheme

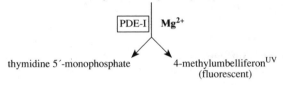

**4-methylumbelliferyl 5′-thymidylate**

PDE-I    $Mg^{2+}$

thymidine 5′-monophosphate    4-methylumbelliferon[UV]
(fluorescent)

### Staining Solution[1]
A. 50 m$M$ Tris–HCl buffer, pH 9.0
   1 mg/ml 4-Methylumbelliferyl 5′-thymidylate
   1 m$M$ $MgCl_2$
B. 1.8% Agarose solution (55°C)

### Procedure
Mix equal volumes of A and B solutions and pour the mixture over the gel surface. Incubate the gel at 37°C and monitor under long-wave UV light. The PDE-I activity is seen as fluorescent bands. Record the zymogram or photograph using a yellow filter.

*Notes:* Another fluorogenic substrate, the 4-methylumbelliferyl phenylphosphonate, also may be used for detection of PDE-I activity on electrophoretic gels.[2]

## METHOD 2

### Visualization Scheme

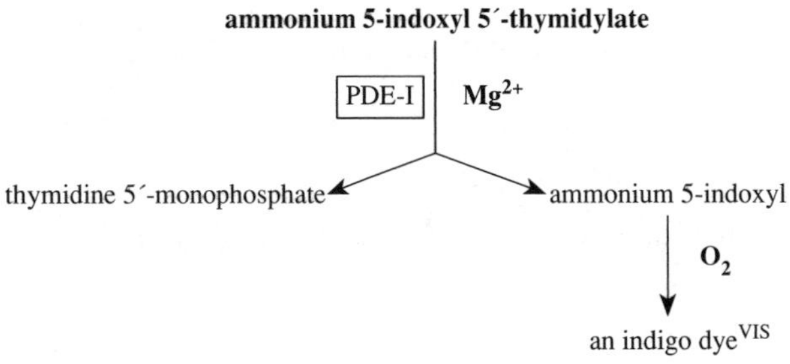

**ammonium 5-indoxyl 5′-thymidylate**

PDE-I    $Mg^{2+}$

thymidine 5′-monophosphate    ammonium 5-indoxyl

$O_2$

an indigo dye[VIS]

### Staining Solution[1]
50 m$M$ Tris–HCl buffer, pH 9.0
0.25 mg/ml Ammonium 5-indoxyl 5′-thymidylate
1 m$M$ $MgCl_2$

### Procedure
Incubate the gel in staining solution at 37°C. Colored bands at sites of PDE-I activity appear after about 8 h of incubation.

*Notes:* Control staining for alkaline phosphatase (3.1.3.1 — ALP) should be made because some ALP isozymes also can hydrolyze ammonium 5-indoxyl 5′-thymidylate.

## METHOD 3

### Visualization Scheme

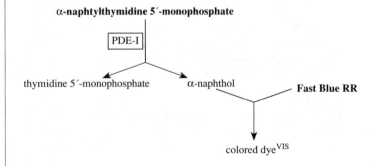

**α-naphtylthymidine 5′-monophosphate**

PDE-I

thymidine 5′-monophosphate    α-naphthol    **Fast Blue RR**

colored dye[VIS]

### Staining Solution[3]
| | |
|---|---:|
| 50 m$M$ Tris–HCl buffer, pH 7.5 | 100 ml |
| Thymidine 5′-monophosphate α-naphthyl ester | 10 mg |
| Fast Blue RR | 100 mg |

### Procedure
Incubate the gel in staining solution in the dark at 37°C until colored bands appear. Wash stained gel with water and fix in 50% glycerol or 3% acetic acid.

*Notes:* Nonspecifically stained bands were observed on PDE-I zymograms obtained using this method after electrophoresis of wheat leaf preparations. These bands were not observed after heating of preparations to 50°C before electrophoresis.[3]

## METHOD 4

### Visualization Scheme

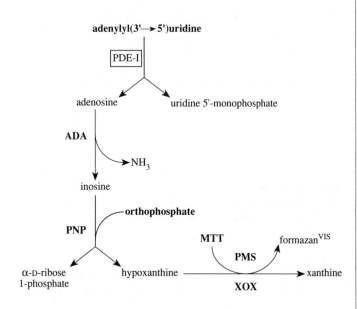

### Staining Solution[4] (modified[5])

A. 10 mg/ml Adenylyl(3′ → 5′)uridine 50 μl
   (in distilled water)

   5 mg/ml PMS 200 μl

   5 mg/ml MTT 200 μl

   Purine-nucleoside phosphorylase (PNP; 10 μl
   Boehringer)

   Xanthine oxidase (XOX; Boehringer) 10 μl

   Adenosine deaminase (ADA; Sigma, Type III) 20 μl

B. 1% Agarose solution in 50 m*M* sodium
   phosphate buffer, pH 8.0 (45°C) 9.5 ml

### Procedure

Mix A and B components of the staining solution and pour the mixture over the gel surface. Incubate the gel in the dark at 37°C until dark blue bands appear. Fix stained gel in 50% ethanol.

*Notes:* An additional gel should be stained in a staining solution lacking adenylyl(3′ → 5′)uridine to identify possible bands of "nothing dehydrogenase" (see 1.X.X.X — NDH).

Adenylyl(3′ → 5′)adenosine also may be used as PDE-I substrate in this method. When it is used, however, bands of spleen exonuclease (see 3.1.16.1 — SE, Method 3) are also developed.

## METHOD 5

### Visualization Scheme

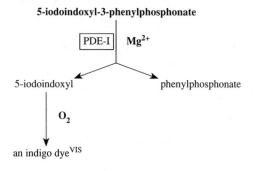

### Staining Solution[6]

50 m*M* Tris–HCl buffer, pH 9.0

1 m*M* MgCl$_2$

1 mg/ml 5-Iodoindoxyl-3-phenylphosphonate

### Procedure

Incubate the gel in staining solution at 37°C until bluish/purplish bands appear (usually for about 10 h).

*Notes:* The substrate 5-iodoindoxyl-3-phenylphosphonate is specific for PDE-I and is not cleaved by alkaline phosphatase, as the other chromogenic substrate, ammonium 5-indoxyl 5′-thymidylate (see above: Method 2, *Notes*).

## OTHER METHODS

When adenylyl(3′ → 5′)uridine is used as PDE-I substrate (see above, Method 4) the product adenosine also can be detected using two coupled reactions catalyzed by auxiliary enzymes, adenosine deaminase and glutamate dehydrogenase (for details see 3.5.4.4 — ADA, Method 2).

## REFERENCES

1. Lo, K. W., Aoyagi, S., and Tsou, K. C., A fluorogenic method for the demonstration of human serum 5′-nucleotide phosphodiesterase isozymes after polyacrylamide gel electrophoresis, *Anal. Biochem.*, 117, 24, 1981.
2. Hawley, D. M., Crisp, M., and Hodes, M. E., The synthesis of 4-methylumbelliferyl phenylphosphonate and its use in an improved method for the zymogram analysis of phosphodiesterase I, *Anal. Biochem.*, 129, 522, 1983.
3. Wolf, G., Rimpau, J., and Lelley, T., Localization of structural and regulatory genes for phosphodiesterase in wheat (*Triticum aestivum*), *Genetics*, 86, 597, 1977.
4. Karn, R. C., Crisp, M., Yount, E. A., and Hodes, M. E., A positive zymogram method for ribonuclease, *Anal. Biochem.*, 96, 464, 1979.
5. Hodes, M. E. and Retz, J. E., A positive zymogram for distinguishing among RNase and phosphodiesterases I and II, *Anal. Biochem.*, 110, 150, 1981.
6. Gangyi, H., The synthesis of 5-iodoindoxyl-3-phenylphosphonate and its use in analysis of phosphodiesterase I, *Anal. Biochem.*, 185, 90, 1990.

## 3.1.4.3 — Phospholipase C; PL

OTHER NAMES    Lipophosphodiesterase I, lecithinase C, *Clostridium welchii* α-toxin, *Clostridium oedematiens* β- and γ-toxins

REACTION    Phosphatidylcholine + $H_2O$ = 1,2-diacylglycerol + choline phosphate

ENZYME SOURCE  Bacteria, protozoa, vertebrates

## METHOD

### Visualization Scheme

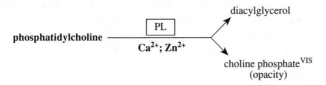

### Staining Solution[1]

A. 20 m$M$ Tris–HCl buffer, pH 7.4
   0.15 $M$ NaCl
   1 m$M$ CaCl$_2$
   1 m$M$ ZnCl$_2$
B. 3% Lecithin (or 20% egg yolk) emulsified in solution A using ultrasonic disintegrator (amplitude 8 μm for 1 to 2 min, 20°C).
C. 2% Agarose solution in solution A (56°C)
D. 1:1 (v/v) Mixture of B and C

### Procedure

Apply solution D to the PAG surface and incubate at 37°C in the humid chamber until opaque bands appear. Record the zymogram or photograph using Kodak photomicrography color film (PCF-36 2483).

*Notes:* The use of decreased concentration of lecithin or egg yolk in the staining solution will result in opacity zones of decreased contrast.

### REFERENCE

1. Smith, C. J. and Wadström, T., Isoelectric focusing in thin layer polyacrylamide gel combined with a zymogram method for detecting enzyme microheterogeneity: sample application, *Anal. Biochem.*, 65, 137, 1975.

## 3.1.4.17 — 3′,5′-Cyclic-nucleotide Phosphodiesterase; CNPE

OTHER NAMES    3′,5′-Cyclic AMP phosphodiesterase

REACTION    Nucleoside 3′,5′-cyclic phosphate + $H_2O$ = nucleoside 5′-phosphate

ENZYME SOURCE  Bacteria, fungi, invertebrates, vertebrates

## METHOD 1

### Visualization Scheme

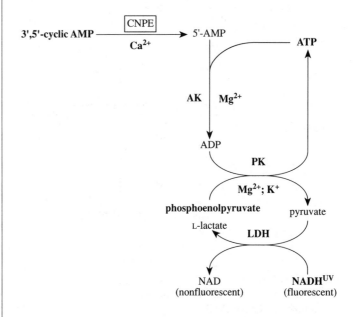

### Staining Solution[1]

| | |
|---|---:|
| A. 0.1 $M$ Tris–HCl buffer, pH 7.9 | 10 ml |
|    3′,5′-Cyclic AMP (monohydrate) | 21 mg |
|    MgSO$_4$·7H$_2$O | 40 mg |
|    KCl | 60 mg |
|    CaCl$_2$·6H$_2$O | 15 mg |
|    ATP (disodium salt, 3H$_2$O) | 7 mg |
|    Phosphoenolpyruvate (potassium salt) | 6 mg |
|    NADH (disodium salt) | 30 mg |
|    Adenylate kinase (AK; 360 U/ml) | 5 μl |
|    Pyruvate kinase (PK; 400 U/ml) | 5 μl |
|    Lactate dehydrogenase (LDH; 2750 U/ml) | 5 μl |
| B. 2% Agar solution (60°C) | 5 ml |

### Procedure

Mix A and B components of the staining solution and pour the mixture over the gel surface. Incubate the gel at 37°C and monitor under long-wave UV light. The areas of CNPE activity are seen as dark (nonfluorescent) bands on a light (fluorescent) background. Record the zymogram or photograph using a yellow filter. When a zymogram that is visible in daylight is required, counterstain the processed gel with MTT/PMS solution to obtain white bands on a blue background.

*Notes:* The bands caused by phosphoenolpyruvate phosphatase activity of alkaline phosphatase (3.1.3.1 — ALP) and/or phosphoglycolate phosphatase (see 3.1.3.18 — PGP, Method 2) can also be developed by this method.

## METHOD 2

### Visualization Scheme

*Stage 1*

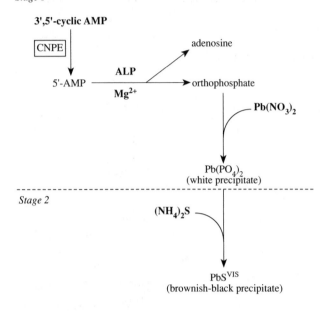

- - - - - - - - - - - - - - - - - - - - - - - - - - - - - - -

*Stage 2*

### Staining Solution[2]
A. 0.32 m$M$ Tris–maleate buffer, pH 7.0
   8 μ$M$ 3′,5′-Cyclic AMP
   0.5 U/ml Alkaline phosphatase (ALP)
   12 m$M$ Pb(NO$_3$)$_2$
   10 μ$M$ MgSO$_4$
B. 5% (NH$_4$)$_2$S

### Procedure
Incubate the gel in solution A at 37°C for 2 h or until bands of white precipitation appear. Wash gel in tap water for 1 h and place in solution B for 2 min. Black bands correspond to localization of CNPE activity in the gel. Wash stained gel in 10 m$M$ sodium acetate, pH 4.0, and store in 50% glycerol.

*Notes:* Solution A may be applied to the gel surface as 1% agarose overlay. 3′,5′-Cyclic GMP may be used as CNPE substrate instead of 3′,5′-cyclic AMP.[3] It should be kept in mind, however, that the bands of phosphodiesterase (EC 3.1.4.35) which are specific to 3′,5′-cyclic GMP can also be developed on CNPE zymograms obtained using cyclic GMP as substrate.

## OTHER METHODS

A. An immunoblotting procedure (for details see Part II) based on the utility of monoclonal antibodies specific to bovine CNPE[4] can also be used for immunohistochemical visualization of the enzyme protein on electrophoretic gels. This procedure is not appropriate for routine laboratory use but may be of great value in special analyses of CNPE.
B. The product 5′-AMP can be hydrolyzed by auxiliary alkaline phosphatase yielding orthophosphate and adenosine (see Method 2 above). The areas of adenosine production can then be detected using additional auxiliary enzymes adenosine deaminase, purine-nucleoside phosphorylase, and xanthine oxidase (e.g., see 3.1.4.1 — PDE-I, Method 4), or using another set of auxiliary enzymes, including adenosine deaminase and glutamate dehydrogenase (see 3.5.4.4 — ADA, Method 2).

## GENERAL NOTES

The enzyme acts on 3′,5′-cyclic AMP, 3′,5′-cyclic dAMP, 3′,5′-cyclic IMP, 3′,5′-cyclic GMP, and 3′,5′-cyclic CMP.

## REFERENCES

1. Monn, E. and Christiansen, R. O., Adenosine 3′,5′-monophosphate phosphodiesterase: multiple molecular forms, *Science*, 173, 540, 1971.
2. Goren, E. N., Hirsch, A. H., and Rosen, O. M., Activity stain for the detection of cyclic nucleotide phosphodiesterase separated by polyacrylamide gel electrophoresis and its application to the cyclic nucleotide phosphodiesterase of beef heart, *Anal. Biochem.*, 43, 156, 1971.
3. Nemoz, G., Prigent, A.-F., and Pacheco, H., Analysis of cyclic nucleotide phosphodiesterase by isoelectric focusing coupled to a specific activity stain, *Anal. Biochem.*, 133, 296, 1983.
4. Hansen, R. S. and Beavo, J. A., Purification of two calcium calmodulin-dependent forms of cyclic nucleotide phosphodiesterase by using conformation specific monoclonal antibody chromatography, *Proc. Natl. Acad. Sci. U.S.A.*, 79, 2788, 1982.

## 3.1.4.37 — Cyclic-CMP Phosphodiesterase; CCPE

OTHER NAMES    2′,3′-Cyclic-nucleotide 3′-phosphodiesterase (recommended name)

REACTION    Nucleoside 2′,3′-cyclic phosphate + $H_2O$ = nucleoside 2′-phosphate

ENZYME SOURCE  Bacteria, vertebrates

## METHOD

### Visualization Scheme

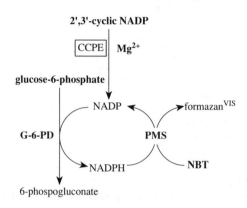

### Staining Solution[1]

A.  200 m$M$ 4-Morpholine–ethanesulfonate buffer, pH 6.1
    60 m$M$ MgCl$_2$
    0.2% Triton X-100
    0.1 m$M$ 2′,3′-Cyclic NADP
    4 mg/ml Glucose-6-phosphate
    0.4 mg/ml NBT
    0.04 mg/ml PMS
    0.7 U/ml Glucose-6-phosphate dehydrogenase (G-6-PD)
B.  1% Agarose solution (55°C)

### Procedure

Mix equal volumes of A and B components of the staining solution and pour the mixture over the gel surface. Incubate the gel in the dark at 37°C until dark blue bands appear. Fix stained gel in 50% ethanol.

*Notes:*  The enzyme is not water-soluble; therefore, sample preparation and electrophoresis should be made in the presence of SDS or a mixture of Triton X-100, CHAPS, and urea. Thus, before staining the gel should be made free of detergents by washing.

    The brain enzyme acts on 2′,3′-cyclic AMP more rapidly than on the CMP or UMP derivatives. The liver enzyme acts on 2′,3′-cyclic CMP more rapidly than on the purine derivatives. Just this latter enzyme has been called cyclic-CMP phosphodiesterase.

    The method described above was developed to detect the enzyme from myelin of the mammalian nervous system. Hydrolytic activity of bacterial enzyme and mammalian enzyme from other tissues towards 2′,3′-cyclic NADP is very low.

### REFERENCE

1.  Bradbury, J. M. and Thompson, R. J., Photoaffinity labeling of central-nervous-system myelin, *Biochem. J.*, 221, 361, 1984.

## 3.1.4.40 — CMP–sialate Hydrolase; CMP-SH

OTHER NAMES    CMP-*N*-acylneuraminate phosphodiesterase (recommended name)

REACTION    CMP-*N*-acylneuraminate + $H_2O$ = CMP + *N*-acylneuraminate

ENZYME SOURCE  Vertebrates

## METHOD

### Visualization Scheme

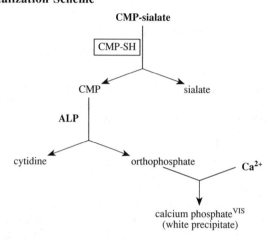

### Staining Solution[1]

A.  0.15 $M$ Tris–HCl buffer, pH 9.0
    5 m$M$ CaCl$_2$
    0.1% Triton X-100
    3 U/ml Alkaline phosphatase (ALP)
B.  60 m$M$ CMP–sialic acid

### Procedure

Cover the surface of electrophorized PAG dropwise with solution A (0.03 ml/cm$^2$) and allow solution to enter the gel. Then apply solution B in the same way and incubate the gel in a humid chamber at 37°C. View the gel against a dark background. White bands of calcium phosphate precipitation are visible after 15 to 120 min of incubation. Store stained gel in 50 m$M$ glycine–KOH, pH 10.0, 5 m$M$ Ca$^{2+}$, either at 5°C or at room temperature in the presence of an antibacterial agent. Gel can be photographed by reflected light against a dark background.

*Notes:*  The precipitated calcium phosphate can be converted to brownish-black lead sulfide (for details see 3.1.3.1 — ALP, Method 7) or subsequently stained with Alizarin Red S.

    The method may be used only when electrophoresis is carried out in a phosphate-free buffer system.

## OTHER METHODS

Several other methods of detection of orthophosphate produced by auxiliary enzyme alkaline phosphatase are also available (see 3.1.3.1 — ALP, Methods 5, 6, and 8 and 3.1.3.2 — ACP, Method 4).

### REFERENCE

1.  Van Dijk, W., Lasthuis, A.-M., Koppen, P. L., and Muilerman, H. G., A universal and rapid spectrophotometric assay of CMP–sialic acid hydrolase and nucleoside-diphosphosugar pyrophosphatase activities and detection in polyacrylamide gels, *Anal. Biochem.*, 117, 346, 1981.

## 3.1.4.X — Nonspecific Phosphodiesterase; NSPDE

REACTION          Hydrolyses bis(p-nitrophenyl) phosphate

ENZYME SOURCE  Bacteria, invertebrates, vertebrates

## METHOD

### Visualization Scheme

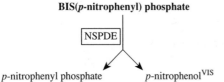

BIS(p-nitrophenyl) phosphate

NSPDE

p-nitrophenyl phosphate       p-nitrophenol[VIS]

### Staining Solution[1]

A. Bis(p-nitrophenyl) phosphate (disodium salt)    470 mg
    $H_2O$    125 ml
B. 0.5 M Sodium acetate buffer, pH 5.7    30 ml
    0.3% Tween 80    9 ml
    $H_2O$    15 ml
C. A mixture of solution A (4 ml) and solution B (5 ml)

### Procedure

Cover the gel with Whatman No. 1 filter paper saturated with staining solution (solution C). Wrap covered gel in Saran Wrap and aluminum foil and incubate at 37°C for 2 h. Drain the gel surface and cover with 0.1 M NaOH. Yellow bands appear immediately at the sites of NSPDE action. The yellow color can be preserved for a few hours if the gel is enclosed in Saran Wrap.

### REFERENCE

1. Hodes, M. E., Crisp, M., and Gelb, E., Electrophoresis of acid phosphohydrolase isozymes on Cellogel, *Anal. Biochem.,* 80, 239, 1977.

## 3.1.6.1. — Arylsulfatase; ARS

OTHER NAMES    Sulfatase

REACTION          Phenol sulfate + $H_2O$ = phenol + sulfate

ENZYME SOURCE  Bacteria, fungi, green algae, plants, invertebrates, vertebrates

## METHOD 1

### Visualization Scheme

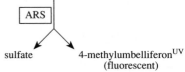

4-methylumbelliferyl sulfate

ARS

sulfate       4-methylumbelliferon[UV]
             (fluorescent)

### Staining Solution[1]

0.5 M Sodium acetate buffer, pH 5.6    2 ml
4-Methylumbelliferyl sulfate    8.8 mg

### Procedure

Cover the gel surface with staining solution and incubate at 37°C in a humid chamber for 1 h. Then fix gel in 10% formalin for 4 min and immerse in 0.25 M sodium carbonate–glycin buffer, pH 10.0, for 4 min. The sites of ARS activity appear as bright fluorescent bands when viewed under long-wave UV light.

*Notes:* Gels electrophorized in tris–glycine buffer, pH 8.4 to 8.6, can display fluorescent bands caused by nonenzymatic cleavage of 4-methylumbelliferyl sulfate. To prevent this staining artifact the use of acid electrophoretic buffers with pH below 6.0 is recommended. Gels electrophorized in acid buffers do not display staining artifacts when stained using 4-methylumbelliferyl derivatives as fluorogenic substrates.[2]

## METHOD 2

### Visualization Scheme

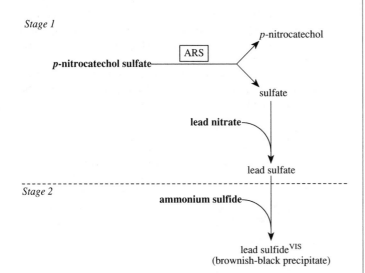

*Stage 1*

*Stage 2*

### Staining Solution[3]

A. 50 m$M$ Sodium acetate buffer, pH 5.5          100 ml
    $p$-Nitrocatechol sulfate          300 mg
    24% Lead nitrate          2 ml
B. 1% Ammonium sulfide          5 ml

### Procedure

Incubate the gel in solution A for 1 to 2 h, then add solution B and wait for dark bands to appear. Rinse stained gel with 10 m$M$ sodium acetate, pH 4.0, and store in 50% glycerol.

*Notes:* The brownish-black lead sulfide precipitate will go into solution if the pH rises above 5.7.

### REFERENCES

1. Rattazzi, M. C., Marks, J. S., and Davidson, R. G., Electrophoresis of arylsulfatase from normal individuals and patients with metachromatic leukodystrophy, *Am. J. Hum. Genet.*, 25, 310, 1973.
2. Chang, P. L., Ballantyne, S. R., and Davidson, R. G., Detection of arylsulfatase A activity after electrophoresis in polyacrylamide gels: problems and solutions, *Anal. Biochem.*, 97, 36, 1979.
3. Vallejos, C. E., Enzyme activity staining, in *Isozymes in Plant Genetics and Breeding, Part A*, Tanskley, S. D. and Orton, T. J., Eds., Elsevier, Amsterdam, 1983, 469.

| OTHER NAMES | Phosphodiesterase II, 3′-exonuclease, spleen phosphodiesterase |
|---|---|
| REACTION | Exonucleolytic cleavage in the 5′- to 3′-direction to yield 3′-phosphomononucleotides |
| ENZYME SOURCE | Vertebrates |

## METHOD 1

### Visualization Scheme

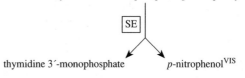

thymidine 3′-monophosphate-*p*-nitrophenyl

thymidine 3′-monophosphate      *p*-nitrophenol[VIS]

### Staining Solution[1]

A. Thymidine 3′-monophosphate–*p*-nitrophenyl
    (ammonium salt)          276 mg
    $H_2O$          1 ml
B. 0.5 $M$ Ammonium acetate buffer, pH 5.7      16.7 ml
    4 m$M$ EDTA (sodium salt)      8.33 ml
    1% Tween 80      0.05 ml
    $H_2O$      14.67 ml
C. A mixture of solution B with 0.25 ml of solution A

### Procedure

Cover the gel with Whatman No. 1 filter paper saturated with staining solution (solution C). Wrap covered gel in Saran Wrap and aluminum foil and incubate at 37°C for 90 to 120 min. Drain the gel surface and cover with 0.1 $M$ NaOH. Yellow bands appear immediately at the sites of SE action. The yellow color can be preserved for a few hours if the gel is enclosed in Saran Wrap.

## METHOD 2

### Visualization Scheme

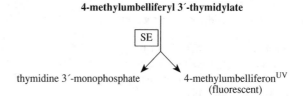

4-methylumbelliferyl 3′-thymidylate

thymidine 3′-monophosphate      4-methylumbelliferon[UV] (fluorescent)

### Staining Solution[2]

2 m$M$ Water solution of 4-methylumbelliferyl 3′-thymidylate

### Procedure

Incubate the gel electrophorized in an alkaline buffer system in the staining solution at 37°C and monitor under long-wave UV light. The areas of SE activity are seen as fluorescent bands. Record the zymogram or photograph using a yellow filter.

## METHOD 3

### Visualization Scheme

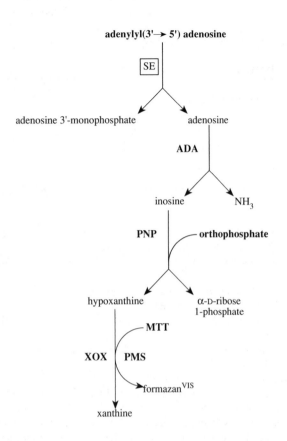

adenylyl(3' → 5') adenosine

SE

adenosine 3'-monophosphate          adenosine

**ADA**

inosine          NH₃

**PNP**          **orthophosphate**

hypoxanthine          α-D-ribose 1-phosphate

**MTT**

**XOX**          **PMS**

formazan^VIS

xanthine

### Staining Solution[3]

| | | |
|---|---|---|
| A. 10 mg/ml Adenylyl(3′ → 5′)adenosine (in distilled water) | 50 µl | |
| 5 mg/ml PMS | 200 µl | |
| 5 mg/ml MTT | 200 µl | |
| Purine-nucleoside phosphorylase (PNP; Boehringer) | 10 µl | |
| Xanthine oxidase (XOX; Boehringer) | 10 µl | |
| Adenosine deaminase (ADA; Sigma, Type III) | 20 µl | |
| B. 1% Agarose solution in 50 m$M$ sodium phosphate buffer, pH 8.0 (45°C) | 9.5 ml | |

### Procedure

Mix A and B components of the staining solution and pour the mixture over the gel surface. Incubate the gel in the dark at 37°C until dark blue bands appear. Fix stained gel in 50% ethanol.

*Notes:* Phosphodiesterase I (see 3.1.4.1 — PDE-I, Method 4) can also be developed on SE zymograms obtained by this method. However, PDE-I bands do not develop on SE zymograms obtained by this method when other dinucleoside monophosphates (UpA or CpA) are used as substrates. Moreover, only PDE-I bands develop when ApU is used as substrate.

An additional gel should be stained in a staining solution lacking the dinucleoside monophosphate to identify "nothing dehydrogenase" (see 1.X.X.X — NDH) bands, which can also develop on SE zymograms obtained by this method.

### REFERENCES

1. Hodes, M. E., Crisp, M., and Gelb, E., Electrophoresis of acid phosphohydrolase isozymes on Cellogel, *Anal. Biochem.,* 80, 239, 1977.
2. Hawley, D. M., Tsou, K. C., and Hodes, M. E., Preparation, properties, and uses of two fluorogenic substrates for the detection of 5′- (venom) and 3′- (spleen) nucleotide phosphodiesterases, *Anal. Biochem.,* 117, 18, 1981.
3. Hodes, M. E. and Retz, J. E., A positive zymogram for distinguishing among RNase and phosphodiesterases I and II, *Anal. Biochem.,* 110, 150, 1981.

| OTHER NAMES | Pancreatic DNase, DNase, thymonuclease |
|---|---|
| REACTION | Endonucleolytic cleavage to 5′-phosphodinucleotide and 5′-phosphooligonucleotide end = products |
| ENZYME SOURCE | Bacteria, fungi, plants, invertebrates, vertebrates |

## METHOD

### Visualization Scheme

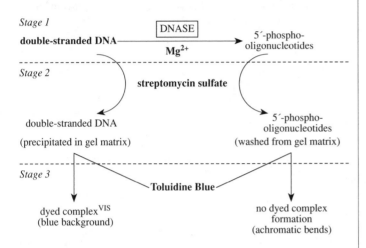

*Stage 1*

**double-stranded DNA** ——— DNASE / $Mg^{2+}$ ——→ 5′-phospho-oligonucleotides

*Stage 2*

**streptomycin sulfate**

double-stranded DNA
(precipitated in gel matrix)

5′-phospho-oligonucleotides
(washed from gel matrix)

*Stage 3*

**Toluidine Blue**

dyed complex[VIS]
(blue background)

no dyed complex
formation
(achromatic bends)

### Staining Solution[1]

A. 20 m$M$ Veronal–acetate buffer, pH 7.0
 0.1% Calf thymus DNA
 40 m$M$ $MgSO_4$

B. 2% Agarose solution (50°C)

C. 10 m$M$ Veronal–acetate buffer, pH 7.0
 1.5% Streptomycin sulfate

D. 0.125% Toluidine Blue
 0.5% Acetic acid

E. 2.5% Glycerol
 20% Methanol
 5% Acetic acid

### Procedure

Mix equal volumes of A and B solutions and form a 1-mm-thick reactive agarose plate. Apply electrophorized gel to reactive agarose plate and incubate in a humid chamber at 40°C for 90 min. Wash reactive agarose plate in solution C for 60 to 90 min and stain in solution D for 10 min. Wash stained agarose plate in solution E. Areas of DNASE activity are seen as achromatic bands on a blue background.

*Notes:* Pyronin G may be used instead of Toluidine Blue, resulting in light red staining of a DNA-containing gel.[2] Methyl Green:DNA dyed substrate complex also may be used to detect DNASE.[3] Native DNA may be specifically stained by the fluorogenic stain, ethidium bromide.[4-6]

Incorporation of DNA substrate directly into a running gel raises the sensitivity of negative stain methods considerably.[7] However, positively charged DNASE molecules could not be separated in electrophoretic gels containing DNA because they would bind to the negatively charged DNA. In this situation the use of SDS–containing PAG is recommended.[4] After denaturation with SDS and separation in SDS–PAG containing DNA, many DNASE isozymes recover activity when SDS–PAGs are subsequently incubated in appropriate buffers without SDS.

The sensitivity with which DNASE activity can be detected after SDS–PAG electrophoresis varies widely, depending upon the particular SDS preparation used for electrophoresis. Sensitivity of detection is greatly increased by using buffered 25% isopropanol, rather than buffer alone, to wash SDS from SDS–PAG after electrophoresis.[8]

The method described above is not specific. The bands of some other DNases with endonucleolytic activity also can be developed on DNASE zymograms.

Identification of DNASEs which display preference for double-stranded or single-stranded DNA can also be accomplished by electrophoresis in gels containing native and denatured DNA.[4]

Human urine DNase-I contains a few sialic acid residues. Desialylation of the enzyme by sialidase treatment of enzyme preparations before electrophoresis simplifies the enzyme pattern, the number of secondary isozyme bands being reduced.[6]

## REFERENCES

1. Berges, J. and Uriel, J., Mise en evidence des activites ribonucleasiques et deoxyribonucleasiques apres electrophorese en acrylamide-agarose, *Biochimie*, 53, 303, 1971.
2. van Loon, L. C., Polynucleotide–acrylamide gel electrophoresis of soluble nucleases from tobacco leaves, *FEBS Lett.*, 51, 266, 1975.
3. Hodes, M. E., Crisp, M., and Gelb, E., Electrophoresis of acid phosphohydrolase isozymes on Cellogel, *Anal. Biochem.*, 80, 239, 1977.
4. Rosenthal, A. L. and Lacks, S. A., Nuclease detection in SDS–polyacrylamide gel electrophoresis, *Anal. Biochem.*, 80, 76, 1977.
5. Kim, H. S. and Liao, T.-H., Isoelectric focusing of multiple forms of DNase in thin layers of polyacrylamide gel and detection of enzymatic activity with a zymogram method following separation, *Anal. Biochem.*, 119, 96, 1982.
6. Yasuda, T., Mizuta, K., Ikehara, Y., and Kishi, K., Genetic analysis of human deoxyribonuclease I by immunoblotting and the zymogram method following isoelectric focusing, *Anal. Biochem.*, 183, 84, 1989.
7. Brown, T. L., Yet, M.-G., and Wold, F., Substrate-containing gel electrophoresis: sensitive detection of amylolytic, nucleolytic, and proteolytic enzymes, *Anal. Biochem.*, 122, 164, 1982.
8. Blank, A., Sugiyama, R. H., and Dekker, C. A., Activity staining of nucleolytic enzymes after sodium dodecyl sulfate–polyacrylamide gel electrophoresis: use of aqueous isopropanol to remove detergent from gels, *Anal. Biochem.*, 120, 267, 1982.

OTHER NAMES     RNase O, RNase D

REACTION     Endonucleolytic cleavage to 5′-phospho-monoester. Cleaves multimeric tRNA precursor at the spacer region; involved also in processing of precursor rRNA, hnRNA, and early T7-mRNA. Also cleaves double-stranded RNA.

ENZYME SOURCE    Bacteria, fungi

## METHOD

### Visualization Scheme

*Stage 1: Enzyme reaction*

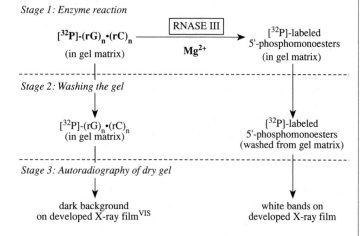

*Stage 2: Washing the gel*

*Stage 3: Autoradiography of dry gel*

### Reaction Mixture[1]
A. The [$^{32}$P]-labeled double-stranded $(rG)_n \cdot (rC)_n$ (300,000 to 400,000 cpm/20 ml gel mixture) is incorporated into the running SDS–PAG mixture before polymerization
B. 40 m$M$ Tris–HCl buffer, pH 8.0
   0.1 m$M$ EDTA
   10 m$M$ MgCl$_2$
   0.1 m$M$ Dithiothreitol
   75 m$M$ NaCl
C. Methanol:acetic acid:water; 5:1:5 (v/v)

### Procedure

*Stages 1, 2.* Upon completion of electrophoresis, subject the gel containing double-stranded RNA (see Reaction mixture, A) to a preliminary washing at room temperature with two changes of 300 ml water for 90 min, with gentle shaking. Then incubate the gel with 300 ml of reaction mixture (solution B). After 1 h of incubation at room temperature, replace the solution by 300 ml fresh solution of B and incubate the gel, with gentle shaking, at 37°C for a further 18 to 40 h.

*Stage 3.* After incubation, soak the gel in solution C for 30 min at room temperature, dry gel, and subject it to autoradiography using Kodirex film (Kodak). Autoradiography is completed in 1 d.

White bands on the developed X-ray film correspond to localization of RNASE III activity in the gel.

*Notes:* The sensitivity of the method can be increased by using buffered 25% isopropanol to wash detergent from the gel after electrophoresis.[2]

Some nonspecific endoribonucleases degrading RNA–DNA hybrids (e.g., see 3.1.26.4 — CTRH) can also be developed on RNASE III autoradiograms obtained using this method.[1]

### REFERENCES

1. Huet, J., Sentenac, A., and Fromageot, P., Detection of nucleases degrading double helical RNA and of nucleic acid–binding proteins following SDS–gel electrophoresis, *FEBS Lett.,* 94, 28, 1978.
2. Blank, A., Sugiyama, R. H., and Dekker, C. A., Activity staining of nucleolytic enzymes after sodium dodecyl sulfate-polyacrylamide gel electrophoresis: use of aqueous isopropanol to remove detergent from gels, *Anal. Biochem.,* 120, 267, 1982.

OTHER NAMES    Endoribonuclease H (calf thymus), RNase H

REACTION    Endonucleolytic cleavage to 5′-phosphomonoester; acts on RNA–DNA hybrids

ENZYME SOURCE  Bacteria, fungi, plants, vertebrates

## METHOD

### Visualization Scheme

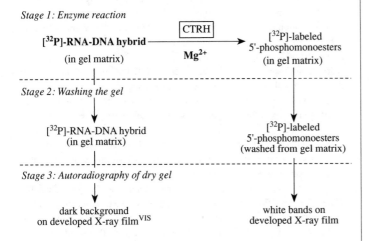

*Stage 1: Enzyme reaction*

[$^{32}$P]-RNA-DNA hybrid →(CTRH, $Mg^{2+}$)→ [$^{32}$P]-labeled 5′-phosphomonoesters (in gel matrix)

(in gel matrix)

*Stage 2: Washing the gel*

[$^{32}$P]-RNA-DNA hybrid (in gel matrix)      [$^{32}$P]-labeled 5′-phosphomonoesters (washed from gel matrix)

*Stage 3: Autoradiography of dry gel*

dark background on developed X-ray film$^{VIS}$      white bands on developed X-ray film

### Reaction Mixture[1]

A. The [$^{32}$P]-labeled RNA–DNA hybrids (300,000 to 400,000 cpm/20 ml gel mixture) are incorporated into the running SDS–PAG mixture before polymerization. Synthetic [$^{32}$P]-labeled $(rA)_n \cdot (dT)_n$ and $(rG)_n \cdot (dC)_n$ are used as substrates

B. 40 m$M$ Tris–HCl buffer, pH 8.0
   0.1 m$M$ EDTA
   10 m$M$ MgCl$_2$
   0.1 m$M$ Dithiothreitol
   75 m$M$ NaCl

C. Methanol:acetic acid:water; 5:1:5 (v/v)

### Procedure

*Stages 1, 2.* Upon completion of electrophoresis, subject the gel containing RNA–DNA hybrids (see Reaction Mixture, A) to a preliminary washing at room temperature with two changes of 300 ml water for 90 min, with gentle shaking. Then incubate the gel with 300 ml of Reaction Mixture (solution B). After 1 h of incubation at room temperature, replace the solution by 300 ml fresh solution B and incubate the gel, with gentle shaking, at 37°C for a further 18 to 40 h.

*Stage 3.* After incubation, soak the gel in solution C for 30 min at room temperature, dry gel, and subject it to autoradiography using Kodirex film (Kodak). Autoradiography is completed in 1 d.

White bands on the developed X-ray film correspond to localization of CTRH activity in the gel.

*Notes:* The sensitivity of CTRH detection may be increased by using buffered 25% isopropanol to wash detergent from the gel after electrophoresis (e.g., see 3.1.21.1 — DNASE, *Notes*).

### REFERENCE

1. Huet, J., Sentenac, A., and Fromageot, P., Detection of nucleases degrading double helical RNA and of nucleic acid–binding proteins following SDS–gel electrophoresis, *FEBS Lett.,*, 94, 28, 1978.

OTHER NAMES    Pancreatic ribonuclease (recommended name), RNase A, RNase B, RNase I, pancreatic RNase

REACTION    Endonucleolytic cleavage to 3′-phosphomononucleotides and 3′-phosphooligonucleotides ending in Cp or Up with 2′,3′-cyclic phosphate intermediates

ENZYME SOURCE    Bacteria, fungi, plants, invertebrates, vertebrates

## METHOD 1

### Visualization Scheme

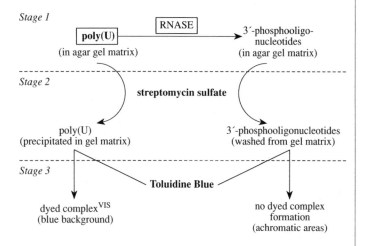

### Staining Solution[1]

A. 50 m$M$ Veronal–acetate buffer, pH 7.0
   10 m$M$ EDTA
   0.01% Poly(U) or 1% yeast RNA
B. 2% Agarose solution (50°C)
C. 10 m$M$ Veronal–acetate buffer, pH 7.0
   1.5% Streptomycin sulfate
D. 0.125% Toluidine Blue
   0.5% Acetic acid
E. 2.5% Glycerin
   20% Methanol
   5% Acetic acid

### Procedure

Mix equal volumes of A and B solutions and form a 1-mm-thick reactive agarose plate. Apply electrophorized gel to the reactive agarose plate and incubate in a humid chamber at 40°C for 90 min. Wash reactive agarose plate in solution C for 60 to 90 min and stain in solution D for 10 min. Wash stained agarose plate in solution E. Areas of RNASE activity are seen as achromatic bands on a blue background.

*Notes:*    Pyronin B and Acridine Orange may be used instead of Toluidine Blue to stain RNA.

Substrate solution may be applied on Whatman No. 1 filter paper when electrophoresis is carried out in acetate cellulose gel. After incubation, the acetate cellulose gel is fixed in a cold mixture of 25% ethanol and 5% acetic acid for 30 min, stained in a mixture of 2% aqueous Pyronin B (10 ml), 0.4 $M$ sodium acetate (45 ml), and 0.4 $M$ acetic acid (45 ml) for 15 min, and destained in a mixture of equal volumes of 0.4 $M$ sodium acetate and acetic acid. The gel is further destained in methanol:water:acetic acid (5:5:1) for 5 min and placed in the acetate–acetic acid destaining solution. The procedure results in a uniform cranberry stain except at the sites of RNASE action.[2]

RNA substrate may be included directly into running PAG before polymerization.[3] In this case the RNASE inhibitor (2 m$M$ copper chloride) should also be added to the running gel. After electrophoresis the gel is preincubated in an appropriate buffer to remove RNASE inhibitor and then placed in an appropriate buffer for a period sufficient for the enzyme action and stained with Toluidine Blue as described above.

Ribosomal RNA-containing SDS–PAG can be stained using the fluorogenic dye ethidium bromide. RNASE activity results in dark (nonfluorescent) bands visible in UV light on a light (fluorescent) background of the gel.[4] Sensitivity of RNASE detection in RNA-containing SDS–PAG is greatly increased by using buffered 25% isopropanol, rather than buffer alone, to wash detergent from electrophorized PAG.[5]

It was found that optimal RNA concentration in 1% agarose reactive plate is 2 mg/ml. Fixation of an incubated agarose reactive plate in 0.5 $N$ HCl (30 min) and subsequent washing in 0.5% acetic acid before staining with Toluidine Blue gives better results than the procedure described above.[6]

The method is not specific. The bands of some other RNASEs with endonucleolytic activity can also be developed on ribonuclease I zymograms.

## METHOD 2

### Visualization Scheme

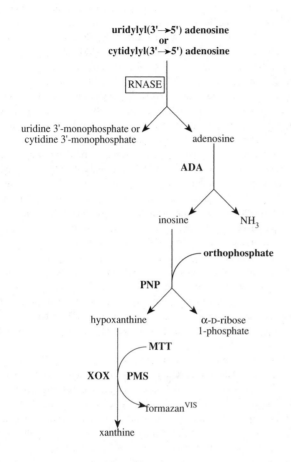

### Staining Solution[7,8]

A. 10 mg/ml Uridylyl($3' \rightarrow 5'$)adenosine,      50 µl
 or cytidylyl($3' \rightarrow 5'$)adenosine,
 in distilled water
 5 mg/ml PMS      200 µl
 5 mg/ml MTT      200 µl
 Purine-nucleoside phosphorylase (PNP;      10 µl
 Boehringer)
 Xanthine oxidase (XOX; Boehringer)      10 µl
 Adenosine deaminase (ADA; Sigma, Type III)      20 µl
B. 1% Agarose solution in 50 m$M$ sodium      9.5 ml
 phosphate buffer, pH 8.0 (45°C)

### Procedure

Mix A and B components of the staining solution and pour the mixture over the gel surface. Incubate the gel in the dark at 37°C until dark blue bands appear. Fix stained gel in 50% ethanol.

*Notes:* Phosphodiesterase II (see 3.1.16.1 — SE) can also be developed on RNASE zymograms obtained by this method. However, phosphodiesterase II bands are also developed by this method when adenylyl($3' \rightarrow 5'$)adenosine is used as substrate, whereas RNASE activity bands are not. These differences in substrate specificity may be used for identification of RNASE and phosphodiesterase II bands on the zymograms obtained by the method described above.

A control gel should also be stained in a staining solution lacking the dinucleoside monophosphates and the auxiliary enzymes to identify "nothing dehydrogenase" (see 1.X.X.X — NDH) bands, which also can develop in the presence of PMS and MTT.

### OTHER METHODS

A. When UpA or CpA are used as RNASE substrates, the product adenosine can also be detected using two auxiliary enzymes: the adenosine deaminase (to convert adenosine into inosine and ammonia) and the glutamate dehydrogenase (to convert ammonia and exogenous 2-oxoglutarate and NADH into L-glutamate and NAD). Gel areas, where conversion of NADH into NAD occurs, are visible in long-wave UV light as dark bands on the fluorescent background of the gel (for details see 3.5.4.4 — ADA, Method 2). An additional gel should be stained for phosphodiesterase II as described above (see Method 2, *Notes*).

B. An auxiliary enzyme, 3′-nucleotidase, may be used to detect 3′-phosphomononucleotides produced by RNASE (for details see 3.1.3.6 — 3′-N).

### GENERAL NOTES

Proteins, such as albumin, can penetrate the RNA-containing overlay and give false RNASE bands on negative zymograms obtained using Method 1.[7] This has not been observed nor would it be expected to occur in the positive zymogram Method 2 or in "Other Methods" (see above), since these methods rely on the production of adenosine or 3′-phosphomononucleotide for the staining reaction to occur.

### REFERENCES

1. Berges, J. and Uriel, J., Mise en evidence des activites ribonucleasiques et deoxyribonucleasiques apres electrophorese en acrylamide–agarose, *Biochimie*, 53, 303, 1971.
2. Hodes, M. E., Crisp, M., and Gelb, E., Electrophoresis of acid phosphohydrolase isozymes on Cellogel, *Anal. Biochem.,* 80, 239, 1977.
3. Randles, J. W., Ribonuclease isozymes in Chinese cabbage, systematically infected with turnip yellow mosaic virus, *Virology*, 36, 556, 1968.
4. Rosenthal, A. L. and Lacks, S. A., Nuclease detection in SDS–polyacrylamide gel electrophoresis, *Anal. Biochem.,* 80, 76, 1977.
5. Blank, A., Sugiyama, R. H., and Dekker, C. A., Activity staining of nucleolytic enzymes after sodium dodecyl sulfate–polyacrylamide gel electrophoresis: use of aqueous isopropanol to remove detergent from gels, *Anal. Biochem.,* 120, 267, 1982.
6. Thomas, J. M. and Hodes, M. E., Improved method for ribonuclease zymogram, *Anal. Biochem.,* 113, 343, 1981.
7. Karn, R. C., Crisp, M., Yount, E. A., and Hodes, M. E., A positive zymogram method for ribonuclease, *Anal. Biochem.,* 96, 464, 1979.
8. Hodes, M. E. and Retz, J. E., A positive zymogram for distinguishing among RNase and phosphodiesterases I and II, *Anal. Biochem.,* 110, 150, 1981.

OTHER NAMES          Glycogenase

REACTION             Endohydrolysis of 1,4-α-D-glucosidic linkages
                     in polysaccharides containing three or more
                     1,4-α-linked D-glucose units

ENZYME SOURCE   Bacteria, fungi, plants, invertebrates, verte-
                brates

## METHOD 1

### Visualization Scheme

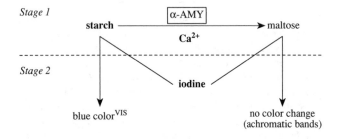

### Staining Solution[1]
A.  50 mM Sodium acetate buffer, pH 5.6                 100 ml
    1 M CaCl₂                                              2 ml
B.  10 mM I₂
    14 mM KI

### Procedure
Incubate electrophorized starch gel (or PAG containing 0.5%
soluble starch) in solution A at 37 to 50°C for 1 h. Discard solution
A, wash gel with distilled water, and stain in an appropriate
volume of solution B. The areas of enzyme activity develop on a
dark blue background of the gel as light blue or translucent bands,
depending on incubation time and the enzyme activity. Discard
solution B and rinse stained gel with water. Record or photograph
zymogram as quickly as possible.

*Notes:*   PAG and acetate cellulose gels can be negatively stained for α-AMY
activity by a two-step procedure using an agar overlay[2] or ultrathin agarose
plate[3] containing soluble starch and KI–iodine solution.

Dyed substrates, Amylopectin Azure[4] and Amylose Azure,[5] also may
be used to obtain the negative α-AMY zymograms by a one-step procedure.
These substrates should be applied to the gel surface as 1% agar overlays.

Amylase-sensitive test paper prepared using Procion Red MX2B-amy-
lopectin is recommended for rapid detection of α-AMY activity on polyacrylamide gels.[6,7] This method gives negative α-AMY zymograms and is sensitive enough to detect the low levels of α-AMY found in urine and serum
and could thus be used to detect α-AMY isozymes in clinical samples.

It should be kept in mind that some negatively stained bands on α-AMY
zymograms obtained using the methods described above may be caused by
phosphorolytic activity of phosphorylase (see 2.4.1.1 — PHOS, Method 3)
when electrophoresis or staining procedures are carried out in the presence
of phosphate-containing buffers.[8,9] Calcium chloride (0.02 M final concentration) inhibits phosphorolytic digestion of the starch by phosphorylase.

No reliable differences can be detected between α-AMY and β-amylase
(β-AMY; EC 3.2.1.2) activities with the negative staining procedures given
above. However, plant α- and β-AMY activities can be discerned when they
are present in the same gel. α-AMY tolerates a short exposure to 70°C, is
insensitive to mercury, copper, and silver. It is activated by calcium, and
inactivated by low pH (below 3.6). β-AMY is heat labile, sensitive to
mercury, copper, and silver, and is not activated by calcium. It tolerates acidic
pH (below 3.6).[2] When a starch–iodine system is used to obtain plant amylase
zymograms, α-AMY activity areas are seen as light or light bluish bands on
a solid blue background, while β-AMY activity areas are seen as reddish
bands on a solid blue background.[10]

When the starch–iodine method is used to detect α-AMY from animal
serum or some plant tissues, additional negatively stained bands not associated with amylase activity also can be developed. It was established that some
plant albumins are responsible for these "false" activity bands.[11] This is due
to the ability of some proteins to preclude the formation of the starch–iodine
complex. The most probable reason for the inhibitory effect of albumins on
the starch–iodine reaction is the presence of free sulfhydryl groups in albumin molecules. These groups reduce iodine presented in a staining solution
into iodide so that no starch–iodine colored complex can be formed in gel
areas occupied by (–SH)-rich protein molecules.

## METHOD 2

### Visualization Scheme

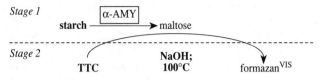

*Stage 1*

starch $\xrightarrow{\boxed{\alpha\text{-AMY}}}$ maltose

- - - - - - - - - - - - - - - - - - - - - - - - - - - - - - - - - - - - - - - - - - - -

*Stage 2*

TTC $\qquad$ **NaOH;** $\qquad$ formazan[VIS]
$\qquad\qquad$ **100°C**

### Staining Solution[12]

A. 0.2 *M* Sodium acetate buffer, pH 5.0 $\qquad$ 100 ml
   Soluble starch (dissolved in the $\qquad$ 0.2 g
   buffer by heating)
B. 2,3,5-Triphenyltetrazolium chloride (TTC) $\qquad$ 0.1 g
   1 *N* NaOH $\qquad$ 100 ml

### Procedure

Incubate electrophorized PAG in solution A at 37°C for 30 min, keeping the gel on a glass plate, surface down. Heat solution B using a water bath. Immediately after the staining solution B starts to boil, dip gel into the solution by keeping gel surface down and heat for 3 to 4 min until red-colored bands appear. Immediately after heating, the gel should be washed with 7.5% acetic acid.

*Notes:* To reduce nonspecific staining of the gel background, treat the gel with 0.1 *M* iodoacetamine for 5 min before staining with solution B.

The use of thin (0.8 mm) PAG is preferable for the detection of α-AMY activity by this method.

## REFERENCES

1. Siepmann, R. and Stegemann, H., Enzym-elektrophorese in einschluß-polymerisaten des acrylamids. A. Amylasen, phosphorylasen, *Z. Naturforsch.*, 22b, 949, 1967.
2. Frydenberg, O. and Nielsen, G., Amylase isozymes in germinating barley seeds, *Hereditas*, 54, 123, 1966.
3. Höffelmann, M., Kittsteiner-Eberle, R., and Schreier, P., Ultrathin-layer agar gels: a novel print technique for ultrathin-layer isoelectric focusing of enzymes, *Anal. Biochem.*, 128, 217, 1983.
4. Schiwara, H.-W., Detection of isoamylases with amylopectin azure as a substrate, *Z. Klin. Chem. Klin. Biochem.*, 11(7), 319, 1973.
5. Rinderknecht, H., Wilding, P., and Haverback, B. J., A new method for the determination of α-amylase, *Experientia*, 23, 805, 1967.
6. Whitehead, P. H. and Kipps, A. E., A test paper for detecting saliva stains, *J. Forens. Sci. Soc.*, 15, 39, 1975.
7. Burdett, P. E., Kipps, A. E., and Whitehead, P. H., A rapid technique for the detection of amylase isoenzymes using an enzyme sensitive "test-paper", *Anal. Biochem.*, 72, 315, 1976.
8. Brewer, G, J., *An Introduction to Isozyme Techniques*, Academic Press, New York, 1970, 133.
9. Vallejos, C. E., Enzyme activity staining, in *Isozymes in Plant Genetics and Breeding, Part A*, Tanskley, S. D. and Orton, T. J., Eds., Elsevier, Amsterdam, 1983, 469.
10. Chao, S. F. and Scandalios, J. G., Identification and genetic control of starch-degrading enzymes in maize endosperm, *Biochem. Genet.*, 3, 537, 1969.
11. Zimniak-Przybylska, Z. and Przybylska, J., Interference of *Pisum* seed albumins with detecting amylase activity on electropherograms: an apparent relationship between protein patterns and amylase zymograms, *Genet. Pol.*, 17, 133, 1976.
12. Mukasa, H., Shimamura, A., and Tsumori, H., Direct activity stains for glycosidase and glucosyltransferase after isoelectric focusing in horizontal polyacrylamide gel layers, *Anal. Biochem.*, 123, 276, 1982.

OTHER NAMES    Endo-1,4-β-glucanase

REACTION    Endohydrolysis of 1,4-β-D-glucosidic linkages in cellulose, lichenin, and cereal β-D-glucans

ENZYME SOURCE   Bacteria, fungi, plants, invertebrates

## METHOD 1

### Visualization Scheme

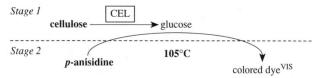

### Staining Solution[1]
   A. 0.1 *M* Acetate buffer, pH 5.0
      0.4% Carboxymethylcellulose
   B. 1% *p*-Anisidine hydrochloride (ethanol solution)

### Procedure

Spray the gel with solution A, cover with a sheet of Whatman No. 1 chromatographic paper and incubate at 37°C for 10 to 20 min. After incubation dry the paper at 105°C, spray with solution B and dry again. The areas of enzyme localization and liberation of reducing sugar are seen as positively stained bands on the paper print.

*Notes:* The inclusion of inert polymers into substrate solution A is desirable to raise the viscosity. The areas of enzymatically produced reducing sugars can also be positively stained using triphenyl tetrazolium chloride.[2] For example, see 3.2.1.1 — α-AMY, Method 2.

## METHOD 2

### Visualization Scheme

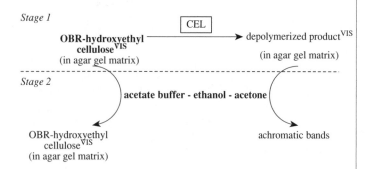

### Staining Solution[3]
   A. OBR (Ostazin Brilliant Red             150 mg
      H-3B)–hydroxyethyl cellulose
      H₂O                                     10 ml
   B. 3% Agar solution in 0.2 *M* acetate      20 ml
      buffer, pH 4.5 (60°C)
   C. 0.05 *M* Acetate buffer, pH 5.4–96% ethanol–acetone; 1:2:1
      (v/v)

### Procedure

Mix A and B solutions and pour the mixture between two polyester sheets mounted on glass plates and separated by plastic spacer bars (0.75 mm). Lay electrophorized gel on an agar gel containing dyed substrate, which is preheated to about 40°C over a hot plate, and incubate at room temperature until the first most active enzyme zones become visible. Separate agar layer from electrophoretic gel and dip into solution C. The achromatic zones of CEL activity develop as a result of solubilization of the depolymerized colored substrate. The duration of the washing in solution C (3 to 20 h) depends on the extent of substrate depolymerization.

A part of the enzyme-released dyed fragments of OBR–hydroxyethyl cellulose stains areas occupied by the enzyme on electrophoretic gel but with a lower color contrast and poor sharpness in comparison with achromatic bands developed on destained agar replica.

*Notes:* A carboxymethyl cellulose–containing agar replica preincubated with electrophorized gel may be negatively stained for CEL activity with Congo Red.[2,4,5] Electrophorized PAG containing carboxymethyl cellulose and preincubated in an appropriate buffer may then be negatively stained for CEL activity with iodine solution.[6] The inclusion of the substrate into running PAG is preferable because the separated CEL isozymes do not need to diffuse out of the gel and therefore isozymes with slight differences in mobility can be readily distinguished. To prevent enzymatic hydrolysis of the substrate during electrophoresis the use of denaturing SDS–PAG is recommended.

OBR-hydroxyethyl cellulose is commercially available (Sigma), but it can be easily prepared under laboratory conditions using hydroxyethyl cellulose and Ostazin Brilliant Red H-3B.[7]

## METHOD 3

### Visualization Scheme

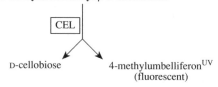

### Staining Solution[8]
   0.1 *M* Succinate buffer, pH 5.8
   1 m*M* 4-Methylumbelliferyl β-D-cellobioside

### Procedure

Apply the staining solution to the gel surface on filter-paper overlay and incubate the gel at 37°C in a humid chamber. Light (fluorescent) bands of CEL activity are visible under long-wave UV light. Record the zymogram or photograph using a yellow filter.

*Notes:* The method is based on cellobiohydrolase activity of CEL from some sources (e.g., *Clostridium*).

## METHOD 4

### Visualization Scheme

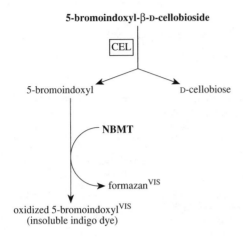

**5-bromoindoxyl-β-D-cellobioside**

CEL

5-bromoindoxyl → → D-cellobiose

NBMT

→ formazan^VIS

oxidized 5-bromoindoxyl^VIS
(insoluble indigo dye)

### Staining Solution[9]

| | | |
|---|---|---|
| A. | 5-Bromoindoxyl-β-D-cellobioside | 5 mg |
| | Nitro blue monotetrazolium chloride (NBMT) | 20 mg |
| | Dimethylformamide | 0.5 ml |
| B. | 0.1 *M* Sodium acetate buffer, pH 5.0 | 20 ml |

### Procedure

Mix A and B components of the staining solution and incubate the gel in the resulting mixture at 40°C in the dark until dark blue bands appear. The time of development is 2 to 15 h, depending on the concentration of the active enzyme in the gel.

*Notes:*  The staining solution can be used many times.

The product 5-bromoindoxyl can also be coupled with diazonium salts (e.g., Fast Blue B or Fast Red TR). However, there is a high background level with these azo dyes.

## REFERENCES

1. Eriksson, K.-E. and Petterson, B., Zymogram technique for detection of carbohydrates, *Anal. Biochem.*, 56, 618, 1973.
2. Bartley, T. D., Murphy-Holland, K., and Eveleigh, D. E., A method for the detection and differentiation of cellulase components in polyacrylamide gels, *Anal. Biochem.*, 140, 157, 1984.
3. Biely, P., Markovič, O., and Mislovičová, D., Sensitive detection of endo-1,4-β-glucanases and endo-1,4-β-xylanases in gels, *Anal. Biochem.*, 144, 147, 1985.
4. Beguin, P., Detection of cellulase activity in polyacrylamide gels using Congo red–stain agar replicas, *Anal. Biochem.*, 131, 333, 1983.
5. Bertheau, Y., Madgidi-Hervan, E., Kotoujansky, A., Nguyen-The, C., Andro, T., and Coleno, A., Detection of depolymerase isoenzymes after electrophoresis or electrofocusing, or in titration curves, *Anal. Biochem.*, 139, 383, 1984.
6. Goren, R. and Huberman, M., A simple and sensitive staining method for the detection of cellulase isozymes in polyacrylamide gels, *Anal. Biochem.*, 75, 1, 1976.
7. Biely, P., Mislovičová, D., and Toman, R., Soluble chromogenic substrates for the assay of endo-1,4-β-xylanases and endo-1,4-β-glucanases, *Anal. Biochem.*, 144, 142, 1985.
8. Schwarz, W. H., Bronnenmeier, K., Gräbnitz, F., and Staudenbauer, W. L., Activity staining of cellulases in polyacrylamide gels containing mixed linkage β-glucans, *Anal. Biochem.*, 164, 72, 1987.
9. Chernoglazov, V. M., Ermolova, O. V., Vozny, Y. V., and Klyosov, A. A., A method for detection of cellulases in polyacrylamide gels using 5-bromoindoxyl-β-D-cellobioside: high sensitivity and resolution, *Anal. Biochem.*, 182, 250, 1989.

## 3.2.1.6 — Endo-1,3(4)-β-glucanase; EG

OTHER NAMES    Endo-1,3-β-glucanase, laminarinase

REACTION    Endohydrolysis of 1,3- or 1,4-linkages in β-D-glucans when the glucose residue whose reducing group is involved in the linkage to be hydrolyzed is itself substituted at C-3

ENZYME SOURCE  Bacteria, invertebrates

## METHOD

### Visualization Scheme

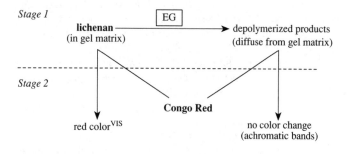

### Staining Solution[1]
A. 0.1 *M* Succinate buffer, pH 5.8
    10 m*M* Dithiothreitol
B. 1 mg/ml Congo Red in 0.1 *M* Tris–HCl buffer, pH 8.0
C. 1 *M* NaCl

### Procedure
Wash electrophorized SDS–PAG containing 0.1% lichenan (a mixed β-1,4- and β-1,3-linked glucan) five times for at least 30 min with cold solution A to remove SDS. Then place gel in 0.1 *M* succinate buffer (pH 5.8) and incubate for 30 to 60 min at 37 to 60°C. After incubation rinse gel in water and place in solution B for 10 min at room temperature. Destain gel in solution C for another 10 min. Achromatic or light yellowish activity bands are visible on a deep red background of the gel.

*Notes:*  Barley β-glucan may also be used as EG substrate instead of lichenan.

    Both mixed linkage β-glucans are suitable for the simultaneous detection of β-glucanases with specificities either for β-1,4- (see 3.2.1.4 — CEL), β-1,3- (see 3.2.1.39 — LAM) and β-1,3-1,4- (3.2.1.6 — EG) linkages. Therefore, it is advisable to perform parallel runs with substrate gels containing either carboxymethyl cellulose (substrate for CEL) or laminarin (substrate for LAM).

### REFERENCE
1. Schwarz, W. H., Bronnenmeier, K., Gräbnitz, F., and Staudenbauer, W. L., Activity staining of cellulases in polyacrylamide gels containing mixed linkage β-glucans, *Anal. Biochem.*, 164, 72, 1987.

## 3.2.1.8 — Endo-1,4-β-xylanase; EX

REACTION    Endohydrolysis of 1,4-β-D-xylosidic linkages in xylans

ENZYME SOURCE  Bacteria, fungi, plants, invertebrates

## METHOD

### Visualization Scheme

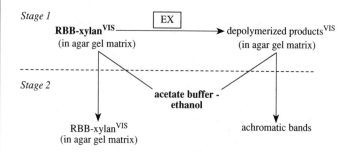

### Staining Solution[1]
A. RBB (Remazol Brilliant Blue R)–xylan    150 mg
    H₂O    10 ml
B. 3% Agar solution in 0.2 *M* acetate buffer,    20 ml
    pH 4.6 (60°C)
C. 0.05 *M* Acetate buffer, pH 5.4–96% ethanol;
    1:2 (v/v)

### Procedure
Prepare solution A by heating at 60 to 70°C and mix with solution B. Pour the mixture between two polyester sheets mounted on glass plates and separated by plastic spacer bars (0.75 mm) to form a 0.75-mm-thick reactive agar plate. Lay electrophorized gel on an agar gel containing dyed substrate, which is preheated to about 40°C over a hot plate, and incubate at room temperature until the enzyme zones become clearly visible against a white light. Then dip agar replica into solution C for 3 to 20 h. The enzyme-degraded substrate zones are destained and appear as pale blue or almost colorless areas on a blue background of the agar replica.

*Notes:*  The dyed substrate RBB–xylan is commercially available from Sigma Chemical Company, but it can be easily prepared in the laboratory.[2]

### REFERENCES
1. Biely, P., Markovič, O., and Mislovičová, D., Sensitive detection of endo-1,4-β-glucanases and endo-1,4-β-xylanases in gels, *Anal. Biochem.*, 144, 147, 1985.
2. Biely, P., Mislovičová, D., and Toman, R., Soluble chromogenic substrates for the assay of endo-1,4-β-xylanases and endo-1,4-β-glucanases, *Anal. Biochem.*, 144, 142, 1985.

OTHER NAMES     Limit dextrinase, isomaltase, sucrase-isomaltase

REACTION     Hydrolysis of 1,6-β-D-glucosidic linkages in isomaltose and dextrins produced from starch and glycogen by α-amylase

ENZYME SOURCE   Fungi, plants, invertebrates, vertebrates

## METHOD 1

### Visualization Scheme

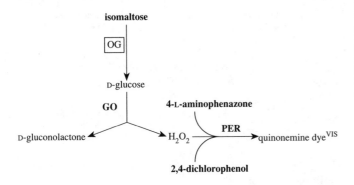

### Staining Solution[1]

A. 2 *M* Sodium phosphate buffer, pH 6.0
    25 m*M* Isomaltose
B. 2,4-Dichlorophenol (sulfonated)
C. 10 U/ml Glucose oxidase (GO)
    10 U/ml Peroxidase (PER)
    0.5 mg/ml 4-L-Aminophenazone
D. 1.6% Agarose solution (60°C)

### Procedure

Mix 0.75 ml A with 0.5 ml B, 2.5 ml C, and 6.25 ml D. Pour the mixture over the gel surface and incubate at 37°C until colored bands appear. Record or photograph the zymogram because the stain is not permanent.

*Notes:* Preparations of glucose oxidase and peroxidase should be catalase-free. If they are not, NaN$_3$ should be included in the stain to inhibit catalase activity.

    Other methods may be used to detect hydrogen peroxide via the linked peroxidase reaction (see 1.11.1.7 — PER).

## METHOD 2

### Visualization Scheme

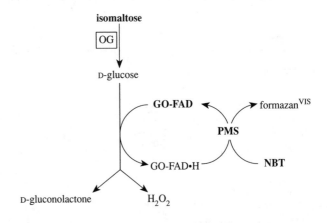

### Staining Solution[1]

A. 2 *M* Sodium phosphate buffer, pH 6.0     1 ml
    H$_2$O     4 ml
    PMS     2 mg
    NBT     5 mg
    Isomaltose     43 mg
    Glucose oxidase (GO)     100 units
B. 2% Agarose solution (60°C)     5 ml

### Procedure

Mix A and B components of the staining solution and pour the mixture over the gel surface. Incubate the gel at 37°C in the dark until dark blue bands appear. Fix stained gel in 50% ethanol or 5% acetic acid.

## OTHER METHODS

A. The product D-glucose may also be detected using linking enzymes hexokinase and NAD(P)-dependent glucose-6-phosphate dehydrogenase in couple with the PMS/MTT (see 3.2.1.26 — FF, Method 5).
B. An immunoblotting procedure (for details see Part II) based on the utility of monoclonal antibodies specific to the rat enzyme[2] can be used for immunohistochemical visualization of the enzyme protein on electrophoretic gels. This procedure is not practical; however, it may be indispensable in special immunogenetic analyses of OG.

## REFERENCES

1. Finlayson, S. D., Moore, P. A., Johnston, J. R., and Berry, D. R., Two staining methods for selectively detecting isomaltase and maltase activity in electrophoretic gels, *Anal. Biochem.*, 186, 233, 1990.
2. Hauri, H. P., Quaroni, A., and Isselbacher, K. J., Monoclonal antibodies to sucrase-isomaltase — probes for the study of postnatal development and biogenesis of the intestinal microvillus membrane, *Proc. Natl. Acad. Sci. U.S.A.*, 77, 6629, 1980.

## 3.2.1.11 — Dextranase; DEX

REACTION      Endohydrolysis of 1,6-α-D-glucosidic linkages in dextran

ENZYME SOURCE    Bacteria, fungi, plants, invertebrates, vertebrates

## METHOD

### Visualization Scheme

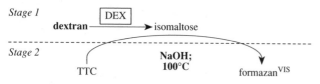

*Stage 1*

dextran —[DEX]→ isomaltose

*Stage 2*

TTC     **NaOH; 100°C**     formazan[VIS]

### Staining Solution[1]
A. 0.2 *M* Sodium acetate buffer, pH 5.0       100 ml
     Dextran T 10 (Pharmacia)              0.1 g
B. 2,3,5-Triphenyltetrazolium chloride (TTC)    0.1 g
     1 *N* NaOH                        100 ml

### Procedure
Incubate electrophorized PAG at 37°C for 30 min, keeping the gel on a glass plate, surface down, in a beaker of an appropriate size which contains solution A. Heat solution B in another beaker in a water bath. Immediately after the staining solution B starts to boil, dip gel into the solution by keeping gel surface down and heat for 3 to 4 min until red-colored bands appear. Wash stained gel with 7.5% acetic acid. Too much heating causes the gel background to be stained pink.

*Notes:*    The use of thin (0.8 mm) PAG is preferable for the detection of DEX activity by this method.

     To reduce nonspecific staining of the gel background, treat the gel with 0.1 *M* iodoacetamine for 5 min before staining with solution B.

## OTHER METHODS

Two linking enzymes, isomaltase and glucose oxidase, may be used in couple with the PMS/NBT system to detect the product isomaltose (see 3.2.1.10 — OG, Method 2).

## REFERENCE
1. Mukasa, H., Shimamura, A., and Tsumori, H., Direct activity stains for glycosidase and glucosyltransferase after isoelectric focusing in horizontal polyacrylamide gel layers, *Anal. Biochem.*, 123, 276, 1982.

## 3.2.1.15 — Polygalacturonase; PG

OTHER NAMES     Pectin depolymerase, pectinase

REACTION      Random hydrolysis of 1,4-α-D-galactosiduronic linkages in pectate and other galacturonans

ENZYME SOURCE    Bacteria, fungi, plants

## METHOD

### Visualization Scheme

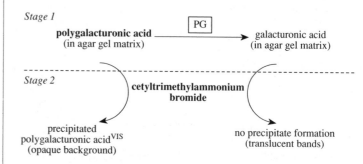

*Stage 1*

**polygalacturonic acid** (in agar gel matrix) —[PG]→ galacturonic acid (in agar gel matrix)

*Stage 2*

**cetyltrimethylammonium bromide**

precipitated polygalacturonic acid[VIS] (opaque background)      no precipitate formation (translucent bands)

### Staining Solution[1]
A. 0.1 *M* Citrate buffer, pH 5.0
     1.5% Agar
     0.5% Polygalacturonic acid (sodium salt)
B. 1% Cetyltrimethylammonium bromide

### Procedure
Prepare solution A by heating in a boiling water bath; cool to 50°C and pour over the surface of electrophorized PAG preincubated in 0.1 *M* citrate buffer, pH 5.0, for 20 min. Incubate overlayed gel at 37°C for 2 to 3 h. Remove agar overlay and place it in solution B. The areas of PG activity appear as translucent bands on an opaque background of the reactive agar plate.

*Notes:*    Bands of polygalacturonate lyase (see 4.2.2.2 — PGL) and galacturan 1,4-α-galacturonidase (see 3.2.1.67 — GG) activities also can develop on PG zymograms obtained by this method. The main difference in substrate specificity of the three enzymes possessing polygalacturonase activity is the ability of PG to hydrolyze pectin (PGL and GG do not act on this polysaccharide). This difference may be used to identify PG activity bands.

## REFERENCE
1. Nguyen-The, C., Bertheau, Y., and Coleno, A., Étude des isoenzymes de polygalacturonases, d'endoglucanases de *Rhizopus* spp. et *Mucor* spp. et différenciation d'isolats dans le sud-est de la France, *Can. J. Bot.*, 62, 2670, 1984.

## 3.2.1.17 — Lysozyme; LZ

**OTHER NAMES**       Muramidase

**REACTION**       Hydrolysis of 1,4-β-linkages between
*N*-acetylmuramic acid and *N*-acetyl-D-glu-
cosamine residues in a peptidoglycan and between *N*-acetyl-D-glucosamine residues in
chitodextrin

**ENZYME SOURCE**  Plants, vertebrates

## METHOD

### Visualization Scheme

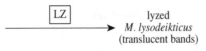

*Micrococcus lysodeikticus*
**in agarose gel matrix**[VIS]      →  [LZ]  →      lyzed
(opaque background)                    *M. lysodeikticus*
(translucent bands)

### Staining Solution[1]

A. 2% Agarose solution in 0.06 *M* phosphate buffer, pH 6.2
(55°C)
B. 0.12% Suspension of *Micrococcus lysodeikticus* in 0.06 *M*
phosphate buffer, pH 6.2

### Procedure

Mix equal volumes of solution A and suspension B and pour the
mixture over the gel surface. Incubate the gel at 37°C until translucent bands appear. Fix developed agarose overlay in 10% acetic
acid.

*Notes:*  Some chitinases (EC 3.2.1.14) also display the activity defined in
LZ.

### REFERENCE

1. Azen, E. A., Genetic polymorphism of basic proteins from parotid
saliva, *Science*, 176, 673, 1972.

## 3.2.1.18 — Sialidase; SIA

**OTHER NAMES**       Neuraminidase

**REACTION**       Hydrolysis of 2,3-, 2,6-, and 2,8-glycosidic
linkages joining terminal nonreducing *N*- or
*O*-acylneuraminyl residues to galactose, *N*-
acethylhexosamine, or *N*- or *O*-acylated
neuraminyl residues in oligosaccharides, glycoproteins, glycolipids, or colominic acid

**ENZYME SOURCE**  Cells infected by some viruses, bacteria, vertebrates

## METHOD

### Visualization Scheme

2′-(4-methylumbelliferyl)-α-D-*N*-acetylneuraminic acid

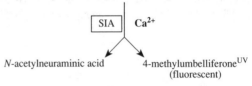

[SIA]   Ca²⁺

*N*-acetylneuraminic acid          4-methylumbelliferone[UV]
(fluorescent)

### Staining Solution[1]

0.2 *M* Acetate buffer, pH 5.0
5 m*M* CaCl₂
0.5 m*M* 2′-(4-Methylumbelliferyl)-α-D-*N*-acetylneuraminic
acid

### Procedure

Preincubate electrophorized gel in 0.2 *M* acetate buffer, pH 5.0,
containing 5 m*M* CaCl₂. Apply the staining solution to the gel
surface with a filter paper and incubate the gel at room temperature for 15 to 30 min in a humid chamber. The areas of SIA
activity are seen in long-wave UV light as fluorescent bands.
Record the zymogram or photograph using a yellow filter.

*Notes:*  In case of low sialidase activity, treat the processed gel for 2 min
with 0.133 *M* glycine buffer, pH 10.0, containing 60 m*M* NaCl and 40 m*M*
Na₂CO₃ to intensify the fluorescence.

### OTHER METHODS

A. Methoxyphenyl-α-D-*N*-acetylneuraminic acid may be used as a
chromogenic substrate for SIA. After enzymatic action the
methoxyphenol released should be coupled with a diazonium
salt, yielding an insoluble dye.
B. An immunoblotting procedure (for details see Part II) based on
the utility of monoclonal antibodies specific to the influenza-A
virus enzyme[2] also can be used for immunohistochemical visualization of the enzyme protein on electrophoretic gels. This
procedure is unsuitable for routine laboratory use, but may be of
value in special analyses of SIA.

## GENERAL NOTES

The advantages of the fluorescent method are the commercial availability of the substrate and the visualization of the product after a single reaction step.

The bacterial enzyme releases essentially all of the sialic acid from a variety of substrates. The enzyme from some bacteria (e.g., *Vibrio cholerae*) requires $Ca^{2+}$ for activity. The mammalian enzyme is less efficient in that it only releases 20 to 30% of the sialic acid from most substrates.

## REFERENCES

1. Berg, W., Gutschker-Gdaniec, G., and Schauer, R., Fluorescent staining of sialidases in polyacrylamide gel electrophoresis and ultrathin-layer isoelectric focusing, *Anal. Biochem.*, 145, 339, 1985.
2. Webster, R. G., Kendal, A. P., and Gerhard, W., Analysis of antigenic drift in recently isolated influenza-A (HINI) viruses using monoclonal antibody preparations, *Virology*, 96, 258, 1979.

OTHER NAMES    Maltase, glucoinvertase, glucosidosucrase, maltase-glucoamylase

REACTION    Hydrolysis of terminal, nonreducing 1,4-linked α-D-glucose residues with release of α-D-glucose

ENZYME SOURCE    Bacteria, fungi, plants, invertebrates, vertebrates

## METHOD 1

### Visualization Scheme

**4-methylumbelliferyl α-D-glucoside**

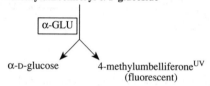

α-D-glucose    4-methylumbelliferone[UV]
(fluorescent)

### Staining Solution[1]

| | |
|---|---|
| 0.1 *M* Citrate buffer, pH 4.0 | 20 ml |
| 4-Methylumbelliferyl α-D-glucoside | 10 mg |

### Procedure

Apply the staining solution to the gel surface with a filter paper and incubate the gel at 37°C in a humid chamber. Remove filter paper after 30 to 60 min and view gel under long-wave UV light. Areas of α-GLU activity are seen as fluorescent bands. Record the zymogram or photograph using a yellow filter.

*Notes:*    Fluorescence of α-GLU activity bands can be enhanced by spraying the gel with ammonia after removal of the filter-paper overlay.

## METHOD 2

### Visualization Scheme

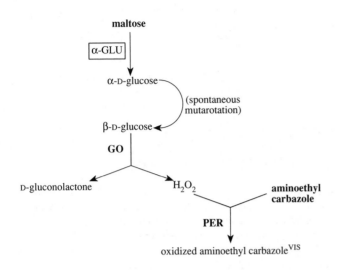

### Staining Solution[1]

A. 0.1 *M* Citrate buffer, pH 5.0                                    10 ml
   Maltose (optional)                                               50 mg
   1000 U/ml Glucose oxidase (GO)                                   50 μl
   2500 U/ml Peroxidase (PER)                                       50 μl
   25 mg/ml 3-Amino-9-ethyl carbazole                                2 ml
      (dissolved in acetone)
B. 2% Agar solution (60°C)                                          12 ml

### Procedure

Mix A and B components of the staining solution and pour the mixture over the gel surface. Incubate the gel at 37°C until reddish-brown bands appear. Fix stained agar overlay in 7% acetic acid and dry on a filter paper sheet or on a glass plate of appropriate size.

*Notes:*  *o*-Dianisidine hydrochloride may be used instead of aminoethyl carbasole. It should be remembered, however, that this redox dye is carcinogenic.

The product D-glucose may be detected using glucose oxidase in couple with the PMS/NBT (e.g., see 3.2.1.10 — OG, Method 2).

## METHOD 3

### Visualization Scheme

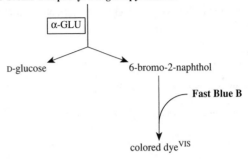

### Staining Solution[2]

A. 50 m*M* Potassium phosphate buffer, pH 6.9
   1 m*M* EDTA
B. 50 m*M* Potassium phosphate buffer, pH 6.9                       10 ml
   6-Bromo-2-naphthyl α-D-glucopyranoside                            5 mg
      (dissolved in minimal volume of dimethyl
      sulfoxide)
C. 50 m*M* Potassium phosphate buffer, pH 6.9                        2 ml
   Fast Blue B                                                      20 mg

### Procedure

Soak electrophorized gel in solution A for 5 min and place in solution B at room temperature for 15 min. Then add solution C. Colored bands of α-GLU activity appear after 3 to 5 min. Fix stained gel in 8% acetic acid–25% ethanol.

### OTHER METHODS

A. An immunoblotting procedure (for details see Part II) based on the utility of monoclonal antibodies specific to the human enzyme[3] can be used for immunohistochemical visualization of the enzyme protein on electrophoretic gels. This procedure is unsuitable for routine laboratory use but may be of great value in special analyses of α-GLU.

B. The product glucose can be detected using linking enzymes hexokinase and NAD(P)-dependent glucose-6-phosphate dehydrogenase in couple with the PMS/MTT system (see 2.7.1.1 — HK).

### GENERAL NOTES

Sucrose α-glucosidase (see 3.2.1.48 — SG) activity bands also can be detected by all the methods described above. In contrast to α-GLU, this enzyme hydrolyzes isomaltose. This difference may be used to differentiate SG and α-GLU bands.

### REFERENCES

1. Harris, H. and Hopkinson, D. A., *Handbook of Enzyme Electrophoresis in Human Genetics*, North-Holland, Amsterdam (Loose leaf with supplements in 1977 and 1978), 1976.
2. Spielman, L. L. and Mowshowitz, D. B., A specific stain for α-glucosidases in isoelectric focusing gels, *Anal. Biochem.*, 120, 66, 1982.
3. Hilkens, J., Tager, J. M., Buijs, F., Brouwer-Kelder, B., Van Thienen, G. M., Tegelaers, F. P., and Hilgers, J., Monoclonal antibodies against human acid α-glucosidase, *Biochim. Biophys. Acta*, 678, 7, 1981.

225

OTHER NAMES      Gentiobiase, cellobiase, amygdalase

REACTION         Hydrolysis of terminal, nonreducing β-D-glucose residues with release of β-D-glucose

ENZYME SOURCE    Bacteria, fungi, red algae, plants, invertebrates, vertebrates

## METHOD 1

### Visualization Scheme

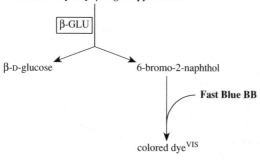

**6-bromo-2-naphthyl β-D-glucopyranoside**

β-GLU

β-D-glucose        6-bromo-2-naphthol

— Fast Blue BB

colored dye[VIS]

### Staining Solution[1]

| | |
|---|---|
| 50 m$M$ Phosphate buffer, pH 6.5 | 70 ml |
| Polyvinylpyrrolidone | 1.6 g |
| 6-Bromo-2-naphthyl β-D-glucopyranoside (dissolved in 10 ml of acetone) | 50 mg |
| Fast Blue BB | 100 mg |

### Procedure

Incubate the gel in staining solution in the dark at 37°C for 2 to 3 h or until blue bands appear. Rinse gel with water and fix in 50% glycerol.

## METHOD 2

### Visualization Scheme

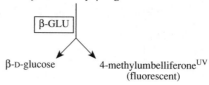

**4-methylumbelliferyl β-D-glucoside**

β-GLU

β-D-glucose        4-methylumbelliferone[UV]
(fluorescent)

### Staining Solution*

| | |
|---|---|
| 0.1 $M$ Phosphate buffer, pH 5.0 | 20 ml |
| 4-Methylumbelliferyl β-D-glucoside | 10 mg |

### Procedure

Lay a piece of filter paper saturated with the staining solution on top of the gel. Incubate the gel for 30 to 60 min at 37°C. Remove filter paper and view the gel under long-wave UV light. Areas of β-GLU activity are seen as fluorescent bands. Record the zymogram or photograph using a yellow filter.

*Notes:* Fluorescence of β-GLU activity bands can be enhanced by spraying the gel with ammonia.

## OTHER METHODS

A. Two linked reactions catalyzed by auxiliary enzymes glucose oxidase and peroxidase, coupled with redox dyes aminoethyl carbazole or *o*-dianisidine hydrochloride, can be used to detect the product β-D-glucose (e.g., see 3.2.1.20 — α-GLU, Method 2).

B. The product D-glucose also can be detected using auxiliary enzyme glucose oxidase in couple with the PMS/NBT system (e.g., see 3.2.1.10 — OG, Method 2).

## REFERENCE

1. Stuber, C. W., Goodman, M. M., and Johnson, F. M., Genetic control and racial variation of β-glucosidase isozymes in maize (*Zea mays* L.), *Biochem. Genet.*, 15, 383, 1977.

---

\*  Adapted from 3.2.1.20—α-GLU, Method 1.

OTHER NAMES     Melibiase

REACTION        Hydrolysis of terminal, nonreducing α-D-ga-
                lactose residues in α-D-galactosides, including
                galactose oligosaccharides, galactomannans,
                and galactolipids

ENZYME SOURCE   Bacteria, fungi, plants, vertebrates

## METHOD 1

### Visualization Scheme

**4-methylumbelliferyl α-D-galactoside**

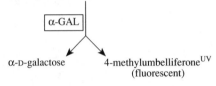

α-D-galactose        4-methylumbelliferone[UV]
                     (fluorescent)

### Staining Solution ¹ (modified)

| | |
|---|---|
| 0.2 *M* Phosphate–citrate buffer, pH 5.0 | 10 ml |
| 4-Methylumbelliferyl α-D-galactoside | 10 mg |

### Procedure

Lay a piece of filter paper saturated with the staining solution on
top of the gel. Incubate the gel for 30 to 60 min at 37°C. Remove
filter paper and view the gel under long-wave UV light.

*Notes:*  Spray the gel with ammonia to enhance fluorescence.

## METHOD 2

### Visualization Scheme

**α-naphthyl α-D-galactopyranoside**

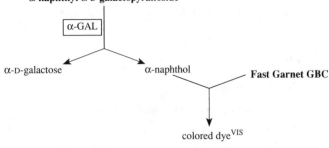

α-D-galactose        α-naphthol        **Fast Garnet GBC**

colored dye[VIS]

### Staining Solution²

| | |
|---|---|
| 0.1 *M* Sodium acetate buffer, pH 5.0 | 100 ml |
| 1% α-Naphthyl α-D-galactopyranoside (in acetone) | 3 ml |
| Fast Garnet GBC | 100 mg |

### Procedure

Incubate the gel in staining solution in the dark at 30°C until
colored bands appear. Rinse gel with water and fix in 50% glycerol.

*Notes:*  Fast Blue B or Fast Blue RR can be used instead of Fast Garnet
GBC. 6-Bromo-2-naphthyl α-D-galactopyranoside may also be used as substrate.

## GENERAL NOTES

Phosphate, citrate, acetate, and phosphate-citrate buffers (pH 4.0
to 7.0) are usually used to detect α-GAL from different sources.
    The enzyme appears to be inactivated by storage in liquid
nitrogen.[3]

## REFERENCES

1. Beutler, E. and Kuhl, W., Biochemical and electrophoretic studies
   of α-galactosidase in normal man, in patients with Fabry's disease
   and in *Equidae, Am. J. Hum. Genet.*, 24, 237, 1972.
2. Vallejos, C. E., Enzyme activity staining, in *Isozymes in Plant
   Genetics and Breeding, Part A*, Tanksley, S. D. and Orton, T. J.,
   Eds., Elsevier, Amsterdam, 1983, 469.
3. Morizot, D. C. and Schmidt, M. E., Starch gel electrophoresis and
   histochemical visualization of proteins, in *Electrophoretic and
   Isoelectric Focusing Techniques in Fisheries Management*,
   Whitmore, D. H., Ed., CRC Press, Boca Raton, FL, 1990, 23.

OTHER NAMES    Lactase

REACTION    Hydrolysis of terminal nonreducing β-D-galactose residues in β-D-galactosides

ENZYME SOURCE    Bacteria, fungi, plants, invertebrates, vertebrates

## METHOD 1

### Visualization Scheme

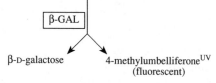

**4-methylumbelliferyl β-D-galactoside**

β-GAL

β-D-galactose    4-methylumbelliferone[UV] (fluorescent)

### Staining Solution[1]

A.  0.5 *M* Acetate buffer, pH 5.0
    3.5 mg/ml 4-Methylumbelliferyl β-D-galactoside
B.  1 *M* Carbonate–bicarbonate buffer, pH 10.0

### Procedure

Apply the staining solution A to the gel surface with filter paper and incubate the gel at 37°C for 30 min. Fluorescent bands of β-GAL activity are seen under long-wave UV light after spraying gel with solution B. Record the zymogram or photograph using a yellow filter.

## METHOD 2

### Visualization Scheme

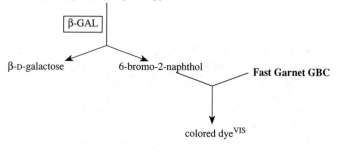

**6-bromo-2-naphthyl β-D-galactopyranoside**

β-GAL

β-D-galactose    6-bromo-2-naphthol    **Fast Garnet GBC**

colored dye[VIS]

### Staining Solution[2]

0.1 *M* Acetate buffer, pH 3.6
1 mg/ml 6-Bromo-2-naphthyl β-D-galactopyranoside
1 mg/ml Fast Garnet GBC

### Procedure

Incubate the gel in staining solution in the dark at 37°C until colored bands appear. Wash gel with water and fix in 50% glycerol.

## METHOD 3

### Visualization Scheme

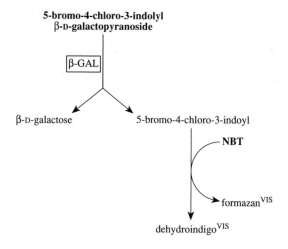

**5-bromo-4-chloro-3-indolyl β-D-galactopyranoside**

β-GAL

β-D-galactose    5-bromo-4-chloro-3-indoyl

NBT

formazan[VIS]

dehydroindigo[VIS]

### Staining Solution[3]

| | |
|---|---:|
| 0.1 *M* Sodium phosphate buffer, pH 7.5 | 95 ml |
| 1% 5-Bromo-4-chloro-3-indolyl β-D-galactopyranoside (in dimethylformamide) | 5 ml |
| NBT | 10 mg |

### Procedure

Incubate the gel in staining solution in the dark at 37°C until dark blue bands appear. Wash gel with water and fix in 25% ethanol.

# METHOD 4

## Visualization Scheme

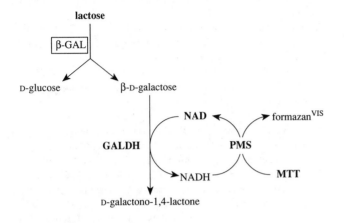

## Staining Solution[4]

A. 0.1 *M* Sodium phosphate buffer, pH 7.0 ... 25 ml
Lactose (glucose-free; Sigma) ... 2 g
NAD ... 25 mg
Galactose dehydrogenase (GALDH; Boehringer) ... 150 µg
MTT ... 5 mg
PMS ... 5 mg

B. 2% Agar solution (60°C) ... 25 ml

## Procedure

Mix A and B components of the staining solution and pour the mixture over the gel surface. Incubate the gel in the dark at 37°C until dark blue bands appear. Fix stained gel in 50% ethanol.

*Notes:* Lactase (EC 3.2.1.108) activity bands can also develop on β-GAL zymograms obtained by this method. This enzyme from intestinal mucosa is isolated as a complex that also catalyzes the reaction of glycosylceramidase (EC 3.2.1.62).

# METHOD 5

## Visualization Scheme

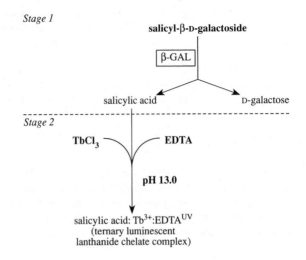

## Staining Solution[5] (adapted)

A. 0.1 *M* Formate buffer, pH 4.0 (see *Notes*)
0.5 m*M* Salicyl-β-D-galactoside (see *Notes*)
1 m*M* MgCl$_2$
1 m*M* Dithiothreitol

B. 0.01 *M* HCl
5 m*M* TbCl$_3$
5 m*M* EDTA (tetrasodium salt)

C. 2.5 *M* Tris, pH 13.0

## Procedure

Apply the substrate solution A to the gel surface with a filter paper or 1% agarose overlay. Incubate the gel at 37°C for 30 min. Remove the first application and apply the next one containing developing solution (one part of solution B, one part of solution C, and three parts of deionized water). Observe luminescent β-GAL bands under 300- to 340-nm UV light and record the zymogram or photograph on Polaroid instant film with a TRP 100 time-resolved photographic camera (Kronem System, Inc., Mississauga, Canada), using a filter combination providing excitation in the range 320 to 400 nm and measuring emission more than 515 nm with a measurement time delay and gate of 440 µsec and 4.1 msec, respectively.

*Notes:* The substrate, salicyl-β-D-galactoside, is not yet commercially available. However, it can be synthesized under laboratory conditions according to the following procedure.[5] To a stirred solution of methyl salicylate (0.304 g in 5 ml of absolute ethanol) add 0.96 ml of 15% sodium ethoxide solution in ethanol under argon. Remove volatile components from the formed precipitate (methyl salicylate sodium salt) on a rotary evaporator. Dry the precipitate by addition of distilled pyridine followed by vacuum evaporation. Add 10 ml of 2 m*M* acetobromo-α-D-galactose in dimethylformamide to 10 m*M* of 2 m*M* methyl salicylate sodium salt in dry distilled dimethylformamide with stirring under argon. Allow the reaction to proceed (with stirring under argon) at room temperature for 9 d. Filter the resulting mixture through a sintered glass funnel and concentrate the filtrate on a rotary evaporator to produce a solid residue. Dissolve the product in dichloromethane–methanol and then chromatograph on a flash silica gel column with 98%

dichloromethane–2% triethylamine as eluting solvent. Pool fractions containing the product with $R_f = 0.60$ and concentrate to produce about 500 mg of salicyl tetra-*O*-acetyl-β-D-galactoside methyl ester, which should then be recrystallized from ethyl acetate–toluene (containing a small amount of hexane) to produce 83 mg of pure product. Dissolve pure salicyl tetra-*O*-acetyl-β-D-galactoside methyl ester (4.82 mg) by stirring in 2 ml 0.1 *M* KOH in methanol with heating in an oil bath at 70°C for 3 h to prepare a stock solution of 5 m*M* salicyl-β-D-galactoside potassium salt.

This substrate is unsuitable for the enzyme with pH-optimum near 7.0. This is probably due to ionization of the carboxyl group, which leaves a negative charge on the substrate molecule and reduces its suitability as a substrate.

## OTHER METHODS

An immunoblotting procedure (for details see Part II) based on the utility of monoclonal antibodies specific to the *E. coli* enzyme[6] can also be used for immunohistochemical visualization of the enzyme protein on electrophoretic gels. This method is unsuitable for routine laboratory use but may be useful in special analyses of β-GAL.

## GENERAL NOTES

The enzyme from some sources (e.g., mouse and human) also hydrolyzes β-D-fucosides and β-D-glucosides.[4,7]

## REFERENCES

1. Grzeschik, K. H., Grzeschik, A. M., Benoff, S., Romeo, G., Siniscalco, M., Van Someren, H., Meera Khan, P., Westerveld, A., and Bootsma, D., X-linkage of human α-galactosidase, *Nature New Biol.*, 240, 48, 1972.

2. Seyedyazdani, R., Floderus, Y., and Lundin, L.-G., Molecular nature of β-galactosidase from different tissues in two strains of the house mouse, *Biochem. Genet.*, 13, 733, 1975.

3. Shows, T. B., Scrafford-Wolff, L. R., Brown, J. A., and Masler, M. H., $G_{M1}$-Gangliosidosis: chromosome 3 assignment of the β-galactosidase-A gene ($βGAL_A$), *Somatic Cell Genet.*, 5, 147, 1979.

4. Ho, M. W., Povey, S., and Swallow, D., Lactase polymorphism in adult British natives: estimating allele frequences by enzyme assays in autopsy samples, *Am. J. Hum. Genet.*, 34, 650, 1982.

5. Evangelista, R. A., Pollak, A., and Templeton, E. F. G., Enzyme-amplified lanthanide luminescence for enzyme detection in bioanalytical assays, *Anal. Biochem.*, 197, 213, 1991.

6. Duncan, R. J., Hewitt, J., and Weston, P. D., Inactivation of β-galactosidase by monoclonal antibodies, *Biochem. J.*, 205, 219, 1982.

7. Seyedyazdani, R. and Lundin, L.-G., Genetic relationship between β-galactosidase and β-fucosidase in the mouse, *Biochem. Genet.*, 12, 441, 1974.

REACTION      Hydrolysis of terminal, nonreducing α-D-mannose residues in α-D-mannosides

ENZYME SOURCE    Fungi, plants, protozoa, invertebrates, vertebrates

## METHOD 1

### Visualization Scheme

**4-methylumbelliferyl α-D-mannopyranoside**

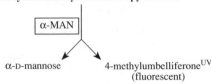

α-D-mannose      4-methylumbelliferone[UV]
(fluorescent)

### Staining Solution[1]

0.05 $M$ Citrate–phosphate buffer, pH 4.0 to 6.0
2 mg/ml 4-Methylumbelliferyl α-D-mannopyranoside

### Procedure

Lay a piece of filter paper saturated with staining solution on top of the gel and incubate at 37°C for 45 min. Remove filter-paper overlay and sprinkle 7.4 $N$ NH₄OH over the gel surface. View gel under long-wave UV light and note zones of enzyme activity as bands of fluorescence. Record the zymogram or photograph through a yellow filter.

## METHOD 2

### Visualization Scheme

***p*-nitrophenyl α-D-mannopyranoside**

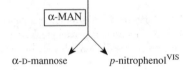

α-D-mannose      *p*-nitrophenol[VIS]

### Staining Solution[2]

25 m$M$ Citrate buffer, pH 4.5
5 m$M$ *p*-Nitrophenyl α-D-mannopyranoside

### Procedure

Preincubate electrophorized gel in 0.2 $M$ acetate buffer, pH 4.9, at room temperature for 30 min and then incubate at 37°C in a staining solution until yellow bands appear. Photograph zymogram using a 436.8-nm interference filter.

## METHOD 3

### Visualization Scheme

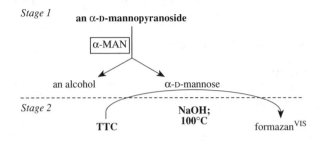

*Stage 1*     **an α-D-mannopyranoside**

α-MAN

an alcohol      α-D-mannose

*Stage 2*      TTC     **NaOH; 100°C**     formazan[VIS]

### Staining Solution[2]

A. 25 m$M$ Citrate buffer, pH 4.5
    5 m$M$ α-D-mannopyranoside (e.g., benzyl α-D-mannopyranoside, methyl α-D mannopyranoside, *p*-nitrophenyl α-D-mannopyranoside)
B. 0.1 $M$ Iodoacetamide
C. 0.1% 2,3,5-Triphenyltetrasolium chloride (TTC)
    0.5 $N$ NaOH

### Procedure

Incubate electrophorized PAG in solution A at room temperature for 30 to 45 min. Rinse gel with water and place in solution B for 5 min. Again, rinse gel with water thoroughly and place in solution C heated in a boiling water bath. Violet bands on a pink background appear after 1 to 2 min. Wash stained gel with water and fix in 7.5% acetic acid.

*Notes:* Treatment of the gel with iodoacetamide is needed to prevent nonspecific reduction of TTC by some nonenzymatic proteins and PAG itself.

### REFERENCES

1. Poenaru, L. and Dreyfus. J.-C., Electrophoretic heterogeneity of human α-mannosidase, *Biochim. Biophys. Acta*, 303, 171, 1973.
2. Gabriel, O. and Wang. S.-F., Determination of enzymatic activity in polyacrylamide gels. I. Enzymes catalyzing the conversion of nonreducing substrates to reducing products, *Anal. Biochem.*, 27, 545, 1969.

OTHER NAMES    Invertase, saccharase, β-h-fructosidase

REACTION    Hydrolysis of terminal nonreducing β-D-fructofuranoside residues in β-D-fructofuranosides

ENZYME SOURCE   Bacteria, fungi, plants

## METHOD 1

### Visualization Scheme

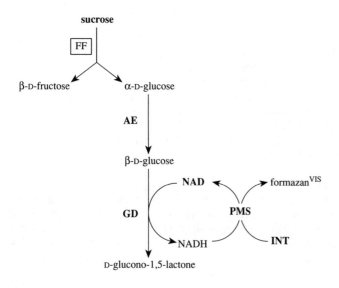

### Staining Solution[1]

    0.12 *M* Sodium phosphate buffer, pH 7.6
    1.3 m*M* NAD
    1.2 m*M* Sucrose
    0.4 m*M* PMS
    0.6 m*M* Iodonitrotetrazolium chloride (INT)
    0.15 *M* NaCl
    2 U/ml Aldose 1-epimerase (AE)
    5 U/ml Glucose dehydrogenase (GD)

### Procedure

Incubate the gel in staining solution in the dark at 37°C until dark brownish-red bands appear. Wash stained gel with water and fix in 50% ethanol.

*Notes:*   Aldose 1-epimerase may be omitted from the staining solution because conversion of α-D-glucose into β-D-glucose can occur as a result of spontaneous mutarotation, although more slowly.

## METHOD 2

### Visualization Scheme

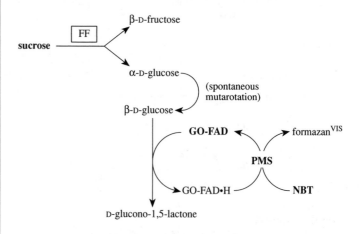

### Staining Solution[2]

    85 m*M* Citrate–phosphate buffer, pH 6.0
    100 m*M* Sucrose
    0.33 mg/ml PMS
    0.33 mg/ml NBT
    10 U/ml Glucose oxidase (GO)

### Procedure

Incubate the gel in the dark at 37°C in staining solution filtered through glass wool until dark blue bands appear. Wash stained gel with water and fix in 50% ethanol.

*Notes:*   Staining solution should be prepared, filtered, and used in complete darkness.

    The main problem concerning the use of glucose oxidase is the presence of varying amounts of FF in most commercial preparations of this enzyme. Only glucose oxidase preparations free of FF activity should be used.

## METHOD 3

### Visualization Scheme

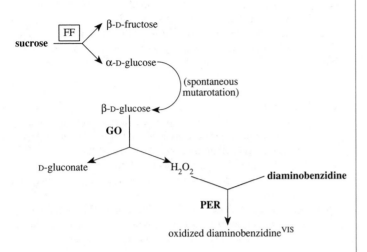

### Staining Solution[2]

85 mM Citrate–phosphate buffer, pH 6.5
100 mM Sucrose
10 U/ml Glucose oxidase (GO)
10 U/ml Peroxidase (PER)
0.30 mg/ml 3,3′-Diaminobenzidine

### Procedure

Incubate the gel at 37°C in staining solution filtered through glass wool until colored bands appear. Wash stained gel with water and fix in 5% acetic acid.

*Notes:* Only glucose oxidase preparations free of FF activity should be used.

Because diaminobenzidine is a carcinogen, its solutions should be handled with extreme care.

## METHOD 4

### Visualization Scheme

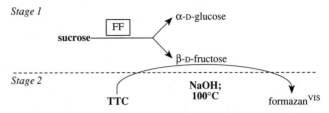

### Staining Solution[3]

A. 0.2 M Acetate buffer, pH 5.0     100 ml
    Sucrose     860 mg
B. 2,3,5-Triphenyltetrazolium chloride (TTC)     100 mg
    1 N NaOH     100 ml

### Procedure

Incubate electrophorized PAG in solution A at 37°C for 30 min and place in solution B heated in a boiling water bath for 1 to 2 h. Red bands appear in gel areas containing β-D-fructose produced by FF. Fix stained gel in 7.5% acetic acid.

*Notes:* To prevent possible nonspecific reduction of triphenyltetrazolium by some proteins and by PAG itself, it is recommended that the gel be treated with 0.1 M iodoacetamide solution for 5 min before being stained in solution B.

## METHOD 5

### Visualization Scheme

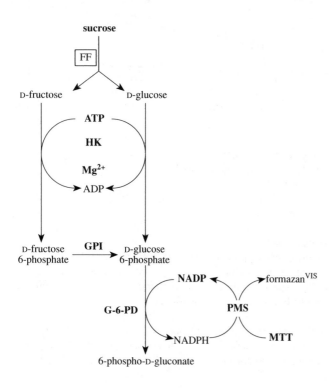

### Staining Solution*

| | |
|---|---|
| A. 0.1 $M$ Tris–HCl buffer, pH 7.0 | 20 ml |
| Sucrose | 300 mg |
| ATP | 40 mg |
| NADP | 20 mg |
| MTT | 10 mg |
| PMS | 1 mg |
| MgCl$_2$·6H$_2$O | 40 mg |
| Hexokinase (HK) | 100 units |
| Glucose-6-phosphate isomerase (GPI) | 80 units |
| Glucose-6-phosphate dehydrogenase (G-6-PD) | 50 units |
| B. 1.5% Agarose solution (55°C) | 20 ml |

### Procedure

Mix A and B components of the staining solution and pour the mixture over the gel surface. Incubate the gel in the dark at 37°C until dark blue bands appear. Fix stained gel in 50% ethanol.

*Notes:* The formazan formation may be doubled by addition of 6-phosphogluconate dehydrogenase to the staining solution. This modified method is supposed to be the most sensitive one among other methods described above.

## GENERAL NOTES

Bands of sucrose α-glucosidase (see 3.2.1.48 — SG) activity can also develop on FF zymograms obtained using the methods described above. This enzyme isolated from intestinal mucosa also displays activity towards isomaltose, while FF does not. This difference in substrate specificity may be used to differentiate the bands of activity caused by these two enzymes hydrolyzing sucrose.

## REFERENCES

1. Babczinski, P., Fractionation of yeast invertase isozymes and determination of enzymatic activity in sodium dodecyl sulfate–polyacrylamide gels, *Anal. Biochem.*, 105, 328, 1980.
2. Faye, L., A new enzymatic staining method for the detection of radish β-fructosidase in gel electrophoresis, *Anal. Biochem.*, 112, 90, 1981.
3. Mukasa, H., Shimamura, A., and Tsumori, H., Direct activity stains for glycosidase and glucosyltransferase after isoelectric focusing in horizontal polyacrylamide gel layers, *Anal. Biochem.*, 123, 276, 1982.

---

*   New; recommended for use.

REACTION      α, α-Trehalose + $H_2O$ = 2 D-glucose

ENZYME SOURCE   Fungi, plants, invertebrates, vertebrates

## METHOD 1

### Visualization Scheme

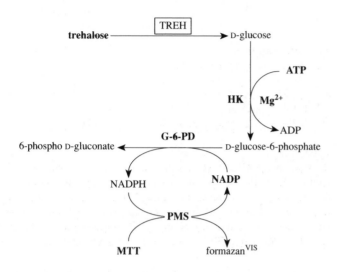

### Staining Solution[1]
A. 0.1 *M* Tris–HCl buffer, pH 7.0
    6 m*M* $MgCl_2$
    1 m*M* ATP
    20 m*M* α, α-Trehalose
    0.2 mg/ml MTT
    0.1 mg/ml PMS
    0.4 m*M* NADP
    1.4 U/ml Hexokinase (HK)
    1.2 U/ml Glucose-6-phosphate dehydrogenase (G-6-PD)
B. 1.5% Agarose solution (55°C)

### Procedure
Mix equal volumes of solutions A and B and pour the mixture over the gel surface. Incubate the gel in the dark at 37°C until dark blue bands appear. Fix stained gel in 50% ethanol.

## METHOD 2

### Visualization Scheme

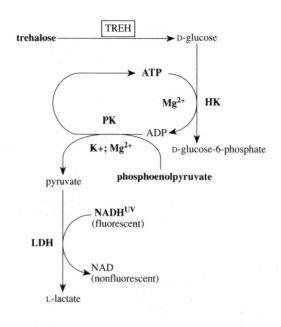

### Staining Solution*
A. 0.2 *M* Tris–HCl buffer, pH 7.0
    30 m*M* α, α-Trehalose
    10 m*M* $MgCl_2$
    0.1 *M* KCl
    1 m*M* ATP
    0.7 mg/ml NADH
    1.5 mg/ml Phosphoenolpyruvate (tricyclohexylammonium salt)
    4.5 U/ml Pyruvate kinase (PK)
    7.5 U/ml Lactate dehydrogenase (LDH)
B. 2% Agarose solution (55°C)

### Procedure
Mix equal volumes of solutions A and B and pour the mixture over the gel surface. Incubate the gel at 37°C and view under long-wave UV light. The areas of TREH activity are seen as dark bands on a fluorescent background. Record the zymogram or photograph using a yellow filter.

*Notes:* When a zymogram that is visible in daylight is required, counterstain the processed gel with MTT/PMS solution. This will result in the development of achromatic bands visible on a blue background of the gel. Fix the negative zymogram in 50% ethanol.

---

\*   New; recommended for use.

## METHOD 3

### Visualization Scheme

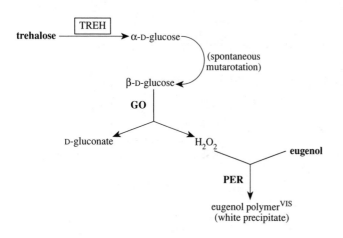

### Staining Solution[2]

50 m*M* Sodium citrate buffer, pH 5.5
6 U/ml Glucose oxidase (GO)
0.9 U/ml Peroxidase (PER)
0.8 m*M* Eugenol

### Procedure

Incubate electrophorized PAG in a staining solution at 37°C until white bands of eugenol polymer deposition appear. Place stained gel in 7.5% acetic acid in 5% methanol for clearing of the gel background. Although sufficient clearing occurs within 4 h (at 23°C), the gel may be exposed to acetic acid–methanol solution overnight to further reduce the background.

*Notes:* Chromogenic peroxidase substrates (e.g., diaminobenzidine, *o*-dianizidine, aminoethyl carbazole) may be used instead of eugenol (e.g., see 3.2.1.26 — FF, Method 3). The use of chromogenic peroxidase substrates will allow application of this method to unclear starch and acetate cellulose gels.

Because glucose oxidase used in this method as an auxiliary enzyme is a FAD-containing flavoprotein, PMS/MTT may be used in the stain instead of peroxidase and eugenol. This substitution will result in the appearance of dark blue bands of TREH activity on a white background of the gel (e.g., see 3.2.1.26 — FF, Method 2).

Aldose 1-epimerase (see 5.1.3.3 — AE) may be added to the staining solution to accelerate spontaneous mutarotation of α-D-glucose to β-D-glucose (e.g., see 3.2.1.26 — FF, Method 1).

Glucose dehydrogenase (EC 1.1.1.47) coupled with the PMS/MTT may be used instead of glucose oxidase to detect the product, β-D-glucose (e.g., see 3.2.1.26 — FF, Method 1).

## METHOD 4

### Visualization Scheme

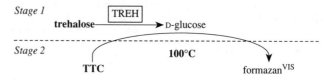

### Staining Solution[3]

A. 0.5 *M* Citrate buffer, pH 5.6
B. 30 m*M* Citrate buffer, pH 5.6
   0.1 *M* α, α-Trehalose
C. 0.1 *M* Iodoacetamide
D. 0.2% 2,3,5-Triphenyltetrasolium chloride (TTC)

### Procedure

Soak electrophorized PAG in solution A for 5 min and incubate in solution B at 30°C for 20 min. Then wash gel with distilled water and immerse in solution C for 5 min. Rinse gel again with water, immerse in solution D (in the dark) and place in a boiling water bath for 4 min. Violet bands appear in gel areas where TREH activity is localized. Fix stained gel in 7.5% acetic acid.

*Notes:* Treatment of the gel with iodoacetamide is needed to prevent nonspecific reduction of TTC by some nonenzymatic proteins and PAG itself.

### REFERENCES

1. Burton, R. S. and La Spada, A., Trehalase polymorphism in *Drosophila melanogaster*, *Biochem. Genet.*, 24, 715, 1986.
2. Killick, K. A. and Wang, L.-W., The localization of trehalase in polyacrylamide gels with eugenol by coupled enzyme assay, *Anal. Biochem.*, 106, 367, 1980.
3. Oliver, M. J., Huber, R. E., and Williamson, J. H., Genetic and biochemical aspects of trehalase from *Drosophila melanogaster*, *Biochem. Genet.*, 16, 927, 1978.

OTHER NAMES    *N*-Acetyl-β-glucosaminidase (recommended name), β-*N*-acetylhexosaminidase

REACTION    Hydrolysis of terminal, nonreducing *N*-acetyl-β-D-glucosamine residues in chitobiose and higher analogs and in glycoproteins

ENZYME SOURCE    Bacteria, plants, invertebrates, vertebrates

## METHOD 1

### Visualization Scheme

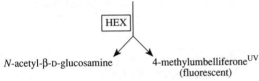

**4-methylumbelliferyl *N*-acetyl-β-D-glucosaminide**

*N*-acetyl-β-D-glucosamine    4-methylumbelliferone[UV] (fluorescent)

### Staining Solution[1]
  A. 1 *M* Sodium citrate buffer, pH 4.0 (or 4.5)
     3 m*M* 4-Methylumbelliferyl *N*-acetyl-β-D-glucosaminide
  B. 2% Agarose solution (60°C)

### Procedure
Mix equal volumes of A and B components of the staining solution and pour the mixture over the gel surface. Incubate the gel at 37°C and monitor under long-wave UV light. The areas of HEX activity appear as fluorescent bands. Spray the processed gel with ammonia to enhance fluorescence. Record the zymogram or photograph using a yellow filter.

*Notes:*    Staining solution (solution A) may be applied to the gel surface with a filter-paper overlay.

## METHOD 2

### Visualization Scheme

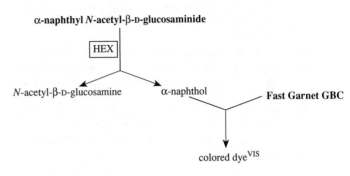

**α-naphthyl *N*-acetyl-β-D-glucosaminide**

*N*-acetyl-β-D-glucosamine    α-naphthol    Fast Garnet GBC

colored dye[VIS]

### Staining Solution[2]
  0.1 *M* Citrate buffer, pH 4.5 to 6.5
  1 mg/ml α-Naphthyl *N*-acetyl-β-D-glucosaminide (dissolved in the buffer by heating)
  1 mg/ml Fast Garnet GBC

### Procedure
Incubate the gel in staining solution in the dark at 37°C until pink bands appear. Wash stained gel with water and fix in 50% glycerol.

*Notes:*    Naphthol A*S*-BI 2-acetamido-2-deoxy-β-D-glucopyranoside (dissolved in ethanol) may be used in the staining solution instead of α-naphthyl *N*-acetyl-β-D-glucosaminide.

## METHOD 3

### Visualization Scheme

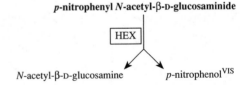

***p*-nitrophenyl *N*-acetyl-β-D-glucosaminide**

*N*-acetyl-β-D-glucosamine    *p*-nitrophenol[VIS]

### Staining Solution[3]
  25 m*M* Citrate buffer, pH 5.5
  5 m*M* *p*-Nitrophenyl *N*-acetyl-β-D-glucosaminide

### Procedure
Rinse electrophorized gel with water and soak in 0.2 *M* acetate buffer (pH 4.9) for 30 min. Incubate the gel in staining solution at room temperature until yellow bands appear. Photograph zymogram using a 436.8-nm interference filter.

## REFERENCES

1. Gilbert, F., Kucherlapati, R., Creagan, R. P., Murnane, M. J., Darlington, G. J., and Ruddle, F. H., Tay-Sachs' and Sandhoff's diseases: the assignment of genes for hexosaminidase A and B to individual human chromosomes, *Proc. Natl. Acad. Sci. U.S.A.*, 72, 263, 1975.
2. Swallow, D. M., Evans, L., Saha, N., and Harris, H., Characterization and tissue distribution of *N*-acetyl hexosaminidase C: suggestive evidence for a separate hexosaminidase locus, *Ann. Hum. Genet.*, 40, 55, 1976.
3. Gabriel, O. and Wang. S.-F., Determination of enzymatic activity in polyacrylamide gels. I. Enzymes catalyzing the conversation of nonreducing substrates to reducing products, *Anal. Biochem.*, 27, 545, 1969.

REACTION        β-D-Glucuronoside + H$_2$O = alcohol + D-glucuronate

ENZYME SOURCE  Bacteria, invertebrates, vertebrates

## METHOD 1

### Visualization Scheme

**4-methylumbelliferyl β-D-glucuronide**

β-GUS

D-glucuronate          4-methylumbelliferone[UV]
(fluorescent)

### Staining Solution[1]

| | |
|---|---|
| 0.5 *M* Tris–citrate buffer, pH 4.5 | 10 ml |
| 4-Methylumbelliferyl β-D-glucuronide | 2 mg |

### Procedure

Apply the staining solution to the gel surface with a filter paper and incubate at 37°C for about 1.5 h. The areas of β-GUS activity are seen under long-wave UV light as fluorescent bands. Record the zymogram or photograph using a yellow filter.

## METHOD 2

### Visualization Scheme

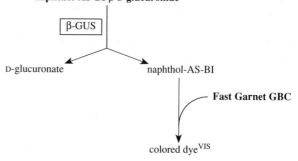

**naphthol-AS-BI β-D-glucuronide**

β-GUS

D-glucuronate          naphthol-AS-BI

Fast Garnet GBC

colored dye[VIS]

### Staining Solution[2]

| | |
|---|---|
| A. 0.2 *M* Sodium acetate–HCl buffer, pH 5.0 | 15 ml |
| Naphthol–A*S*–BI β-D-glucuronide | 10 mg |
| Fast Garnet GBC | 10 mg |
| B. 2% Agar solution (60°C) | 10 ml |

### Procedure

Mix A and B solutions and pour the mixture over the gel surface. Incubate the gel at 37°C in the dark until colored bands of sufficient intensity appear. Wash stained gel in water and fix in 7% acetic acid.

*Notes:* 6-Bromo-2-naphthyl β-D-glucuronide in couple with Fast Blue B can also be used to obtain the positive zymograms of β-GUS.

## METHOD 3

### Visualization Scheme

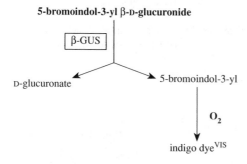

### Staining Solution[3]

| | |
|---|---|
| 0.4 M Acetate buffer, pH 4.5 | 100 ml |
| 5-Bromoindol-3-yl β-D-glucuronide | 45 mg |

### Procedure

Incubate the gel in staining solution at 37°C until dark blue bands appear. Fix stained gel in 10% trichloroacetic acid for 8 h and store in 7% acetic acid.

*Notes:* The indigogenic substrate 5-bromo-4-chloro-3-indolyl β-D-glucuronide may be used in couple with NBT (e.g., see 3.1.3.1 — ALP, Method 2). This combination will give simultaneous formation of blue dehydroindigo dye and blue formazan in gel areas where β-GUS activity is localized.

### REFERENCES

1. Harris, H. and Hopkinson, D. A., *Handbook of Enzyme Electrophoresis in Human Genetics*, North-Holland, Amsterdam (Loose leaf with supplements in 1977 and 1978), 1976.
2. Aebersold, P. B., Winans, G. A., Teel, D. J., Milner, G. B., and Utter, F. M., *Manual for Starch Gel Electrophoresis: A Method for the Detection of Genetic Variation*, NOAA Technical Report NMFS 61, U.S. Dept. of Commerce, National Marine Fisheries Service, Seattle, WA, 1987.
3. Yoshida, K., Iino, N., Koga, I., and Kato, K., Demonstration of β-glucuronidase in disc electrophoresis by means of 5-bromoindol-3-yl-β-D-glucuronide, *Anal. Biochem.*, 58, 77, 1974.

## 3.2.1.35 — Hyaluronoglucosaminidase; HYAL

| | |
|---|---|
| OTHER NAMES | Hyaluronidase |
| REACTION | Random hydrolysis of 1,4-linkages between *N*-acetyl-β-D-glucosamine and D-glucuronate residues in hyaluronate |
| ENZYME SOURCE | Bacteria, invertebrates, vertebrates |

## METHOD

### Visualization Scheme

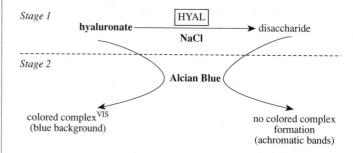

### Staining Solution[1]

A. 50 mM Phosphate–citrate buffer, pH 5.0
   1 mg/ml Hyaluronic acid
   0.15 M NaCl

B. 1% Alcian Blue in 7% acetic acid

### Procedure

Join electrophorized acetate-cellulose strip with a second acetate-cellulose strip soaked in solution A, avoiding the appearance of air bubbles between the strips. Place the strips between two glass plates and incubate at 37°C for 30 min. Dry the substrate-containing strip and stain in solution B for 1 min. Wash stained acetate-cellulose strip with water until achromatic bands appear on a blue background.

*Notes:* Hyaluronic acid may be incorporated directly into running PAG prior to polymerization. After incubation in an appropriate buffer solution, the gel may be negatively stained with "Stains-all".[2]

Two other enzymes possessing hyaluronidase activity can develop on HYAL zymograms obtained by this method. These are hyaluronoglucuronidase (EC 3.2.1.36) and hyaluronate lyase (EC 4.2.2.1). Chondroitinase (EC 4.2.2.4) activity bands can also be developed by this method when an alkaline buffer is used in the stain.

### REFERENCES

1. Herd, J. K., Tschida, J., and Motycka, L., The detection of hyaluronidase on electrophoresis membranes, *Anal. Biochem.*, 61, 133, 1974.
2. Fiszer-Szafarz, B., Hyaluronidase polymorphism detected by polyacrylamide gel electrophoresis. Application to hyaluronidases from bacteria, slime molds, bee, and snake venoms, bovine testes, rat liver lysosomes, and human serum, *Anal. Biochem.*, 143, 76, 1984.

## 3.2.1.37 — Xylan 1,4-β-xylosidase; XX

OTHER NAMES     Xilobiase, β-xylosidase, exo-1,4-β-xylosidase

REACTION     Hydrolysis of 1,4-β-D-xylans to remove successive D-xylose residues from the nonreducing termini

ENZYME SOURCE    Bacteria, fungi, plants

## METHOD

### Visualization Scheme

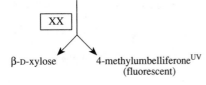

**4-methylumbelliferyl β-D-xyloside**

XX

β-D-xylose     4-methylumbelliferone[UV] (fluorescent)

### Staining Solution[1]
A. 50 mM Sodium acetate buffer, pH 5.5     100 ml
B. 50 mM Sodium acetate buffer, pH 5.5     10 ml
    1% 4-Methylumbelliferyl β-D-xyloside     0.3 ml
    (dissolved in 50% acetone)

### Procedure
Soak electrophorized gel in solution A for 30 to 45 min. Discard solution A and place a piece of filter paper saturated with solution B on top of the gel. Incubate the gel for 30 min to 2 h and view under long-wave UV light for fluorescent bands. Record the zymogram or photograph using a yellow filter. Resolution of the bands will be lost in a short period of time.

### REFERENCE
1. Vallejos, C. E., Enzyme activity staining, in *Isozymes in Plant Genetics and Breeding, Part A*, Tanskley, S. D. and Orton, T. J., Eds., Elsevier, Amsterdam, 1983, 469.

## 3.2.1.39 — Glucan Endo-1,3-β-glucosidase; LAM

OTHER NAMES     Laminarinase, endo-1,3-β-glucanase

REACTION     Hydrolysis of 1,3-β-D-glucosidic linkages in 1,3-β-D-glucans

ENZYME SOURCE    Bacteria, fungi, algae, plants, invertebrates, vertebrates (fishes)

## METHOD 1

### Visualization Scheme

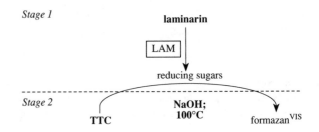

*Stage 1*           **laminarin**

LAM

reducing sugars

*Stage 2*       **NaOH; 100°C**

TTC           formazan[VIS]

### Staining Solution[1]
A. 0.05 M Potassium acetate buffer, pH 5.0     75 ml
B. Laminarin     1 g
    H₂O     75 ml
C. 1.0 M NaOH     100 ml
    2,3,5-Triphenyltetrazolium chloride (TTC)     150 mg

### Procedure
Wash electrophorized PAG with distilled water three times and preincubate in 0.05 M potassium acetate buffer, pH 5.0, for 5 min with slow shaking. Before mixing A and B components of the staining solution, dissolve laminarin in water by heating in a boiling water bath. Incubate the gel in A+B mixture at 40°C for 30 min. Wash gel three times with distilled water and place onto a glass tray containing solution C. Keep the tray in a boiling water bath until red bands appear (about 10 min).

*Notes:* To reduce the pink background, put the gel into 7.5% acetic acid as soon as the bands of interest clearly appear. To avoid breaking the gel, it should be placed in a mixture containing 3% glycerol, 40% methanol, 10% acetic acid, and 47% water (v/v). This mixture, however, destains the gel slowly.

    A control gel should be incubated under the same conditions, except that laminarin is omitted in order to identify nonspecifically stained bands.

## 3.2.1.39—Glucan Endo-1,3-β-glucosidase; LAM (continued)

### METHOD 2

#### Visualization Scheme

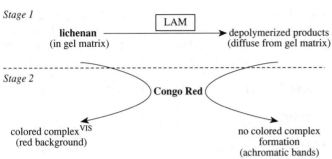

*Stage 1*

lichenan ──── [LAM] ──→ depolymerized products
(in gel matrix)                    (diffuse from gel matrix)

*Stage 2*

Congo Red

colored complex^VIS          no colored complex
(red background)                   formation
                                          (achromatic bands)

#### Staining Solution[2]
A. 0.1 *M* Succinate buffer, pH 5.8
   10 m*M* Dithiothreitol
B. 1 mg/ml Congo Red in 0.1 *M* Tris–HCl buffer, pH 8.0
C. 1 *M* NaCl

#### Procedure
Wash electrophorized SDS–PAG containing 0.1% lichenan (a mixed β-1,4- and β-1,3-linked glucan) five times for at least 30 min with cold solution A to remove detergent. Then submerge gel in 0.1 *M* succinate buffer, pH 5.8, and incubate for 30 to 60 min at 37 to 60°C. After incubation rinse gel in water and place in solution B for 10 min at room temperature. Destain gel in solution C for another 10 min. Achromatic or light yellowish activity bands are visible on a deep red background of the gel.

*Notes:* Barley β-glucan may also be used as LAM substrate instead of lichenan. Both mixed linkage β-glucans are suitable for the simultaneous detection of β-glucanases with specificities either for β-1,4- (see 3.2.1.4 — CEL), β-1,3-, 1,4- (see 3.2.1.6 — EG), or β-1,3- (3.2.1.39 — LAM) linkages. It is therefore advisable to perform parallel runs with substrate gels containing either carboxymethylcellulose (substrate for CEL) or laminarin (substrate for LAM).

#### REFERENCES
1. Pan, S.-Q., Ye, X.-S., and Kuć, J., Direct detection of β-1,3-glucanase isozymes on polyacrylamide electrophoresis and isoelectrofocusing gels, *Anal. Biochem.*, 182, 136, 1989.
2. Schwarz, W. H., Bronnenmeier, K., Gräbnitz, F., and Staudenbauer, W. L., Activity staining of cellulases in polyacrylamide gels containing mixed linkage β-glucans, *Anal. Biochem.*, 164, 72, 1987.

## 3.2.1.41 — α-Dextrin Endo-1,6-α-glucosidase; DEG

OTHER NAMES    Pullulanase, limit dextranase, debranching enzyme, amylopectin 6-glucanohydrolase

REACTION    Hydrolysis of 1,6-α-D-glucosidic linkages in pullulan, amylopectin, and glycogen and in the α- and β-amylase limit dextrins of amylopectin and glycogen

ENZYME SOURCE    Bacteria, plants

### METHOD 1

#### Visualization Scheme

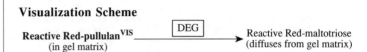

Reactive Red-pullulan^VIS ──── [DEG] ──→ Reactive Red-maltotriose
(in gel matrix)                                  (diffuses from gel matrix)

#### Staining Solution[1]
A. 0.2 *M* Acetate buffer, pH 5.0
   5% Reactive Red–pullulan
B. 4.2% Agar solution (60°C)

#### Procedure
Mix equal volumes of solutions A and B and pour the mixture over the surface of electrophorized gel soaked in 0.2 *M* acetate buffer, pH 5.0, for 10 to 20 min. Incubate the gel at 37°C in a humid chamber until light bands appear on a red background. Fix stained gel in 3% acetic acid.

*Notes:* Reactive Red–pullulan is obtained with the dyestuff covalently bound to pullulan.[2]

## 3.2.1.41 — α-Dextrin Endo-1,6-α-glucosidase; DEG (continued)

### METHOD 2

#### Visualization Scheme

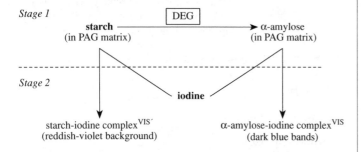

*Stage 1*

starch → DEG → α-amylose
(in PAG matrix)       (in PAG matrix)

*Stage 2*

iodine

starch-iodine complex[VIS']      α-amylose-iodine complex[VIS]
(reddish-violet background)     (dark blue bands)

#### Staining Solution[3]
A. 0.1 *M* Sodium citrate buffer, pH 5.0
B. 14 m*M* Potassium iodide
   10 m*M* Iodine

#### Procedure

Incubate electrophorized PAG containing 0.1% starch in solution A for 5 h and place in solution B. Dark blue bands of DEG activity appear on a reddish-violet background. Record or photograph the zymogram.

*Notes:* Development of DEG activity bands is caused by hydrolysis of the α-1,6-branch linkages of the starch by the enzyme action, resulting in a greater capacity of the unit chain to adopt the helical configuration for iodine complex formation.

    Amylase activity bands (light bands) also develop on DEG zymograms obtained by this method.

    Bands of DEG activity can also develop on phosphorylase zymograms obtained using the backward reaction of the enzyme (see 2.4.1.1 — PHOS, Method 1).

### REFERENCES

1. Yang, S.-S. and Coleman, R. D., Detection of pullulanase in polyacrylamide gels using pullulan-reactive red agar plates, *Anal. Biochem.*, 160, 480, 1987.
2. Rinderknecht, M., Wilding, P., and Haverback, B. J., A new method for the determination of α-amylase, *Experientia*, 23, 805, 1967.
3. Gerbrandy, S. J. and Verleur, J. D., Phosphorylase isoenzymes: localization and occurrence in different plant organs in relation to starch metabolism, *Phytochemistry*, 10, 261, 1971.

## 3.2.1.48 — Sucrose α-Glucosidase; SG

**OTHER NAMES**    Sucrose α-glucohydrolase, sucrase, sucrase isomaltase

**REACTION**    Hydrolysis of sucrose and maltose by an α-D-glucosidase–type reaction; also hydrolyzes isomaltose by an oligo-1,6-glucosidase–type reaction (see 3.2.1.10 — OG)

**ENZYME SOURCE**   Invertebrates, vertebrates

### METHOD 1

#### Visualization Scheme

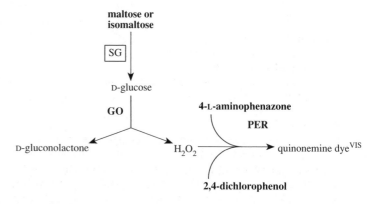

maltose or isomaltose

SG

D-glucose

GO

D-gluconolactone     $H_2O_2$

4-L-aminophenazone
PER
2,4-dichlorophenol

→ quinonemine dye[VIS]

#### Staining Solution[1]
A. 2 *M* Sodium phosphate buffer, pH 6.0
   25 m*M* Maltose or isomaltose
B. 2,4-Dichlorophenol (sulfonated)
C. 10 U/ml Glucose oxidase (GO)
   10 U/ml Peroxidase (PER)
   0.5 mg/ml 4-L-Aminophenazone
D. 1.6% Agarose solution (60°C)

#### Procedure
Mix 0.75 ml A with 0.5 ml B, 2.5 ml C, and 6.25 ml D. Pour the resulting mixture over the gel surface and incubate at 37°C until colored bands appear. Record or photograph zymogram because the stain is not permanent.

*Notes:* Preparations of glucose oxidase and peroxidase should be catalase-free. If they are not, $NaN_3$ should be included in the staining solution to inhibit catalase activity.

    Other methods may be used to detect hydrogen peroxide via peroxidase (see 1.11.1.7 — PER).

## METHOD 2

### Visualization Scheme

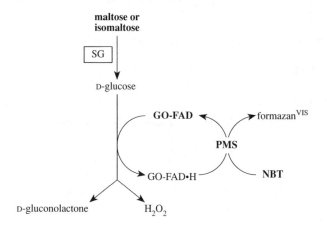

### Staining Solution[1]

A.  2 *M* Sodium phosphate buffer, pH 6.0             1 ml
    $H_2O$                                                   4 ml
    PMS                                             2 mg
    NBT                                           5 mg
    Maltose or isomaltose                 43 mg
    Glucose oxidase (GO)            100 units
B.  2% Agarose solution (60°C)          5 ml

### Procedure

Mix A and B solutions and pour the mixture over the gel surface. Incubate the gel at 37°C in the dark until dark blue bands appear. Fix stained gel in 50% ethanol or 5% acetic acid.

## OTHER METHODS

A. The product D-glucose can also be detected using linking enzymes hexokinase and NAD(P)-dependent glucose-6-phosphate dehydrogenase in couple with the PMS/MTT (e.g., see 2.7.1.1 — HK).

B. An immunoblotting procedure (for details see Part II) based on the utility of monoclonal antibodies specific to the rat enzyme[2] can be used for immunohistochemical visualization of the enzyme protein on electrophoretic gels.

## GENERAL NOTES

α-Glucosidase (see 3.2.1.20 — α-GLU) can also be detected by Methods 1 and 2 described above when maltose is used as substrate. However, in contrast to SG, α-GLU is not able to hydrolyze isomaltose. This difference may be used to differentiate SG and α-GLU activities.

When isomaltose is used as substrate, the oligo-1,6-glucosidase (see 3.2.1.10 — OG) activity bands can also develop on SG zymograms. In contrast to SG, OG is not able to hydrolyze maltose. This distinction may be used to discriminate between these enzymes.

## REFERENCES

1. Finlayson, S. D., Moore, P. A., Johnston, J. R., and Berry, D. R., Two staining methods for selectively detecting isomaltase and maltase activity in electrophoretic gels, *Anal. Biochem.*, 186, 233, 1990.
2. Hauri, H. P., Quaroni, A., and Isselbacher, K. J., Monoclonal antibodies to sucrase-isomaltase-probes for the study of postnatal development and biogenesis of the intestinal microvillus membrane, *Proc. Natl. Acad. Sci. U.S.A.*, 77, 6629, 1980.

## 3.2.1.51 — α-L-Fucosidase; α-FUC

REACTION       α-L-Fucoside + $H_2O$ = alcohol + L-fucoside

ENZYME SOURCE   Bacteria, plants, invertebrates, vertebrates

## METHOD

### Visualization Scheme

**4-methylumbelliferyl α-L-fucoside**

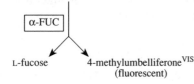

L-fucose      4-methylumbelliferone[VIS]
(fluorescent)

### Staining Solution[1]
A. 0.1 *M* Citrate–phosphate buffer, pH 4.8
    0.2 mg/ml 4-Methylumbelliferyl α-L-fucoside
B. 85 m*M* Glycine–carbonate buffer, pH 10.0

### Procedure

Apply solution A to the gel surface on filter-paper overlay. Incubate the gel in a humid chamber at 37°C for 30 to 60 min and then place in solution B. Fluorescent bands of α-FUC activity are seen under long-wave UV light. Record the zymogram or photograph using a yellow filter.

### REFERENCE

1. Turner, B. M., Beratis, N. G., Turner, V. S., and Hirschhorn, K., Isozyme of human α-L-fucosidase detectable by starch gel electrophoresis, *Clin. Chim. Acta*, 57, 29, 1974.

## 3.2.1.53 — β-*N*-Acetylgalactosaminidase; AGA

OTHER NAMES      β-Galactosaminidase

REACTION            Hydrolysis of terminal nonreducing *N*-acetyl-D-galactosamine residues in *N*-acetyl-β-D-galactosaminides

ENZYME SOURCE   Invertebrates, vertebrates

## METHOD

### Visualization Scheme

**4-methylumbelliferyl *N*-acetyl-β-D-galactosaminide**

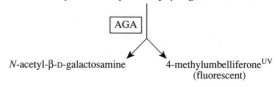

*N*-acetyl-β-D-galactosamine      4-methylumbelliferone[UV]
(fluorescent)

### Staining Solution[1]
A. 0.1 *M* Phosphate–citrate buffer, pH 9.5      15 ml
    4-Methylumbelliferyl *N*-acetyl-β-D-galactosaminide      5 mg
    (dissolved in 0.25 ml of dimethyl sulfoxide)
B. 2% Agar solution (60°C)      10 ml

### Procedure

Mix A and B solutions and pour the mixture over the gel surface. Incubate the gel at 37°C until fluorescent bands visible under long-wave UV light appear. Record the zymogram or photograph using a yellow filter.

### REFERENCE

1. Aebersold, P. B., Winans, G. A., Teel, D. J., Milner, G. B., and Utter, F. M., *Manual for Starch Gel Electrophoresis: A Method for the Detection of Genetic Variation*, NOAA Technical Report NMFS 61, U.S. Dept. of Commerce, National Marine Fisheries Service, Seattle, WA, 1987.

## 3.2.1.55 — α-L-Arabinofuranosidase; AF

**OTHER NAMES**    Arabinosidase, α-arabinosidase

**REACTION**    Hydrolysis of terminal nonreducing α-L-arabinofuranoside residues in α-L-arabinosides

**ENZYME SOURCE**  Bacteria, vertebrates

## METHOD

### Visualization Scheme

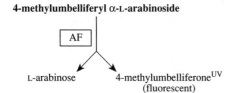

4-methylumbelliferyl α-L-arabinoside

AF

L-arabinose          4-methylumbelliferone[UV]
                     (fluorescent)

### Staining Solution[1]

| | |
|---|---|
| 0.1 *M* Phosphate-citrate buffer, pH 4.0 | 5 ml |
| 4-Methylumbelliferyl α-L-arabinoside | 10 mg |

### Procedure

Apply the staining solution to the gel surface on filter-paper overlay. Incubate the gel at 37°C for 30 to 60 min and then spray with ammonia solution. Fluorescent bands of AF activity are seen under long-wave UV light. Record the zymogram or photograph using a yellow filter.

### REFERENCE

1. Eitner, B. J., α-L-Arabinofuranosidase expression in the blue shark, *Prionace glauca, Isozyme Bull.*, 22, 49, 1989.

## 3.2.1.67 — Galacturan 1,4-α-galacturonidase; GG

**OTHER NAMES**    Poly(galacturonate) hydrolase, exopolygalacturonase

**REACTION**    $(1,4-\alpha\text{-D-Galacturonide})_n + H_2O = (1,4-\alpha\text{-D-galacturonide})_{n-1} + \text{D-galacturonate}$

**ENZYME SOURCE**  Fungi, plants

## METHOD

### Visualization Scheme

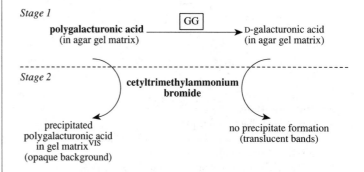

*Stage 1*

polygalacturonic acid ———— GG ————→ D-galacturonic acid
(in agar gel matrix)                    (in agar gel matrix)

*Stage 2*    cetyltrimethylammonium bromide

precipitated                              no precipitate formation
polygalacturonic acid                     (translucent bands)
in gel matrix[VIS]
(opaque background)

### Staining Solution[1]

A.  0.1 *M* Citrate buffer, pH 5.0
    1% Polygalacturonic acid
B.  3% Agarose solution (60°C)
C.  1% Water solution of cetyltrimethylammonium bromide

### Procedure

Mix solutions A and B and pour the mixture over the surface of electrophorized PAG. Incubate PAG at 37°C for 1 to 4 h. Place PAG and substrate-containing agarose plate in solution C. Translucent bands of GG activity appear on the opaque background of the PAG and agarose plate. The bands with high GG activity are more clearly visible on the agarose plate while the bands with low GG activity are more distinct on PAG.

*Notes:*  Two other enzymes with polygalacturonase activity can also be developed on GG zymograms obtained by this method. These are polygalacturonase (see 3.2.1.15 — PG) and polygalacturonate lyase (see 4.2.2.2 — PGL). The main difference in substrate specificity between enzymes with polygalacturonase activity is the ability of PG to hydrolyze pectin; PGL and GG do not act on this polysaccharide. Moreover, PGL displays maximal activity in alkaline conditions while both GG and PG displays optimal activity in acid conditions. These differences can be used to identify GG activity bands.

### REFERENCE

1. Bertheau, Y., Madgidi-Hervan, E., Kotoujansky, A., Nguyen-The, C., Andro, T., and Coleno, A., Detection of depolymerase isoenzymes after electrophoresis or electrofocusing, or in titration curves, *Anal. Biochem.*, 139, 383, 1984.

OTHER NAMES   Exo-cellobiohydrolase

REACTION   Hydrolysis of 1,4-β-D-glucosidic linkages in cellulose and cellotetraose releasing cellobiose from the nonreducing ends of the chain

ENZYME SOURCE   Bacteria, fungi

## METHOD

### Visualization Scheme

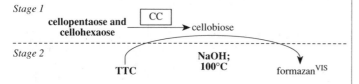

*Stage 1*
cellopentaose and cellohexaose → CC → cellobiose

*Stage 2*
TTC   NaOH; 100°C   formazan[VIS]

### Staining Solution[1]
A. 0.1 *M* Phosphate buffer, pH 5.0 to 6.5
   0.25% Cellopentaose and cellohexaose mixture
B. 0.1 *M* Iodoacetamide
C. 0.1% 2,3,5-Triphenyltetrazolium chloride (TTC)
   0.5 *M* NaOH

### Procedure
Wash electrophorized PAG for 15 min in two changes of 0.1 *M* phosphate buffer, pH 5.0 to 6.5, with gentle shaking. Rinse gel with distilled water and place in solution A for 15 min at 50°C. Rinse gel again with distilled water and place in solution B for 5 min. Then rinse gel again and place in a 2-l beaker containing solution C. Heat the solution over a gas burner with gentle agitation for several minutes until red bands are evident. The heating must be terminated before the appearance of a general red background. Rinse gel immediately with distilled water and soak in several changes of 7.5% acetic acid. The heating and initial storage of the stained gel must be carried out in the dark.

*Notes:*   The bands of cellulase activity (see 3.2.1.4 — CEL) can also develop on CC zymograms obtained by this method. However, CC activity bands do not develop on CEL negative zymograms obtained using carboxymethylcellulose as substrate and Congo Red staining of the poly-β-1,4-glucopyranoside (see 3.2.1.4 — CEL, Method 2, *Notes*). This difference can be used to differentiate the activity bands caused by CEL and CC. Specific detection of the product cellobiose can be performed using cellobiose-specific auxiliary enzymes (see below).

## OTHER METHODS

The product cellobiose can be detected via chromogenic reactions catalyzed by auxiliary enzymes cellobiose dehydrogenase (quinone, EC 1.1.5.1) and cellobiose dehydrogenase (acceptor, EC 1.1.99.18) coupled with the PMS/MTT and DCIP/MTT systems, respectively.

## REFERENCE
1. Bartley, T. D., Murphy-Holland, K., and Eveleigh, D. E., A method for the detection and differentiation of cellulase components in polyacrylamide gels, *Anal. Biochem.*, 140, 157, 1984.

OTHER NAMES    NAD(P) glycohydrolase

REACTION    NAD(P) + H$_2$O = nicotinamide + ADPribose(P)

ENZYME SOURCE    Bacteria, fungi, vertebrates

## METHOD 1

### Visualization Scheme

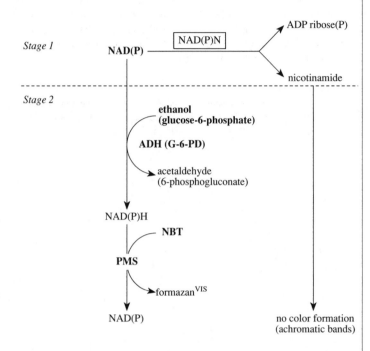

### Staining Solution[1]
A. 50 mM Phosphate buffer, pH 6.5
   0.65 mM NAD or NADP
B. 0.1 M Pyrophosphate buffer, pH 8.8          50 ml
   Ethanol                                      0.3 ml
   NBT                                          10 mg
   PMS                                          1 mg
   Alcohol dehydrogenase (ADH)                  25 units
C. 0.1 M Tris–HCl buffer, pH 8.0                50 ml
   Glucose-6-phosphate (disodium salt)          10 mg
   NBT                                          10 mg
   PMS                                          1 mg
   Glucose-6-phosphate dehydrogenase (G-6-PD)   25 units

### Procedure
Incubate electrophorized gel in solution A at 37°C for 1 to 2 h. Rinse gel with water and counterstain with solution B or C in the dark at 37°C to detect NAD or NADP, respectively. Achromatic bands visible on a blue background of the gel indicate areas occupied by NAD(P)N. Wash negatively stained gel with water and fix in 50% ethanol.

*Notes:* This method gives good results with cellulose acetate gel but can also be applied to PAG and starch gel.

## METHOD 2

### Visualization Scheme

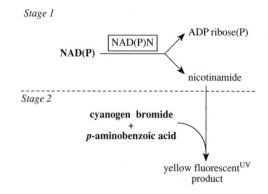

### Staining Solution[2]
A. 0.1 M Phosphate buffer, pH 6.5
   12 mM NAD or NADP
B. 2% (w/v) *p*-Aminobenzoic acid

### Procedure
Incubate electrophorized gel in solution A for 1 to 2 h at 37°C. Place preincubated gel in an atmosphere of cyanogen bromide in a sealed container and spray with solution B. Deep yellow bands, brightly fluorescent under long-wave UV light, indicate gel areas occupied by NAD(P)N activity. Record the zymogram immediately. The bands are visible for a few minutes and then fade.

*Notes:* This method is not as practical as Method 1. It generates very diffuse NAD(P)N activity bands.

### OTHER METHODS

NAD(P)N can also function as a transferase catalyzing the transfer of ADPribose(P) residues to nicotinamide, thus resulting in synthesis of NAD(P). The product NAD(P) can be detected using any NAD(P)-dependent dehydrogenase and MTT/PMS, as described in Method 1 above. This method will result in the development of positively stained bands of NAD(P) activity.

### REFERENCES
1. Ravazzolo, R., Bruzzone, G., Garrè, C., and Ajmar, F., Electrophoretic demonstration and initial characterization of human red cell NAD(P)⁺ase, *Biochem. Genet.*, 14, 877, 1976.
2. Flechner, I., Hirshorn, S., and Bekierkunst, A., A method of localization of soluble NAD–glycohydrolase from mycobacterial extracts after electrophoresis on cellulose acetate, *Life Sci.*, 7, 1327, 1968.

OTHER NAMES     Myrosinase, sinigrinase, sinigrase

REACTION     Thioglucoside + $H_2O$ = thiol + sugar

ENZYME SOURCE  Plants, vertebrates

## METHOD

### Visualization Scheme

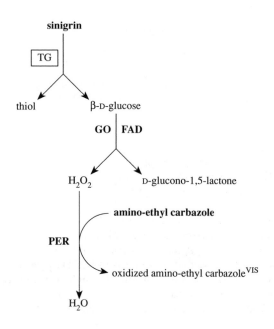

### Staining Solution[1]
A. 0.2 *M* Acetate buffer, pH 5.5       50 ml
   Sinigrin       0.1 g
   FAD       2 mg
   Glucose oxidase (GO)       30 units
   Peroxidase (PER)       5 mg
   3-Amino-9-ethyl carbazole (dissolved       10 mg
    in 2 ml of formamide)
B. 1.5% Agar solution (60°C)       50 ml

### Procedure
Mix A and B components of the staining solution and pour the mixture over the gel surface. Incubate the gel at 37°C in the dark until reddish-brown bands appear. Wash gel with water and fix in 7% acetic acid.

*Notes:* The PMS/NBT system can be used in couple with linking enzyme glucose oxidase to produce blue formazan in gel areas occupied by TG activity (e.g., see 3.2.1.26 — FF, Method 2). Other chromogenic substrates may be used for peroxidase in place of amino-ethyl carbazole (see 1.11.1.7 — PER).

Glucose oxidase used as a linking enzyme is a flavoprotein containing tightly bound FAD molecules. Thus, FAD may be omitted from the staining solution.

## OTHER METHODS

A. The linking enzyme β-D-glucose dehydrogenase in couple with the PMS/INT system may be used to detect the product β-D-glucose (e.g., see 3.2.1.26 — FF, Method 1).
B. The product β-D-glucose may be detected using two reactions catalyzed by auxiliary enzymes, hexokinase and glucose-6-phosphate dehydrogenase, coupled with the PMS/MTT system (e.g., see 3.2.1.28 — TREH, Method 1).

Both these methods, however, should be applied in two-step procedures because of differences in pH-optima between TG (maximal activity at acid conditions) and β-D-glucose dehydrogenase, hexokinase, and glucose-6-phosphate dehydrogenase (maximal activities at alkaline conditions).

### REFERENCE
1. Vaughan, J. G., Gordon, E., and Robinson, D., The identification of myrosinase after the electrophoresis of *Brassica* and *Sinapis* seed proteins, *Phytochemistry*, 7, 1345, 1968.

OTHER NAMES  *S*-Adenosylhomocysteine hydrolase

REACTION  *S*-Adenosyl-L-homocysteine + $H_2O$ = adenosine + L-homocysteine

ENZYME SOURCE  Vertebrates

## METHOD

### Visualization Scheme

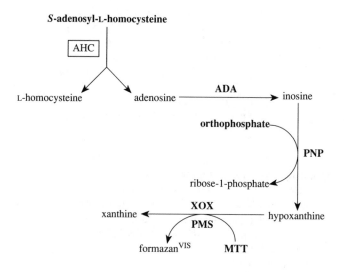

### Staining Solution[1] (adapted)
A. 0.1 *M* Phosphate buffer, pH 7.5
   0.476 µ*M* *S*-Adenosyl-L-homocysteine
   1.33 U/ml Adenosine deaminase (ADA)
   0.033 U/ml Purine-nucleoside phosphorylase (PNP)
   0.033 U/ml Xanthine oxidase (XOX)
   0.1 mg/ml MTT
   0.02 mg/ml PMS
B. 1.5% Agarose solution (55°C)

### Procedure
Mix equal volumes of A and B solutions and pour the mixture over the gel surface. Incubate the gel at 37°C in the dark until dark blue bands appear. Fix stained gel in 50% ethanol.

*Notes:*  This method demonstrates a general approach for visualizing enzymes releasing adenosine.[2]

## OTHER METHODS

A. An immunoblotting procedure (for details see Part II) based on the utility of monoclonal antibodies specific to the human enzyme[3] can be used for immunohistochemical visualization of the enzyme protein on electrophoretic gels. This procedure may be of great value in special analyses of AHC but is unsuitable for routine use in population genetics studies.

B. A method exists which is based on the strong absorbance at 296 nm of a ketimine ring, which is formed by the reaction of the enzymatic product L-homocysteine with 3-bromopyruvate.[4] The AHC activity bands can be detected by gel scanning at 296 nm (one-dimensional spectroscopy procedure). A special optic device constructed for two-dimensional spectroscopy of electrophoretic gels[5] can be used to photograph AHC zymograms obtained by this method.

## REFERENCES
1. Corbo, R. M., Scacchi, R., Palmarino, R., Lucarelli, P., Carapella-De Luca, E., and Businco, L., Detection of heterozygotes in three Italian families with adenosindeaminase deficiency and severe combined immunodeficiency, *Neonatalogica*, 2, 144, 1987.
2. Friedrich, C. A., Chakravarti, S., and Ferrell, R. E., A general method for visualizing enzymes releasing adenosine or adenosine-5′-monophosphate, *Biochem. Genet.*, 22, 389, 1984.
3. Hershfield, M. S. and Francke, U., The human genes for *S*-adenosylhomocysteine hydrolase and adenosine deaminase are syntenic on chromosome 20, *Science*, 216, 739, 1982.
4. Ricci, G., Caccuri, A. M., Lo Bello, M., Solinas, S. P., and Nardini, M., Ketimine rings: useful detectors of enzymatic activities in solution and on polyacrylamide gel, *Anal. Biochem.*, 165, 356, 1987.
5. Klebe, R. J., Mancuso, M. G., Brown, C. R., and Teng, L., Two-dimensional spectroscopy of electrophoretic gels, *Biochem. Genet.*, 19, 655, 1981.

OTHER NAMES    Cytosol aminopeptidase (recommended name), leucine arylaminopeptidase, naphthylamidase, arylamidase

REACTION    Aminoacyl-peptide + $H_2O$ = amino acid + peptide (see also General Notes)

ENZYME SOURCE    Bacteria, fungi, plants, protozoa, invertebrates, vertebrates

## METHOD 1

### Visualization Scheme

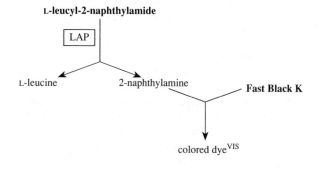

### Staining Solution[1]

| | |
|---|---|
| 0.1 $M$ Phosphate buffer, pH 5.8 | 100 ml |
| L-Leucyl-2-naphthylamide | 40 mg |
| Fast Black K | 60 mg |

### Procedure

Incubate the gel in filtered staining solution in the dark at 37°C until dark blue bands appear. Wash stained gel with water and fix in 7% acetic acid.

*Notes:*   The staining of the gel should be carried out with extreme caution because the product 2-naphthylamine is believed to be a carcinogen that causes bladder tumors.

## METHOD 2

### Visualization Scheme

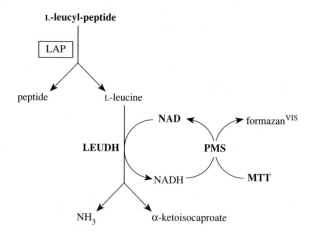

### Staining Solution[2] (adapted)

100 m$M$ Tricine–NaOH buffer, pH 8.3
2 mg/ml L-Leucyl–L-leucyl–L-leucine (or L-leucyl–L-valine, or L-leucyl–glycyl–glycine)
10 U/ml Leucine dehydrogenase (LEUDH)
2 mg/ml NAD
0.4 mg/ml MTT
0.04 mg/ml PMS

### Procedure

Apply the staining solution to gel dropwise. Incubate the gel in a humid chamber in the dark at 37°C until dark blue bands appear. Fix stained gel in 50% ethanol.

*Notes:*   This method is too expensive to be used in large-scale population assays.

Bacterial enzyme, leucine dehydrogenase, displays optimal activity in alkaline conditions while LAP from many sources is most active at pHs below 7.0. Thus, a two-step procedure of LAP detection by this method may sometimes be desirable.

### GENERAL NOTES

The enzyme has low specificity for the amino acid in the *N*-terminus. It does not act on lysyl and arginyl peptides, and it preferentially splits leucine.

### REFERENCES

1. Brewer, G. J., *An Introduction to Isozyme Techniques*, Academic Press, New York, 1970, 100.
2. Takamiya, S., Ohshima, T., Tanizawa, K., and Soda, K., A spectrophotometric method for the determination of aminopeptidase activity with leucine dehydrogenase, *Anal. Biochem.*, 130, 266, 1983.

## 3.4.11.2 — Alanine Aminopeptidase; AAP

OTHER NAMES      Microsomal aminopeptidase (recommended name), aminopeptidase M, aminopeptidase N, particle-bound aminopeptidase, amino-oligopeptidase

REACTION      Aminoacyl-peptide + $H_2O$ = amino acid + oligopeptide (see also *Notes*)

ENZYME SOURCE    Plants, invertebrates, vertebrates

### METHOD

#### Visualization Scheme

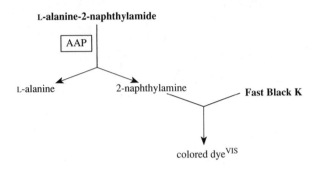

#### Staining Solution[1] (modified)

| | |
|---|---|
| 0.1 *M* Phosphate buffer, pH 5.8 | 100 ml |
| L-Alanine-2-naphthylamide hydrochloride | 30 mg |
| Fast Black K | 50 mg |

#### Procedure

Incubate the gel in filtered staining solution in the dark at 37°C until dark blue bands appear. Wash stained gel with water and fix in 7% acetic acid.

*Notes:* The staining of the gel should be carried out with extreme caution because the product 2-naphthylamine is believed to be a carcinogen that causes bladder tumors.

The enzyme splits α-amino acids (preferentially alanine, not proline) from peptides, amides, and 4-nitroanilides.

### OTHER METHODS

The product L-alanine can be detected using auxiliary NAD-dependent L-alanine dehydrogenase in couple with the PMS/MTT. A two-step procedure of detection should be used because of difference in pH-optima between AAP (about pH 7.0) and L-alanine dehydrogenase (about pH 10.0).

### REFERENCE

1. Okada, Y., Kawamura, K., Kawashima, A., and Mori, M., Hystochemistry and biology of leucine aminopeptidases, *Acta Histochem. Cytochem.*, 8, 265, 1975.

## 3.4.11.3 — Cystyl-aminopeptidase; CAP

OTHER NAMES      Oxytocinase

REACTION      Cystyl-peptide + $H_2O$ = amino acid + peptide

ENZYME SOURCE    Vertebrates

### METHOD 1

#### Visualization Scheme

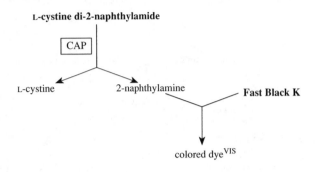

#### Staining Solution[1]

| | |
|---|---|
| 0.2 *M* Tris–maleate buffer, pH 6.0 | 90 ml |
| L-Cystine di-2-naphthylamide (dissolved in 10 ml of dimethylformamide) | 30 mg |
| Fast Black K | 30 mg |

#### Procedure

Incubate the gel in filtered staining solution in the dark until dark blue bands appear. Wash stained gel with water and fix in 7% acetic acid.

*Notes:* Because L-cystine di-2-naphthylamine is a potential carcinogen, solutions of this substrate should be handled with extreme caution.

## METHOD 2

### Visualization Scheme

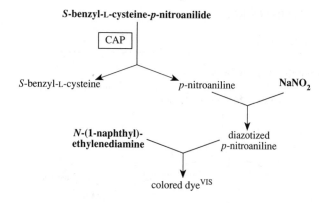

### Staining Solution[2]

A. S-Benzyl-L-cysteine-p-nitroanilide .......... 26 mg
   2-Methoxyethanol ........................... 20 ml
B. 0.1 M Citrate–phosphate buffer, pH 6.0 .... 50 ml
   NaNO₂ ...................................... 50 mg
   N-(1-Naphthyl)-ethylenediamine ............ 10 mg
   dihydrochloride
C. 12.5% Trichloroacetic acid ................ 100 ml

### Procedure

Prepare solution B before use. Use solution A stored at 4°C in a brown bottle. Mix 1 part of solution A with 3 parts of solution B. Incubate the gel in the resulting mixture at 37°C until pink bands appear. Wash gel 1 min with water to remove excass NaNO₂ and substrate. Place gel in solution C. The intensity of the pink bands become maximal 5 to 6 min after treatment with solution C and remains constant for 1 h.

*Notes:* A pink azo dye formed by this method does not precipitate in the gel matrix and thus stable zymograms may not be obtained. The enzymoblotting method was developed to overcome this problem.[3] This method is based on transferring proteins from an electrophoretic gel to a nitrocellulose (NC) membrane, and subsequent staining of membrane-bound enzymes using a procedure very similar to that described above. The enzymoblotting method of detection of enzymes producing *p*-nitroaniline allows one to obtain zymograms that are stable for 16 months when stored between two plastic sheets, sealed with adhesive tape, at –18°C.

## GENERAL NOTES

Both methods are specific for CAP, but Method 2 is more sensitive.

## REFERENCES

1. Kleiner, H. and Brouet-Yager, M., Separation of L-cystinyl-di-2-naphthylamide hydrolase ("oxytocinase") isoenzymes by acrylamide gel electrophoresis of human pregnancy, *Clin. Chim. Acta*, 40, 177, 1972.
2. Van Buul, T. and Van Oudheusden, A. P. M., A specific detection method for multiple forms of cystine aminopeptidase (oxytocinase-isoenzymes) after polyacrylamide gel electrophoresis, *J. Clin. Chem. Clin. Biochem.*, 16, 187, 1978.
3. Ohlsson, B. G., Weström, B. R., and Karlsson, B. W., Enzymoblotting: a method for localizing proteinases and their zymogens using *para*-nitroanilide substrates after agarose gel electrophoresis and transfer to nitrocellulose, *Anal. Biochem.*, 152, 239, 1986.

## 3.4.11.6 — Arginine Aminopeptidase; ARAP

REACTION          L-Arginyl-peptide + H₂O = L-arginine + peptide

ENZYME SOURCE  Plants, invertebrates, vertebrates

## METHOD

### Visualization Scheme

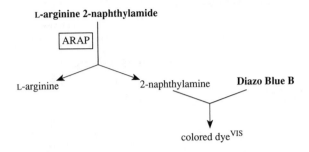

### Staining Solution[1]

| | |
|---|---|
| 0.1 $M$ Phosphate buffer, pH 6.6 | 100 ml |
| L-Arginine 2-naphthylamide | 100 mg |
| Diazo Blue B | 100 mg |

### Procedure

Incubate the gel in filtered staining solution in the dark at 37°C until colored bands appear. Rinse stained gel with water and fix in 5% acetic acid.

*Notes:*  L-Lysine-2-naphthylamide may be used in place of L-arginine-2-naphthylamide and Fast Black K salt in place of Diazo Blue B.

## OTHER METHODS

L-Arginine *p*-nitroanilide and L-Lysine *p*-nitroanilide can be used as ARAP substrates. Enzymatically generated *p*-nitroaniline, which is too faintly colored, can then be diazotized and coupled with *N*-(1-naphthyl)-ethylenediamine to produce a readily visible red azo dye. This method may prove more sensitive than that described above, especially when applied to the enzyme transferred from electrophoretic gel to nitrocellulose membrane (e.g., see 3.4.21.4 — T, Method 3).

## GENERAL NOTES

The enzyme is activated by Cl⁻ ions.

## REFERENCE

1. Okada, Y., Kawamura, K., Kawashima, A., and Mori, M., Hystochemistry and biology of leucine aminopeptidases, *Acta Histochem. Cytochem.*, 8, 265, 1975.

## 3.4.11 or 13... — Peptidases; PEP

OTHER NAMES    Dipeptidases, tripeptidases, aminopeptidases

REACTIONS      1. Dipeptide + H₂O = L-amino acids
                     2. Tripeptide + H₂O = L-amino acid + dipeptide

ENZYME SOURCE  Bacteria, algae, fungi, plants, protozoa, invertebrates, vertebrates

## METHOD 1

### Visualization Scheme

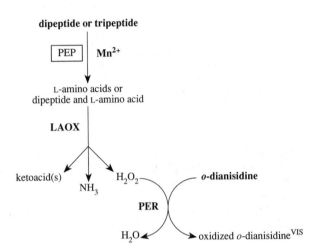

### Staining Solution[1]

| | |
|---|---|
| A. 0.2 $M$ Phosphate buffer, pH 7.5 | 25 ml |
|    *o*-Dianisidine dihydrochloride | 5 mg |
|    Snake venom L-amino acid oxidase (LAOX) | 2-3 units |
|    Peroxidase (PER) | 200 units |
|    0.1 $M$ MnCl₂ | 0.5 ml |
|    Dipeptide (or tripeptide); see *Notes* | 20 mg |
| B. 2% Agar solution (55°C) | 25 ml |

### Procedure

Mix A and B components of the staining solution and pour the mixture over the gel surface. Incubate the gel at 37°C until brown bands appear. Fix stained gel in 50% glycerol.

*Notes:*  *o*-Dianisidine dihydrochloride is a potential carcinogen. Solutions of this chromatogen should be handled with caution. An alternative chromatogen, 3-amino-9-ethyl carbazole, may be used in place of *o*-dianisidine dihydrochloride. However, *o*-dianisidine dihydrochloride usually gives better results. Do not use *o*-dianisidine (without diHCl) or benzidine as acceptors in the coupled peroxidase reaction as these are extremely carcinogenic.

    The staining system in Method 1 depends on the release from the peptide of an L-amino acid that is sensitive to the action of snake venom L-amino acid oxidase. In practice this requires the liberation from the peptide of the following L-amino acids: isoleucine, leucine, methionine, phenylalanine, triptophan, and tyrosine. For example, most of these L-amino acids are effectively oxidized by L-amino acid oxidases from the snakes *Agkistrodon caliginosus* and *Bothrops atrox*. Therefore, this method could be applied to detect peptidases which hydrolyze peptides consisting of the L-amino acids which may be oxidized by an L-amino acid oxidase used. A number of di- and tripeptides are available for use in PEP stains.[2,3] Crude snake venom (about 0.1 to 0.2 mg/ml) is usually used in the staining solution as the source of L-amino acid oxidase.

## METHOD 2

### Visualization Scheme

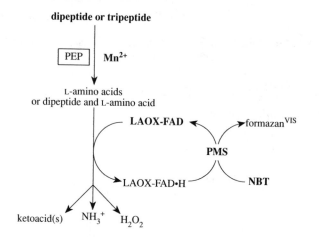

### Staining Solution[4]

| | |
|---|---|
| 50 m$M$ Tris–HCl buffer, pH 8.0 | 10 ml |
| L-Amino acid oxidase (from *Agkistrodon caliginosus*) | 2 units |
| Di- or tripeptide; see *Notes* | 10 mg |
| NBT | 5 mg |
| PMS | 1 mg |

### Procedure

Incubate the gel in staining solution in the dark at 37°C until dark blue bands appear. Wash stained gel with water and fix in 50% ethanol.

*Notes:* The use of NBT gives better results with acetate cellulose and starch gels. For PAGs the use of INT is preferable.

L-Amino acid oxidase from the snake *Agkistrodon caliginosus* is specific to L-phenylalanine, L-tryptophan, L-leucine, L-tyrosine, and L-isoleucine. Therefore, when LAOX from this source is used, the method could be applied to peptidases which hydrolyze peptides consisting of the L-amino acids mentioned above. Other preparations of L-amino acid oxidase with differing substrate specificity are commercially available.

## METHOD 3

### Visualization Scheme

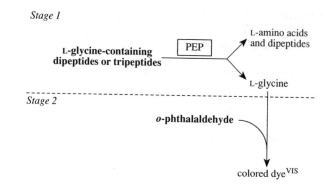

### Staining Solution[5]

A. 2 mg/ml Glycyl-L-leucine, pH 7.8 (adjusted with 0.1 $N$ NaOH)

B. 1:1 (w/v) *o*-Phthalaldehyde in 48% ethanol

### Procedure

Apply solution A to the gel surface on a filter-paper overlay. Incubate the gel at 37°C for 1 h. Remove filter paper and cover gel with solution B. Areas of PEP activity appear as dark green bands.

*Notes:* This method can be applied to detect only those peptidases which hydrolyze L-glycine–containing peptides and produce L-glycine.

## METHOD 4

### Visualization Scheme

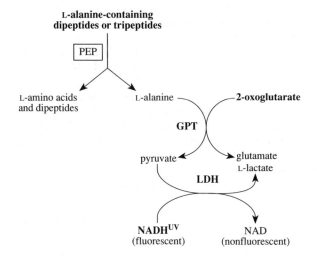

### Staining Solution[6]
| | |
|---|---|
| A. 0.1 $M$ Tris–HCl buffer, pH 7.5 | 25 ml |
| L-Alanine–containing di- or tripeptide (e.g., Ala–Gly, Ala–Ala–Ala) | 15 mg |
| Glutamic–pyruvic transaminase (GPT) | 3.2 units |
| Lactate dehydrogenase (LDH) | 27.5 units |
| NADH (disodium salt) | 10 mg |
| 2-Oxoglutarate (disodium salt) | 20 mg |
| B. 2% Agar solution (55°C) | 25 ml |

### Procedure

Mix A and B components of the staining solution and pour the mixture over the gel surface. Incubate the gel at 37°C and monitor under long-wave UV light. Areas of PEP activity are visible as dark (nonfluorescent) bands on the fluorescent background of the gel. Record the zymogram or photograph using a yellow filter.

*Notes:* This method can be applied to detect only those peptidases which hydrolyze L-alanine–containing peptides and produce L-alanine.

When a final zymogram that is visible in daylight is required, the processed gel can be counterstained with the PMS/MTT solution. This will result in the appearance of achromatic bands on a blue background.

The product L-alanine can be detected using auxiliary NAD-dependent L-alanine dehydrogenase in couple with the PMS/MTT system.

## REFERENCES

1. Lewis, W. H. P. and Harris, H., Human red cell peptidases, *Nature*, 215, 351, 1967.
2. Lewis, W. H. P. and Truslove, G. M., Electrophoretic heterogeneity of mouse erythrocyte peptidases, *Biochem. Genet.*, 3, 493, 1969.
3. Harris, H. and Hopkinson, D. A., *Handbook of Enzyme Electrophoresis in Human Genetics*, North-Holland, Amsterdam (Loose leaf with supplements in 1977 and 1978), 1976.
4. Sugiura, M., Ito, Y., Hirano, K., and Sawaki, S., Detection of dipeptidase and tripeptidase activities on polyacrylamide gel and cellulose acetate gel by the reduction of tetrazolium salts, *Anal. Biochem.*, 81, 481, 1977.
5. Kühnl, P., Anneken, K., and Spielmann, V., PEP A⁹, a new, unstable variant in the peptidase A system, *Hum. Genet.*, 47, 187, 1979.
6. Rapley, S., Lewis, W. H. P., and Harris, H., Tissue distribution, substrate specificities and molecular sizes of human peptidases determined by separate gene loci, *Ann. Hum. Genet.*, 34, 307, 1971.

OTHER NAMES    Prolidase, iminodipeptidase

REACTION    Aminoacyl-L-proline + H$_2$O = amino acid + L-proline

ENZYME SOURCE    Bacteria, vertebrates

## METHOD

### Visualization Scheme

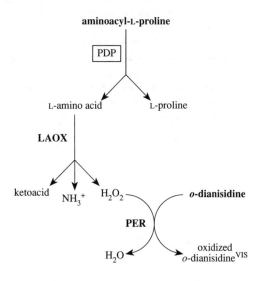

aminoacyl-L-proline

PDP

L-amino acid        L-proline

LAOX

ketoacid    NH$_3^+$    H$_2$O$_2$        *o*-dianisidine

PER

H$_2$O        oxidized *o*-dianisidine$^{VIS}$

### Staining Solution[1]

A.  0.2 *M* Phosphate buffer, pH 7.5    25 ml
    *o*-Dianisidine dihydrochloride    5 mg
    L-Amino acid oxidase (LAOX)    8 units
    Peroxidase (PER)    200 units
    Leucyl-L-proline, or phenylalanyl-proline,    20 mg
       or glycyl-L-proline
B.  2% Agar solution (55°C)    25 ml

### Procedure

Mix A and B solutions and pour the mixture over the gel surface. Incubate the gel at 37°C until brown bands appear. Fix stained gel in 50% glycerol.

*Notes:*  Because *o*-dianisidine dihydrochloride is a potential carcinogen, solutions containing this chromatogen should be handled with caution. Other chromogenic and fluorogenic peroxidase substrates may be used in place of *o*-dianisidine dihydrochloride (see 1.11.1.7 — PER).

## OTHER METHODS

A. The PMS/MTT system can replace the peroxidase system. The FAD which is tightly bound to L-amino acid oxidase is reduced when the enzyme catalyzes the oxidation of L-amino acid. Then MTT is reduced by FADH in the presence of PMS (see 3.4.11 or 13... — PEP, Method 2).

B. *o*-Phthalaldehyde can be used to detect the product L-glycine when glycyl-L-proline is used as substrate for PDP (see 3.4.11 or 13... — PEP, Method 3).

C. Two linked reactions catalyzed by glutamate–pyruvate transaminase and lactate dehydrogenase can be used to detect the product L-alanine when alanyl-L-proline is used as substrate for PDP (see 3.4.11 or 13... — PEP, Method 4).

## REFERENCE

1. Lewis, W. H. P. and Harris, H., Human red cell peptidases, *Nature*, 215, 351, 1967.

## 3.4.16.1 — Serine Carboxypeptidase; SCP

**OTHER NAMES**  Carboxypeptidase C, carboxypeptidase Y, cathepsin A, carboxypeptidase A, carboxypeptidase W

**REACTION**  Peptidyl-L-amino acid + H$_2$O = peptide + L-amino acid (broad specificity)

**ENZYME SOURCE**  Bacteria, fungi, plants, invertebrates, vertebrates

## METHOD

### Visualization Scheme

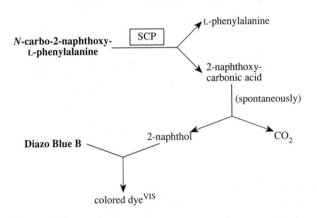

### Staining Solution[1]

| | |
|---|---|
| 0.1 $M$ Tris–HCl buffer, pH 7.0 | 150 ml |
| $N$-Carbo-2-naphthoxy-D,L-phenylalanine | 60 mg |
| Diazo Blue B | 45 mg |
| 25% CaCl$_2$ | 3 drops |
| 10% ZnCl$_2$ | 2 drops |

### Procedure

Incubate the gel in staining solution in the dark at 37°C until colored bands appear. Wash stained gel with water and fix in 50% glycerol.

*Notes:*  The enzyme represents a group of carboxypeptidases with broad specificity and usually with optimum pH of 4.5 to 6.0. It releases different C-terminal amino acids, including L-proline, L-arginine, and L-lysine.

Different $N$-carbobenzoxy amino acids can be used as substrates for SCP. Releasing C-terminal L-amino acids can then be detected using coupled reactions catalyzed by L-amino acid oxidase and peroxidase (e.g., see 3.4.11 or 13... — PEP, Methods 1 and 2).

### REFERENCE

1. Schopf, T. J., Population genetics of bryozoans, in *Biology of Bryozoans*, Woollacott, R. M. and Zimmer, R. L., Eds., Academic Press, New York, 1977, 459.

## 3.4.17.1 — Carboxypeptidase A; CPA

**OTHER NAMES**  Carboxypolypeptidase

**REACTION**  Peptidyl-L-amino acid + H$_2$O = peptide + L-amino acid

**ENZYME SOURCE**  Invertebrates, vertebrates

## METHOD

### Visualization Scheme

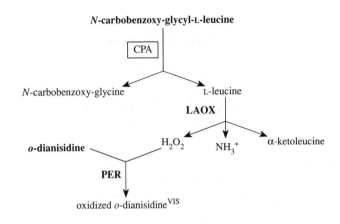

### Staining Solution[1,2]

| | |
|---|---|
| A. 0.2 $M$ Tris–HCl buffer, pH 7.5 | 30 ml |
| $N$-Carbobenzoxy-glycyl-L-leucine | 20 mg |
| Snake venom L-amino acid oxidase (LAOX) | 2 to 3 units |
| Peroxidase (PER Type II, Sigma) | 2 to 3 mg |
| $o$-Dianisidine dihydrochloride | 10 mg |
| B. 2% Agar solution (55°C) | 30 ml |

### Procedure

Mix A and B components of the staining solution and pour the mixture over the gel surface. Incubate the gel at 37°C until brown bands appear. Fix stained gel in 50% glycerol.

*Notes:*  The enzyme releases C-terminal amino acids, with the exception of C-terminal arginine, lysine, and proline (compare with 3.4.16.1 — SCP).

Other $N$-carbobenzoxy blocked dipeptides are commercially available and may be used as substrates for CPA. C-Terminal L-amino acids should be leucine, isoleucine, phenylalanine, tyrosine, methionine, and tryptophan when a linked reaction catalyzed by L-amino acid oxidase is used to detect CPA.

The MTT/PMS system may be used in the staining solution instead of the peroxidase/$o$-dianisidine system (e.g., see 3.4.11 or 13... — PEP, Method 2).

Solutions containing $o$-dianisidine dihydrochloride should be handled with caution because this chromatogen is a potential carcinogen.

The EDTA-containing electrophoretic and staining buffers should not be used because of the inhibitory effect of EDTA on the activity of CPA from some sources. Divalent ions (Ca$^{2+}$, Mg$^{2+}$, Mn$^{2+}$, Co$^{2+}$) may be added to the staining solution to activate CPA from some sources.

### REFERENCES

1. Baker, J. E., Isolation and properties of digestive carboxypeptidases from midguts of larvae of the black carpet beetle *Attagenus megatoma*, *Insect Biochem.*, 11, 583, 1981.
2. Baker, J. E., Application of capillary thin layer isoelectric focusing in polyacrylamide gel to the study of alkaline proteinases in stored-product insects, *Comp. Biochem. Physiol.*, 71B, 501, 1982.

## 3.4.19.3 — 5-Oxoprolyl-peptidase; OPP

**OTHER NAMES**
Pyrrolidone-carboxylate peptidase, pyroglutamyl aminopeptidase, pyroglutamate aminopeptidase

**REACTION**
5-Oxoprolyl-peptide + $H_2O$ = 5-oxoproline + peptide

**ENZYME SOURCE** Bacteria, vertebrates

## METHOD

### Visualization Scheme

**L-pyroglutamic acid-2-naphthylamide**

OPP

L-pyroglutamic acid     2-naphthylamine[UV] (fluorescent)

### Staining Solution[1]
0.1 M Potassium phosphate buffer, pH 7.0
2 mM L-Pyroglutamic acid-2-naphthylamide (dissolved in ethanol)
10 mM 2-Mercaptoethanol
10 mM EDTA

### Procedure
Incubate the gel in staining solution at 30°C for 1 h.
Observe fluorescent bands of OPP activity under UV light. Record the zymogram or photograph using a yellow filter.

*Notes:* The product 2-naphthylamine can be coupled with Fast Blue B (or other diazonium salts) resulting in the formation of colored dye visible in daylight (e.g., see 3.4.21.1 — CT, Method 2). The post-coupling procedure may prove beneficial.

Because 2-naphthylamine derivatives are potential carcinogens, the OPP staining solutions should be handled with extreme caution.

## OTHER METHODS

The substrate L-pyroglutamic acid *p*-nitroanilide can also be used to visualize OPP activity bands on electrophoretic gels. Enzymatically generated *p*-nitroaniline, which is too faintly colored, can then be diazotized and coupled with *N*-(1-naphthyl)-ethylenediamine to produce a readily visible red azo dye. This method may prove more sensitive than that described above, especially when applied to the enzyme transferred from electrophoretic gel to nitrocellulose membrane (e.g., see 3.4.21.4 — T, Method 3).

## REFERENCE
1. Sullivan, J. J., Muchnicky, E. E., Davidson, B. E., and Jago, G. R., Purification and properties of the pyrrolidonecarboxylate peptidase of *Streptococcus falcium*, *Aust. J. Biol. Sci.*, 30, 543, 1977.

## 3.4.21.1 — Chymotrypsin; CT

**OTHER NAMES**
Chymotrypsin A, chymotrypsin B

**REACTION**
Hydrolyzes peptides, amides, and esters, preferentially at the carbonyl end of Tyr-, Trp-, Phe-, Leu-

**ENZYME SOURCE** Invertebrates, vertebrates

## METHOD 1

### Visualization Scheme

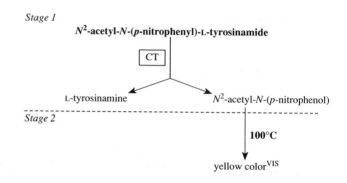

*Stage 1*

$N^2$-acetyl-*N*-(*p*-nitrophenyl)-L-tyrosinamide

CT

L-tyrosinamide     $N^2$-acetyl-*N*-(*p*-nitrophenol)

*Stage 2*

100°C

yellow color[VIS]

### Staining Solution[1]
50 mM Tris–HCl buffer, pH 8.0
5 mM $N^2$-Acetyl-*N*-(*p*-nitrophenyl)-L-tyrosinamide (dissolved in dimethylformamide)

### Procedure
Apply the staining solution to the gel surface on chromatographic paper (Whatman 3MM) overlay and incubate at 40°C for 10 to 15 min. Remove paper overlay and dry it at 100°C. Yellow bands indicate areas of CT activity.

## METHOD 2

### Visualization Scheme

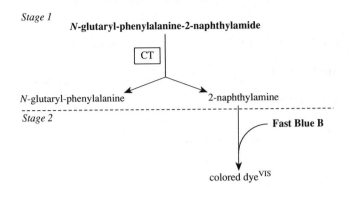

*Stage 1*

**N-glutaryl-phenylalanine-2-naphthylamide**

CT

N-glutaryl-phenylalanine          2-naphthylamine

*Stage 2*

Fast Blue B

colored dye$^{VIS}$

### Staining Solution[2]

A. 50 m$M$ Phosphate buffer, pH 8.0
   0.5 mg/ml N-Glutaryl-phenylalanine-2-naphthylamide (Merck; dissolved in dimethylformamide)

B. 50 m$M$ Phosphate buffer, pH 8.0
   1 mg/ml Fast Blue B (or 2 mg/ml Fast Garnet GBC)

### Procedure

Incubate the gel in solution A at 37°C for 30 min, wash briefly with water to remove excess naphthylamine and place in solution B. After appearance of the orange-red bands transfer gel into water. The color is stable to light and the gel may be stored at room temperature for months.

*Notes:* The post-coupling procedure used for the detection of CT activity has the advantage that the enzyme bands in the gel are rather distinct and bright in color. Furthermore, by using this procedure, a possible inhibitory effect of the diazonium salt on CT activity is avoided. The substrate (amino acid naphthylamide) lends itself well to the post-coupling procedure, since the chromogen (2-naphthylamine) released from the substrate has a great affinity for the protein, and thus, no significant diffusion occurs.

Because the substrate is a 2-naphthylamine derivative and therefore a potential carcinogen, solutions of this substrate should be handled with extreme caution.

## METHOD 3

### Visualization Scheme

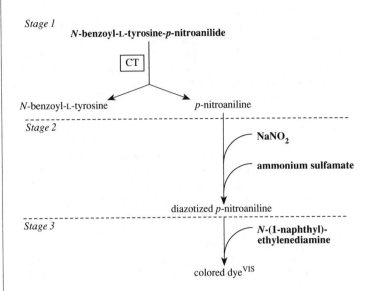

*Stage 1*

**N-benzoyl-L-tyrosine-p-nitroanilide**

CT

N-benzoyl-L-tyrosine          p-nitroaniline

*Stage 2*

NaNO$_2$

ammonium sulfamate

diazotized p-nitroaniline

*Stage 3*

N-(1-naphthyl)-ethylenediamine

colored dye$^{VIS}$

### Staining Solution[3]

A. 0.2 $M$ Tris–HCl buffer, pH 7.8
   0.5 mg/ml N-Benzoyl-L-tyrosine-p-nitroanilide (dissolved in dimethyl sulfoxide)

B. 0.1% NaNO$_2$
   1.0 $M$ HCl

C. 0.5% Ammonium sulfamate
   1.0 $M$ HCl

D. 0.05% N-(1-Naphthyl)-ethylenediamine
   47.5% Ethanol

### Procedure

Immediately after electrophoresis of active CT, cover gel by a nitrocellulose (NC) membrane. Perform blotting by covering the NC membrane with sheets of filter paper and paper towels under pressure (1 kg) for 30 min at room temperature (this time period is optimal for agarose gel). After blotting remove the NC membrane, dry lightly on air, and stain as described below.

For analysis of chymotrypsinogen use the same procedure but before blotting, preincubate the NC membrane for 1 h at room temperature with the activating enzymes enteropeptidase or trypsin (1.0 and 0.1 mg/ml, respectively), dissolved in 0.2 $M$ tris–HCl buffer, pH 7.8, containing 50 m$M$ CaCl$_2$. After blotting, incubate the NC membrane at room temperature in solution A for 60 min. Then diazotize the product p-nitroaniline as follows: put the NC membrane into solution B for 5 min; after another 5 min of incubation in solution C, put the membrane in solution D.

When the developing red-colored bands are of a maximal intensity (usually after 1 to 5 min), take up the NC membrane and allow the solution D to drip off. Put the moist NC membrane between two plastic sheets (overhead film; air bubbles should be avoided), seal with adhesive tape, and store at −18°C.

*Notes:* N-succinyl-L-phenylalanine-*p*-nitroanilide may be used in solution A instead of N-benzoyl-L-tyrosine-*p*-nitroanilide.

A red azo dye formed by this method does not precipitate in the gel. The transfer of the enzyme from the electrophoretic gel to a NC membrane is used to avoid this disadvantage.

If the NC membrane is incubated too long in substrate solution A the product *p*-nitroaniline is produced in such amounts that it is released from proteinase zones on the NC membrane, giving a yellow color to the substrate solution and causing undesirable background staining after diazotation and coupling with N-(1-naphthyl)-ethylenediamine. Therefore, incubation in solution A must be stopped just after the yellow bands have appeared.

## REFERENCES

1. Gertler, A., Tencer, Y., and Tinman, G., Simultaneous detection of trypsin and chymotripsin with 4-nitroanilide substrates on cellulose acetate electropherograms, *Anal. Biochem.*, 54, 270, 1973.
2. Hagenmaier, H. E., Polyacrylamide gel electrophoresis as a method for differentiation of gut proteinases which catalyze the hydrolysis of amino acid naphthylamides, *Anal. Biochem.*, 63, 579, 1975.
3. Ohlsson, B. G., Weström, B. R., and Karlsson, B. W., Enzymoblotting: a method for localizing proteinases and their zymogens using *para*-nitroanilide substrates after agarose gel electrophoresis and transfer to nitrocellulose, *Anal. Biochem.*, 152, 239, 1986.

OTHER NAMES    α-Trypsin, β-trypsin

REACTION    Hydrolyses peptides, amides, and esters at bonds involving the carboxyl group of L-arginine or L-lysine

ENZYME SOURCE   Bacteria, invertebrates, vertebrates

## METHOD 1

### Visualization Scheme

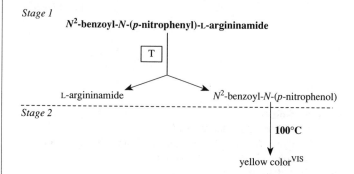

### Staining Solution[1]

     50 m$M$ Tris–HCl buffer, pH 8.0
     5 m$M$ $N^2$-Benzoyl-$N$-(*p*-nitrophenyl)-L-argininamide (dissolved in dimethylformamide)

### Procedure

Apply the staining solution to the gel surface on chromatographic paper (Whatman 3MM) overlay and incubate at 40°C for 10 to 15 min. Remove the paper overlay and dry it at 100°C. Yellow bands indicate areas of T activity.

## METHOD 2

### Visualization Scheme

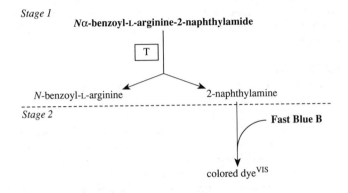

*Stage 1*

$N\alpha$-benzoyl-L-arginine-2-naphthylamide

T

$N$-benzoyl-L-arginine          2-naphthylamine

*Stage 2*

Fast Blue B

colored dye$^{\text{VIS}}$

### Staining Solution[2]
A. 50 m$M$ Phosphate buffer, pH 8.0
   0.5 mg/ml $N\alpha$-Benzoyl-D,L-arginine-2-naphthylamide
   (dissolved in dimethylformamide)
B. 50 m$M$ Phosphate buffer, pH 8.0
   1 mg/ml Fast Blue B (or 2 mg/ml Fast Garnet GBC)

### Procedure
Incubate the gel in solution A at 37°C for 30 min, wash briefly with water to remove excess naphthylamine and place in solution B. After appearance of the orange-red bands transfer gel into water. The color is stable to light and stained gel may be stored at room temperature for months.

*Notes:* The post-coupling procedure used for the detection of T activity has the advantage that the enzyme bands in the gel are rather distinct and bright in color. Furthermore, by using this procedure, a possible inhibitory effect of the diazonium salt on the T activity is avoided. The substrate (amino acid naphthylamide) lends itself well to the post-coupling procedure since the chromogen (2-naphthylamine) released from the substrate has a great affinity for the protein, and thus, no significant diffusion occurs.

Because the substrate is a 2-naphthylamine derivative and therefore a potential carcinogen, solutions of this substrate should be handled with extreme caution.

## METHOD 3

### Visualization Scheme

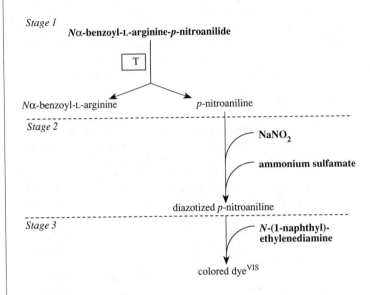

*Stage 1*

$N\alpha$-benzoyl-L-arginine-$p$-nitroanilide

T

$N\alpha$-benzoyl-L-arginine          $p$-nitroaniline

*Stage 2*

NaNO$_2$

ammonium sulfamate

diazotized $p$-nitroaniline

*Stage 3*

$N$-(1-naphthyl)-ethylenediamine

colored dye$^{\text{VIS}}$

### Staining Solution[3]
A. 0.2 $M$ Tris–HCl buffer, pH 7.8
   0.5 mg/ml $N\alpha$-Benzoyl-D,L-arginine-$p$-nitroanilide (Sigma;
   dissolved in buffer at 95°C)
B. 0.1% NaNO$_2$
   1.0 $M$ HCl
C. 0.5% Ammonium sulfamate
   1.0 $M$ HCl
D. 0.05% $N$-(1-Naphthyl)-ethylenediamine (Sigma)
   47.5% Ethanol

### Procedure
Immediately after electrophoresis of active T, cover gel by a nitrocellulose (NC) membrane. Perform the blotting by covering the NC membrane with sheets of filter paper and paper towels under pressure (1 kg) for 30 min at room temperature (this time period is optimal for agarose gel). After blotting, remove the NC membrane, dry lightly in air, and stain as described below.

For analysis of trypsinogen use the same procedure, but before blotting preincubate the NC membrane for 1 h at room temperature with the activating enzyme, enteropeptidase (1.0 mg/ml), dissolved in 0.2 $M$ tris–HCl buffer, pH 7.8, containing 50 m$M$ CaCl$_2$.

After blotting, incubate the NC membrane at room temperature in solution A for 60 min. Then diazotize the product $p$-nitroaniline as follows: put the NC membrane into solution B for 5 min; after another 5 min of incubation in solution C, put the membrane in solution D.

When the developing red-colored bands are of a maximal intensity (usually after 1 to 5 min), take up the NC membrane and allow the solution D to drip off. Put the moist NC membrane between two plastic sheets (overhead film; air bubbles should be avoided), seal with adhesive tape, and store at −18°C.

*Notes:* A red azo dye formed by this method does not precipitate in the gel. The transfer of the enzyme from the electrophoretic gel to a NC membrane is used to avoid this disadvantage.

If the NC membrane is incubated too long in substrate solution A the product *p*-nitroaniline is produced in such amounts that it is released from proteinase zones on the NC membrane, giving a yellow color to the substrate solution and causing undesirable background staining after diazotation and coupling with *N*-(1-naphthyl)-ethylenediamine. Therefore, incubation in solution A must be stopped just after the yellow bands have appeared.

## OTHER METHODS

A. Trypsin can also be detected via the hydrogen ion formed during the tryptic hydrolysis of the substrate protamine sulfate by means of the color change of the pH indicator Phenol Red. In order to remove electrophoretic buffer, which can interfere with pH change, the electrophoretic gel should be washed with 1 m$M$ borate, pH 8.0, for 2 to 5 min prior to being placed in contact with substrate-containing agarose plate. Substrate–agarose consists of 0.01% Phenol Red, 20 m$M$ CaCl$_2$, 1 m$M$ borate, pH 8.0, 10 mg/ml protamine sulfate, and 1% agarose. Sites of trypsin activity are indicated by a color change.[4]

B. Trypsin can be detected by bioautography (for more details see Part II) by placing an electrophoretic gel in contact with indicator agar containing 1.5% Bacto-agar, 1 mg/ml protamine sulfate in *E. coli* minimal medium (see Appendix A-1) and 0.01 OD/ml exponentially growing Arg H$^-$ arginine-required *E. coli*. Bands of growing *E. coli* are observed 3 h after initiation of the assay at locations where L-arginine is generated by trypsin in the electrophoretic gel.[4]

C. Two-dimensional spectroscopy of electrophoretic gels (for more details see Part II) permits detection of trypsin activity bands by purely optical means.[4] In this procedure trypsin is detected using substrates α-*N*-benzoyl-L-arginine ethyl ester (BAEE), or α-*N*-benzoyl-L-arginine-*p*-nitroanilide (BAPNA), or α-*N*-benzoyl-L-arginine 7-amido-4-methyl-coumarin (BAAMC). All reactions are carried out by placing an electrophoretic gel in contact with 1% substrate–agarose plate containing 0.1 $M$ tris–HCl buffer (pH 8.0), 20 m$M$ CaCl$_2$, 5 m$M$ BAEE (or 2.5 m$M$ BAPNA, or 0.05 m$M$ BAAMC). When BAPMC is used as substrate, the product is detected due to the fluorescence excited at 313 nm and emitted at 420 nm. When BAEE and BAPNA are used as substrates, the product formation is detected due to the absorption at 253 nm and 392 nm, respectively. A special optical device permits one to take a photograph of the developed agarose overlay.

## GENERAL NOTES

Two-dimensional spectroscopy and bioautography methods are not widely used because they are too complex. It should be pointed out, however, that the bioautographic method is one of the most sensitive and detects about 0.04 units of T activity towards BAEE per band.

## REFERENCES

1. Gertler, A., Tencer, Y., and Tinman, G., Simultaneous detection of trypsin and chymotripsin with 4-nitroanilide substrates on cellulose acetate electropherograms, *Anal. Biochem.*, 54, 270, 1973.
2. Hagenmaier, H. E., Polyacrylamide gel electrophoresis as a method for differentiation of gut proteinases which catalyze the hydrolysis of amino acid naphthylamides, *Anal. Biochem.*, 63, 579, 1975.
3. Ohlsson, B. G., Weström, B. R., and Karlsson, B. W., Enzymoblotting: a method for localizing proteinases and their zymogens using *para*-nitroanilide substrates after agarose gel electrophoresis and transfer to nitrocellulose, *Anal. Biochem.*, 152, 239, 1986.
4. Klebe, R. J., Mancuso, M. G., Brown, C. R., and Teng, L., Two-dimensional spectroscopy of electrophoretic gels, *Biochem. Genet.*, 19, 655, 1981.

## 3.4.21.5 — Thrombin; THR

OTHER NAMES    Fibrinogenase

REACTION    Preferential cleavage at the carbonyl end of L-Arg

ENZYME SOURCE  Vertebrates

## METHOD

### Visualization Scheme

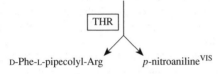

D-**Phe-L-pipecolyl-Arg-***p***-nitroanilide**

THR

D-Phe-L-pipecolyl-Arg     *p*-nitroaniline[VIS]

### Staining Solution[1]

  A. 0.1 *M* Sodium barbital buffer, pH 7.75
    0.2 *M* NaCl
    3.4 m*M* CaCl$_2$
    1.4 m*M* MgCl$_2$
    2 m*M* D-Phe-L-pipecolyl-Arg-*p*-nitroanilide
  B. 3% Agarose solution (60°C)

### Procedure

Mix equal volumes of solutions A and B and pour the mixture over the gel surface. Incubate the gel at 37°C until yellow bands appear.

*Notes:* The product *p*-nitroaniline is usually too faint to be directly visualized in the gel and is registrated spectrophotometrically at 405 nm. When *p*-nitroaniline is diazotized and coupled with naphthylethylenediamine a readily visible red azo dye is formed. Unfortunately, this dye does not precipitate in the gel. However, by using a method based on the transfer of enzymes from electrophoretic gel to an immobilizing matrix of nitrocellulose, this disadvantage can be overcome.[2] The example of application of this method is given above (see 3.4.21.4 — T, Method 3).

### REFERENCES

  1. Wagner, O. F., Bergmann, I., and Binder, B. R., Chromogenic substrate autography: a method for detection, characterization, and quantitative measurement of serine proteases after sodium dodecyl sulfate–polyacrylamide gel electrophoresis or isoelectric focusing in polyacrylamide gels, *Anal. Biochem.*, 151, 7, 1985.
  2. Ohlsson, B. G., Weström, B. R., and Karlsson, B. W., Enzymoblotting: a method for localizing proteinases and their zymogens using *para*-nitroanilide substrates after agarose gel electrophoresis and transfer to nitrocellulose, *Anal. Biochem.*, 152, 239, 1986.

## 3.4.21.10 — Acrosin; ACR

OTHER NAMES    Acrosomal proteinase

REACTION    Hydrolysis of Arg- and Lys-bonds; preferential cleavage Arg–Xaa ≫ Lys–Lys ≫ Lys–Xaa

ENZYME SOURCE  Invertebrates, vertebrates

## METHOD

### Visualization Scheme

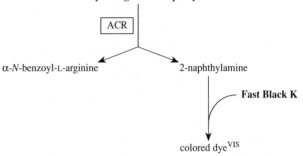

α-*N*-**benzoyl-L-arginine-2-naphthylamide**

ACR

α-*N*-benzoyl-L-arginine    2-naphthylamine

**Fast Black K**

colored dye[VIS]

### Staining Solution[1]

  A. 0.1 *M* Phosphate buffer, pH 7.5
    0.9 mg/ml Fast Black K
  B. 0.1 *M* Phosphate buffer, pH 7.5
    1.25 mg/ml α-*N*-Benzoyl-D,L-arginine-2-naphthylamide (dissolved in dimethyl sulfoxide)
    0.85 mg/ml Fast Black K

### Procedure

Wash electrophorized gel in filtered solution A at 37°C for 3 to 5 min and then transfer to filtered solution B. Incubate the gel in solution B at 37°C in the dark until blue bands appear. Wash stained gel in water and fix in 7% acetic acid.

*Notes:* Fast Garnet GBC and Fast Blue B can also be used as coupling dyes. The most stable dye is obtained, however, with Fast Black K.

    Because the substrate is a 2-naphthylamine derivative and therefore a potential carcinogen, solutions of this substrate should be handled with extreme caution.

    The method described above is not specific for ACR. However, this trypsin-like proteinase occurs only in spermatozoa (in acrosomes) and thus can be easily identified based on its tissue specificity.

### OTHER METHODS

α-*N*-Benzoyl-L-arginine-*p*-nitroanilide can also be used as a chromogenic substrate for ACR. Enzymatically released *p*-nitroaniline, which is too faintly colored, can then be diazotized and coupled with *N*-(1-naphthyl)ethylenediamine to produce a readily visible red azo dye. This method may prove more sensitive than that described above, especially when applied to the enzyme transferred from electrophoretic gel to nitrocellulose membrane (e.g., see 3.4.21.4 — T, Method 3).

### REFERENCE

  1. Garner, D. L., Improved zymographic detection of bovine acrosin, *Anal. Biochem.*, 67, 688, 1975.

OTHER NAMES     Plasminogen activator (recommended name)

REACTION        Preferential cleavage of Arg–Val bonds in plasminogen and conversion of plasminogen into plasmin

ENZYME SOURCE   Bacteria, vertebrates

## METHOD 1

### Visualization Scheme

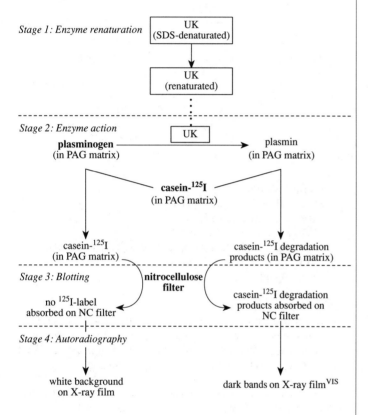

*Stage 1: Enzyme renaturation*

UK (SDS-denatured)

UK (renaturated)

*Stage 2: Enzyme action*

UK

**plasminogen** (in PAG matrix) ⟶ plasmin (in PAG matrix)

**casein-$^{125}$I** (in PAG matrix)

casein-$^{125}$I (in PAG matrix)          casein-$^{125}$I degradation products (in PAG matrix)

*Stage 3: Blotting*     **nitrocellulose filter**

no $^{125}$I-label absorbed on NC filter          casein-$^{125}$I degradation products absorbed on NC filter

*Stage 4: Autoradiography*

white background on X-ray film          dark bands on X-ray film$^{VIS}$

### Substrate-Containing PAG[1]

Electrophoresis of UK is carried out according to Laemmli[2] in SDS–PAG containing 0.08% casein-$^{125}$I (specific activity 6 to 7 × $10^4$ cpm/µg) and 46 µg/ml plasminogen.

## Procedure

*Stage 1.* Shake electrophorized SDS–PAG gently in cold 2.5% Triton X-100 for 60 min at 4°C, rinse thoroughly with water and shake again in 0.1 *M* tris–HCl, pH 8.1, for 10 min.

*Stage 2.* Incubate washed PAG for 2 h at 37°C in a humid chamber.

*Stage 3.* Wash nitrocellulose filter (0.45 µm, Schleicher and Schull) in water and then in 0.1 *M* tris–HCl, pH 8.1. Remove excess liquid by blotting on Whatman 3MM paper and then lay the filter in a dish. Dip incubated PAG in 0.1 *M* tris–HCl, pH 8.1, for about 5 s, mount on nitrocellulose filter, and blot for 60 min at 37°C in a humid chamber. Shake blotted filter in phosphate-buffered saline solution for 60 min at room temperature and remove excess liquid by blotting on Whatman 3MM paper.

*Stage 4.* Dry blotted and washed nitrocellulose filter, cover with Saran wrap, and expose to X-ray film (Kodak, X-omat, RP-2) at –70°C for 5 to 48 h.

Dark bands on developed X-ray film correspond to the position of UK in PAG.

*Notes:* Washed and incubated PAG can also be stained with Coomassie brilliant blue to develop achromatic bands of UK activity on a blue gel background. However, autoradiographic detection is about 10 times more sensitive as compared with the Coomassie staining procedure.

The sensitivity and accuracy of autoradiographic detection are higher when SDS and iodinated substrate of high quality are used.

Autoradiographic detection is especially advantageous for crude samples containing proteins comigrating with UK. Such proteins develop on the Coomassie-stained PAG as dark bands which interfere with or completely mask achromatic zones of UK.

## METHOD 2

### Visualization Scheme

**pyroglutamyl-Gly-Arg-*p*-nitroanilide**

| UK |

pyroglutamyl-Gly-Arg        *p*-nitroaniline [VIS]

### Staining Solution[3]
A.  0.1 *M* Sodium barbital buffer, pH 7.75
    0.2 *M* NaCl
    3.4 m*M* CaCl₂
    1.4 m*M* MgCl₂
    0.9 m*M* Pyroglutamyl-Gly-Arg-*p*-nitroanilide
B.  3% Agarose solution (60°C)

### Procedure
Mix equal volumes of A and B solutions and pour the mixture onto a prewarmed glass plate to give a 2-mm-thick gel. Place electrophorized SDS–PAG (washed as described in Method 1) on top of substrate-containing agarose gel and incubate at 37°C in a moist chamber for up to 12 h. Areas of UK activity appear as yellow bands in the agarose gel. Record the zymogram or scan on a densitometer at 405 nm.

*Notes:*  This method was used to visualize UK after electrophoresis of purified enzyme preparations and, perhaps, is not as specific as Method 1.

The chromogenic substrate H-D-Ile-Pro-Arg-*p*-nitroanilide may also be used.

The product *p*-nitroaniline is usually too faint-colored, but when it is diazotized and coupled with *N*-(1-naphthyl)-ethylenediamine, a readily visible red azo dye is formed. This dye, however, does not precipitate in the gel. To overcome this disadvantage a method may be used which is based on transferring proteins from electrophoretic gel to a nitrocellulose membrane[4] (the example of application of this method is 3.4.21.4 — T, Method 3).

## OTHER METHODS

An immunoblotting procedure (for details see Part II) based on the utility of monoclonal antibodies specific to the human enzyme[5] can also be used for immunohistochemical visualization of the enzyme protein on electrophoretic gels. This procedure is too complex for routine laboratory use but may be of great value in special analyses of UK.

### REFERENCES
1.  Miskin, R. and Soreq, H., Sensitive autoradiographic quantification of electrophoretically separated proteases, *Anal. Biochem.*, 118, 252, 1981.
2.  Laemmli, U. K., Cleavage of structural proteins during the assembly of the head of bacteriophage T4, *Nature*, 227, 680, 1970.
3.  Wagner, O. F., Bergmann, I., and Binder, B. R., Chromogenic substrate autography: a method for detection, characterization, and quantitative measurement of serine proteases after sodium dodecyl sulfate–polyacrylamide gel electrophoresis or isoelectric focusing in polyacrylamide gels, *Anal. Biochem.*, 151, 7, 1985.
4.  Ohlsson, B. G., Weström, B. R., and Karlsson, B. W., Enzymoblotting: a method for localizing proteinases and their zymogens using *para*-nitroanilide substrates after agarose gel electrophoresis and transfer to nitrocellulose, *Anal. Biochem.*, 152, 239, 1986.
5.  Kaltoft, K., Nielsen, L. S., Zeuthen, J., and Dan, K., Monoclonal antibody that specifically inhibits a human MR 52000 plasminogen activating enzyme, *Proc. Natl. Acad. Sci. U.S.A.*, 79, 3720, 1982.

OTHER NAMES    Kallikrein, kininogenin, serum kallikrein, kininogenase, arginine esterase

REACTION    Cleaves Lys–Arg and Arg–Ser bonds in kininogen to produce bradykinin; hydrolyzes ester bonds in acyl- and benzoyl-arginine esters

ENZYME SOURCE   Vertebrates

## METHOD 1

### Visualization Scheme

N-α-benzoyl-L-arginine ethyl ester

PKK

N-α-benzoyl-L-arginine     ethanol

NAD ← → formazan$^{VIS}$

**ADH**       **PMS**

NADH    NBT

acetaldehyde

### Staining Solution[1]

| | |
|---|---|
| 80 mM Tris–EDTA–borate buffer, pH 9.2 | 150 ml |
| N-α-Benzoyl-L-arginine ethyl ester | 250 mg |
| NAD | 100 mg |
| PMS | 1 mg |
| NBT | 30 mg |
| KCN | 1 mg |
| Alcohol dehydrogenase (ADH; suitable for determination of ethanol; Sigma) | 1500 units |
| CaCl$_2$ | 300 mg |

### Procedure

Incubate the gel in staining solution in the dark at 37°C until dark blue bands appear. Fix stained gel in 7% acetic acid.

*Notes:* Bands of trypsin activity can also be developed by this method. These bands, however, can be easily identified by adding a soybean trypsin inhibitor in the staining solution.

## METHOD 2

### Visualization Scheme

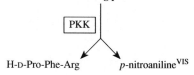

**H-D-Pro-Phe-Arg-*p*-nitroanilide**

PKK

H-D-Pro-Phe-Arg     *p*-nitroaniline$^{VIS}$

### Staining Solution[2]

A. 0.1 *M* Sodium barbital buffer, pH 7.75
    0.2 *M* NaCl
    3.4 mM CaCl$_2$
    1.4 mM MgCl$_2$
    2.4 mM H-D-Pro-Phe-Arg-*p*-nitroanilide
B. 3% Agarose solution (60°C)

### Procedure

Mix equal volumes of A and B solutions and pour the mixture onto a prewarmed glass plate to give a 2-mm-thick gel. Place electrophorized SDS–PAG (washed in an excess volume of 2.5% Triton X-100 for 50 min and rinsed with distilled water for 15 min) on top of substrate-containing agarose gel and incubate at 37°C in a moist chamber for up to 12 h. Areas of PKK activity appear as yellow bands in the agarose gel. Record the zymogram or scan on a densitometer at 405 nm.

*Notes:* The chromogenic substrate H-D-Val-Leu-Arg-*p*-nitroanilide can also be used to detect tissue kallikrein (E.C. 3.4.21.35).

The product *p*-nitroaniline is usually too faint-colored, but when it is diazotized and coupled with *N*-(1-naphthyl)-ethylenediamine, a readily visible red azo dye is formed. However, this dye does not precipitate in the gel. To overcome this disadvantage a method which is based on transferring proteins from electrophoretic gel to a nitrocellulose membrane and subsequent staining of the membrane-bound enzyme was developed[3] (the example of application of this method is 3.4.21.4 — T, Method 3).

The method described above was used to visualize PKK after electrophoresis of purified enzyme preparations of plasma and tissue (urine) kallikreins from human and mouse. Its specificity was not tested in detail.

## GENERAL NOTES

The enzyme activates coagulation factors XII, VII, and plasminogen. It is formed from prekallikrein by factor XIIa or XIIf.

## REFERENCES

1. Fujimoto, Y., Moriya, H., Yamaguchi, K., and Moriwaki, C., Detection of arginine esterase of various kallikrein preparations on gellified electrophoretic media, *J. Biochem. (Tokyo)*, 71, 751, 1972.
2. Wagner, O. F., Bergmann, I., and Binder, B. R., Chromogenic substrate autography: a method for detection, characterization, and quantitative measurement of serine proteases after sodium dodecyl sulfate–polyacrylamide gel electrophoresis or isoelectric focusing in polyacrylamide gels, *Anal. Biochem.*, 151, 7, 1985.
3. Ohlsson, B. G., Weström, B. R., and Karlsson, B. W., Enzymoblotting: a method for localizing proteinases and their zymogens using *para*-nitroanilide substrates after agarose gel electrophoresis and transfer to nitrocellulose, *Anal. Biochem.*, 152, 239, 1986.

OTHER NAMES    Pancreatic elastase (recommended name), pancreatopeptidase E, pancreatic elastase 1

REACTION    Preferentially cleaves bonds at the carboxyl of Gly, Ala, Val, Leu, Ile; hydrolyzes elastin

ENZYME SOURCE  Bacteria, fungi, vertebrates

## METHOD 1

### Visualization Scheme

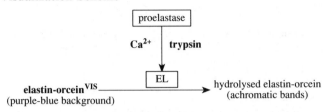

### Substrate-Containing Reactive Plate[1]

To prepare substrate-containing reactive agarose plate, grind elastin–Orcein crystals (100 mg) in a mortar with 1 ml of 20 m$M$ tris–HCl buffer, pH 8.8. Wash the particles twice with the same buffer by centrifugation until a colorless supernatant is obtained to remove contaminating dye-bound polypeptides. Suspend the pelleted particles in 1 ml of the buffer and mix with 49 ml of 2% agarose solution in 20 m$M$ tris–HCl buffer, pH 8.8 (60°C). Pour the mixture onto a glass plate of an appropriate size. After solidification, the substrate-containing agarose reactive plate is ready for use.

### Procedure

Activate proelastase in electrophorized gel by incubating the gel for 30 min at 37°C in 20 m$M$ tris–HCl (pH 8.2), 20 m$M$ CaCl$_2$, 50 µg/ml trypsin. After incubation wash gel twice with 20 m$M$ tris–HCl buffer, pH 8.8, to remove excess trypsin. Then blot gel with filter paper and lay onto substrate-containing reactive plate. Incubate the electrophoretic gel/reactive plate combination at 37°C for 2 h or until colorless bands appear on the purple-blue background of the reactive agarose plate. Fix stained reactive plate in 3% acetic acid.

*Notes:*  Without activation of the proenzyme with trypsin, no EL activity could be detected.

Only a small part of the substrate complex usually is broken down as a result of EL activity so that it is worthwhile to regain the remaining part of the particles from agarose gel. To achieve this, agarose gel containing elastin–Orcein should be liquefied at 70°C by heating in a water bath. The pH of the solution should be lowered to 3 by addition of HCl. The color of the particles changes reversibly from purple-blue at pH 8.8 to pink at pH 3. Under this acid condition, an agarose solution stays liquid at room temperature, and the elastine-Orcein particles can easily be spun down by centrifugation for 2 min at 5000 g. The isolated elastine–Orcein should then be suspended in buffer, washed twice by centrifugation, and stored in a refrigerator.

Elastin–Congo Red can also be used as colored substrate complex to obtain the negative EL zymograms.

## METHOD 2

### Visualization Scheme

**N-succinyl-Ala-Ala-Ala-p-nitroanilide**

EL

*N*-succinyl-Ala-Ala-Ala             *p*-nitroaniline[VIS]

### Substrate-Containing Reactive Plate[2]

Prepare 0.125 $M$ stock solution of *N*-succinyl-L-Ala-L-Ala-L-Ala-*p*-nitroanilide (SAPNA) in *N*-methylpirrolidone by heating at 60°C for 10 min and stirring. Store this solution at 4°C in a dark bottle. Prepare the 1.5 m$M$ substrate solution just before use by dilution of the stock solution with 0.2 $M$ tris–HCl, pH 8.0. Suspend agar in 0.2 $M$ tris–HCl, pH 8.0 (1.5% w/v), heat to 100°C to liquefy, and cool to 60°C. Add 1.5 m$M$ substrate solution to the agar solution (10 µl/ml) and stir for 3 min at 60°C. Pour the resulting mixture onto a preheated (45°C) glass plate of an appropriate size and allow to solidify. Use substrate-containing reactive plate immediately or store in an air-tight bag at 4°C.

### Procedure

Treat electrophorized PAG with trypsin to convert proelastase into elastase as described in Method 1. Apply the reactive plate on top of PAG, ensuring that no air bubbles are trapped between the two slabs. Incubate the PAG/reactive plate combination at 37°C in a humid box. Bands of yellow reaction product (*p*-nitroaniline) appear almost immediately. When the bands are well developed, record, photograph, or scan the zymogram on a densitometer at 405 nm immediately, since the yellow bands increase progressively in intensity.

*Notes:*  The product *p*-nitroaniline can be diazotized and coupled with *N*-(1-naphthyl)-ethylenediamine resulting in a readily visible red azo dye. However, this dye does not precipitate in the gel. To overcome this disadvantage, the method of nitrocellulose enzyme blotting may be used[3] (for example, see 3.4.21.4 — T, Method 3).

## GENERAL NOTES

Method 1 is highly specific for EL; however, the considerable time necessary for developing the zymogram in this procedure enhances the potential risk that enzyme bands placed closely together could mix with each other by diffusion. This method has a detection limit of 0.5 µg of EL per band after incubation at 37°C overnight. The same amount of EL can be detected with Method 2 within a few minutes. It should be taken into account, however, that Method 2 can also detect some elastase-like esterases cleaving SAPNA but not elastin. Such esterases may occur in certain biological fluids, e.g., human synovial fluid.

### REFERENCES

1. Dijkhof, J. and Poort, C., Visualization of proelastase in polyacrylamide gels, *Anal. Biochem.*, 83, 315, 1977.
2. Gardi, C. and Lungarella, G., Detection of elastase activity with a zymogram method after isoelectric focusing in polyacrylamide gel, *Anal. Biochem.*, 140, 472, 1984.
3. Ohlsson, B. G., Weström, B. R., and Karlsson, B. W., Enzymoblotting: a method for localizing proteinases and their zymogens using *para*-nitroanilide substrates after agarose gel electrophoresis and transfer to nitrocellulose, *Anal. Biochem.*, 152, 239, 1986.

OTHER NAMES    Submandibular proteinase A (recommended name), esteroprotease A

REACTION    Hydrolysis of proteins by cleavage of arginyl bonds; hydrolysis of ester bonds in acetyl-methionine and tosyl-arginine esters

ENZYME SOURCE    Vertebrates (mammalian submandibular gland)

## METHOD 1

### Visualization Scheme

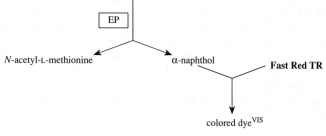

*N*-acetyl-L-methionine α-naphthyl ester

*N*-acetyl-L-methionine     α-naphthol     **Fast Red TR**

colored dye$^{VIS}$

### Staining Solution[1]

66.6 m$M$ Phosphate buffer, pH 6.5

0.75 m$M$ *N*-Acetyl-L-methionine α-naphthyl ester (dissolved in dimethyl sulfoxide)

1.5 mg/ml Fast Red TR

### Procedure

Dissolve the substrate in a minimal volume of dimethyl sulfoxide, and then dissolve the dye in the buffer. Add the substrate solution to the dye solution under vigorous stirring. Incubate the gel in the resulting mixture at room temperature until red-brown bands appear. Fix stained gel in 50% glycerol or 3% acetic acid.

## METHOD 2

### Visualization Scheme

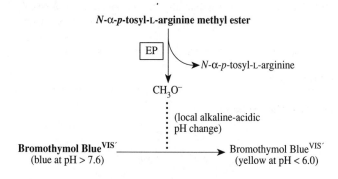

*N*-α-*p*-tosyl-L-arginine methyl ester

EP

→ *N*-α-*p*-tosyl-L-arginine

$CH_3O^-$

(local alkaline-acidic pH change)

Bromothymol Blue$^{VIS'}$            Bromothymol Blue$^{VIS'}$
(blue at pH > 7.6)                                    (yellow at pH < 6.0)

### Staining Solution[2]

A.  50 m$M$ Tris–EDTA-borate buffer, pH 8.6     10 ml
     Bromothymol Blue     100 mg

B.  N-α-*p*-Tosyl-L-arginine methyl ester     100 mg
     $H_2O$     10 ml

### Procedure

Place electrophorized acetate cellulose gel horizontally and cover with solution A. After 1 min blot gel and cover with solution B. The areas of EP activity appear as yellow bands on a blue background of the gel. Record or photograph zymogram.

### GENERAL NOTES

Both methods described above are not specific for EP. Additional bands caused by esteroprotease E develop on the zymograms obtained by Method 1. Method 2 develops activity bands of both EP and esteroprotease, called "tamase".[3] Activity bands caused by different esteroproteases can be identified by using both methods in parallel, based on different substrate specificities of these esteroproteases as indicated in the table below:

| Substrates | Esteroproteases | | |
| --- | --- | --- | --- |
|  | EP | Esteroprotease E | "Tamase" |
| *N*-Acetyl-L-methionine α-naphthyl ester | + | + | – |
| N-α-Tosyl-L-arginine methyl ester | + | – | + |

### REFERENCES

1. Schaller, E. and Von Deimling, O., Methionine-α-naphthyl ester, a useful chromogenic substrate for esteroproteases of the mouse submandibular gland, *Anal. Biochem.*, 93, 251, 1979.
2. Skow, L. C., Genetic variation at a locus (TAM-1) for submaxillary gland protease in the mouse and its location on chromosome 7, *Genetics*, 90, 713, 1978.
3. Otto, J. and Von Deimling, O., Prt-4 and Prt-5: new constituents of a gene cluster on chromosome 7 coding for esteroproteases in the submandibular gland of the house mouse (*Mus musculus*), *Biochem. Genet.*, 19, 431, 1981.

OTHER NAMES    Proteolytic enzymes, proteases, endopeptidases, peptidyl-peptide hydrolases. The enzymes of sub-subclasses 3.4.21 (serine proteinases) have an active center histidine and serine involved in the catalytic process; those of 3.4.22 (cysteine, or thyol, proteinases) have a cysteine in the active center; those of 3.4.23 have a pH-optimum below 5, due to the involvement of an acidic residue in the catalytic process (aspartic, or acidic, proteinases); and those of 3.4.24 are metalloproteins using a metal ion in the catalytic mechanism (metalloproteinases).

REACTIONS    Attack all denatured and many native proteins and catalyze endohydrolysis of peptide bonds; do not have a substrate specificity in the ordinary sense. Many proteinases have a very close but not entirely identical specificity. The products resulting from their action on the same protein as substrate differ quantitatively and qualitatively.

ENZYME SOURCE    Bacteria, fungi, plants, invertebrates, vertebrates

## GENERAL PRINCIPLES OF DETECTION

Many methods are developed for the detection of PROT activity on electrophoretic gels. The majority of them are based on incorporation of specific proteins (usually denaturated) directly into separating gels or agarose gels that are held in contact with electrophoretic gels. After incubation, substrate-containing gels are treated with protein-precipitating agents (e.g., trichloroacetic acid or acetic acid–methanol–water mixture) and stained for general proteins with Amidoblack or Coomassie Brilliant Blue dyes. The most frequently used PROT substrates are casein,[1-3] hemoglobin,[1,3,4] bovine serum albumin,[5,6] gelatin,[7,8] and keratin.[9] Commercial photographic sheet films containing a thin, uniform layer of gelatin were shown to be a very convenient and highly sensitive form of substrate for PROT.[10] Before use, a sheet film should be cleared with a nonhardening fixing solution in total darkness, washed thoroughly, and dried.

Proteinases can also be detected by incubating electrophoretic gels with colored substrates such as cytochrome *c*,[11] elastin–Orcein,[12] or Azocoll.[13] All these methods are negative, i.e., they develop achromatic PROT bands on a colored background. The exception is the so-called "caseogram" method, which produces positively stained PROT bands.[3] Many PROT have been electrophoretically studied using the detection methods listed above: chymotrypsins (EC 3.4.21.1–2), trypsin (EC 3.4.21.4), thrombin (EC 3.4.21.5), plasmin (EC 3.4.21.7), urokinase (EC 3.4.21.31), elastases (EC 3.4.21.36–37), cathepsin B (EC 3.4.22.1), papain (EC 3.4.22.2), ficin (EC 3.4.22.3), bromelain (EC 3.4.22.4), pepsins (EC 3.4.23.1–3), chymosin (EC 3.4.23.4), cathepsin D (EC 3.4.23.5), microbial aspartic proteases (all EC 3.4.23.6), collagenase (EC 3.4.24.3), thermolysin (EC 3.4.24.4), euphorbain (EC 3.4.99.7), keratin hydrolase (EC 3.4.99...) and others.

Another approach in detecting PROT activities is the use of chromogenic peptide substrates containing the terminal groups 2-naphthylamide, 1- or 2-naphthyl esters, ethyl or methyl esters, and *p*-nitroanilide. Naphthylamine and naphthols liberated as a result of PROT action are then coupled to a suitable diazonium salt (e.g., Fast Black K, Fast Blue B, Fast Garnet GBC, Fast Red TR) to generate an insoluble azo dye. The use of derivatives of 4-methoxy-2-naphthylamine, which complexes much more quickly with diazonium salts than does 2-naphthylamine, reduces the problem of diffusion during color development. Besides that, when a post-coupling technique is used, the progress of enzyme action towards those substrates can be assessed from time to time by viewing the gel under long-wave UV light, where the blue bands of fluorescent reaction product, 1-methoxy-3-naphthylamine, are visible.[14] Peptide substrates containing the terminal groups 2-naphthylamide and a naphthyl ester are not always as specific and sensitive as substrates containing the *p*-nitroanilide group.[15] The enzymatically released yellow-colored *p*-nitroaniline is observed visually or registered spectrophotometrically at 405 nm. However, *p*-nitroaniline is usually too faintly colored to be readily observed on the gel, but when diazotized and coupled with naphthylethylenediamine, a clearly visible red azo dye is formed. This dye does not precipitate in a gel matrix and preservation of zymograms is not possible. However, when the "enzymoblotting" method (based on transferring enzymes from electrophoretic gel to nitrocellulose membrane) is used, the colored reaction products may be bound to nitrocellulose, thus increasing both the sensitivity and the resolution of the method and providing zymograms that are stable for a long time when stored frozen.[15] Peptides containing the ethyl ester terminal group are used as substrates for esteroproteases. Ethanol liberated as a result of enzyme action is then detected using alcohol dehydrogenase and the PMS/MTT system.[16] Substrates containing the ethyl ester terminal group liberate the $CH_3O^-$ acidic ion, which causes local pH change in the gel areas where esteroprotease activities are localized. The alkaline–acidic pH change is then detected via the indicator dye Bromothymol Blue.[17] Peptides containing the 4-methylcoumarin terminal group can also be used as fluorogenic substrates for PROT detection. A number of chromogenic substrates suitable for PROT activity detection on electrophoretic gels are now commercially available. Some of them are listed below:

| Chromogenic Substrates | Proteinases |
| --- | --- |
| N-Acetyl-L-methionine α-Naphthyl ester | Submandibular esteroprotease A |
| N²-Acetyl-N-(p-nitrophenyl)-L-tyrosinamide* | Chymotrypsin |
| N-α-Benzoyl-D,L-arginine-β-naphthylamide | Trypsin |
| N-α-Benzoyl-L-arginine ethyl ester | Plasma kallikrein |
| N-α-Benzoyl-D,L-arginine-p-nitroanilide | Trypsin |
| N²-Benzoyl-N-(p-nitrophenyl)-L-argininamide* | Trypsin |
| N-Benzoyl-Phe-Val-Arg-p-nitroanilide | Thrombin, trypsin, reptilase |
| N-Benzoyl-Pro-Phe-Arg-p-nitroanilide | Plasma kallikrein, thrombin-like proteinase (*Agkistrodon contortrix*) |
| N-Benzoyl-L-tyrosine-p-nitroanilide | Chymotrypsin |
| N-CBZ-Ala–Arg–Arg-4-methoxy-β-naphthylamide** | Kathepsin B |
| N-CBZ-Gly-Gly-Arg-β-naphthylamide | Human serum trypsin |
| N-CBZ-Gly-Gly-Leu-p-nitroanilide | Subtilisin |
| N-CBZ-Leu-Leu-Glu-β-naphthylamide | Cation-sensitive proteinase |

## Chromogenic Substrates (continued)

| Chromogenic Substrates (continued) | Proteinases |
|---|---|
| N-CBZ-Pro-Phe-His-Leu-Leu-Val-Tyr-Ser β-naphthylamide | Renin |
| pGlu-Gly-Arg-p-nitroanilide*** | Urokinase |
| pGlu-Phe-Leu-p-nitroanilide | Papain, ficin, bromelain |
| N-Glutaryl-phenylalanine-β-naphthylamide | Chymotrypsin |
| H-D-Ile-Pro-Arg-p-nitroanilide | Human epidermal keratin hydrolase |
| D-Phe-L-pipecolyl-Arg-p-nitroanilide | Thrombin |
| H-D-Pro-Phe-Arg-p-nitroanilide | Plasma kallikrein |
| N-Succinyl-Ala-Ala-Ala-p-nitroanilide | Elastase |
| N-Succinyl-Ala-Ala-Pro-Leu-p-nitroanilide | Elastase |
| N-Succinyl-Ala-Ala-Pro-Phe-p-nitroanilide | Chymotrypsin, human leukocyte cathepsin G |
| N-Succinyl-phenylalanine-p-nitroanilide | Chymotrypsin |
| N-α-p-Tosyl-L-arginine methyl ester | Tamase, submandibular esteroprotease A |
| N-p-Tosyl-Gly-Pro-Arg-p-nitroanilide | Thrombin |
| N-p-Tosyl-Gly-Pro-Lys-p-nitroanilide | Plasmin |
| H-D-Val-Leu-Arg-p-nitroanilide | Tissue kallikrein |

* Yellow p-nitrophenol is liberated from the product after treatment of the gel at high temperature (100°C).
** CBZ, "carbobenzoxy".
*** pGLU, "pyroglutamyl".

Usually it is not possible to attribute the bands developed using chromogenic peptide substrates to any one proteinase with certainty except when purified enzymes are electrophorized. In some cases, however, specific PROT can be identified using certain chromogenic substrates in couple with specific inhibitors and taking into account such information as pH-optimum, tissue specificity, the preference to cleave peptide bonds only at certain few amino acids, existence of a proenzyme, and differences in proenzyme-activating agents.

The detection methods that may be considered as semispecific for certain proteinases are given separately (see 3.4.21.1 — CT; 3.4.21.4 — T; 3.4.21.5 — THR; 3.4.21.10 — ACR; 3.4.21.31 — UK; 3.4.21.34 — PKK; 3.4.21.36 — EL; 3.4.21.40 — EP; 3.4.23.1-3 — P).

The only way to specifically detect certain proteinases on electrophoretic gels is to use specific antibodies and labeled anti-antibodies, i.e., to use the immunoblotting procedure (for details see Part II). This procedure was successfully applied towards human uropepsinogen (see 3.4.23.1-3 — P, Other Methods).

## GENERAL NOTES

Many PROT exist in proenzyme forms and are converted into active enzymes only under certain conditions. For example, plasminogen is converted into plasmin by urokinase; activation of proelastase is under trypsin control; pepsinogen is converted into pepsin in acid conditions (0.1 $M$ HCl). In normal tissues, the active forms of many PROT are under control of tissue proteinase inhibitors. The examples are keratin hydrolase and urokinase.[9]

Cysteine (or thyol) PROT require thyol reagents (e.g., cysteine) for their stability. So, cysteine is usually included in extraction and staining solutions when these proteinases are analyzed.

Staining of aspartic (or acid) PROT is carried out at pH below 5 (usually at pH 2.5 to 3.5).

When a protein substrate is incorporated directly into the separating gel, the use of SDS–PAG is recommended to denature PROT and to prevent their action during the electrophoresis. After completion of electrophoresis, SDS should be removed by washing the gel in 2.5% Triton X-100 to renature PROT. Subsequent equilibration of the gel in an appropriate buffer is also needed for optimal PROT activity.

Because 2-naphthylamide derivatives are potential carcinogens, their solutions should be handled with extreme caution.

## REFERENCES

1. Andary, T. J. and Dabich, D., A sensitive polyacrylamide disc gel method for detection of proteinases, *Anal. Biochem.*, 57, 457, 1974.
2. Höfelmann, M., Kittsteiner-Eberle, R., and Schreier, P., Ultrathin-layer agar gels: a novel print technique for ultrathin-layer isoelectric focusing of enzymes, *Anal. Biochem.*, 128, 217, 1983.
3. Foltmann, B., Szecsi, P. B., and Tarasova, N. I., Detection of proteases by clotting of casein after gel electrophoresis, *Anal. Biochem.*, 146, 353, 1985.
4. Kaminski, E. and Bushuk, W., Detection of multiple forms of proteolytic enzymes by starch–gel electrophoresis, *Can. J. Biochem.*, 46, 1317, 1968.
5. Hanley, W. B., Boyer, S. H., and Naughton, M. A., Electrophoretic and functional heterogeneity of pepsinogen in several species, *Nature*, 209, 996, 1966.
6. Herd, J. K. and Motycka, L., Detection of proteolytic enzymes in agar electrophoresis, *Anal. Biochem.*, 53, 514, 1973.
7. Foissy, H. A., A method for demonstrating bacterial proteolytic isoactivities after electrophoresis in acrylamide gels, *J. Appl. Bacteriol.*, 37, 133, 1974.
8. Every, D., Quantitative measurement of protease activities in slab polyacrylamide gel electrophoretograms, *Anal. Biochem.*, 116, 519, 1981.
9. Hibino, T., Purification and characterization of keratin hydrolase in psoriatic epidermis: application of keratin–agarose plate and keratin–polyacrylamide enzymography methods, *Anal. Biochem.*, 147, 342, 1985.
10. Burger, W. C. and Schroeder, R. L., A sensitive method for detecting endopeptidases in electrofocused thin-layer gels, *Anal. Biochem.*, 71, 384, 1976.
11. Ward, C. W., Detection of proteolytic enzymes in polyacrylamide gels, *Anal. Biochem.*, 74, 242, 1976.
12. Dijkhof, J. and Poort, C., Visualization of proelastase in polyacrylamide gels, *Anal. Biochem.*, 83, 315, 1977.
13. Lynn, K. R. and Clevette-Radford, N. A., Staining for protease activity on polyacrylamide gels, *Anal. Biochem.*, 117, 280, 1981.
14. Mort, J. S. and Leduc, M., A simple, economical method for staining gels for cathepsin B–like activity, *Anal. Biochem.*, 119, 148, 1982.
15. Ohlsson, B. G., Weström, B. R., and Karlsson, B. W., Enzymoblotting: a method for localizing proteinases and their zymogens using *para*-nitroanilide substrates after agarose gel electrophoresis and transfer to nitrocellulose, *Anal. Biochem.*, 152, 239, 1986.
16. Fujimoto, Y., Morija, H., Yamaguchi, K., and Moriwaki, C., Detection of arginine esterase of various kallikrein preparations on gellified electrophoretic media, *J. Biochem.* (Tokyo), 71, 751, 1972.
17. Skow, L. C., Genetic variation at a locus (TAM-1) for submaxillary gland protease in the mouse and its location on chromosome 7, *Genetics*, 90, 713, 1978.

OTHER NAMES    Pepsin A (EC 3.4.23.1), pepsin B (EC 3.4.23.2), pepsin C (EC 3.4.23.3)

REACTIONS    Pepsin A:   preferential cleavage at Phe-, Leu-

Pepsin B:  more restricted specificity than pepsin A; degradation of gelatin; little activity with hemoglobin as substrate

Pepsin C:  more restricted specificity than pepsin A; high activity toward hemoglobin

ENZYME SOURCE  Vertebrates

## METHOD

### Visualization Scheme

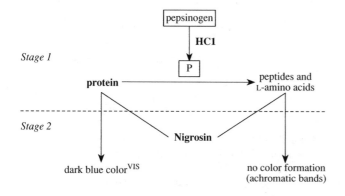

### Staining Solution[1]
A. 0.06 *N* HCl, pH 1.4
   0.65% Bovine hemoglobin
B. 10% Acetic acid in 50% methanol
C. 0.2 mg/ml Nigrosin in solution B

### Procedure
Immerse gel in solution A for 10 min and then place in a humid chamber and incubate at 37°C for 1 h. Immerse incubated gel in solution B for 18 h to fix the undigested protein and to wash away products of degradation. Stain gel in solution C and wash in solution B to remove unbound Nigrosin. The gel areas occupied by P are indicated by achromatic bands visible on a dark blue background.

*Notes:*  Other proteins, e.g., bovine serum albumin, can be used in place of hemoglobin, and Amidoblack can be used in place of Nigrosine.[2]

Some proteinases with pepsin-like activity (e.g., cathepsin D) can also be detected by this method. The bands caused by other then pepsin proteinase activities can, in some cases, be identified by omitting the stage of treating the gel with HCl.

## OTHER METHODS

The immunoblotting procedure was used to detect human uropepsinogen after PAG electrophoresis using polyclonal rabbit anti-uropepsinogen antibodies and commercial preparation of peroxidase-labeled goat anti-rabbit immunoglobulin.[3] This method is highly specific; however, its application is very limited.

### REFERENCES
1. Harris, H. and Hopkinson, D. A., *Handbook of Enzyme Electrophoresis in Human Genetics*, North-Holland, Amsterdam (Loose leaf with supplements in 1977 and 1978), 1976.
2. Hanley, W. B., Boyer, S. H., and Naughton, M. A., Electrophoretic and functional heterogeneity of pepsinogen in several species, *Nature*, 209, 996, 1966.
3. Kishi, K. and Yasuda, T., Newly characterized genetic polymorphism of uropepsinogen group A (PGA) using both isoelectric focusing and immunoblotting, Hum. Genet., 75, 209, 1987.

## 3.5.1.1 — Asparaginase; ASP

OTHER NAMES    Asparaginase II

REACTION    L-Asparagine + $H_2O$ = L-aspartate + $NH_3$

ENZYME SOURCE   Bacteria, green alga, fungi, invertebrates, vertebrates

## METHOD

### Visualization Scheme

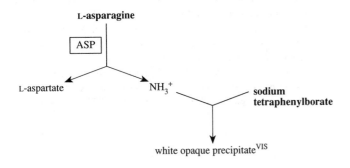

### Staining Solution[1]
  A. 0.2 *M* Tris–phosphate buffer, pH 8.0      20 ml
      L-Asparagine      52 mg
      Sodium tetraphenylborate      70 mg
  B. 2% Agar solution      20 ml

### Procedure
Mix A and B solutions and pour the mixture over the surface of electrophorized PAG. Incubate the gel at 37°C in a humid chamber until white opaque bands appear.

*Notes:*   All solutions used for ASP electrophoresis and detection should be made using bidistilled water lacking ammonia.

### OTHER METHODS

A. The areas of ammonia production can be detected using the backward reaction of a linking enzyme, glutamate dehydrogenase (e.g., see 3.5.4.4 — ADA, Method 2). Dark (nonfluorescent) bands of the enzyme activity are observed on a light (fluorescent) background in long-wave UV light.

B. The local pH change due to the production of ammonia can be detected using the pH indicator dye Phenol Violet (e.g., see 3.5.4.4 — ADA, Method 3), the NBT (or MTT)/dithiothreitol system (e.g., see 3.5.3.1 — ARG, Method 1), or neutral $AgNO_3$ solution containing photographic developers (e.g., see 3.5.1.5 — UR, Method 2).

C. The areas of L-aspartate production can be detected using two linking enzymes, glutamic–oxaloacetic transaminase and malate dehydrogenase (e.g., see 2.6.1.1 — GOT, Method 2). Dark (nonfluorescent) bands of ASP activity are visible in long-wave UV light on the light (fluorescent) background of the gel.

D. Positive tetrazolium staining of the areas of L-aspartate production can be achieved by using two linking enzymes, glutamic–oxaloacetic transaminase and glutamate dehydrogenase (e.g., see 2.6.1.1 — GOT, Method 4).

### REFERENCE
1. Pajdak, E. and Pajdak, W., A simple and sensitive method for detection of L-asparaginase by polyacrylamide gel electrophoresis, *Anal. Biochem.*, 50, 317, 1972.

## 3.5.1.2 — Glutaminase; GLUT

REACTION    L-Glutamine + $H_2O$ = L-glutamate + $NH_3$

ENZYME SOURCE   Bacteria, fungi, invertebrates, vertebrates

## METHOD

### Visualization Scheme

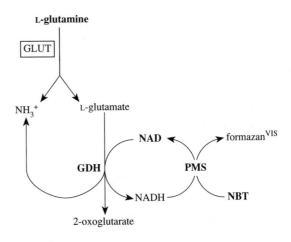

### Staining Solution[1]
0.1 *M* Potassium phosphate buffer, pH 7.1
15 m*M* L-Glutamine
20 U/ml Glutamate dehydrogenase (GDH)
2 mg/ml NAD
2 mg/ml NBT
0.04 mg/ml PMS

### Procedure
Incubate the gel in staining solution in the dark at 37°C until dark blue bands appear. Fix stained gel in 50% ethanol.

*Notes:*   Use L-glutamine that is free of L-glutamate, or purify crude L-glutamine using a Dowex 1-C1 column.

### OTHER METHODS

A. The local pH change due to the production of ammonia can be detected using the pH indicator dye Phenol Violet (e.g., see 3.5.4.4 — ADA, Method 3), the NBT (or MTT)/dithiothreitol system (e.g., see 3.5.3.1 — ARG, Method 1), or neutral $AgNO_3$ solution containing photographic developers (e.g., see 3.5.1.5 — UR, Method 2).

B. Tetraphenylborate can also be used to detect ammonia ions produced by GLUT (see 3.5.1.1 — ASP). This method is applicable only to transparent electrophoretic gels.

### REFERENCE
1. Davis, J. N. and Prusiner, S., Stain for glutaminase activity, *Anal. Biochem.*, 54, 272, 1973.

REACTION        Urea + $H_2O$ = $CO_2$ + $2NH_3$

ENZYME SOURCE  Bacteria, fungi, plants, vertebrates

## METHOD 1

### Visualization Scheme

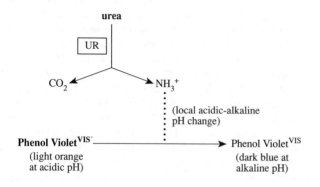

### Staining Solution[1]

| | |
|---|---:|
| Urea | 5 g |
| Agar | 1 g |
| Phenol Violet (saturated water solution) | 10 ml |
| $H_2O$ | 90 ml |

### Procedure

Dissolve the components of the staining solution by heating in a boiling water bath, cool the solution to 45°C, and pour over the gel surface. Incubate the gel at 37°C until dark blue bands appear on a light orange background of the gel. Record or photograph the zymogram.

*Notes:*  Electrode and gel buffers used for UR electrophoresis should be of minimal ionic strength.

## METHOD 2

### Visualization Scheme

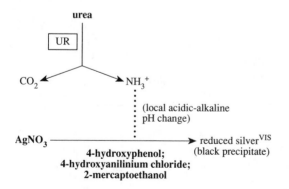

### Staining Solution[2]

A. 10 m*M* 2-Mercaptoethanol
B. 10 m*M* 2-Mercaptoethanol
   250 m*M* Urea
C. 0.2 mg/ml 4-Hydroxyphenol
   0.2 mg/ml 4-Hydroxyanilinium chloride (freshly prepared and
     adjusted to pH 8.0 ± 0.1 by 0.25 *M* NaOH)
D. 2 mg/ml $AgNO_3$

### Procedure

After electrophoresis, immerse PAG sequentially in 100 ml of solution A (30 min: 10 min × three changes), solution B (3 min), and solution C (2 min) under continuous shaking. Wash gel quickly (15 s) with 100 ml glass-distilled water to eliminate solution C from both the gel surface and the container, and immerse in 100 ml of solution D. The UR activity bands become visible at this last step, the faintest ones requiring about 5 min. After this period of time only the background increases. This undesirable process can be prevented by immersing the gel in 5% (v/v) acetic acid. However, the developed bands show a tendency to bleach in this solution. Thus, the stained and fixed gel is recommended to be washed with abundant glass-distilled water and then dried or photographed.

*Notes:*  Using this method, 0.015 units of UR per band can be detected.

## OTHER METHODS

A. The areas of ammonia production can also be detected using the backward reaction of a linking enzyme, glutamate dehydrogenase (e.g., see 3.5.4.4 — ADA, Method 2). Dark (nonfluorescent) bands of enzyme activity are observed on a light (fluorescent) background in long-wave UV light.
B. The areas of ammonia production can also be detected using tetraphenylborate (see 3.5.1.1 — ASP). This method is applicable only to transparent electrophoretic gels.
C. The local pH change due to the production of ammonia can also be detected using the NBT (or MTT)/dithiothreitol system (e.g., see 3.5.3.1 — ARG, Method 1).

### REFERENCES

1. Daly, M. P. and Tully, E. R., Detection of ammonia-producing enzymes after electrophoresis: a screening procedure for adenosine deaminase in blood, *Biochem. Soc. Trans.*, 5, 1756, 1977.
2. Martin de Llano, J. J., Garcia-Segura, J. M., and Gavilanes, J. G., Selective silver staining of urease activity in polyacrylamide gels, *Anal. Biochem.*, 177, 37, 1989.

OTHER NAMES    Dehydropeptidase II, histozyme, hippuricase, benzamidase, acylase I

REACTION    $N$-Acyl-L-amino acid + $H_2O$ = fatty acid anion + L-amino acid

ENZYME SOURCE    Bacteria, fungi, vertebrates

## METHOD

### Visualization Scheme

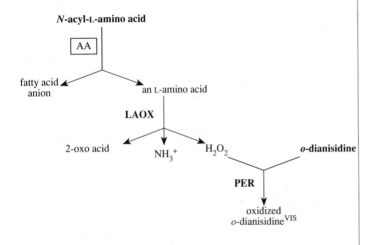

### Staining Solution[1]

| | |
|---|---|
| 0.3 $M$ Sodium phosphate buffer, pH 7.5 | 5 ml |
| $N$-Acetyl-L-methionine (or $N$-formyl-L-methionine) | 10 mg |
| L-Amino acid oxidase (LAOX; crude snake venom from *Agkistrodon piscivorus* or *Crotalus adamanteus*) | 3 mg |
| Peroxidase (PER) | 3 mg |
| $o$-Dianisidine dihydrochloride | 5 mg |
| 12.5 m$M$ MnCl$_2$ | 0.2 ml |

### Procedure

Apply the staining solution to the surface of electrophorized acetate cellulose or starch gel and incubate in a humid chamber at 37°C until brown bands appear. Fix stained gel in 7% acetic acid.

*Notes:* When acetate cellulose gel is used for AA electrophoresis, only about 10 µg of protein (2 to 5 µl of cell extract) is needed to detect the enzyme activity bands by this method.

## OTHER METHODS

A. A bioautographic procedure can also be used to visualize AA activity bands on electrophoretic gels.[2] The principle of bioautography is the visualization of an enzyme by a zone of bacterial growth that results when an auxotrophic bacterium is supplied with a product of the enzyme (see Part II for details). This procedure has its own limitations (e.g., to produce optimal banding patterns, conditions must be maintained that do not interfere either with bacterial growth or with enzyme activity) and is not as practical as the method described above.

B. A procedure for spectrophotometric detection of AA activity bands on electrophoretic PAG has also been developed.[3] The method is based on the use of $N$-acetyl-L-cysteine as substrate and on the strong absorbance at 296 nm of a ketimine ring which is formed by the reaction of the enzymatic product (L-cysteine) with 3-bromopyruvate. The procedure allows one to visualize up to about 1 to 10 mU of the enzyme, but it also is not practical because it requires the use of a scanning spectrophotometer or a special optic device used for two-dimensional spectroscopy of electrophoretic gels.[4]

## REFERENCES

1. Qavi, H. and Kit, S., Electrophoretic patterns of aminoacylase-1 (ACY-1) isozymes in vertebrate cells and histochemical procedure for detecting ACY-1 activity, *Biochem. Genet.*, 18, 669, 1980.
2. Naylor, S. L., Shows, T. B., and Klebe, R. J., Bioautographic visualization of aminoacylase-1: assignment of the structural gene ACY-1 to chromosome 3 in man, *Somat. Cell Genet.*, 5, 11, 1979.
3. Ricci, G., Caccuri, A. M., Lo Bello, M., Solinas, S. P., and Nardini, M., Ketimine rings: useful detectors of enzymatic activities in solution and on polyacrylamide gel, *Anal. Biochem.*, 165, 356, 1987.
4. Klebe, R. J., Mancuso, M. G., Brown, C. R., and Teng, L., Two-dimensional spectroscopy of electrophoretic gels, *Biochem. Genet.*, 19, 655, 1981.

| | |
|---|---|
| REACTION | Pantetheine + $H_2O$ = cysteamine + pantothenate |
| | Also acts on a variety of pantetheine derivatives |
| ENZYME SOURCE | Vertebrates (mammals) |

## METHOD

### Visualization Scheme

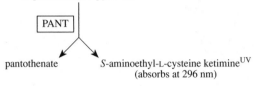

**S-pantetheine 3-pyruvate**

PANT

pantothenate      S-aminoethyl-L-cysteine ketimine[UV] (absorbs at 296 nm)

### Staining Solution[1]
 0.1 $M$ Phosphate buffer, pH 8.0
 4 m$M$ S-Pantetheine 3-pyruvate

### Procedure
Incubate electrophorized PAG in the staining solution at 20°C for 30 min, wash with water, and scan at 296 nm using a scanning spectrophotometer (e.g., Beckman gel scanner apparatus).

*Notes:* The method is semiquantitative. After a 30-min incubation the intensity of the peak observed on photometric scan is proportional to the amount of enzyme applied on the gel, in the range of 0.001 to 0.01 U.

    Two-dimensional spectrograms of processed PAGs can also be obtained using a special optical device constructed for two-dimensional spectroscopy of electrophoretic gels.[2]

### REFERENCES
 1. Ricci, G., Caccuri, A. M., Lo Bello, M., Solinas, S. P., and Nardini, M., Ketimine rings: useful detectors of enzymatic activities in solution and on polyacrylamide gel, *Anal. Biochem.*, 165, 356, 1987.
 2. Klebe, R. J., Mancuso, M. G., Brown, C. R., and Teng, L., Two-dimensional spectroscopy of electrophoretic gels, *Biochem. Genet.*, 19, 655, 1981.

| | |
|---|---|
| OTHER NAMES | β-Lactamase (recommended name), cephalosporinase |
| REACTION | β-lactam + $H_2O$ = substituted β-amino acid |
| ENZYME SOURCE | Bacteria |

## METHOD

### Visualization Scheme

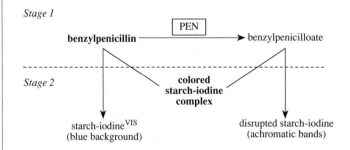

*Stage 1*

**benzylpenicillin** ⟶ PEN ⟶ benzylpenicilloate

*Stage 2*      **colored starch-iodine complex**

starch-iodine[VIS] (blue background)      disrupted starch-iodine (achromatic bands)

### Staining Solution[1]
 A. 10 m$M$ Potassium phosphate buffer, pH 7.0
     0.5 $M$ NaCl
     100 mg/ml Benzylpenicillin
 B. 0.25 $M$ $I_2$
     1.25 $M$ KI
 C. 2% Starch soluble for iodometry (Fisher Scientific); dissolved in distilled water by heating and stirring

### Procedure
Add 1 part of solution B to 100 parts of freshly prepared solution C. Dip a strip of Whatman 3MM paper in starch–iodine solution and hang to dry overnight. Store prepared strips in a dark, cool, and dry place before use.

    Place electrophorized PAG on a glass plate of an appropriate size and cover with a strip of Whatman 3MM paper soaked in solution A. Apply a second glass plate, avoiding formation of air bubbles, press down firmly and evenly, and incubate at room temperature for 8 to 10 min. Remove the top glass plate and the first paper application. Cover gel with starch–iodine paper saturated with solution A and press down firmly and evenly with another glass plate. Invert gel with glass plates and observe white bands of PEN activity on a dark blue background. Mark the position of achromatic bands and the "origin" on a glass plate by a marker.

*Notes:* This method is based on the ability of penicilloic acid, produced by PEN, to reduce $I_2$ and hence to decolorize the starch–iodine complex.

## OTHER METHODS

An immunoblotting procedure (for details see Part II) based on the utility of antibodies specific to the *E. coli* enzyme and [125]I-protein A as a radiolabel for anti-antibodies is also available.[1] This procedure, however, is more time-consuming and labor-intensive in comparison to that described above.

### REFERENCE
 1. Tai, P. C., Zyk, N., and Citri, N., *In situ* detection of β-lactamase activity in sodium dodecyl sulfate–polyacrylamide gels, *Anal. Biochem.*, 144, 199, 1985.

## 3.5.2.11 — L-Lysine lactamase; LL

**REACTION**    L-Lysine 1,6-lactam + $H_2O$ = L-lysin

**ENZYME SOURCE**  Bacteria

## METHOD

### Visualization Scheme

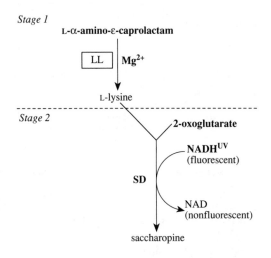

### Staining Solution[1] (adapted)
A.  0.05 $M$ Tris–HCl buffer, pH 9.0
    0.3 m$M$ $MgCl_2$
    2.5 m$M$ L-α-Amino-ε-caprolactam
B.  2% Agar solution (60°C)
C.  0.1 $M$ Potassium phosphate buffer, pH 6.8
    0.3 m$M$ NADH
    2.5 m$M$ 2-Oxoglutarate
    1 U/ml Saccharopine dehydrogenase (NAD, L-lysine–
    forming) (SD)

### Procedure
Mix equal volumes of A and B solutions and pour the mixture over the gel surface. Incubate the gel at 37°C for 30 to 60 min. Remove agar overlay. Apply solution C to the gel surface on a filter-paper overlay and incubate for 20 to 30 min at 37°C in a moist chamber. View gel under long-wave UV light. Dark (nonfluorescent) bands of LL activity are visible on a light (fluorescent) background. Record the zymogram or photograph using a yellow filter.

*Notes:*  Lysine lactamase shows maximum reactivity at a pH value about 9.0 and the rate of substrate hydrolysis declines markedly below pH values of 8.0. Saccharopine dehydrogenase has a narrow pH-optimum at 6.0 to 7.0. The use of a two-step staining procedure allows one to avoid the problem of different pH-optima of the two enzymes.

### REFERENCE
1.  Laber, B. and Amrhein, N., A spectrophotometric assay for *meso*-diaminopimelate decarboxylase and L-α-amino-ε-caprolactam hydrolase, *Anal. Biochem.*, 181, 297, 1989.

## 3.5.3.1 — Arginase; ARG

**OTHER NAMES**    Arginine amidinase, canavanase

**REACTION**        L-Arginine + $H_2O$ = L-ornithine + urea

**ENZYME SOURCE**  Bacteria, fungi, plants, invertebrates, vertebrates

## METHOD 1

### Visualization Scheme

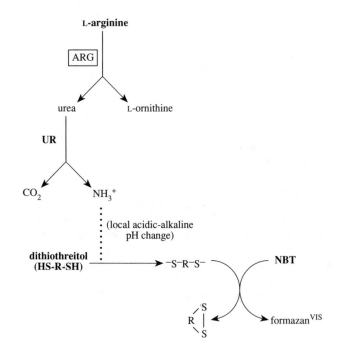

### Staining Solution[1]
| | |
|---|---:|
| A.  2 mg/ml Urease (UR; Sigma, type VI) | 1 ml |
| 0.85 $M$ L-Arginine (pH 6.8) | 2 ml |
| 0.1 $M$ Dithiothreitol | 0.6 ml |
| 1.3% NBT | 0.3 ml |
| B.  2% Agar solution (45°C) | 15 ml |

### Procedure
Mix A and B components of the staining solution and pour the mixture over the gel surface. Incubate the gel at 37°C until dark blue bands appear. Wash stained gel with water and fix in 50% ethanol.

*Notes:*  All solutions used for ARG electrophoresis and detection should be made using bidistilled water lacking ammonia. Electrode and gel buffers used for ARG electrophoresis should be of minimal ionic strength.

## 3.5.3.1 — Arginase; ARG (continued)

### METHOD 2

#### Visualization Scheme

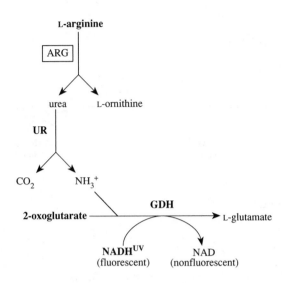

#### Staining Solution[2]

| | |
|---|---:|
| 0.1 $M$ Tris–HCl buffer, pH 7.6 | 5 ml |
| Urease (UR; Sigma, type VI) | 20 units |
| 2-Oxoglutarate | 25 mg |
| NADH | 10 mg |
| Glutamate dehydrogenase (GDH; Sigma, 500 units/ml) | 50 µl |

#### Procedure

Apply the staining solution to the gel surface on filter-paper overlay and incubate at 37°C until dark (nonfluorescent) bands visible under long-wave UV light on a light (fluorescent) background appear.

### OTHER METHODS

The areas of ammonia production can also be detected using the pH indicator dye Phenol Violet (e.g., see 3.5.4.4 — ADA, Method 3), sodium tetraphenylborate (e.g., see 3.5.1.1 — ASP), and neutral $AgNO_3$ solution containing photographic developers (e.g., see 3.5.1.5 — UR, Method 2).

### GENERAL NOTES

The enzyme activity (at least in mammals) is inhibited by citrate and borate. Thus, electrophoretic and staining buffers containing these substances are unsuitable for ARG electrophoresis and detection.

The enzyme from some sources is activated by manganese ions.

### REFERENCES

1. Farron, F., Arginase isozymes and their detection by catalytic staining in starch gel, *Anal. Biochem.*, 53, 264, 1973.
2. Nelson, R. L., Povey, S., Hopkinson, D. A., and Harris, H., The detection after electrophoresis of enzymes involved in ammonia metabolism using L-glutamate dehydrogenase as a linking enzyme, *Biochem. Genet.*, 15, 1023, 1977.

## 3.5.4.3 — Guanine Deaminase; GDA

| | |
|---|---|
| OTHER NAMES | Guanase, guanine aminase |
| REACTION | Guanine + $H_2O$ = xanthine + $NH_3$ |
| ENZYME SOURCE | Invertebrates, vertebrates |

### METHOD

#### Visualization Scheme

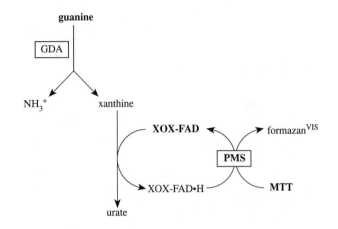

#### Staining Solution[1]

A. 0.2 $M$ Tris–HCl buffer, pH 7.6

| | |
|---|---:|
| | 20 ml |
| 1 mg/ml Guanine (prepared by dissolving 50 mg guanine in 10 ml warm 0.1 $N$ NaOH and made up to 50 ml with water) | 3 ml |
| 4 U/ml Xanthine oxidase (XOX) | 25 µl |
| MTT | 7.5 mg |
| PMS | 2.5 mg |
| B. 2% Agar solution (60°C) | 25 ml |

#### Procedure

Mix A and B components of the staining solution and pour the mixture over the gel surface. Incubate overlayed gel in the dark at 37°C until dark blue bands appear. Fix zymogram in 50% ethanol.

### OTHER METHODS

A. The areas of ammonia production can be detected using the backward reaction of a linking enzyme, glutamate dehydrogenase (e.g., see 3.5.3.1 — ARG, Method 2). Dark (nonfluorescent) bands of GDA activity are observed on a light (fluorescent) background of the gel in long-wave UV light.

B. The areas of ammonia production can also be detected using sodium tetraphenylborate, which precipitates in the presence of ammonia ions resulting in the formation of white opaque bands visible in PAG (see 3.5.1.1 — ASP).

C. The local pH change due to the production of ammonia can be detected using the pH indicator dye Phenol Violet (e.g., see 3.5.4.4 — ADA, Method 3), the NBT (or MTT)/dithiothreitol system (e.g., see 3.5.3.1 — ARG, Method 1), and neutral $AgNO_3$ solution containing photographic developers (e.g., see 3.5.1.5 — UR, Method 2).

### REFERENCE

1. Harris, H. and Hopkinson, D. A., *Handbook of Enzyme Electrophoresis in Human Genetics*, North-Holland, Amsterdam (Loose leaf with supplements in 1977 and 1978), 1976.

REACTION        Adenosine + H₂O = inosine + NH₃

ENZYME SOURCE   Bacteria, fungi, protozoa, invertebrates, vertebrates

## METHOD 1

### Visualization Scheme

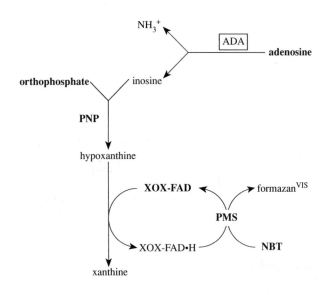

### Staining Solution[1]

A. 0.05 *M* Phosphate buffer, pH 7.5                    25 ml
   Adenosine                                            20 mg
   NBT                                                   5 mg
   PMS                                                   5 mg
   Xanthine oxidase (XOX)                               0.08 unit
   Purine-nucleoside phosphorylase (PNP)                0.08 unit
B. 2% Agar solution (60°C)                              25 ml

### Procedure
Mix A and B components of the staining solution and pour the mixture over the gel surface. Incubate the gel in the dark at 37°C until dark blue bands appear. Fix stained gel in 50% ethanol.

## METHOD 2

### Visualization Scheme

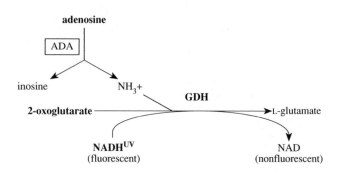

### Staining Solution[2]
0.1 *M* Tris–HCl buffer, pH 7.6                    5 ml
Adenosine                                         30 mg
2-Oxoglutarate                                    25 mg
NADH                                              10 mg
500 U/ml Glutamate dehydrogenase (GDH)            50 µl

### Procedure
Apply the staining solution to the gel surface on filter-paper overlay and incubate at 37°C until dark (nonfluorescent) bands visible in long-wave UV light appear on a light (fluorescent) background. Photograph developed gel using a yellow filter.

*Notes:*   To make ADA bands visible in daylight, cover the processed gel with a second filter-paper overlay containing PMS and MTT (or NBT). Achromatic bands corresponding to nonfluorescent areas visible in UV light appear almost immediately. The negative zymogram may be stored in 50% ethanol or 3% acetic acid.

## METHOD 3

### Visualization Scheme

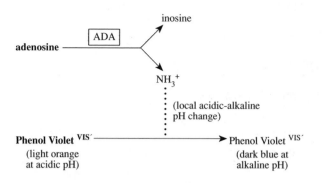

### Staining Solution[3]

| | |
|---|---|
| Adenosine | 1 g |
| Phenol Violet (saturated water solution) | 10 ml |
| Agar | 1 g |

### Procedure

Dissolve components of the staining solution at 100°C and cool to 45°C. Pour the mixture over the gel surface and incubate until dark blue bands appear on a light orange background.

*Notes:* All solutions used for ADA electrophoresis and detection should be made using bidistilled water lacking ammonia. Electrode and gel buffers should be of minimal ionic strength.

## OTHER METHODS

A. The areas of ammonia production can also be detected using sodium tetraphenylborate, which precipitates in the presence of ammonia ions, resulting in the formation of white opaque bands visible in PAG (e.g., see 3.5.1.1 — ASP).

B. The local pH change due to the production of ammonia can be detected using the NBT (MTT)/dithiothreitol system (e.g., see 3.5.3.1 — ARG, Method 1) and neutral $AgNO_3$ solution containing photographic developers (e.g., see 3.5.1.5 — UR, Method 2).

C. A bioautographic procedure (for details see Part II) for ADA location in electrophoretic gels has also been developed.[4] However, this procedure is more complex and less practical than any one of those described above.

## REFERENCES

1. Spencer, N., Hopkinson, D. A., and Harris, H., Adenosine deaminase polymorphism in man, *Ann. Hum. Genet.*, 32, 9, 1968.
2. Nelson, R. L., Povey, S., Hopkinson, D. A., and Harris, H., The detection after electrophoresis of enzymes involved in ammonia metabolism using L-glutamate dehydrogenase as a linking enzyme, *Biochem. Genet.*, 15, 1023, 1977.
3. Daly, M. P. and Tully, E. R., Detection of ammonia-producing enzymes after electrophoresis: a screening procedure for adenosine deaminase in blood, *Biochem. Soc. Trans.*, 5, 1756, 1977.
4. Naylor, S. L., Bioautographic visualization of enzymes, in *Isozymes. Current Topics in Biological and Medical Research, Vol. 4*, Rattazzi, M. C., Scandalios, J. M., and Whitt, G. S., Eds., Alan R. Liss, New York, 1980, 69.

## 3.5.4.5 — Cytidine Deaminase; CDA

REACTION          Cytidine + $H_2O$ = uridine + $NH_3$

ENZYME SOURCE  Bacteria, vertebrates

## METHOD 1

### Visualization Scheme

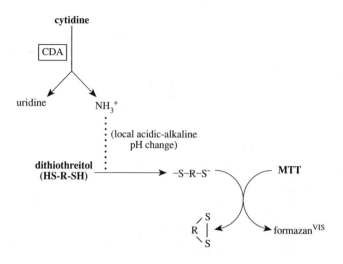

### Staining Solution[1]

| | | |
|---|---|---|
| A. | Cytidine | 15 mg |
| | 0.3% Dithiothreitol | 1 ml |
| | 5 MTT | 0.3 ml |
| | $H_2O$ | 10 ml |
| B. | 2% Agar solution (60°C) | 10 ml |

### Procedure

Mix A and B components of the staining solution and pour the mixture over the gel surface. Incubate the gel at 37°C until dark blue bands appear. Fix stained gel in 50% ethanol.

*Notes:* This method requires that the electrophoretic gel be only minimally buffered, since staining is dependent on the ability of thiol groups in dithiothreitol to reduce a tetrazolium dye nonenzymatically when there is a rise in pH. All solutions used for CDA electrophoresis and detection should be made using bidistilled water lacking ammonia.

## METHOD 2

### Visualization Scheme

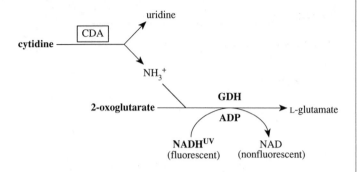

### Staining Solution[2]

| | |
|---|---|
| 0.1 $M$ Tris–HCl buffer, pH 7.6 | 5 ml |
| Cytidine | 40 mg |
| Dithiothreitol | 10 mg |
| ADP (disodium salt) | 10 mg |
| 2-Oxoglutarate | 25 mg |
| NADH | 10 mg |
| 500 U/ml Glutamate dehydrogenase (GDH) | 50 μl |

### Procedure

Apply the staining solution to the gel surface on filter-paper overlay and incubate at 37°C until dark (nonfluorescent) bands visible in long-wave UV light appear on a light (fluorescent) background. Record or photograph developed gel using a yellow filter.

*Notes:* To make CDA bands visible in daylight, cover the processed gel with filter paper soaked in PMS/MTT solution. Achromatic CDA bands appear on a blue background of the gel almost immediately. Fix negatively stained gel in 50% ethanol.

### OTHER METHODS

A. The areas of ammonia production can be detected using sodium tetraphenylborate, which precipitates in the presence of ammonia ions, resulting in the formation of white opaque bands visible in PAG (see 3.5.1.1 — ASP).

B. The local pH change due to the production of ammonia can also be detected using pH indicator dye Phenol Violet (e.g., see 3.5.4.4 — ADA, Method 3) and neutral AgNO₃ solution containing photographic developers (e.g., see 3.5.1.5 — UR, Method 2).

### REFERENCES

1. Teng, Y.-S., Anderson, J. E., and Giblett, E. R., Cytidine deaminase: a new genetic polymorphism demonstrated in human granulocytes, *Am. J. Hum. Genet.*, 27, 492, 1975.
2. Nelson, R. L., Povey, S., Hopkinson, D. A., and Harris, H., The detection after electrophoresis of enzymes involved in ammonia metabolism using L-glutamate dehydrogenase as a linking enzyme, *Biochem. Genet.*, 15, 1023, 1977.

## 3.5.4.6 — AMP Deaminase; AMPDA

**OTHER NAMES** Adenylate deaminase, adenylic acid deaminase, AMP aminase

**REACTION** $AMP + H_2O = IMP + NH_3$

**ENZYME SOURCE** Bacteria, fungi, vertebrates

## METHOD 1

### Visualization Scheme

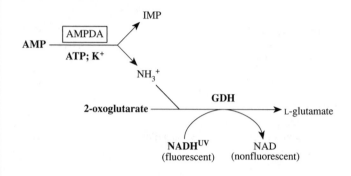

### Staining Solution

| | |
|---|---|
| 0.1 $M$ Tris–HCl buffer, pH 7.6 | 5 ml |
| AMP (disodium salt; 6H₂O) | 100 mg |
| ATP (disodium salt; 3H₂O) | 10 mg |
| KCl | 40 mg |
| 2-Oxoglutaric acid (neutralized) | 25 mg |
| NADH | 10 mg |
| 500 U/ml Glutamate dehydrogenase (GDH) | 50 μl |

### Procedure

Apply the staining solution to the gel surface on filter-paper overlay. Incubate covered gel in a humid chamber at 37°C and monitor under long-wave UV light. Dark (nonfluorescent) bands visible on a light (fluorescent) background indicate areas of AMPDA activity. Photograph developed gel using a yellow filter.

*Notes:* To make AMPDA bands visible in daylight, cover the processed gel with a second filter-paper overlay saturated with the PMS/MTT solution. Achromatic bands visible on a blue background appear almost immediately. Fix negatively stained gel in 50% ethanol or 3% acetic acid.

To increase the apparent affinity of the enzyme for AMP, ATP is included in the stain.

## METHOD 2

### Visualization Scheme

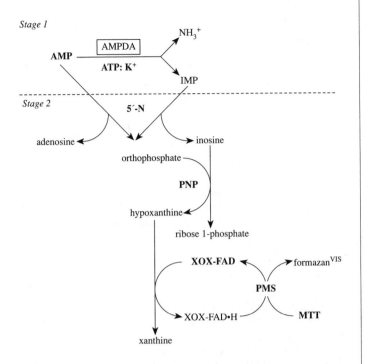

### Staining Solution[2]

A. 0.1 *M* Tris–HCl buffer, pH 7.8 — 10 ml
   AMP (disodium salt; $6H_2O$) — 200 mg
   ATP (disodium salt; $3H_2O$) — 10 mg
   KCl — 40 mg
B. 2% Agar solution (60°C) — 20 ml
C. 0.1 *M* Tris–HCl buffer, pH 7.8 — 10 ml
   100 U/mg 5′-Nucleotidase (5′-N) — 1 mg
   4 U/ml Xanthine oxidase (XOX) — 10 µl
   25 U/ml Purine-nucleoside phosphorylase
     (PNP) — 10 µl
   MTT — 2.5 mg
   PMS — 2.5 mg

### Procedure

Mix A with 10 ml B and pour the mixture over the gel surface. Incubate the gel at 37°C for 3 h. Remove first agar overlay. Mix C with remaining 10 ml B and pour over the gel surface. Incubate the gel with second agar overlay at 37°C in the dark until dark blue bands appear. Fix stained gel in 50% ethanol.

*Notes:* Additional bands caused by adenosine deaminase activity (see 3.5.4.4 — ADA, Method 1) can also be developed by this method. This is due to production of adenosine by the linking enzyme 5′-nucleotidase. Adenosine is then converted by endogenous ADA into inosine, which is detected as a result of the action of two other linking enzymes (PNP and XOX) present in the staining solution. Thus, when this method is used, a control staining for ADA should also be made in parallel with AMPDA staining.

To increase the apparent affinity of the enzyme for AMP, ATP and $K^+$ are included in the stain.

## METHOD 3

### Visualization Scheme

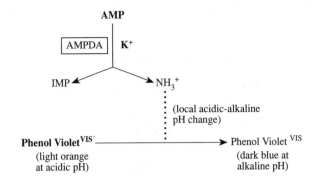

### Staining Solution[3]

A. AMP — 250 mg
   KCl — 550 mg
   Phenol Violet (saturated water solution) — 5 ml
   $H_2O$ — 20 ml
B. 2% Agar solution (60°C) — 25 ml

### Procedure

Mix A and B components of the staining solution and pour the mixture over the gel surface. Incubate overlayed gel at room temperature or at 37°C until dark blue bands appear on a light orange background. Record or photograph the zymogram.

*Notes:* This method requires that electrophoretic gel be only minimally buffered. All solutions should be prepared using bidistilled water lacking ammonia.

## OTHER METHODS

A. The local pH change due to the production of ammonia can also be detected using the NBT (or MTT)/dithiothreitol system (e.g., see 3.5.4.5 — CDA, Method 1) or neutral $AgNO_3$ solution containing photographic developers (e.g., see 3.5.1.5 — UR, Method 2).

B. The areas of ammonia production can be detected using sodium tetraphenylborate, which precipitates in the presence of ammonia ions, resulting in the formation of white opaque bands visible in PAG (e.g., see 3.5.1.1 — ASP).

### REFERENCES

1. Nelson, R. L., Povey, S., Hopkinson, D. A., and Harris, H., The detection after electrophoresis of enzymes involved in ammonia metabolism using L-glutamate dehydrogenase as a linking enzyme, *Biochem. Genet.*, 15, 1023, 1977.
2. Anderson, J. E., Teng, Y.-S., and Giblett, E. R., Stains for six enzymes potentially applicable to chromosomal assignment by cell hybridization, *Cytogenet. Cell Genet.*, 14, 465, 1975.
3. Daly, M. P. and Tully, E. R., Detection of ammonia-producing enzymes after electrophoresis: a screening procedure for adenosine deaminase in blood, *Biochem. Soc. Trans.*, 5, 1756, 1977.

## 3.6.1.1 — Inorganic Pyrophosphatase; PP

OTHER NAMES     Pyrophosphatase

REACTION        Pyrophosphate + H₂O = 2 orthophosphate

ENZYME SOURCE   Bacteria, fungi, plants, invertebrates, vertebrates

## METHOD 1

### Visualization Scheme

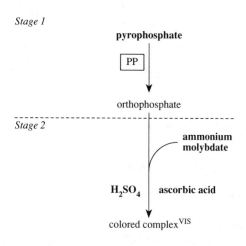

### Staining Solution[1]

A. 0.05 $M$ Tris–HCl buffer, pH 7.8        12.5 ml
   0.02 $M$ Pyrophosphate                  12.5 ml
   0.2 $M$ MgCl₂                           1.25 ml
B. 2% Agar solution (60°C)                 50 ml
C. Ascorbic acid                           2.5 g
   2.5% Ammonium molybdate in 4 $N$ H₂SO₄  25 ml

### Procedure

Mix solution A with 25 ml of solution B and pour the mixture over the gel surface. Incubate the gel with agar overlay for 30 to 60 min. Remove agar overlay. Mix solution C with remaining 25 ml of solution B and pour over the gel surface. Dark blue bands visible on a light blue background appear after 1 to 5 min. Record the zymogram or photograph because after about 1 h the PP bands disappear.

*Notes:*  To obtain permanent PP zymograms with colored bands stable for several months, the Malachite Green–phosphomolybdate method should be used.[2] In this method the first stage of PP activity detection is the same as described above. The second stage is treatment of the gel with orthophosphate detection solution, which is prepared as follows. Initially stock solutions of 0.045% Malachite Green (oxalate salt) and 4.2% ammonium molybdate in 4 $N$ HCl are prepared using deionized water. Then 90 ml of the Malachite Green solution and 30 ml of the ammonium molybdate solution are mixed for 20 min at room temperature, after which the mixture is passed through a Whatman No. 5 filter and 2.4 ml of 2% sterox (a detergent diluent used in flame photometry) are added. This stock solution may be prepared in advance and stored at 4°C for a week. The orthophosphate detection solution is prepared by mixing 60 ml of stock solution with 40 ml of deionized water immediately prior to use. After treatment with this solution, color development is usually complete in 10 to 20 min. Stained gel is washed with several changes of water and stored in water or 5% acetic acid, 20% ethanol. The color is stable for several months. The only restriction related to the use of the Malachite Green is prevention of color formation when a citrate-containing staining buffer is used.

## METHOD 2

### Visualization Scheme

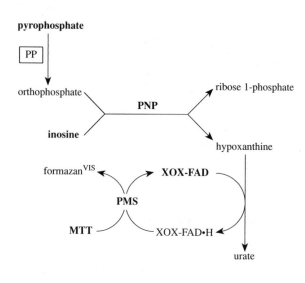

### Staining Solution[3] (adapted)

A. 0.01 $M$ Tris–HCl buffer, pH 7.5              23 ml
   0.1 $M$ Inosine                               2 ml
   0.75 U/ml Xanthine oxidase (XOX)              10 µl
   1.67 U/ml Purine-nucleoside phosphorylase     250 µl
   (PNP)
   MTT                                           10 mg
   PMS                                           3 mg
B. 2% Agarose solution (60°C)                    25 ml

### Procedure

Mix A and B components of the staining solution and pour the mixture over the gel surface. Incubate the gel in the dark at 37°C until dark blue bands appear. Fix stained gel in 50% ethanol.

### OTHER METHODS

Some other methods of orthophosphate detection are also available (e.g., see 3.1.3.1 — ALP, Methods 6 and 7).

### GENERAL NOTES

Orthophosphate should not be used as a component of any buffer used for electrophoresis or staining of PP.

### REFERENCES

1. Fisher, R. A., Turner, B. M., Dorkin, H. L., and Harris, H., Studies of human erythrocyte inorganic pyrophosphatase, *Ann. Hum. Genet.*, 37, 341, 1974.
2. Zlotnick, G. W. and Gottlieb, M., A sensitive staining technique for the detection of phosphohydrolase activities after polyacrylamide gel electrophoresis, *Anal. Biochem.*, 153, 121, 1986.
3. Klebe, R. J., Schloss, S., Mock, L., and Link, C. R., Visualization of isozymes which generate inorganic phosphate, *Biochem. Genet.*, 19, 921, 1981.

OTHER NAMES     Adenylpyrophosphatase, ATP monophosphatase, triphosphatase, ATPase

REACTION     ATP + H₂O = ADP + orthophosphate

ENZYME SOURCE    Bacteria, fungi, plants, protozoa, invertebrates, vertebrates

## METHOD 1

### Visualization Scheme

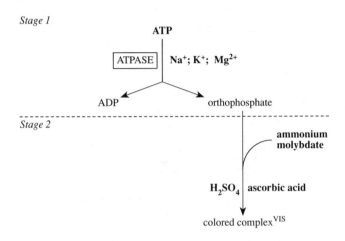

*Stage 1*

ATP

ATPASE   Na⁺; K⁺; Mg²⁺

ADP     orthophosphate

*Stage 2*

ammonium molybdate

H₂SO₄   ascorbic acid

colored complex$^{VIS}$

### Staining Solution[1] (modified)

A. 0.1 *M* Tris–HCl buffer, pH 7.6
    0.1 *M* NaCl
    20 m*M* KCl
    6 m*M* MgCl₂
    1.5 m*M* ATP
B. 1.5% Agar solution (60°C)
C. 100 mg/ml Ascorbic acid
    2.5% Ammonium molybdate in 4 *N* H₂SO₄

### Procedure

Mix equal volumes of A and B solutions and pour the mixture over the gel surface. Incubate the gel 1 to 2 h at 37°C. Remove first agar overlay. Mix equal volumes of solutions B and C and pour over the gel surface. Dark blue bands visible on a light blue background appear after 1 to 5 min. Record or photograph zymogram because after about 1 h the ATPASE bands disappear.

*Notes:*   To obtain permanent ATPASE zymograms with colored bands stable for several months, the Malachite Green–phosphomolybdate method should be used (e.g., see 3.6.1.1 — PP, Method 1, *Notes*).

    Orthophosphate should not be used as a component of any buffer used for electrophoresis or staining of ATPASE by methods based on orthophosphate detection.

## METHOD 2

### Visualization Scheme

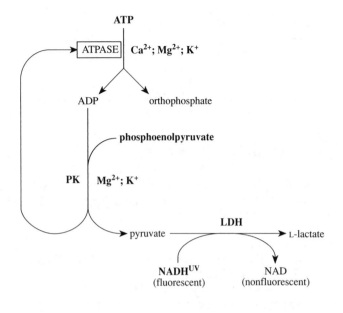

ATP

ATPASE   Ca²⁺; Mg²⁺; K⁺

ADP     orthophosphate

**phosphoenolpyruvate**

PK   Mg²⁺; K⁺

LDH

pyruvate     L-lactate

NADH$^{UV}$ (fluorescent)     NAD (nonfluorescent)

### Staining Solution*

| | |
|---|---:|
| 0.1 *M* Tris–HCl buffer, pH 7.6 | 5 ml |
| ATP | 30 mg |
| Phosphoenolpyruvate (trisodium salt) | 6 mg |
| NADH | 6 mg |
| Pyruvate kinase (PK) | 30 units |
| Lactate dehydrogenase (LDH) | 50 units |
| CaCl₂ | 10 mg |
| MgCl₂ | 10 mg |
| KCl | 20 mg |

### Procedure

Apply the staining solution to the gel surface on filter paper or dropwise and incubate at 37°C until dark (nonfluorescent) bands visible in long-wave UV light appear on a light (fluorescent) background. Record or photograph zymogram using a yellow filter.

*Notes:*   Areas of phosphoenolpyruvate phosphatase activity of alkaline phosphatase (see 3.1.3.1 — ALP, General Notes) and phosphoglycolate phosphatase (see 3.1.3.18 — PGP, Method 2) can also be detected by this method. These areas can be identified by incubating control gel with staining solution lacking ATP and PK.

    A similar staining procedure was used for detection of Mg²⁺-dependent ATPASE in brain /eye extracts of poeciliid fishes.[2]

---

*   New; recommended for use.

## OTHER METHODS

A. An immunoblotting procedure (for details see Part II) based on the utility of monoclonal antibodies specific to the barley enzyme[3] can also be used for immunohistochemical visualization of the enzyme protein on electrophoretic gels.

B. The product orthophosphate can be detected enzymatically using two linking enzymes purine-nucleoside phosphorylase and xanthine oxidase coupled with the PMS/MTT system (e.g., see 3.6.1.1 — PP, Method 2).

C. Some other nonenzymatic methods of orthophosphate detection are also available (see 3.1.3.1 — ALP, Methods 6 and 7; 3.1.3.2 — ACP, Method 5).

## GENERAL NOTES

Many enzymes previously listed under this number are now listed separately as EC 3.6.1.32–39. Some of these enzymes can also be detected by methods described above.

## REFERENCES

1. Brewer, G, J., *An Introduction to Isozyme Techniques*, Academic Press, New York, 1970, 129.
2. Morizot, D. C. and Schmidt, M. E., Starch gel electrophoresis and histochemical visualization of proteins, in *Electrophoretic and Isoelectric Focusing Techniques in Fisheries Management*, Whitmore, D. H., Ed., CRC Press, Boca Raton, 1990, 23.
3. Chin, J. J., Monoclonal antibodies that immunoreact with a cation stimulated plant membrane ATPase, *Biochem. J.*, 203, 51, 1982.

## 3.6.1.7 — Acylphosphatase; AP

REACTION      Acylphosphate + $H_2O$ = fatty acid anion + orthophosphate

ENZYME SOURCE    Vertebrates

## METHOD

### Visualization Scheme

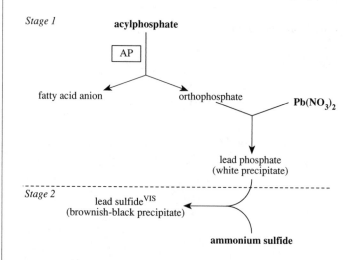

### Staining Solution[1]

A. 0.1 *M* Sodium acetate buffer, pH 5.3     8 ml
    0.05 *M* Acetyl phosphate (dissolved in     5 ml
     0.1 *M* acetate buffer, pH 5.3)
    $H_2O$ (deionized)     8 ml
B. 2% $Pb(NO_3)_2$     4 ml
C. 1% Ammonium sulfide

### Procedure

Add solution B to solution A with stirring. After standing for about 5 min centrifuge the mixture for 5 min at 1500 *g* to remove the white precipitate formed and transfer the supernatant to a transparent plastic tray. Rinse electrophorized PAG with deionized water and place in the tray. Incubate the gel at room temperature with gentle rocking until white bands of lead phosphate are seen when the gel is viewed against a black background. Then wash PAG for 30 to 40 min in repeatedly changed deionized water and immerse in solution C. Brownish-black bands appear after about 10 min, which indicate areas of AP activity. Rinse stained gel with deionized water and fix in 5% methanol/7.5% acetic acid.

*Notes:* Benzoyl phosphate and carbamoyl phosphate can also be used as substrates.

## OTHER METHODS

A. Ammonium molybdate (e.g., see 3.1.3.1 — ALP, Method 5) or Malachite Green–ammonium molybdate (e.g., see 3.1.3.2 — ACP, Method 4) methods can also be used to detect the product orthophosphate.

B. Orthophosphate can also be detected using linking enzymes purine nucleoside phosphorylase and xanthine oxidase in couple with the PMS/NBT system (e.g., see 3.1.3.1 — ALP, Method 8).

## REFERENCE

1. Mizuno, Y., Ohba, Y., Fujita, H., Kanesaka, Y., Tamura, T., and Shiokawa, H., Activity staining of acylphosphatase after gel electrophoresis, *Anal. Biochem.*, 183, 46, 1989.

| | |
|---|---|
| OTHER NAMES | Inosine triphosphatase, ITPase |
| REACTION | Nucleoside triphosphate + $H_2O$ = nucleotide + pyrophosphate |
| ENZYME SOURCE | Vertebrates |

## METHOD

### Visualization Scheme

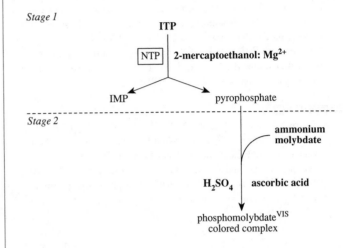

### Staining Solution[1]

A. 0.2 *M* Tris–HCl buffer, pH 7.6 — 10 ml
   Inosine triphosphate (trisodium salt) — 20 mg
   0.1 *M* $MgCl_2$ — 10 ml
   2-Mercaptoethanol — 0.2 ml
B. Ascorbic acid — 1 g
   2.5% Ammonium molybdate in 4 *N* $H_2SO_4$ — 20 ml
C. 2% Agar solution (60°C) — 20 ml

### Procedure

Apply solution A to the gel surface on filter-paper overlay and incubate at 37°C for 1 to 2 h. Remove filter-paper overlay. Mix solutions B and C and pour the mixture over the gel surface. Blue bands of NTP activity appear after 1 to 5 min. Record or photograph zymogram because the bands are ephemeral.

*Notes:* Buffer systems used for electrophoresis and staining NTP should be orthophosphate-free.

## 3.6.1.19 — Nucleoside-triphosphatase Phosphatase; NTP (continued)

### OTHER METHODS

A. The calcium pyrophosphate method can also be used to detect NTP activity in transparent gels.[2] This method is based on the formation of white calcium pyrophosphate precipitate in gel areas where pyrophosphate-releasing enzymes are localized (e.g., see 2.7.7.9 — UGPP, Method 3).

B. Pyrophosphate can be detected by fluorogenic (or chromogenic) enzymatic methods which use at least three linked enzymatic reactions sequentially catalyzed by bacterial pyrophosphate-fructose-6-phosphate 1-phosphotransferase, aldolase, and glycerol-3-phosphate dehydrogenase (or glyceraldehyde-3-phosphate dehydrogenase). For details see 2.7.1.90 — PFPPT.

C. The product IMP can be detected using an auxiliary enzyme, NAD-dependent IMP dehydrogenase, in couple with the PMS/MTT system (see 1.1.1.205 — IMPDH).

### REFERENCES

1. Harris, H. and Hopkinson, D. A., *Handbook of Enzyme Electrophoresis in Human Genetics*, North-Holland, Amsterdam (Loose leaf with supplements in 1977 and 1978), 1976.
2. Nimmo, H. G. and Nimmo, G. A., A general method for the localization of enzymes that produce phosphate, pyrophosphate, or $CO_2$ after polyacrylamide gel electrophoresis, *Anal. Biochem.*, 121, 17, 1982.

## 3.6.1.X — Nucleoside-diphosphosugar Pyrophosphatase; NDP

REACTION    Nucleoside diphosphosugar + $H_2O$ = nucleotide + sugar 1-phosphate

ENZYME SOURCE   Vertebrates

### METHOD

**Visualization Scheme**

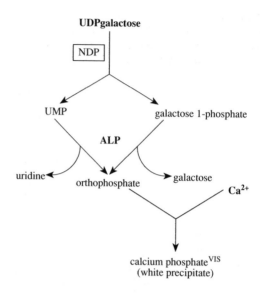

### Staining Solution[1]
A.  0.15 $M$ Tris–HCl buffer, pH 9.0
     5 m$M$ CaCl$_2$
     0.1% Triton X-100
     3 U/ml Alkaline phosphatase (ALP; Boehringer, type I)
B.  60 m$M$ UDPgalactose

### Procedure
Apply solution A to the surface of electrophorized PAG dropwise and allow the solution to enter the gel for 15 min. Then apply solution B and incubate the gel in a humid chamber at 37°C until opaque bands visible against a dark background appear. When an activity stain of sufficient intensity is obtained, store the gel in 50 m$M$ glycine–KOH buffer, pH 10, 5 m$M$ Ca$^{2+}$ at 5°C or at room temperature in the presence of an antibacterial agent. Stained gel can be photographed by reflected light against a dark background.

*Notes:*   The precipitated calcium phosphate can be subsequently stained with Alizarin Red S. This does not increase the sensitivity of the staining method although it is of advantage for more opaque gel systems, such as starch.[2]

   UDP–*N*-acetylglucosamine and UDPglucuronate can also be used as substrates. Several other methods may be used to detect the product orthophosphate (e.g., see 3.1.3.1 — ALP).

## REFERENCES

1. Van Dijk, W., Lasthuis, A.-M., Koppen, P. L., and Muilerman, H. G., A universal and rapid spectrophotometric assay of CMP–sialic acid hydrolase and nucleoside-diphosphosugar pyrophosphatase activities and detection in polyacrylamide gels, *Anal. Biochem.*, 117, 346, 1981.
2. Nimmo, H. G. and Nimmo, G. A., A general method for the localization of enzymes that produce phosphate, pyrophosphate, or $CO_2$ after polyacrylamide gel electrophoresis, *Anal. Biochem.*, 121, 17, 1982.

**4.1.1.1 — Pyruvate Decarboxylase; PDC**

OTHER NAMES    α-Carboxylase, pyruvic decarboxylase, α-ketoacid carboxylase

REACTION    2-Oxo acid = aldehyde + $CO_2$

ENZYME SOURCE  Bacteria, fungi, plants, vertebrates

## METHOD 1

### Visualization Scheme

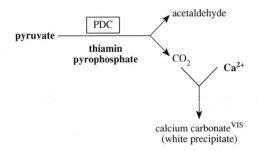

### Staining Solution[1]
100 m$M$ Tris–HCl buffer, pH 8.5
5 m$M$ Sodium pyruvate
67 m$M$ Thiamin pyrophosphate
2 m$M$ $Ca^{2+}$

### Procedure
Soak electrophorized PAG in 100 m$M$ tris–HCl buffer, pH 8.5, at 37°C for 20 to 30 min and transfer to staining solution. Incubate the gel at room temperature until opaque bands visible against a dark background appear. Store stained gel in 50 m$M$ glycine–KOH, pH 10.0, at 5°C or at room temperature in the presence of an antibacterial agent.

*Notes:* It was supposed that this method is not adequate for PDC detection because the enzyme has almost no activity at pH above 7.0, loses its cofactor (thiamin pyrophosphate) rapidly at pH above 8.0, and displays a tendency to denature at room temperature under alkaline conditions.[2] It was also pointed out that at acid pH (6.0 to 6.2) optimal for PDC activity the formation of calcium carbonate is questionable.

## 4.1.1.1 — Pyruvate Decarboxylase; PDC (continued)

### METHOD 2

#### Visualization Scheme

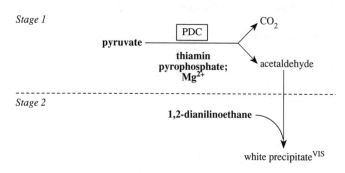

*Stage 1*

pyruvate — [PDC] — $CO_2$

thiamin pyrophosphate; $Mg^{2+}$ — acetaldehyde

*Stage 2*

1,2-dianilinoethane

white precipitate[VIS]

#### Staining Solution[2]

A. 0.3 *M* Sodium citrate buffer, pH 6.0
   30 m*M* Sodium pyruvate
   5 m*M* $MgSO_4$
   5 m*M* Thiamin pyrophosphate

B. 100 mg 1.2-Dianilinoethane dissolved in 10 ml of glacial acetic acid and total volume adjusted to 35 ml with water

#### Procedure

Incubate electrophorized PAG in 200 ml of solution A at room temperature for 50 min and then add 3 ml of solution B. Opaque bands clearly visible against a dark background appear after 5 to 15 min. Wash stained gel with water and photograph.

*Notes:* The method is very sensitive and allows detection of about 10 mU of PDC activity per band.

A high concentration of staining buffer is used to overcome the alkaline pH of electrophoretic gel.

### OTHER METHODS

NAD-dependent aldehyde dehydrogenase in couple with the PMS/NBT system can also be used to detect the product acetaldehyde.[2] This method is of advantage when PDC electrophoresis is carried out in opaque gels, e.g., acetate cellulose or starch. However, the difference of pH-optima for PDC (6.0) and aldehyde dehydrogenase (8.0) does not allow staining of PDC activity bands using a one-step procedure. So, zymograms obtained by this method display more diffuse PDC bands than do zymograms obtained by Method 2.

### REFERENCES

1. Nimmo, H. G. and Nimmo, G. A., A general method for the localization of enzymes that produce phosphate, pyrophosphate, or $CO_2$ after polyacrylamide gel electrophoresis, *Anal. Biochem.*, 121, 17, 1982.
2. Zehender, H., Trescher, D., and Ullrich, J., Activity stain for pyruvate decarboxylase in polyacrylamide gels, *Anal. Biochem.*, 135, 16, 1983.

## 4.1.1.15 — Glutamate Decarboxylase; GDC

OTHER NAMES — ʟ-Glutamic acid decarboxylase, ʟ-glutamic decarboxylase

REACTION — ʟ-Glutamate = 4-aminobutanoate + $CO_2$

ENZYME SOURCE — Bacteria, plants, vertebrates

### METHOD

#### Visualization Scheme

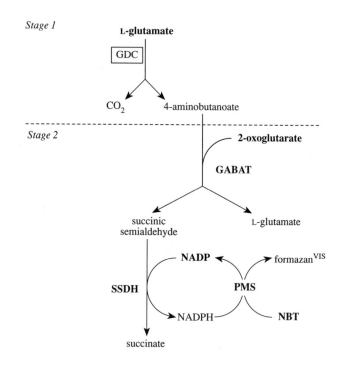

*Stage 1*

**ʟ-glutamate**

[GDC]

$CO_2$     4-aminobutanoate

*Stage 2*     **2-oxoglutarate**

**GABAT**

succinic semialdehyde     ʟ-glutamate

NADP ← → formazan[VIS]

**SSDH**     **PMS**

NADPH     **NBT**

succinate

#### Staining Solution[1]

| | |
|---|---:|
| A. 0.2 *M* Citrate buffer, pH 4.7 | 40 ml |
| 20 m*M* ʟ-Glutamic acid in 0.2 *M* citrate buffer, pH 4.7 | 5 ml |
| B. 1.0 *M* Tris–HCl buffer, pH 8.0 | 40 ml |
| NADP | 10 mg |
| PMS | 1.5 mg |
| NBT | 25 mg |
| 0.7% 2-Mercaptoethanol in 1.0 M tris–HCl buffer, pH 8.0 | 0.5 ml |
| 0.02 *M* 2-Oxoglutaric acid in 1.0 M tris–HCl buffer, pH 8.0 | 1 ml |
| GABASE: a mixture of 4-aminobutyrate aminotransferase (GABAT; EC 2.6.1.19) and succinate-semialdehyde dehydrogenase (SSDH; EC 1.2.1.16) | 1 ml |

## 4.1.1.15 — Glutamate Decarboxylase; GDC (continued)

### Procedure

Incubate the gel in solution A at 37°C for 30 min and then place in solution B. Incubate the gel in solution B in the dark at 37°C until dark blue bands appear. Wash stained gel in water and fix in 50% ethanol.

*Notes:* Both enzymes, GDC and auxiliary GABAT, require pyridoxal 5′-phosphate as a cosubstrate. However, usually there is no need to add the cosubstrate in the staining solution because both enzymes contain sufficient quantities of pyridoxal 5′-phosphate bound to the enzyme molecules.

Buffers containing Cl⁻ should not be used for electrophoresis because Cl⁻ anions competitively inhibit GDC activity.

Several methods suitable for detection of carbonate ions also may be applied to visualize GDC activity bands (for details see Part II). However, all these methods work well only at alkaline pHs, which are not compatible with the acidic pHs optimal for GDC activity. Thus, the use of these methods requires that GDC visualization be carried out in a two-step procedure.

### REFERENCE

1. Akers, E. and Aronson, J. N., Detection on polyacrylamide gels of L-glutamic acid decarboxylase activities from *Bacillus thuringiensis*, *Anal. Biochem.*, 39, 535, 1971.

## 4.1.1.20 — Diaminopimelate Decarboxylase; DAPD

REACTION    *meso*-2,6-Diaminoheptanedioate = L-lysine + $CO_2$

ENZYME SOURCE   Bacteria, plants

## METHOD

### Visualization Scheme

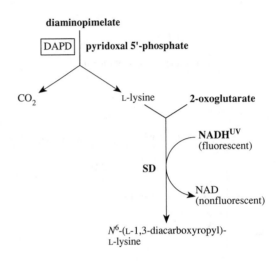

### Staining Solution[1] (adapted)

- 100 µ$M$ Potassium phosphate buffer, pH 6.8
- 1 µ$M$ EDTA
- 1 µ$M$ 2,3-Dimercaptopropanol
- 0.1 µ$M$ Pyridoxal 5′-phosphate
- 0.3 µ$M$ NADH
- 4 µ$M$ *meso*-2,6-Diaminopimelate
- 2.5 µ$M$ 2-Oxoglutarate
- 0.1 U/ml Saccharopine dehydrogenase (NAD, L-lysine–forming) (SD)

### Procedure

Apply the staining solution to the gel surface on filter-paper overlay and incubate the gel at 37°C in a moist chamber. After 20 to 30 min of incubation monitor gel under long-wave UV light. Dark (nonfluorescent) bands of DAPD are visible on a light (fluorescent) background. Record the zymogram or photograph using a yellow filter.

*Notes:* When a zymogram that is visible in daylight is required, counterstain the processed gel with MTT/PMS solution to develop white bands of DAPD on a blue background. Fix negatively stained gel in 50% ethanol.

### GENERAL NOTES

The enzyme is a pyridoxal-phosphate protein.

### REFERENCE

1. Laber, B. and Amrhein, N., A spectrophotometric assay for *meso*-diaminopimelate decarboxylase and L-α-amino-ε-caprolactam hydrolase, *Anal. Biochem.*, 181, 297, 1989.

OTHER NAMES    Dopa decarboxylase, tryptophan decarboxy-lase, hydroxytryptophan decarboxylase

REACTION    L-Tryptophan = tryptamine + $CO_2$

ENZYME SOURCE  Bacteria, invertebrates, vertebrates

## METHOD

### Visualization Scheme

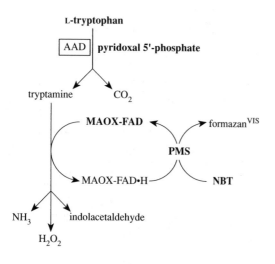

### Staining Solution[1]

0.05 *M* Phosphate buffer, pH 7.6
0.1 mg/ml Pyridoxal 5′-phosphate
0.4 mg/ml NBT
0.04 mg/ml PMS
0.4 mg/ml L-Tryptophan (or L-tyrosin, or dihydroxyphenylalanine)
Monoamine oxidase (MAOX; EC 1.4.3.4; the enzyme concentration is determined experimentally)

### Procedure

Incubate the gel in staining solution in the dark at 37°C until dark blue bands appear. Wash stained gel in water and fix in 50% ethanol.

## OTHER METHODS

A. The calcium carbonate precipitation method[2] may be used to detect the product carbon dioxide (for example see 4.1.1.1 — PDC, Method 1). Phosphate-containing buffers must not be used in this case because calcium ions also interact with phosphate, resulting in the formation of calcium phosphate precipitate all over the gel.

B. The product carbon dioxide can also be detected using a linked reaction catalyzed by phosphoenolpyruvate carboxylase in couple with a diazonium salt (see 4.1.1.31 — PEPC, Method), or using two linked reactions sequentially catalyzed by phosphoenolpyruvate carboxylase and malate dehydrogenase (see 4.1.1.31 — PEPC; Other Methods, B).

## REFERENCES

1. Antonas, K. N., Coulson, W. F., and Jepson, J. B., A monoamine oxidase–tetrazolium reaction for locating aromatic amino acid decarboxylases in electrophoretic media, *Biochem. J.*, 121, 38, 1971.
2. Nimmo, H. G. and Nimmo, G. A., A general method for the localization of enzymes that produce phosphate, pyrophosphate, or $CO_2$ after polyacrylamide gel electrophoresis, *Anal. Biochem.*, 121, 17, 1982.

REACTION    Orthophosphate + oxaloacetate = $H_2O$ + phos-
            phoenolpyruvate + $CO_2$

ENZYME SOURCE  Bacteria, fungi, plants, vertebrates

## METHOD

### Visualization Scheme

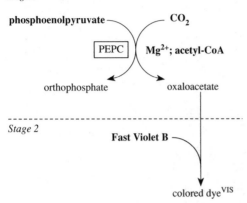

*Stage 1*

phosphoenolpyruvate — $CO_2$

PEPC    $Mg^{2+}$; acetyl-CoA

orthophosphate    oxaloacetate

- - - - - - - - - - - - - - - - - - - - - - - - - - - - -

*Stage 2*

Fast Violet B —

colored dye$^{VIS}$

### Staining Solution[1]
A. 100 m$M$ Tris–HCl buffer, pH 8.5
   3 m$M$ Phosphoenolpyruvate
   5 m$M$ $MgCl_2$
   20 m$M$ $KHCO_3$
   0.5 m$M$ Acetyl-CoA (or propionyl-CoA)
B. 1 mg/ml Fast Violet B salt

### Procedure
Incubate the gel in solution A at room temperature for 30 min, wash in distilled water, and place in solution B. Incubate the gel in the dark until colored bands appear. Wash stained gel in water and fix in 50% glycerol or 5% acetic acid.

*Notes:*  The plant enzyme is not activated by acetyl-CoA (or propionyl-CoA). Thus, when the enzyme from a plant source is detected, this expensive ingredient may be excluded from the staining solution.[2]

Fast Blue B or BB salts can also be used in place of Fast Violet B salt.

The two-step post-coupling procedure (as shown on the scheme) is recommended when a diazonium salt has an inhibitory effect on PEPC activity. If there is no obvious inhibition, a one-step detection procedure is preferable because it reduces diffusion of the product oxaloacetate and results in the development of sharper and more distinct bands.

## OTHER METHODS

A. A general method of detection of orthophosphate[3] may also be used to detect PEPC activity. This method involves two linking enzymes, purine-nucleoside phosphorylase and xanthine oxidase, coupled with the PMS/MTT system (e.g., see 3.6.1.1 — PP, Method 2). It should be kept in mind that gel areas occupied by phosphoenolpyruvate phosphatase (see 3.1.3.18 — PGP; Method 2, *Notes*) can also be developed by this method.
B. The product oxaloacetate can be detected using the auxiliary enzyme malate dehydrogenase. This method results in the appearance of dark (nonfluorescent) bands of PEPC visible on a light (fluorescent) background in long-wave UV light (e.g., see 2.6.1.1 — GOT, Method 2).

## REFERENCES
1. Scrutton, M. C. and Fatebene, F., An assay system for localization of pyruvate and phosphoenolpyruvate carboxylase activity on polyacrylamide gels and its application to detection of these enzymes in tissue and cell extracts, *Anal. Biochem.*, 69, 247, 1975.
2. Brown, A. H. D., Nevo, E., Zohary, D., and Dagan, O., Genetic variation in natural populations of wild barley (*Hordeum spontaneum*), *Genetica*, 49, 97, 1978.
3. Klebe, R. J., Schloss, S., Mock, L., and Link, C. R., Visualization of isozymes which generate inorganic phosphate, *Biochem. Genet.*, 19, 921, 1981.

OTHER NAMES — Fructose-bisphosphate aldolase (recommended name), fructose-1,6-bisphosphate triosephosphate-lyase

REACTION — D-Fructose-1,6-bisphosphate = glycerone phosphate + D-glyceraldehyde 3-phosphate

ENZYME SOURCE — Bacteria, fungi, plants, protozoa, invertebrates, vertebrates

## METHOD 1

### Visualization Scheme

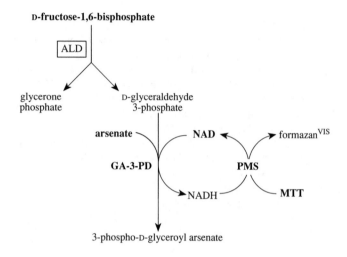

### Staining Solution[1]

A. 0.1 $M$ Tris–HCl buffer, pH 8.0 — 25 ml
Fructose-1,6-bisphosphate — 100 mg
NAD — 20 mg
Sodium arsenate — 60 mg
Glyceraldehyde-3-phosphate dehydrogenase — 50 µl
  (GA-3-PD; 800 U/ml)
MTT — 7.5 mg
PMS — 2.5 mg
B. 2% Agar solution (60°C) — 25 ml

### Procedure

Mix A and B components of the staining solution and pour the mixture over the gel surface. Incubate the gel in the dark at 37°C until dark blue bands appear. Fix stained gel in 50% ethanol.

*Notes:* The linking enzyme triose-phosphate isomerase may be added to the staining solution to convert glycerone phosphate into D-glyceraldehyde 3-phosphate and thus to enhance the staining of low-activity ALD isozymes.[2]

The PMS and MTT may be omitted from the staining solution and fluorescent bands of ALD activity observed in long-wave UV light.[3]

## METHOD 2

### Visualization Scheme

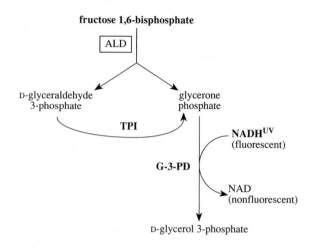

### Staining Solution[4]

0.1 $M$ Tris–HCl buffer, pH 7.8
1.1 m$M$ NADH
2.5 m$M$ Fructose-1,6-bisphosphate
1.5 U/ml Glycerol-3-phosphate dehydrogenase (G-3-PD)
111 U/ml Triose-phosphate isomerase (TPI)

### Procedure

Cover the gel surface with a filter paper and flood with the staining solution. Incubate covered gel at 37°C and monitor under long-wave UV light. Dark (nonfluorescent) bands on a light (fluorescent) background indicate areas of ALD activity localization. Record the zymogram or photograph using a yellow filter.

*Notes:* This method is the most sensitive among the ALD activity detection methods so far described.

The linking enzyme triose-phosphate isomerase can be omitted where ALD activity is high.

To develop ALD bands visible in daylight, treat the processed gel with the PMS/MTT mixture. White bands visible on a blue background appear almost immediately.

## METHOD 3

### Visualization Scheme

**fructose 1-phosphate**

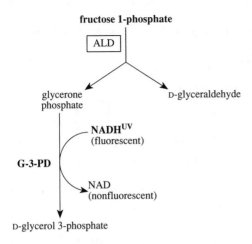

### Staining Solution[1]

| | |
|---|---|
| 0.1 *M* Tris–HCl buffer, pH 8.0 | 25 ml |
| Fructose 1-phosphate (disodium salt) | 25 mg |
| NADH (disodium salt) | 10 mg |
| Glycerol-3-phosphate dehydrogenase (G-3-PD; 80 U/ml) | 50 µl |

### Procedure

Apply the staining solution to the gel surface on filter paper. Incubate overlayed gel in a humid chamber at 37°C and view under long-wave UV light. Dark (nonfluorescent) bands visible on a light (fluorescent) background indicate areas of ALD activity. Record the zymogram or photograph using a yellow filter.

*Notes:* Some ALD isozymes (e.g., human liver ALD-B) catalyze the breakdown of fructose 1-phosphate to glyceraldehyde and glycerone phosphate. The method described above was developed to detect just such ALD isozymes.

## OTHER METHODS

The silver method may be used to detect orthophosphate liberated from the products glycerone phosphate and glyceraldehyde 3-phosphate after treatment with iodacetamide.[5] This method is not widely used because the intermediary orthophosphate is readily diffusable.

## REFERENCES

1. Harris, H. and Hopkinson, D. A., *Handbook of Enzyme Electrophoresis in Human Genetics*, North-Holland, Amsterdam (Loose leaf with supplements in 1977 and 1978), 1976.
2. Richardson, B. J., Baverstock, P. R., and Adams, M., *Allozyme Electrophoresis: A Handbook for Animal Systematics and Population Studies*, Academic Press, Sydney, 1986, 167.
3. Susor, W. A. and Rutter, W. J., Method for the detection of pyruvate kinase, aldolase, and other pyridine nucleotide linked enzyme activities after electrophoresis, *Anal. Biochem.*, 43, 147, 1971.
4. Anderson, J. E. and Giblett, E. R., Intraspecific red cell enzyme variation in the pigtailed macaque (*Macaca nemestrina*), *Biochem. Genet.*, 13, 189, 1975.
5. Pietruszko, R. and Baron, D. N., A staining procedure for demonstration of multiple forms of aldolase, *Biochim. Biophys. Acta*, 132, 203, 1967.

## 4.1.2.15 — Phospho-2-dehydro-3-deoxyheptonate Aldolase; PDDA

OTHER NAMES    Phospho-2-keto-3-deoxyheptonate aldolase, DHAP synthase, KDPH synthetase

REACTION    7-Phospho-2-dehydro-3-deoxy-D-*arabino*-heptonate + orthophosphate = phosphoenolpyruvate + D-erythrose 4-phosphate + $H_2O$

ENZYME SOURCE    Bacteria, fungi

## METHOD

### Visualization Scheme

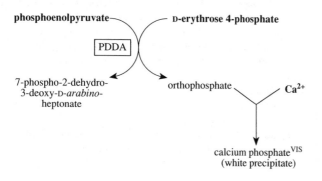

### Staining Solution[1]

50 m$M$ Glycine–KOH buffer, pH 10.0
0.1 m$M$ Phosphoenolpyruvate
0.1 m$M$ Erythrose 4-phosphate
10 m$M$ Ca$^{2+}$

### Procedure

Incubate electrophorized PAG in the staining solution at 37°C until opaque bands visible against a dark background appear. Store stained gel in 50 m$M$ glycine–KOH, pH 10.0, 5 m$M$ Ca$^{2+}$ at 5°C or at room temperature in the presence of an antibacterial agent (e.g., sodium azide).

*Notes:*    The areas of calcium phosphate precipitation may be counterstained with Alizarin Red S. This does not increase the sensitivity of the method but would be of advantage for opaque gels such as acetate cellulose or starch.

## OTHER METHODS

The enzymatic method of detection of the product orthophosphate[2] can also be adapted to visualize PDDA activity in electrophoretic gels. This method is based on reactions catalyzed by two linking enzymes, purine-nucleoside phosphorylase and xanthine oxidase, in couple with the PMS/MTT system (e.g., see 3.6.1.1 — PP, Method 2).

### REFERENCES

1. Nimmo, H. G. and Nimmo, G. A., A general method for the localization of enzymes that produce phosphate, pyrophosphate, or CO$_2$ after polyacrylamide gel electrophoresis, *Anal. Biochem.*, 121, 17, 1982.
2. Klebe, R. J., Schloss, S., Mock, L., and Link, C. R., Visualization of isozymes which generate inorganic phosphate, *Biochem. Genet.*, 19, 921, 1981.

## 4.1.3.1 — Isocitrate Lyase; IL

OTHER NAMES    Isocitrase, isocitritase, isocitratase

REACTION    D-Isocitrate = succinate + glyoxylate

ENZYME SOURCE    Bacteria, fungi, plants, protozoa

## METHOD

### Visualization Scheme

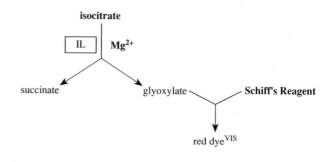

### Staining Solution[1]

A. 50 m$M$ Potassium phosphate buffer, pH 7.5
   1 m$M$ EDTA
   3 m$M$ MgCl$_2$
   30 m$M$ Dithiothreitol
   10 m$M$ D,L-Isocitrate
B. Schiff's Reagent (see *Notes*)

### Procedure

Incubate electrophorized PAG in a mixture of 50 ml A and 3 ml B at 37°C. Dark red bands appear after 20 to 30 min of incubation. Record or photograph zymogram.

*Notes:*    Prepare modified Schiff's Reagent as follows: add 500 ml of warm distilled water to 0.25 g of fuchsin (basic); mix thoroughly and filtrate. Add to the filtered solution 5 ml of 1 $N$ HCl and then 0.125 ml of concentrated HCl. Finally add to the mixture 0.5 g of sodium metabisulfite. Store solution in a dark glass bottle at 4°C.

This method requires control staining of an additional gel in a mixture lacking isocitrate and MgCl$_2$ to be sure that developed bands are really caused by IL activity.

## OTHER METHODS

The product glyoxylate can be detected by a negative fluorescent method using NADH–dependent glyoxylate reductase (EC 1.1.1.26) as a linking enzyme. When using this method it should be taken into account that commercially available glyoxylate reductase from spinach leaves display optimal activity at pH 6.4 while IL pH optimum is above 7.0. Thus, the detection of IL by this method should be carried out in a two-step procedure.

### REFERENCE

1. Reeves, H. C. and Volk, M. J., Determination of isocitrate lyase activity in polyacrylamide gels, *Anal. Biochem.*, 48, 437, 1972.

OTHER NAMES    Malate condensing enzyme, glyoxylate transacetylase, malate synthetase

REACTION    L-Malate + CoA = acetyl-CoA + $H_2O$ + glyoxylate

ENZYME SOURCE  Bacteria, fungi, plants

## METHOD

### Visualization Scheme

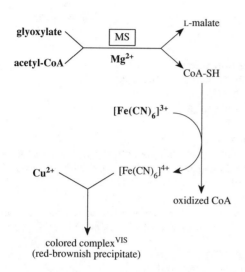

### Staining Solution[1]

| | |
|---|---|
| 30 m$M$ Phosphate buffer, pH 7.6 | 7.5 ml |
| 100 m$M$ Sodium phosphotartrate | 2.5 ml |
| 50 m$M$ $CuSO_4$ | 2.5 ml |
| 15 m$M$ Potassium ferricyanide | 12.5 ml |
| 25 m$M$ $MgCl_2$ | 25 ml |
| 10 m$M$ Acetyl-CoA | 2.5 ml |
| 50 m$M$ Sodium glyoxylate | 5 ml |

### Procedure

Incubate electrophorized gel in a staining solution at 37°C for 30 to 60 min. Reddish-brown bands indicate areas of MS activity.

*Notes:*  This method and some others (see below) based on the detection of free sulfhydril group of the product CoA require the control staining of an additional gel in staining solution lacking glyoxylate to identify bands of acetyl-CoA hydrolase (see 3.1.2.1 — ACoAH).

## OTHER METHODS

A. PAG prepared using *N*-[5-(hydroxyethyl)dithio-2-nitrobenzoyla-minoethyl]acrylamide (iodide) can be used to visualize MS activity bands. The method is based on the reduction of disulfide bonds of the chromogenic group (dithio-2-nitrobenzene) by thiol reagents including CoA-SH produced by MS (e.g., see 3.1.1.7 — ACHE, Method 2). Free dithiobis(2-nitrobenzoic acid) can also be used (e.g., see 1.6.4.2 — GSR, Method 3).

B. The product CoA-SH can be detected using redox indicator 2,6-dichlorophenolindophenol coupled with the tetrazolium system (e.g., see 4.1.3.7 — CS).

C. Reaction of a linking enzyme, NAD-dependent malate dehydrogenase, coupled with the PMS/MTT system, can be used to detect the product L-malate (see 1.1.1.37 — MDH, Method 1).

### REFERENCE

1. Volk, M. J., Trelease, R. N., and Reeves, H. C., Determination of malate synthase activity in polyacrylamide gels, *Anal. Biochem.*, 58, 315, 1974.

OTHER NAMES    Citrase (pro-3S)-lyase (recommended name), citrase, citratase, citritase, citridensmolase, citrate aldolase

REACTION    Citrate = acetate + oxaloacetate

ENZYME SOURCE  Bacteria

## METHOD 1

### Visualization Scheme

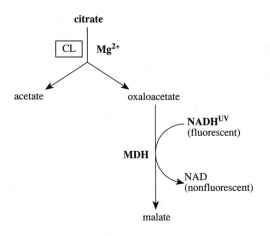

### Staining Solution[1] (adapted)

| | |
|---|---:|
| 0.1 $M$ Tris–HCl buffer, pH 8.0 | 16 ml |
| Citric acid (trisodium salt) | 50 mg |
| 0.2 $M$ MgCl$_2$ | 50 µl |
| Malate dehydrogenase (MDH) | 55 units |
| NADH | 10 mg |

### Procedure
Apply the staining solution to the gel surface on filter-paper overlay. Incubate the gel at 37°C and monitor under long-wave UV light. Dark (nonfluorescent) bands visible on a light (fluorescent) background indicate areas of CL activity. Record the zymogram or photograph using a yellow filter.

*Notes:*   The processed gel can be counterstained with the PMS/MTT solution and achromatic bands observed on a blue background of the gel. Fix negatively stained gel in 50% ethanol.

## METHOD 2

### Visualization Scheme

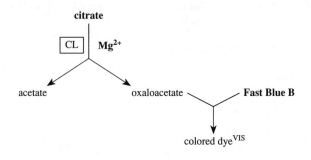

### Staining Solution*

| | |
|---|---:|
| 0.1 $M$ Tris–citrate buffer, pH 7.6 | 100 ml |
| MgCl$_2$·6H$_2$O | 50 mg |
| Fast Blue B salt | 100 mg |

### Procedure
Incubate the gel in staining solution in the dark at 37°C until brown bands appear. Wash stained gel with water and fix in 7% acetic acid.

*Notes:*   This method is less expensive in comparison to the former one. It may be preferable when a double stain of the same gel is made.

### REFERENCE
1. Slaughter, C. A., Hopkinson, D. A., and Harris, H., The distribution and properties of aconitase isozymes in man, *Ann. Hum. Genet.*, 40, 385, 1977.

---

* New; recommended for use.

OTHER NAMES     Citrate (si)-synthase (recommended name), condensing enzyme, citrate condensing enzyme, citrogenase, oxaloacetate transacetase

REACTION     Citrate + CoA = acetyl-CoA + $H_2O$ + oxaloacetate

ENZYME SOURCE     Bacteria, fungi, plants, invertebrates, vertebrates

## METHOD

### Visualization Scheme

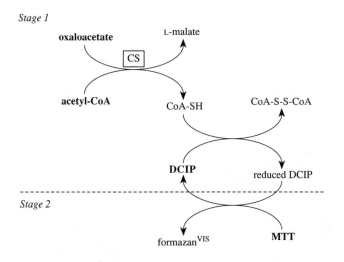

*Stage 1*

*Stage 2*

### Staining Solution[1]
A. 100 m$M$ Tris–HCl buffer, pH 7.6     125 µl

    10 m$M$ Oxaloacetate in 100 m$M$ tris–HCl     50 µl
    buffer, pH 7.6

    10 m$M$ Acetyl-CoA in 100 m$M$ tris–HCl     25 µl
    buffer, pH 7.6

    2,6-Dichlorophenolindophenol (DCIP)     0.3 mg

B. 0.5 mg/ml MTT in 100 m$M$ tris–HCl
    buffer, pH 7.6

### Procedure
Apply solution A dropwise to electrophorized acetate cellulose gel and incubate at room temperature in a moist chamber for 10 to 15 min or until white bands of CS activity appear on a blue gel background. Then counterstain gel with solution B to obtain purple CS bands on a white background. Remove excess DCIP and MTT by extensive washing of the gel with water. Fix stained gel in 50% ethanol.

## OTHER METHODS

A. PAG prepared using *N*-[5-(hydroxyethyl)dithio-2-nitro-benzoylaminoethyl]acrylamide (iodide) can be used to visualize CS activity bands. The method is based on the reduction of disulfide bonds of the chromogenic group (dithio-2-nitrobenzene) by thiol reagents, including CoA-SH produced by CS (e.g., see 3.1.1.7 — ACHE, Method 2). Free 2-nitrobenzoic acid can also be used (e.g., see 1.6.4.2 — GSR, Method 3).

B. The ferricyanide method developed for detection of malate synthase (see 4.1.3.2 — MS) can also be adapted for visualization of CS activity bands.

## REFERENCE
1. Craig, I., A procedure for the analysis of citrate synthase (EC 4.1.3.7) in somatic cell hybrids, *Biochem. Genet.*, 9, 351, 1973.

REACTION          Chorismate + $NH_3$ (or L-glutamine) = anthranilate + pyruvate + (L-glutamate)

ENZYME SOURCE  Bacteria

## METHOD

### Visualization Scheme

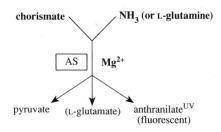

### Staining Solution[1]
A. For detection of $NH_3$-dependent AS activity:
   50 m$M$ Triethanolamine–HCl buffer, pH 8.3
   0.34 m$M$ Chorismate
   50 m$M$ Ammonium sulfate
   5 m$M$ $MgCl_2$
   2 m$M$ 2-Mercaptoethanol
B. For detection of glutamine-dependent AS activity:
   50 m$M$ Potassium phosphate buffer, pH 7.4
   0.34 m$M$ Chorismate
   5 m$M$ L-Glutamine
   5 m$M$ $MgCl_2$

### Procedure
Depending on what AS activity should be detected, incubate electrophorized PAG in the staining solution A or B at 37°C for 10 to 30 min and view fluorescent bands in long-wave UV light. Record the developed gel or photograph using Corning No. 18 filters and a Wratten 2B filter.

## OTHER METHODS

The product of glutamine-dependent AS activity, L-glutamate, may be detected using the linking enzyme NAD(P)-dependent glutamate dehydrogenase in couple with the PMS/MTT system (e.g., see 3.5.1.2 — GLUT).

## GENERAL NOTES

The native enzyme in some bacteria exists as a complex with anthranilate phosphoribozyltransferase (EC 2.4.2.18) which can use either L-glutamine or $NH_3$. The AS separated from the complex uses $NH_3$ only.

## REFERENCE
1. Grove, T. H. and Levy, H. R., Fluorescent assay of anthranilate synthetase–anthranilate 5-phosphoribozylpyrophosphate phosphoribozyltransferase enzyme-complex on polyacrylamide gels, *Anal. Biochem.*, 65, 458, 1975.

OTHER NAMES     Carbonate dehydratase (recommended name)

REACTION          $H_2CO_3 = CO_2 + H_2O$

ENZYME SOURCE  Fungi, green algae, plants, invertebrates, vertebrates

## METHOD 1

### Visualization Scheme

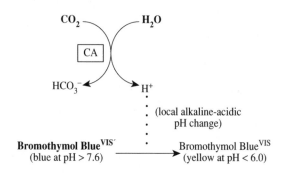

### Staining Solution[1]
A. 0.1 $M$ Veronal buffer, pH 9.0
   0.1% Bromothymol Blue
B. $CO_2$

### Procedure
Soak electrophorized gel in solution A for about 10 min. Blot gel with filter paper and place in a tank containing dry ice, or pass a stream of $CO_2$ over the gel surface. Yellow bands on a blue background appear rapidly and then fade. Record the zymogram as quickly as possible.

*Notes:*   Drawing on the gel (using a felt-tip pen) in the position of the major isozymes will allow permanent positions to be noted after the bands have faded.

    It is possible to restain gel by repeating the procedure described above.

    Phenol Red pH-indicator dye (yellow at pH <6.8; red at pH >8.2) may be used in place of Bromothymol Blue.[2] Bromocressol Blue, a pH indicator, becomes fluorescent at low pHs and also is used to detect CA activity.[3]

## METHOD 2

### Visualization Scheme

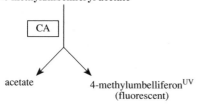

**4-methylumbelliferyl acetate**

acetate      4-methylumbelliferon[UV]
(fluorescent)

### Staining Solution[4]

| | |
|---|---|
| 0.1 $M$ Phosphate buffer, pH 6.5 | 25 ml |
| 4-Methylumbelliferyl acetate | 2.5 mg |
| (dissolved in a few drops of acetone) | |

### Procedure

Apply the staining solution to the gel surface on a filter-paper overlay and inspect gel under long-wave UV light after 5 to 10 min of incubation at 37°C. Fluorescent bands indicate the areas of CA activity. Record the zymogram or photograph using a yellow filter.

*Notes:* The fluorogenic substrate fluoresceine diacetate can also be used in place of 4-methylumbelliferyl acetate. Different isozymes can display different activity towards these synthetic substrates, e.g., human red cell $CA_I$ isozyme preferentially cleaves 4-methylumbelliferyl acetate, whereas $CA_{II}$ is more specific to fluoresceine diacetate.[4]

Some esterase isozymes (see 3.1.1... — EST) can also be visualized by this method. To identify CA activity bands, the CA-specific Method 1 (see above) should be used initially. Specific CA inhibitors can also be used to distinguish CA from esterase. The most commonly used inhibitors (and their concentrations) are acetazolamide ($7.8 \times 10^{-9}$ $M$), sulfanilamide ($1.3 \times 10^{-5}$ M), sodium azide ($3.9 \times 10^{-5}$ $M$), and sodium chloride ($5.6 \times 10^{-2}$ $M$).[5]

## METHOD 3

### Visualization Scheme

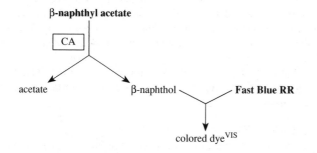

**β-naphthyl acetate**

acetate      β-naphthol ⟍    **Fast Blue RR**

colored dye[VIS]

### Staining Solution[1]

| | |
|---|---|
| 0.1 $M$ Phosphate buffer, pH 7.2 | 100 ml |
| β-Naphthyl acetate (dissolved in | 20 mg |
| a few drops of acetone) | |
| Fast Blue RR salt | 50 mg |

### Procedure

Incubate the gel in staining solution in the dark at 37°C until red bands appear. Wash gel with water and fix in 7% acetic acid.

*Notes:* Esterase (3.1.1.... — EST) activity bands also are visualized by this method. Thus, the control staining of an additional gel should be made initially using CA-specific Method 1 (see above) to identify true CA activity bands. The use of CA-specific inhibitors is also recommended in order to distinguish CA from esterase activity (see Method 2, *Notes*).

## OTHER METHODS

A. CA activity bands may be detected on electrophorized PAG by using conductivity measurements. In areas of CA activity the conductivity increases due to $CO_2$ hydration.[6]

B. The "positive" fluorescent stain based on specific binding of the fluorochrome, 5-(dimethylamino)naphthalene-1-sulfonamide (DNSA), with CA molecules is also available.[7] In this method DNSA (2.5 mg) is initially dissolved in 0.1 $N$ NaOH (10 ml) and then mixed with 10 m$M$ tris–sulfate, pH 8.9 (190 ml). This mixture (from 0.1 to 0.5 ml) is mixed with crude enzyme preparation (2 ml) and incubated for 15 min. Pretreated preparations are electrophorized as usual. After completion of electrophoresis the gel is viewed under long-wave UV light for fluorescent CA bands.

C. The immunoblotting procedure (for details see Part II) based on the utility of monoclonal antibodies specific to the human and cow enzyme[8] can also be used for immunohistochemical visualization of the enzyme protein on electrophoretic gels. This procedure is not quite appropriate for large-scale population studies but it may be of great value in specific analyses of CA.

## REFERENCES

1. Tashian, R. E., The esterases and carbonic anhydrases in human erythrocytes, in *Biochemical Methods in Red Cell Genetics*, Yunis, J. J., Ed., Academic Press, New York, 1969, 307.

2. Richardson, B. J., Baverstock, P. R., and Adams, M., *Allozyme Electrophoresis: A Handbook for Animal Systematics and Population Studies*, Academic Press, Sydney, 1986, 171.

3. Patterson, B. D., Atkins, C. A., Graham, D., and Wills, R. B. H., Carbonic anhydrase: a new method of detection on polyacrylamide gels using low-temperature fluorescence, *Anal. Biochem.*, 44, 388, 1971.

4. Hopkinson, D. A., Coppock, J. S., Mühlemann, M. F., and Edwards, Y. H., The detection and differentiation of the products of the human carbonic anhydrase loci, $CA_I$ and $CA_{II}$, using fluorogenic substrates, *Ann. Hum. Genet.*, 38, 155, 1974.

5. Bundy, H. F. and Coté, S., Purification and properties of carbonic anhydrase from *Chlamidomonas reinhardii*, *Phytochemistry*, 19, 253, 1980.

6. Wiedner, G., Simon, B., and Thomas, L., Carbonic anhydrase (carbonate dehydratase): new method of detection on polyacrylamide gels by using conductivity measurements, *Anal. Biochem.*, 55, 93, 1973.

7. Drescher, D. G., Purification of blood carbonic anhydrase and specific detection of carbonic anhydrase isozymes on polyacrylamide gels with 5-dimethylaminonaphthalene-1-sulfonamide (DNSA), *Anal. Biochem.*, 90, 349, 1978.

8. Erickson, R. P., Kay, G., Hewett-Emmett, D., Tashian, R. E., and Claflin, J. L., Cross-reactions among carbonic anhydrase-I, anhydrase-II, and anhydrase-III studied by binding tests and with monoclonal antibodies, *Biochem. Genet.*, 20, 809, 1982.

OTHER NAMES      Fumarase

REACTION      L-Malate = fumarate + $H_2O$

ENZYME SOURCE      Bacteria, fungi, plants, protozoa, invertebrates, vertebrates

## METHOD 1

### Visualization Scheme

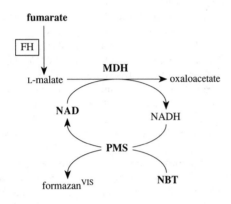

### Staining Solution[1]

| | |
|---|---|
| 25 m$M$ Phosphate buffer, pH 7.1 | 100 ml |
| Potassium fumarate | 770 mg |
| NAD | 80 mg |
| Malate dehydrogenase (MDH) | 200 units |
| NBT | 30 mg |
| PMS | 1 mg |

### Procedure

Incubate the gel in staining solution in the dark at 37°C until dark blue bands appear. Wash stained gel in water and fix in 50% ethanol.

*Notes:* Staining solution can also be applied as 1% agar overlay.

## METHOD 2

### Visualization Scheme

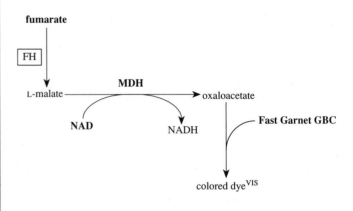

### Staining Solution[2]

| | | |
|---|---|---|
| A. | 0.2 $M$ Tris–HCl buffer, pH 8.0 | 20 ml |
| | 100 mg/ml Fumaric acid (pH 8.0) | 2 ml |
| | 50 mg/ml NAD | 1 ml |
| | Fast Garnet GBC | 120 mg |
| | Malate dehydrogenase (MDH) | 80 units |
| B. | 2% Agar solution (60°C) | 20 ml |

### Procedure

Mix A and B components of the staining solution and pour the mixture over the gel surface. Incubate the gel in the dark at 37°C until colored bands appear. Wash stained gel in water and fix in 3% acetic acid.

*Notes:* Where enzyme activity is weak, greater sensitivity may be obtained using a post-coupling technique: apply liquid staining solution (solution A) lacking Fast Garnet GBC to the gel, incubate the gel for 15 to 30 min, and then add Fast Garnet GBC.

### GENERAL NOTES

Method 1 is more frequently used and is more sensitive than Method 2. The latter method may be preferable when a double stain of the same gel is made. This method does not allow the staining of artifact bands caused by "nothing dehydrogenase" (see 1.X.X.X — NDH).

Maleic and citric acids concurrently inhibit FH. Thus, electrophoretic and staining buffers containing these substances should not be used.

### REFERENCES

1. Shaw, C. R. and Prasad, R., Starch gel electrophoresis of enzymes: a compilation of recipes, *Biochem. Genet.*, 4, 297, 1970.
2. Richardson, B. J., Baverstock, P. R., and Adams, M., *Allozyme Electrophoresis: A Handbook for Animal Systematics and Population Studies*, Academic Press, Sydney, 1986, 178.

OTHER NAMES    Aconitate hydratase (recommended name)

REACTION    Citrate = *cis*-aconitate + $H_2O$; also converts isocitrate into *cis*-aconitate

ENZYME SOURCE    Bacteria, fungi, plants, invertebrates, vertebrates

## METHOD 1

### Visualization Scheme

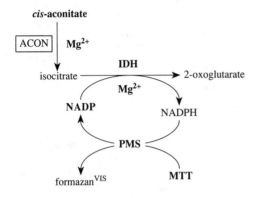

### Staining Solution[1]

A. 
| | |
|---|---|
| 0.2 *M* Tris–HCl buffer, pH 8.0 | 20 ml |
| 20 mg/ml *cis*-Aconitic acid (pH 8.0) | 5 ml |
| $MgCl_2 \cdot 6H_2O$ | 150 mg |
| NADP | 10 mg |
| PMS | 1.5 mg |
| MTT | 7 mg |
| Isocitrate dehydrogenase (IDH) | 10 units |

B. 
| | |
|---|---|
| 2% Agar solution (60°C) | 25 ml |

### Procedure

Mix A and B components of the staining solution and pour the mixture over the gel surface. Incubate the gel in the dark at 37°C until dark blue bands appear. Fix stained gel and/or agar overlay in 50% ethanol.

## METHOD 2

### Visualization Scheme

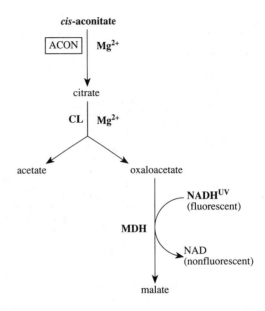

### Staining Solution[2]

| | |
|---|---|
| 0.1 *M* Tris–HCl buffer, pH 8.0 | 16 ml |
| *cis*-Aconitic acid (neutralized) | 20 mg |
| 0.2 *M* $MgCl_2$ | 50 µl |
| Citrate lyase (CL) | 38 units |
| Malate dehydrogenase (MDH) | 55 units |
| NADH | 10 mg |

### Procedure

Apply the staining solution to the gel surface on a filter-paper overlay and incubate at 37°C. Monitor gel under long-wave UV light. Dark (nonfluorescent) bands on a light (fluorescent) background indicate areas of ACON activity. Record the zymogram or photograph using a yellow filter.

*Notes:* To make ACON bands visible in daylight, counterstain the processed gel with the PMS/MTT solution. Achromatic ACON bands will appear on a blue background almost immediately. Fix stained gel in 50% ethanol.

### GENERAL NOTES

Magnesium ions are included in the staining solutions given in both methods to shift the reaction equilibrium towards citrate and isocitrate. *cis*-Aconitic acid may form the *trans* isomer upon prolonged storage. Thus, the use of fresh preparations of this substrate is recommended.

### REFERENCES

1. Shaw, C. R. and Prasad, R., Starch gel electrophoresis of enzymes: a compilation of recipes, *Biochem. Genet.*, 4, 297, 1970.
2. Slaughter, C. A., Hopkinson, D. A., and Harris, H., The distribution and properties of aconitase isozymes in man, *Ann. Hum. Genet.*, 40, 385, 1977.

## 4.2.1.9 — Dihydroxy-acid Dehydratase; DHAD

REACTION     2,3-Dihydroxy-3-methylbutanoate = 2-oxo-3-methylbutanoate + $H_2O$

ENZYME SOURCE  Bacteria, fungi

## METHOD

### Visualization Scheme

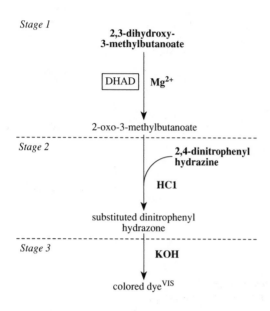

*Stage 1*

**2,3-dihydroxy-3-methylbutanoate**

DHAD  **$Mg^{2+}$**

2-oxo-3-methylbutanoate

*Stage 2*

**2,4-dinitrophenyl hydrazine**

**HCl**

substituted dinitrophenyl hydrazone

*Stage 3*    **KOH**

colored dye$^{VIS}$

### Staining Solution[1]
A. 50 m$M$ Tris–HCl buffer, pH 7.8
   5 m$M$ $MgSO_4$
B. 0.5 $M$ 2,3-Dihydroxy-3-methylbutanoate (sodium salt)
C. 0.025% 2,4-Dinitrophenyl hydrazine
   0.5 $N$ HCl
D. 10% KOH

### Procedure
Incubate electrophorized PAG in solution A at 37°C for 5 min and then add solution B to 5 m$M$ final concentration of 2,3-dihydroxy-3-methylbutanoate and incubate the gel further at 37°C with gentle shaking for 30 min. Transfer gel into solution C and incubate at room temperature for 20 min with occasional agitation. Finally, transfer gel into solution D. Brown bands, at the positions of the DHAD, begin to develop rapidly and reach maximum intensity in 30 min. Record the zymogram or photograph quickly, because the brown bands gradually become blurred and fade upon storage in the KOH.

*Notes:*  The substrate, 2,3-dihydroxy-3-methylbutanoate (or DL-α,β-dihydroxyisovalerate) is not yet commercially available and should be synthesized in the laboratory.

    3-Hydroxy-2-naphthoic acid hydrazide can also be used to detect the carbonyl ketonic group of the product 2-oxo-3-methylbutanoate (or α-ketoisovalerate). The hydrazones formed can then be cross-linked with each other by a tetrazonium salt (see 2.7.1.40 — PK, Method 3).

### REFERENCE
1. Kuo, C. F., Mashino, T. and Fridovich, I., An activity stain for dihydroxy-acid dehydratase, *Anal. Biochem.*, 164, 526, 1987.

## 4.2.1.11 — Enolase; ENO

OTHER NAMES    Phosphopyruvate hydratase, 2-phosphoglycerate dehydratase

REACTION    2-Phospho-D-glycerate = phosphoenolpyruvate + $H_2O$

ENZYME SOURCE  Bacteria, fungi, plants, invertebrates, vertebrates

## METHOD 1

### Visualization Scheme

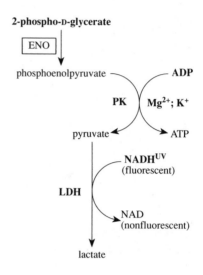

**2-phospho-D-glycerate**

ENO

phosphoenolpyruvate    **ADP**

**PK**  **$Mg^{2+}$; $K^+$**

pyruvate    **ATP**

**NADH$^{UV}$** (fluorescent)

**LDH**

NAD (nonfluorescent)

lactate

### Staining Solution[1]
  38 m$M$ Triethanolamine buffer, pH 7.5
  7.7 m$M$ $MgSO_4$
  3.2 m$M$ EDTA
  1.8 m$M$ ADP
  1.0 m$M$ NADH
  67 m$M$ KCl
  1 m$M$ 2-Phospho-D-glycerate
  1.5 U/ml Pyruvate kinase (PK)
  3.6 U/ml Lactate dehydrogenase (LDH)

### Procedure
Apply the staining solution to the gel surface on a filter-paper overlay and incubate at 37°C for 1 h. Monitor gel under long-wave UV light. Dark (nonfluorescent) bands on a light (fluorescent) background indicate areas of ENO activity. Record the zymogram or photograph using a yellow filter.

*Notes:*  To make ENO bands visible in daylight, counterstain the processed gel with the PMS/MTT solution. Achromatic ACON bands will appear on a blue background almost immediately. Fix stained gel in 50% ethanol.

    3-Phospho-D-glycerate and phosphoglycerate mutase (see 5.4.2.1 — PGLM) may be included in the staining mixture instead of 2-phospho-D-glycerate.[2]

## METHOD 2

### Visualization Scheme

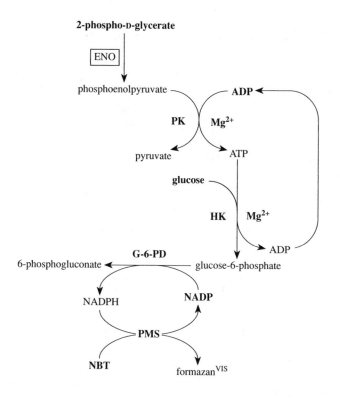

**2-phospho-D-glycerate**

ENO

phosphoenolpyruvate — ADP

PK    Mg²⁺

pyruvate    ATP

**glucose**

HK    Mg²⁺

ADP

G-6-PD

6-phosphogluconate ← glucose-6-phosphate

NADPH    NADP

PMS

NBT    formazan^VIS

### Staining Solution[3]

50 m$M$ Tris–HCl buffer, pH 7.5
2 m$M$ MgCl$_2$
1 m$M$ Glucose
0.1 m$M$ ADP
20 m$M$ AMP
0.5 m$M$ NADP
4 U/ml Pyruvate kinase (PK)
3 U/ml Hexokinase (HK)
1.4 U/ml Glucose-6-phosphate dehydrogenase (G-6-PD)
0.4 mg/ml NBT
1.4 m$M$ 2-Phospho-D-glycerate
0.024 mg/ml PMS

### Procedure

Apply the staining solution to the gel surface dropwise and incubate at 37°C in the dark until dark blue bands appear. Fix stained gel in 50% ethanol.

*Notes:* The appearance of adenylate kinase (see 2.7.4.3 — AK) activity bands is prevented by inclusion of excess AMP and by use of catalytic levels of ADP, the latter being regenerated by hexokinase. Omission of AMP and use of higher concentration of ADP leads to the appearance of extra bands, which are not dependent on the presence of 2-phospho-D-glycerate and are due to adenylate kinase.

## OTHER METHODS

A spectrophotometric procedure for the qualitative and quantitative estimation of ENO on polyacrylamide gels is described.[4] The procedure is based upon the acid hydrolysis (at 100°C) of the product phosphoenolpyruvate to pyruvate, which is then treated with phenylhydrazine and detected as phenylhydrazone by spectrophotometric scanning of PAG at 325 nm.

### REFERENCES

1. Rider, C. C. and Taylor, C. B., Enolase isoenzymes in rat tissues: electrophoretic, chromatographic, immunological and kinetic properties, *Biochim. Biophys. Acta*, 365, 285, 1974.
2. Harris, H. and Hopkinson, D. A., *Handbook of Enzyme Electrophoresis in Human Genetics*, North-Holland, Amsterdam (Loose leaf with supplements in 1977 and 1978), 1976.
3. Hullin, D. A. and Thompson, R. J., An improved nonfluorescent stain for enolase activity on cellulose acetate strips, *Anal. Biochem.*, 82, 240, 1977.
4. Sharma, H. K. and Rothstein, M., A new method for the detection of enolase activity on polyacrylamide gels, *Anal. Biochem.*, 98, 226, 1979.

## 4.2.1.13 — L-Serine Dehydratase; L-SD

OTHER NAMES    Serine deaminase, L-hydroxyaminoacid dehydratase

REACTION    L-Serine + $H_2O$ = pyruvate + $NH_3$ + $H_2O$

ENZYME SOURCE  Bacteria, fungi, invertebrates, vertebrates

## METHOD

### Visualization Scheme

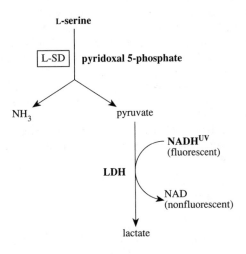

### Staining Solution[1]
A. 0.1 *M* Potassium phosphate buffer, pH 8.0
   0.05 m*M* Pyridoxal 5-phosphate
   1 m*M* NADH
   3.5 U/ml Lactate dehydrogenase (LDH)
   0.15 *M* L-Serine
B. 3% Agar solution (60°C)

### Procedure
Mix 19 ml of solution A with 5 ml of solution B and pour the mixture over the gel surface. Incubate the gel at 30°C for 10 to 15 min and observe nonfluorescent bands on a fluorescent background under long-wave UV light. Record the zymogram or photograph using a yellow filter.

*Notes:* The bands of threonine dehydratase (see 4.2.1.16 — TD) from some sources can also be developed by this method.

## OTHER METHODS

Several methods are also available to detect the product ammonia (e.g., see 4.2.1.16 — TD, Other Methods). However, all these methods are usually less sensitive and not as practical as the method described above.

### REFERENCE
1. Yanagi, S., Tsutsumi, T., Saheki, S., Saheki, K., and Yamamoto, N., Novel and sensitive activity stains on polyacrylamide gel of serine and threonine dehydratase and ornithine aminotransferase, *Enzyme*, 28, 400, 1982.

## 4.2.1.16 — Threonine Dehydratase; TD

OTHER NAMES    Threonine deaminase, L-serine dehydratase, serine deaminase

REACTION    L-Threonine + $H_2O$ = 2-oxobutanoate + $NH_3$ + $H_2O$

ENZYME SOURCE  Bacteria, fungi, invertebrates, vertebrates

## METHOD 1

### Visualization Scheme

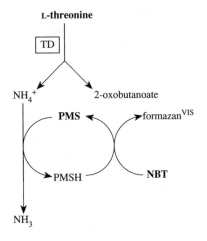

### Staining Solution[1]
0.1 *M* Phosphate buffer, pH 8.0
20 m*M* L-Threonine
0.2 mg/ml PMS
1 mg/ml NBT

### Procedure
Incubate the gel in staining solution in the dark at 37°C until dark blue bands appear. Fix gel in 50% ethanol.

*Notes:* Pyridoxal 5-phosphate may be added to the staining solution and electrophoretic buffer to enhance TD activity.

## METHOD 2

### Visualization Scheme

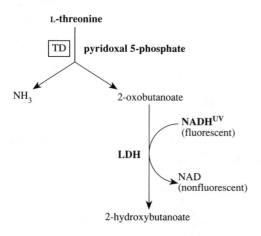

### Staining Solution[2]

A.  0.1 $M$ Potassium phosphate buffer, pH 8.0
   0.05 m$M$ Pyridoxal 5-phosphate
   1 m$M$ NADH
   3.5 U/ml Lactate dehydrogenase (LDH)
   0.15 $M$ L-Threonine
B.  3% Agar solution (60°C)

### Procedure

Mix 19 ml of solution A with 5 ml of solution B and pour the mixture over the gel surface. Incubate the gel at 30°C for 10 to 15 min and observe dark (nonfluorescent) bands under long-wave UV light. Record the zymogram or photograph using a yellow filter.

*Notes:* The method is based on the ability of LDH to use 2-oxobutanoate as a substrate in the backward reaction. It is about two orders more sensitive than Method 1.

## OTHER METHODS

A.  The areas of ammonia production may be detected in UV light using the backward reaction of linking enzyme glutamate dehydrogenase (e.g., see 3.5.3.1 — ARG, Method 2).
B.  The areas of ammonia production may also be visualized using sodium tetraphenylborate which precipitates in the presence of ammonia ions, resulting in the formation of white opaque bands visible in PAG (e.g., see 3.5.1.1 — ASP).
C.  The local pH change due to production of ammonia may be detected using the pH indicator dye, Phenol Violet (e.g., see 3.5.4.4 — ADA, Method 3), the NBT (or MTT)/dithiothreitol system (e.g., see 3.5.3.1 — ARG, Method 1), or neutral AgNO$_3$ solution containing photographic developers (see 3.5.1.5 — UR, Method 2).

## GENERAL NOTES

The enzyme from some sources can use L-serine as substrate and thus be functionally identical to L-serine dehydratase (see 4.2.1.13 — L-SD).

## REFERENCES

1. Feldberg, R. S. and Datta, P., Threonine deaminase: a novel activity stain on polyacrylamide gels, *Science*, 170, 1414, 1970.
2. Yanagi, S., Tsutsumi, T., Saheki, S., Saheki, K., and Yamamoto, N., Novel and sensitive activity stains on polyacrylamide gel of serine and threonine dehydratase and ornithine aminotransferase, *Enzyme*, 28, 400, 1982.

## 4.2.1.20 — Tryptophan Synthase; TS

OTHER NAMES    Tryptophan desmolase

REACTION    L-Serine + indoleglycerol-phosphate = L-tryptophan + glyceraldehyde 3-phosphate

ENZYME SOURCE    Bacteria, fungi, plants

## METHOD

### Visualization Scheme

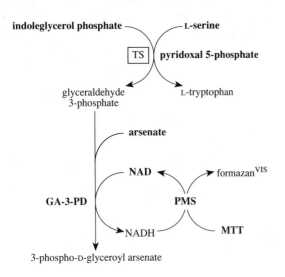

### Staining Solution[1] (modified)

| | | |
|---|---|---|
| A. | 0.05 $M$ Tris–HCl buffer, pH 7.8 | 25 ml |
| | Indoleglycerol-phosphate | 30 mg |
| | L-Serine | 30 mg |
| | Pyridoxal 5-phosphate | 30 mg |
| | Sodium arsenate | 100 mg |
| | Glyceraldehyde-3-phosphate dehydrogenase (GA-3-PD) | 90 units |
| | NAD | 30 mg |
| | MTT | 8 mg |
| | PMS | 1 mg |
| B. | 2% Agar solution (60°C) | 25 ml |

### Procedure

Mix A and B components of the staining solution and pour the mixture over the gel surface. Incubate the gel in the dark at 37°C until dark blue bands appear. Fix stained gel in 50% ethanol.

*Notes:* The enzyme also catalyzes the conversion of L-serine and indole into L-tryptophan and $H_2O$ and of indoleglycerol-phosphate into indole and glyceraldehyde 3-phosphate.

### REFERENCE

1. Crawford, I. P., Ito, J., and Hatanaka, M., Genetic and biochemical studies of enzymatically active subunits of *E. coli* tryptophan synthetase, *Ann. NY Acad. Sci.*, 151, 171, 1968.

## 4.2.1.22 — Serine Sulfhydrase; SS

OTHER NAMES    Cystathionine β-synthase (recommended name), β-thionase, methylcysteine synthase

REACTIONS    1. L-Serine + L-homocysteine = cystathionine + $H_2O$

2. L-cysteine + $H_2O$ = L-serine + $H_2S$

3. See *Notes*

ENZYME SOURCE    Fungi, vertebrates

## METHOD

### Visualization Scheme

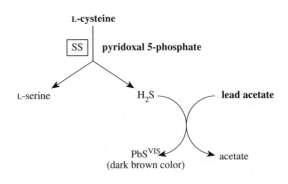

### Staining Solution[1]

0.1 $M$ Sodium phosphate buffer, pH 7.8
20 m$M$ L-Cysteine
50 m$M$ 2-Mercaptoethanol
0.1 m$M$ Pyridoxal 5-phosphate
0.2 m$M$ Lead acetate

### Procedure

Incubate the gel in the staining solution at 37°C until dark brown bands appear. Record or photograph zymogram.

*Notes:* The enzyme is a multifunctional pyridoxal-phosphate protein which catalyzes β-replacement reactions between L-serine, L-cysteine, cysteine thioether, or some other β-substituted α-L-amino acids and a variety of mercaptans.

### REFERENCE

1. Willhardt, I. and Wiederanders, B., Activity staining of cystathionine-β-synthetase and related enzymes, *Anal. Biochem.*, 63, 263, 1975.

## 4.2.1.24 — Porphobilinogen Synthase; PBGS

OTHER NAMES    Aminolevulinate dehydratase

REACTION    5-Aminolevulinate = porphobilinogen + H$_2$O

ENZYME SOURCE  Bacteria, plants, vertebrates

## METHOD

### Visualization Scheme

*Stage 1*

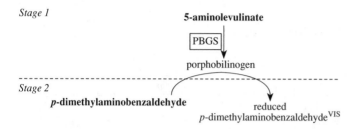

### Staining Solution[1]

A. 0.1 *M* Potassium phosphate, pH 7.2
   13 m*M* 5-Aminolevulinic acid
   15 m*M* Reduced glutathione (or 2 m*M* dithiothreitol)
B. Erlich's reagent:

   1. *p*-Dimethylaminobenzaldehyde          0.1 g
      Acetic acid                             3.4 ml
   2. 0.25 *M* HgCl$_2$                        1 ml
      70% Perchloric acid                     1.6 ml

### Procedure

Apply solution A to the gel surface on a filter-paper overlay and incubate at 37°C for 2 to 3 h. Remove filter paper and rinse gel with water. Place gel in solution B and incubate until pink bands appear.

*Notes:*   HgCl$_2$ is added to Erlich's reagent to oxidize reducing agents before reaction between porphobilinogen and *p*-dimethylaminobenzaldehyde. Dithioerythritol may be included in solution A in place of reduced glutathione or dithiothreitol.[2]

## OTHER METHODS

The immunoblotting procedure (for details see Part II) based on the utility of monoclonal antibodies specific to the spinach enzyme[3] can also be used for immunohistochemical visualization of the enzyme protein on electrophoretic gels. This procedure is expensive, time-consuming, and thus unsuitable for routine laboratory use. Monoclonal antibodies, however, may be of great value in special analyses of PBGS.

### REFERENCES

1. Battistuzzi, G., Petrucci, R., Silvagni, L., Urbani, F. R., and Caiola, S., δ-Aminolevulinate dehydratase: a new genetic polymorphism in man, *Ann. Hum. Genet.*, 45, 223, 1981.
2. Meera Khan, P., Rijken, H., Wijnen, J. Th., Wijnen, L. M. M., and De Boer, L. E. M., Red cell enzyme variation in the orang utan: electrophoretic characterization of 45 enzyme systems in cellogel, in *The Orang Utan. Its Biology and Conservation*, De Boer, L. E. M., Ed., Dr. W. Junk Publishers, The Hague, 1982, 61.
3. Liedgens, W., Grutzmann, R., and Schneider, H. A., Highly efficient purification of the labile plant enzyme 5-aminolevulinate dehydratase (E.C. 4.2.1.24) by means of monoclonal antibodies, *Z. Naturforsch.*, 35, 958, 1980.

## 4.2.1.46 — dTDPglucose 4,6-Dehydratase; TDPGD

REACTION    dTDPglucose = dTDP-4-dehydro-6-deoxy-D-glucose + H$_2$O

ENZYME SOURCE  Bacteria

## METHOD

### Visualization Scheme

*Stage 1*

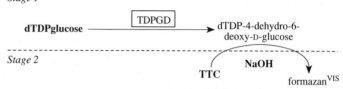

### Staining Solution[1]

A. 20 m*M* Tris–HCl buffer, pH 8.0
   3 m*M* dTDPglucose
B. 0.1% 2,3,5-Triphenyl tetrazolium chloride (TTC)
   1 *N* NaOH

### Procedure

Rinse electrophorized gel in distilled water and incubate in solution A at 37°C for 20 min. Rinse gel again thoroughly and put in freshly prepared solution B. Incubate the gel in this solution in the dark until violet bands appear on a pink background. Fix stained gel in 7% acetic acid.

*Notes:*   The method is based on the ability of the product dTDP-4-dehydro-6-deoxy-D-glucose to reduce TTC in the presence of alkali.

### REFERENCE

1. Gabriel, O. and Wang, S.-F., Determination of enzymatic activity in polyacrylamide gels. I. Enzymes catalyzing the conversion of nonreducing substrates to reducing products, *Anal. Biochem.*, 27, 545, 1969.

## 4.2.1.49 — Urocanate Hydratase; UH

OTHER NAMES      Urocanase

REACTION      4,5-Dihydro-4-oxo-5-imidazolepropanoate = urocanate + $H_2O$

ENZYME SOURCE   Bacteria, vertebrates

## METHOD

### Visualization Scheme

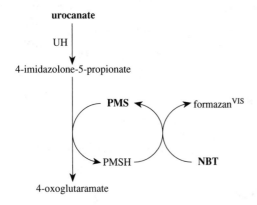

### Staining Solution[1]
A. 0.1 $M$ Phosphate buffer, pH 7.0
   0.01 mg/ml PMS
   0.04 mg/ml NBT
B. 0.1 $M$ Phosphate buffer, pH 7.0
   0.01 mg/ml PMS
   0.04 mg/ml NBT
   10 m$M$ Urocanate

### Procedure
Incubate the gel in solution A in the dark at room temperature for 45 min and then place in solution B. Dark blue bands indicating UH activity appear after 20 to 60 min. Fix stained gel in 50% ethanol.

### REFERENCE
1. Bell, M. V. and Hassall, H., A method for the detection of urocanase on polyacrylamide gels and its use with crude cell extracts of *Pseudomonas*, *Anal. Biochem.*, 75, 436, 1976.

## 4.2.2.2 — Polygalacturonate Lyase; PGL

OTHER NAMES      Pectate lyase (recommended name), pectate transeliminase

REACTION      Eliminative cleavage of pectate to give oligosaccharides with 4-deoxy-α-D-gluc-4-enuronosyl groups at their nonreducing ends

ENZYME SOURCE   Bacteria

## METHOD

### Visualization Scheme

*Stage 1*

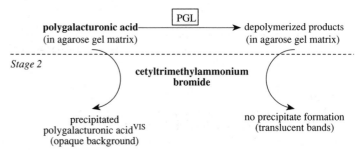

### Staining Solution[1]
A. 0.1 $M$ Tris–HCl buffer, pH 8.6
   1% Polygalacturonic acid
B. 3% Agar solution (60°C)
C. 1% Cetyltrimethylammonium bromide

### Procedure
Mix equal volumes of A and B solutions and form a reactive agarose plate of an appropriate size. Rinse electrophorized PAG in 10 volumes of 0.05 $M$ tris–HCl buffer, pH 8.6. Place reactive agarose plate on top of PAG and incubate at 37°C for 1 to 4 h. Put PAG and reactive agarose plate in solution C. The areas of PGL appear on PAG and agarose plate as translucent bands visible on an opaque background. Photograph developed gel against a black background.

*Notes:* The areas of high PGL activity are more clearly displayed on reactive agarose plate while areas of low PGL activity are more clearly manifested on PAG.

     In principle, areas of galacturan 1,4-α-galacturonidase (see 3.2.1.67 — GG) activity can also be developed by the method described above; however, this enzyme displays maximal activity at pH 5.0.

     Another enzyme, polygalacturonase (see 3.2.1.15 — PG), can also display its activity on PGL zymograms. However, in contrast to PGL, polygalacturonase also hydrolyzes pectin. This difference may be used to identify bands caused by PGL and PG.

### REFERENCE
1. Bertheau, Y., Madgidi-Hervan, E., Kotoujansky, A., Nguyen-The, C., Andro, T., and Coleno, A., Detection of depolymerase isoenzymes after electrophoresis or electrofocusing, or in titration curves, *Anal. Biochem.*, 139, 383, 1984.

## 4.3.1.8 — Uroporphyrinogen-I Synthase; UPS

OTHER NAMES    Porphobilinogen deaminase (recommended name), hydroxymethylbilane synthase, pre-uroporphyrinogen synthase

REACTION    4 Porphobilinogen + $H_2O$ = uroporphyrinogen-I + 4 $NH_3$

ENZYME SOURCE  Vertebrates

## METHOD

### Visualization Scheme

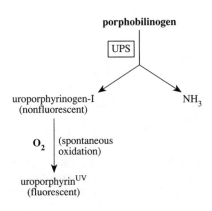

### Staining Solution[1]
    0.1 $M$ Tris–HCl buffer, pH 8.2
    90 m$M$ Porphobilinogen

### Procedure
Incubate the gel in staining solution in the dark at 45°C until red fluorescent bands become visible under long-wave UV light. Expose gel to light and air for several minutes to complete the conversion of uroporphyrinogen to uroporphyrin. Record the zymogram or photograph using a yellow filter.

*Notes:*   Staining solution may be applied to the gel surface on cellulose acetate membrane and the final concentration of porphobilinogen reduced to 0.5 m$M$.[2]

## OTHER METHODS

A. Areas of ammonia production may be detected in UV light using the backward reaction of the linking enzyme glutamate dehydrogenase (e.g., see 3.5.4.4 — ADA, Method 2).

B. The product ammonia may be visualized using sodium tetraphenylborate, which is precipitated in the presence of ammonia ions resulting in the formation of white opaque bands visible in PAG (see 3.5.1.1 — ASP).

C. The local pH change due to production of ammonia may be detected using the pH indicator dye, Phenol Violet (e.g., see 3.5.4.4 — ADA, Method 3), the NBT (or MTT)/dithiothreitol system (e.g., see 3.5.3.1 — ARG, Method 1), or neutral $AgNO_3$ solution containing photographic developers (see 3.5.1.5 — UR, Method 2).

## REFERENCES

1. Meisler, M. H. and Carter, L. C., Rare structural variants of human and murine uroporphyrinogen I synthase, *Proc. Natl. Acad. Sci. U.S.A.*, 77, 2848, 1980.
2. Veser, J., Preparative free solution isoelectric focusing of human erythrocyte uroporphyrinogen I synthase in an ampholyte pH gradient, *Anal. Biochem.*, 182, 217, 1989.

## 4.3.2.1 — Argininosuccinate Lyase; ASL

OTHER NAMES    Argininosuccinase

REACTION    L-Argininosuccinate = fumarate + L-arginine

ENZYME SOURCE  Bacteria, fungi, plants, vertebrates

## METHOD 1

### Visualization Scheme

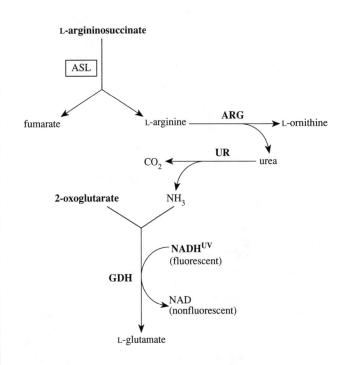

### Staining Solution[1]

| | |
|---|---:|
| 0.1 $M$ Tris–HCl buffer, pH 7.6 | 5 ml |
| L-Argininosuccinic acid (Ba salt) | 50 mg |
| Arginase (ARG) | 40 units |
| Urease (UR) | 20 units |
| 2-Oxoglutarate | 25 mg |
| NADH | 10 mg |
| Glutamate dehydrogenase (GDH) | 25 units |

### Procedure
Apply the staining solution to gel on a filter-paper overlay. Incubate the gel at 37°C and monitor for defluorescent zones under long-wave UV light. Record the zymogram or photograph using a yellow filter.

## METHOD 2

### Visualization Scheme

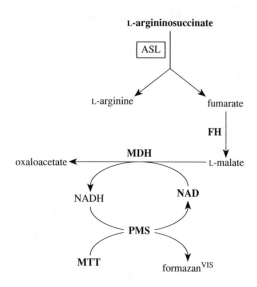

### Staining Solution*

A. 0.1 *M* Phosphate buffer, pH 7.5                 25 ml
   L-Argininosuccinic acid (Ba salt)               50 mg
   NAD                                             25 mg
   Malate dehydrogenase (MDG)                   30 units
   Fumarate hydratase (FH)                       60 units
   PMS                                              1 mg
   MTT                                              8 mg
B. 2% Agarose solution (60°C)                       25 ml

### Procedure

Mix A and B components of the staining solution and pour the mixture over the gel surface. Incubate the gel at 37°C in the dark until dark blue bands appear. Fix stained gel in 50% ethanol.

## METHOD 3

### Visualization Scheme

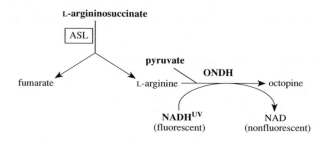

### Staining Solution*

0.1 *M* Phosphate buffer, pH 7.5                   10 ml
L-Argininosuccinic acid (Ba salt)                 50 mg
NADH                                              10 mg
Octopine dehydrogenase (ONDH)                  10 units
Sodium pyruvate                                   30 mg

### Procedure

Apply the staining solution to gel on a filter-paper overlay. Incubate the gel at 37°C and monitor for defluorescent zones under long-wave UV light. Record the zymogram or photograph using a yellow filter.

*Notes:* Lactate dehydrogenase activity bands can also be developed by this method. Therefore, an additional gel should be stained for LDH (see 1.1.1.27 — LDH; Other Methods, A) as control.

### OTHER METHODS

A bioautographic method (for details see Part II) for ASL detection on electrophoretic gel is also available.[2] However, this method is not as practical as the methods described above.

### REFERENCES

1. Nelson, R. L., Povey, S., Hopkinson, D. A., and Harris, H., Detection after electrophoresis of enzymes involved in ammonia metabolism using L-glutamate dehydrogenase as a linking enzyme, *Biochem. Genet.*, 15, 1023, 1977.
2. Naylor, S. L., Klebe, R. J., and Shows, T. B., Argininosuccinic aciduria: assignment of the argininosuccinate lyase gene to the pter→q22 region of human chromosome 7 by bioautography, *Proc. Natl. Acad. Sci. U.S.A.*, 75, 6159, 1978.

---

\* New; recommended for use.

\* New; recommended for use.

OTHER NAMES   Lactoylglutathione lyase (recommended name), methylglyoxalase, aldoketomutase, ketone-aldehyde mutase

REACTION   *S*-Lactoylglutathione = glutathione + methylglyoxal

ENZYME SOURCE   Fungi, invertebrates, vertebrates

## METHOD 1

### Visualization Scheme

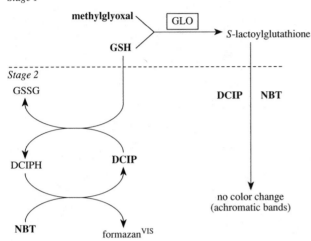

### Staining Solution[1]
A.  0.2 *M* Phosphate buffer, pH 6.8
    257 m*M* Methylglyoxal
    16.3 m*M* Glutathione (reduced; GSH)
    2.4 m*M* NBT
B.  0.1 *M* Tris–HCl buffer, pH 7.0 to 8.0
    0.06 m*M* 2,6-Dichlorophenolindophenol (DCIP)

### Procedure
Incubate the gel in solution A at 37°C for 15 to 45 min and then place in solution B. Achromatic bands indicating areas of GLO activity develop on a blue background of the gel. Fix stained gel in 50% ethanol.

*Notes:*   This method was developed for starch gel. When it was applied to acetate cellulose gel with solution B prepared using tris–HCl buffer, pH 7.8, dark blue bands were observed at the sites of GLO activity when negatively stained gel was left in a moist chamber at room temperature.[2] This reversal is pH-dependent, because, at pH levels higher than 8.0, white bands appear against a blue background also on acetate cellulose gel.

A modified method which uses PMS instead of DCIP is also available.[3]

## METHOD 2

### Visualization Scheme

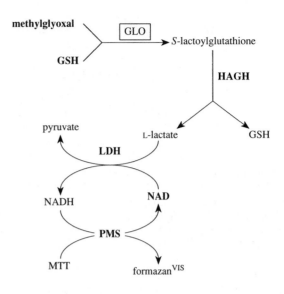

### Staining Solution[3]
A.  0.2 *M* Phosphate buffer, pH 6.7                       25 ml
    Methylglyoxal (40% water solution)                     0.5 ml
    Glutathione (reduced; GSH)                             30 mg
    Hydroxyacylglutathione hydrolase (HAGH)                5 units
    Lactate dehydrogenase (LDH)                            20 units
    NAD                                                    25 mg
    PMS                                                    1 mg
    MTT                                                    8 mg
B.  2% Agarose solution (60°C)                             25 ml

### Procedure
Mix A and B components of the staining solution and pour the mixture over the gel surface. Incubate the gel at 37°C in the dark until dark blue bands appear. Fix stained gel in 50% ethanol.

*Notes:*   The method usually gives substantial staining of the gel background. This problem can be avoided by omission of PMS and MTT from the staining solution and viewing the gel for fluorescent bands under long-wave UV lamp.

## METHOD 3

### Visualization Scheme

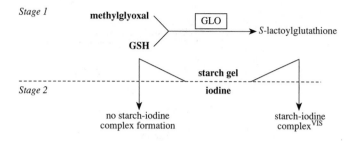

*Stage 1*   methylglyoxal

GLO ⟶ *S*-lactoylglutathione

GSH

starch gel

*Stage 2*   iodine

no starch-iodine complex formation

starch-iodine complex[VIS]

### Staining Solution[4]

A.  0.2 *M* Phosphate buffer, pH 6.7 .......... 12 ml
    Glutathione (reduced; GSH) .......... 40 mg
    Methylglyoxal (40% water solution) .......... 0.5 ml
B.  0.7% Agar solution (45°C) .......... 30 ml
    1% Iodine in 1% KI solution .......... 1.3 ml

### Procedure

Apply solution A to the surface of the starch gel on a filter-paper overlay and incubate the gel at 37°C for 40 min. Remove filter paper and blot gel carefully to remove excess solution A, then pour solution B over the gel surface. Intense blue bands appear almost immediately in areas of GLO location due to starch–iodine complex formation. Record the zymogram or photograph, because staining is not stable.

*Notes:*   Starch gel preincubated with solution A may be further developed by placing it in a tank containing some crystals of iodine.[5]

This method is applicable to starch gels or PAGs containing soluble starch.

### REFERENCES

1.  Kömpf, J., Bissbort, S., Gussmann, S., and Ritter, H., Polymorphism of red cell glyoxalase I (EC 4.4.1.5): a new genetic marker in man, *Humangenetik*, 27, 141, 1975.
2.  Meera Khan, P. and Doppert, B. A., Rapid detection of glyoxalase I (GLO) on cellulose acetate gel and the distribution of GLO variants in a Dutch population, *Hum. Genet.*, 34, 53, 1976.
3.  Bagster, I. A. and Parr, C. W., Human erythrocyte glyoxalase I polymorphism, *J. Physiol.*, 256, 56P, 1976.
4.  Parr, C. W., Bagster, I. A., and Welch, S. G., Human red cell glyoxalase I polymorphism, *Biochem. Genet.*, 15, 109, 1977.
5.  Pflugshaupt, R., Scherz, R., and Bütler, R., Human red cell glyoxalase I polymorphism in the Swiss population: phenotype frequences and simplified technique, *Hum. Hered.*, 28, 235, 1978.

OTHER NAMES   Cysteine S-conjugate β-lyase

REACTION   RS–CH$_2$–CH(NH$_3^+$)COO$^-$ = RSH + pyruvate + ammonia; RH may represent aromatic compounds such as 4-bromobenzene and 2,4-dinitrobenzene

ENZYME SOURCE   Vertebrates

## METHOD 1

### Visualization Scheme

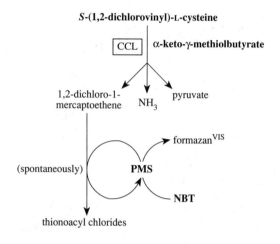

*S*-(1,2-dichlorovinyl)-L-cysteine

CCL | α-keto-γ-methiolbutyrate

1,2-dichloro-1-mercaptoethene      NH$_3$      pyruvate

(spontaneously)      PMS      formazan[VIS]

NBT

thionoacyl chlorides

### Staining Solution[1]

0.1 *M* Potassium phosphate buffer, pH 7.2
2 m*M* *S*-(1,2-Dichlorovinyl)-L-cysteine
0.5 m*M* α-Keto-γ-methiolbutyrate
0.1 m*M* PMS
1 m*M* NBT

### Procedure

Wash electrophorized PAG twice with distilled water and incubate in the staining solution in the dark at 37°C until dark blue bands appear. Fix stained gel in 50% ethanol.

*Notes:*   Each of two identical subunits of CCL contains one equivalent of tightly bound pyridoxal 5′-phosphate. α-Keto-γ-methiolbutyrate is added to ensure maintenance of the enzyme in the pyridoxal 5′-phosphate form. In the absence of α-keto-γ-methiolbutyrate, activity of CCL is greatly reduced. This is because with *S*-(1,2-dichlorovinyl)-L-cysteine as substrate the enzyme catalyzes competing β-elimination (the products are pyruvate, ammonia, and an unstable thiol) and transamination (the product is *S*-(1,2-dichlorovinyl)-3-mercapto-2-oxopropionate) reactions. During the transamination reaction, the enzyme is converted to the pyridoxamine phosphate form, which cannot catalyze the β-elimination reaction. The added α-keto-γ-methiolbutyrate converts the pyridoxamine phosphate form of CCL to the pyridoxal phosphate form which is competent to catalyze β-elimination reaction.[2]

The mechanism of reduction of NBT is not known in detail. It may be more complex than a simple electron transfer from the sulfhydryl of the 1,2-dichloro-1-mercaptoethene via PMS molecules.

Faint bands caused by L-2-hydroxy acid oxidase (see 1.1.3.15 — GOX, General Notes) can also be developed by this method. Thus, an additional gel should be stained for GOX as a control.

## METHOD 2

### Visualization Scheme

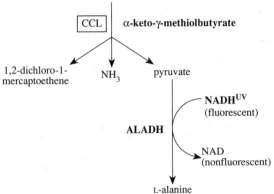

S-(1,2-dichlorovinyl)-L-cysteine

CCL  α-keto-γ-methiolbutyrate

1,2-dichloro-1-mercaptoethene  NH₃  pyruvate

NADH^UV (fluorescent)

ALADH

NAD (nonfluorescent)

L-alanine

### Staining Solution[1] (adapted)
0.1 *M* Tris–HCl buffer, pH 8.0
1 m*M* α-Keto-γ-methiolbutyrate
2 m*M* S-(1,2-Dichlorovinyl)-L-cysteine
1 m*M* NADH
7 U/ml Alanine dehydrogenase (ALADH)

### Procedure
Apply the staining solution to the gel surface with filter paper or 1% agar overlay and incubate at 37°C. Monitor gel under long-wave UV light for dark (nonfluorescent) bands visible on a light (fluorescent) background. Photograph developed gel using a yellow filter.

*Notes:* This method is an adaptation of the spectrophotometric method used for detection of CCL activity in sections of PAG.

Lactate dehydrogenase (EC 1.1.1.27) is unsuitable as a linking enzyme for detection of the product pyruvate because it displays good activity towards α-keto-γ-methiolbutyrate.

## GENERAL NOTES

The cystosolic form of CCL from rat kidney was shown to be identical to a soluble form of glutamine transaminase K (see 2.6.1.64 — GTK).[2]

## REFERENCES
1. Abraham, D. G. and Cooper, A. J. L., Glutamine transaminase K and cysteine S-conjugate β-lyase activity stains, *Anal. Biochem.*, 197, 421, 1991.
2. Cooper, A. J. L. and Anders, M. W., Glutamine transaminase K and cysteine conjugate β-lyase, *Ann. NY Acad. Sci.*, 585, 118, 1990.

## 4.6.1.3 — 3-Dehydroquinate Synthase; DQS

REACTION  7-Phospho-3-deoxy-*arabino*-heptulosonate = 3-dehydroquinate + orthophosphate

ENZYME SOURCE  Bacteria, fungi

## METHOD

### Visualization Scheme

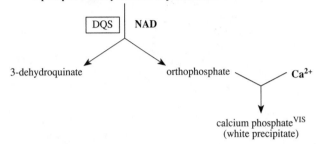

**7-phospho-3-deoxy-*arabino*-heptulosonate**

DQS  NAD

3-dehydroquinate  orthophosphate  Ca²⁺

calcium phosphate^VIS (white precipitate)

### Staining Solution[1]
50 m*M* Glycine–KOH buffer, pH 10.0
1 m*M* 7-Phospho-3-deoxy-*arabino*-heptulosonate
50 μ*M* NAD
10 m*M* Ca²⁺

### Procedure
Incubate electrophorized PAG in the staining solution at 37°C until opaque bands visible against a dark background appear. Store stained gel in 50 m*M* glycine–KOH, pH 10.0, 5 m*M* Ca²⁺ at 5°C or at room temperature in the presence of an antibacterial agent (e.g., sodium azide).

*Notes:* The areas of calcium phosphate precipitation can be counterstained with Alizarin Red S. This does not increase the sensitivity of the method but would be of advantage for opaque gels such as acetate cellulose or starch.

## OTHER METHODS

The enzymatic method of detection of the product orthophosphate can also be used.[2] This method is based on reactions catalyzed by two linking enzymes, purine-nucleoside phosphorylase and xanthine oxidase, coupled with PMS/MTT (e.g., see 3.6.1.1 — PP, Method 2).

## GENERAL NOTES

The enzyme from *Neurospora* is a part of the multienzyme complex "*arom*".

## REFERENCES
1. Nimmo, H. G. and Nimmo, G. A., A general method for the localization of enzymes that produce phosphate, pyrophosphate, or CO₂ after polyacrylamide gel electrophoresis, *Anal. Biochem.*, 121, 17, 1982.
2. Klebe, R. J., Schloss, S., Mock, L., and Link, C. R., Visualization of isozymes which generate inorganic phosphate, *Biochem. Genet.*, 19, 921, 1981.

## 4.6.1.4 — Chorismate Synthase; CHOS

REACTION $O^5$-(1-Carboxyvinyl)-3-phosphoshikimate = chorismate + orthophosphate

ENZYME SOURCE  Bacteria, fungi

## METHOD

### Visualization Scheme

$O^5$-(1-carboxyvinyl)-3-phosphoshikimate

CHOS   NADPH; FMN

chorismate          orthophosphate          $Ca^{2+}$

calcium phosphate$^{VIS}$
(white precipitate)

### Staining Solution[1]
100 m$M$ Tris–HCl buffer, pH 8.0
50 µ$M$ 3-Enolpyruvylshikimate-5-phosphate
0.5 m$M$ NADPH
10 µ$M$ FMN
10 m$M$ $Ca^{2+}$

### Procedure
Incubate electrophorized PAG in a staining solution at 37°C until opaque bands visible against a dark background appear. Store stained gel in 50 m$M$ glycine–KOH, pH 10.0, 5 m$M$ $Ca^{2+}$ at 5°C or at room temperature in the presence of an antibacterial agent (e.g., sodium azide).

*Notes:*   The areas of calcium phosphate precipitation can be counterstained with Alizarin Red S. This would be of advantage for opaque gels such as acetate cellulose or starch.

## GENERAL NOTES

The enzyme from *Neurospora* is a part of the multienzyme complex "*arom*" and is active only in the complex with NADPH-dependent flavine reductase. The purified enzyme requires $Mg^{2+}$, FAD, or FMN and diaphorase for its activity.

## REFERENCE
1. Nimmo, H. G. and Nimmo, G. A., A general method for the localization of enzymes that produce phosphate, pyrophosphate, or $CO_2$ after polyacrylamide gel electrophoresis, *Anal. Biochem.*, 121, 17, 1982.

## 5.1.3.1 — Ribulose-phosphate 3-Epimerase; RPE

OTHER NAMES   Phosphoribulose epimerase

REACTION   D-Ribulose 5-phosphate = D-xylulose 5-phosphate

ENZYME SOURCE  Bacteria, fungi, vertebrates

## METHOD

### Visualization Scheme

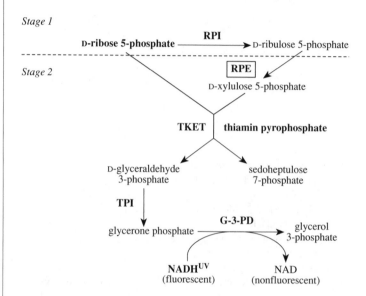

*Stage 1*

D-ribose 5-phosphate  —RPI→  D-ribulose 5-phosphate

*Stage 2*

RPE

D-xylulose 5-phosphate

TKET   thiamin pyrophosphate

D-glyceraldehyde          sedoheptulose
3-phosphate              7-phosphate

TPI

glycerone phosphate  —G-3-PD→  glycerol 3-phosphate

NADH$^{UV}$                    NAD
(fluorescent)              (nonfluorescent)

### Staining Solution[1]
| | |
|---|---|
| A. 0.1 $M$ Tris–HCl buffer, pH 8.0 | 10 ml |
| 0.1 $M$ $MgCl_2$ | 40 ml |
| 0.25% Thiamin pyrophosphate (pH 7.0) | 40 ml |
| Transketolase (TKET) | 1 unit |
| Triose-phosphate isomerase (TPI) | 50 units |
| Glycerol-3-phosphate dehydrogenase (G-3-PD) | 17 units |
| NADH | 20 mg |
| B. D-Ribose 5-phosphate | 10 mg |
| Ribose-5-phosphate isomerase (RPI) | 50 units |
| $H_2O$ | 0.5 ml |
| C. 2% Agar solution (55°C) | 100 ml |

### Procedure
Prepare solution B and incubate at room temperature for 15 min before addition to solution A. Mix A and B solutions and add solution C. Pour the resulting mixture over the gel surface and incubate at 37°C until dark (nonfluorescent) bands visible in long-wave UV light appear on a light (fluorescent) background. Record the zymogram or photograph using a yellow filter.

## OTHER METHODS

To obtain zymograms with RPE activity bands visible in daylight, glyceraldehyde-3-phosphate dehydrogenase (1.2.1.12 — GA-3-PD), sodium arsenate, NAD, PMS, and MTT should be included in solution A in place of TPI, G-3-PD, and NADH (e.g., see 5.4.2.7 — PPM, Method 1).

## REFERENCE

1. Spencer, N. and Hopkinson, D. A., Biochemical genetics of the pentose phosphate cycle: human ribose 5-phosphate isomerase (RPI) and ribulose 5-phosphate 3-epimerase (RPE), *Ann. Hum. Genet.*, 43, 335, 1980.

OTHER NAMES    Mutarotase, aldose mutarotase

REACTION    α-D-Glucose = β-D-glucose

ENZYME SOURCE   Fungi, vertebrates (kidney)

## METHOD

### Visualization Scheme

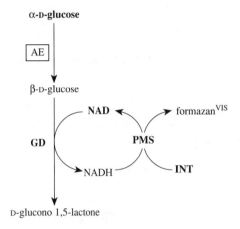

### Staining Solution[1] (adapted)

| | |
|---|---|
| A. 0.2 *M* Sodium phosphate buffer, pH 7.6 | 20 ml |
| α-D-Glucose | 100 mg |
| β-D-Glucose dehydrogenase (GD; EC 1.1.1.47) | 150 units |
| NAD | 25 mg |
| MTT (or INT) | 8 mg |
| PMS | 1 mg |
| B. 1.5% Agarose solution (55°C) | 20 ml |

### Procedure

Mix A and B components of the staining solution and pour the mixture over the gel surface. Incubate the gel in the dark at room temperature until dark blue bands appear. Fix stained gel in 50% ethanol.

*Notes:* It is important to use α-D-glucose preparations that are free of the β-anomer.

## OTHER METHODS

Two coupled reactions catalyzed by the auxiliary enzymes glucose oxidase and peroxidase can be used to detect the product β-D-glucose. Since glucose oxidase is an FAD-containing enzyme, the product β-D-glucose can also be detected using auxiliary glucose oxidase in couple with the MTT/PMS system (e.g., see 1.1.3.4 — GO).

## REFERENCE

1. Babczinsky, P., Fractionation of yeast invertase isozymes and determination of enzymatic activity in sodium dodecyl sulfate–polyacrylamide gels, *Anal. Biochem.*, 105, 328, 1980.

| | |
|---|---|
| OTHER NAMES | Phosphotriose isomerase, triosephosphate mutase |
| REACTION | D-Glyceraldehyde 3-phosphate = glycerone phosphate |
| ENZYME SOURCE | Bacteria, fungi, plants, invertebrates, vertebrates |

## METHOD 1

### Visualization Scheme

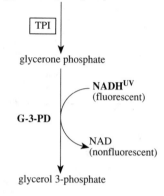

### Staining Solution[1]

| | |
|---|---|
| A. 0.1 *M* Triethanolamine–HCl buffer, pH 8.0 (containing 5 m*M* EDTA) | 20 ml |
| 30 m*M* D,L-Glyceraldehyde 3-phosphate (see *Notes*) | 2 ml |
| NADH | 20 mg |
| Glycerol-3-phosphate dehydrogenase (G-3-PD) | 16 units |
| B. 2% Agar solution (60°C) | 20 ml |

### Procedure

Mix A and B solutions and pour over the gel surface. Incubate the gel at 37°C until dark (nonfluorescent) bands visible in long-wave UV light appear on a light (fluorescent) background. Record the zymogram or photograph using a yellow filter.

*Notes:* D,L-Glyceraldehyde 3-phosphate (free acid) is commercially available; however, it is not sufficiently stable (stability studies indicate decomposition of as much as 10% in 3 d when exposed to room temperature). D-Glyceraldehyde 3-phosphate diethyl acetal (dicyclohexylammonium salt) available from Sigma is the more practical preparation, but it is very expensive. The optimal way is to generate D,L-glyceraldehyde 3-phosphate from the relatively cheap diethyl acetal barium salt, or from fructose-1,6-diphosphate using aldolase (see 1.2.1.12 — GA-3-PD, Method 1).

## METHOD 2

### Visualization Scheme

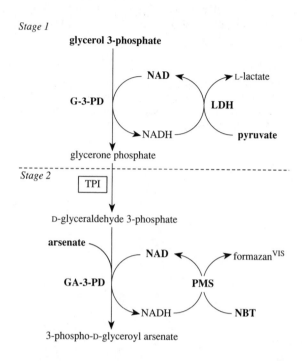

### Staining Solution[2] (modified)

| | |
|---|---|
| A. 0.1 *M* Tris–HCl buffer, pH 8.5 | 20 ml |
| α-Glycerophosphate | 600 mg |
| NAD | 20 mg |
| Glycerol-3-phosphate dehydrogenase (G-3-PD) | 20 units |
| Sodium pyruvate | 200 mg |
| Lactate dehydrogenase (LDH) | 60 units |
| B. Solution A (prepared as described in Procedure) | 20 ml |
| NAD | 20 mg |
| PMS | 1 mg |
| MTT | 8 mg |
| Sodium arsenate | 70 mg |
| Glyceraldehyde-3-phosphate dehydrogenase (GA-3-PD) | 40 units |
| C. 2% Agar solution (55°C) | 20 ml |

### Procedure

Incubate solution A at 37°C for 2 h and then stop reaction by dropwise addition of concentrated HCl until pH is 2.0. Readjust solution A to pH 8.0 with NaOH. Prepare solution B and mix with solution C. Pour the resulting mixture over the gel surface and incubate the gel at 37°C in the dark until dark blue bands appear. Fix stained gel in 50% ethanol.

## 5.3.1.1 — Triose-phosphate Isomerase; TPI (continued)

*Notes:* The bands of G-3-PD and LDH also develop on TPI zymograms obtained by this method. Therefore, control stainings of two additional gels are necessary to identify activity bands caused by these two dehydrogenases.

A stable lithium salt of dihydroxyacetone phosphate (glycerone phosphate) is now available from Sigma Chemical Company. The use of this preparation in place of solution A makes control staining for G-3-PD and LDH activities unnecessary.[3]

### REFERENCES

1. Harris, H. and Hopkinson, D. A., *Handbook of Enzyme Electrophoresis in Human Genetics*, North-Holland, Amsterdam (Loose leaf with supplements in 1977 and 1978), 1976.
2. Shaw, C. R. and Prasad, R., Starch gel electrophoresis of enzymes: a compilation of recipes, *Biochem. Genet.*, 4, 297, 1970.
3. Aebersold, P. B., Winans, G. A., Teel, D. J., Milner, G. B., and Utter, F. M., *Manual for Starch Gel Electrophoresis: A Method for the Detection of Genetic Variation*, NOAA Technical Report NMFS 61, U.S. Dept. of Commerce, National Marine Fisheries Service, Seattle, WA, 1987.

## 5.3.1.6 — Ribose-5-phosphate Isomerase; RPI

OTHER NAMES    Phosphopentoisomerase, phosphoriboisomerase

REACTION    D-Ribose 5-phosphate = D-ribulose 5-phosphate

ENZYME SOURCE   Bacteria, plants, invertebrates, vertebrates

## METHOD

### Visualization Scheme

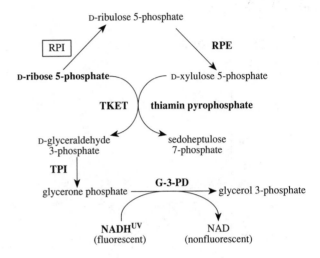

### Staining Solution[1]

A.   0.1 *M* Tris–HCl buffer, pH 8.0    5 ml
    0.1 *M* MgCl$_2$    20 ml
    0.25% Thiamin pyrophosphate (pH 7.0)    20 ml
    Transketolase (TKET)    0.5 unit
    D-Ribose 5-phosphate    5 mg
    Ribulose-phosphate 3-epimerase (RPE)    0.5 unit
    Triose-phosphate isomerase (TPI)    25 units
    Glycerol-3-phosphate dehydrogenase (G-3-PD)    8.5 units
    NADH    10 mg
B.   2% Agar solution (55°C)    45 ml

### Procedure

Mix A and B components of the staining solution and pour the mixture over the gel surface. Incubate the gel at 37°C until dark (nonfluorescent) bands visible in long-wave UV light appear on a light (fluorescent) background. Record the zymogram or photograph using a yellow filter.

*Notes:* To obtain a zymogram with RPI activity bands visible in daylight, glyceraldehyde-3-phosphate dehydrogenase (1.2.1.12 — GA-3-PD), sodium arsenate, NAD, PMS, and MTT should be included in solution A in place of TPI, G-3-PD, and NADH.

### REFERENCE

1. Spencer, N. and Hopkinson, D. A., Biochemical genetics of the pentose phosphate cycle: human ribose 5-phosphate isomerase (RPI) and ribulose 5-phosphate 3-epimerase (RPE), *Ann. Hum. Genet.*, 43, 335, 1980.

## 5.3.1.8 — Mannose-6-phosphate Isomerase; MPI

OTHER NAMES    Phosphomannose isomerase, phosphohexomutase, phosphohexoisomerase

REACTION    D-Mannose 6-phosphate = D-fructose 6-phosphate

ENZYME SOURCE    Bacteria, fungi, plants, invertebrates, vertebrates

## METHOD

### Visualization Scheme

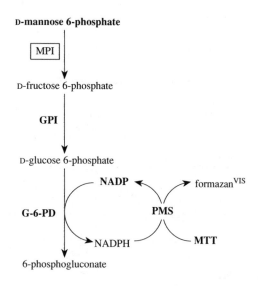

### Staining Solution[1]

| A. 0.35 $M$ Tris–HCl buffer, pH 8.0 | 10 ml |
|---|---|
| Mannose 6-phosphate (Ba salt; 3H$_2$O) | 10 mg |
| PMS | 0.8 mg |
| MTT | 3 mg |
| NADP | 5 mg |
| Glucose-6-phosphate isomerase (GPI) | 3.5 units |
| Glucose-6-phosphate dehydrogenase (G-6-PD; see *Notes*) | 1.5 units |
| B. 1.5% Agar solution (55°C) | 20 ml |

### Procedure

Mix A and B components of the staining solution and pour the mixture over the gel surface. Incubate the gel in the dark at 37°C until dark blue bands appear. Fix stained gel in 50% ethanol.

*Notes:*   The use of the NAD-dependent form of the linking enzyme G-6-PD (available from Sigma) is preferable because substitution of NAD for NADP in the staining solution results in a cost saving.

### REFERENCE

1. Nichols, E. A. and Ruddle, F. H., A review of enzyme polymorphisms, linkage and electrophoretic conditions for mouse and somatic cell hybrids in starch gels, *J. Histochem. Cytochem.*, 21, 1066, 1973.

## 5.3.1.9 — Glucose-6-phosphate Isomerase; GPI

OTHER NAMES    Phosphohexose isomerase, phosphohexomutase, oxoisomerase, hexosephosphate isomerase, phosphosaccharomutase, phosphoglucoisomerase, phosphohexoisomerase

REACTION    D-Glucose 6-phosphate = D-fructose 6-phosphate

ENZYME SOURCE    Bacteria, fungi, plants, protozoa, invertebrates, vertebrates

## METHOD

### Visualization Scheme

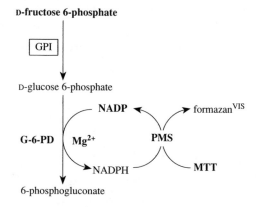

### Staining Solution[1] (modified)

| A. 0.1 $M$ Tris–HCl buffer, pH 8.5 | 25 ml |
|---|---|
| NADP | 10 mg |
| MTT | 7 mg |
| PMS | 1 mg |
| MgCl$_2$ (6H$_2$O) | 40 mg |
| D-Fructose 6-phosphate (Ba salt) | 20 mg |
| Glucose-6-phosphate dehydrogenase (G-6-PD; see *Notes*) | 10 units |
| B. 2% Agar solution (60°C) | 25 ml |

### Procedure

Mix A and B components of the staining solution and pour the mixture over the gel surface. Incubate the gel in the dark at 37°C until dark blue bands appear. Fix stained gel in 50% ethanol.

*Notes:*   The use of the NAD-dependent form of the linking enzyme G-6-PD (available from Sigma) is preferable because substitution of NAD for NADP in the staining solution results in a cost saving. The use of G-6-PD immobilized into the gel matrix is recommended when PAG is used for GPI electrophoresis.[2]

### REFERENCES

1. De Lorenzo, R. J. and Ruddle, F. H., Genetic control of two electrophoretic variants of glucosephosphate isomerase, *Biochem. Genet.*, 3, 151, 1969.
2. Harrison, A. P., The detection of hexokinase, glucosephosphate isomerase and phosphoglucomutase activities in polyacrylamide gels after electrophoresis: a novel method using immobilized glucose 6-phosphate dehydrogenase, *Anal. Biochem.*, 61, 500, 1974.

## 5.4.2.1 — Phosphoglycerate Mutase; PGLM

OTHER NAMES    Phosphoglyceric acid mutase, phosphoglycerate phosphomutase, phosphoglyceromutase

REACTION    2-Phospho-D-glycerate = 3-phospho-D-glycerate (also see General Notes)

ENZYME SOURCE    Bacteria, fungi, plants, invertebrates, vertebrates

## METHOD 1

### Visualization Scheme

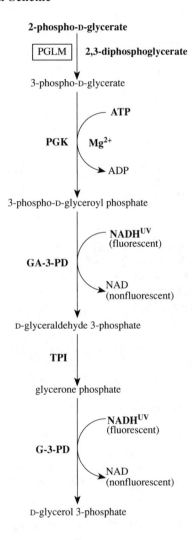

### Staining Solution[1]

A. 0.2 $M$ Tris–HCl buffer, pH 8.0      20 ml
   2-Phospho-D-glycerate (Na$_3$ salt; 6H$_2$O)      30 mg
   2,3-Diphosphoglycerate (pentacyclohexyl ammonium salt; 4H$_2$O)      15 mg
   Phosphoglycerate kinase (PGK)      60 units
   Glyceraldehyde-3-phosphate dehydrogenase (GA-3-PD)      100 units
   NADH      10 mg
   MgCl$_2$ (6H$_2$O)      12 mg
   EDTA (Na$_2$ salt; 2H$_2$O)      30 mg
   Triose-phosphate isomerase (TPI)      100 units
   Glycerol-3-phosphate dehydrogenase (G-3-PD)      40 units
B. 2% Agar solution (55°C)      20 ml

### Procedure

Mix A and B solutions and pour the mixture over the gel surface. Incubate the gel at 37°C until dark (nonfluorescent) bands visible in long-wave UV light appear on a light (fluorescent) background. Record the zymogram or photograph using a yellow filter.

*Notes:* Auxiliary enzymes TPI and G-3-PD are used to intensify the progress of NADH into NAD conversion. These enzymes may be omitted from the staining solution when preparations with high PGLM activity are analyzed.

## METHOD 2

### Visualization Scheme

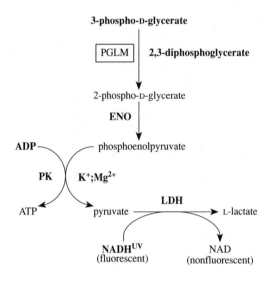

### Staining Solution[2]

0.17 $M$ Tris–HCl buffer, pH 8.0      10 ml
3-Phospho-D-glycerate (Na$_3$ salt)      10 mg
2,3-Diphosphoglycerate (pentacyclohexyl ammonium salt; 4H$_2$O)      8 mg
ADP (Na$_2$ salt)      15 mg
NADH      10 mg
MgCl$_2$ (6H$_2$O)      40 mg
KCl      30 mg
Enolase (ENO)      10 units
Pyruvate kinase (PK)      10 units
Lactate dehydrogenase (LDH)      15 units

### Procedure

Apply the staining solution to the gel surface on a filter-paper overlay and incubate the gel at 37°C until dark (nonfluorescent) bands visible in long-wave UV light appear on a light (fluorescent) background. Record the zymogram or photograph using a yellow filter.

## GENERAL NOTES

The 2,3-diphosphoglycerate (DPG) may be firmly attached to the enzyme molecule during the catalytic cycle, or in other cases may be released so that free DPG is required as an activator. The enzyme from mammals and yeast requires DPG while the enzyme from wheat, rice, insects, and some fungi has maximum activity in the absence of DPG.

Some mammalian PGLM isozymes also catalyze the reactions of bisphosphoglycerate phosphatase (see 3.1.3.13 — BPGP) and bisphosphoglycerate mutase (see 5.4.2.4 — BPGM). Comparative electrophoretic studies showed that in mammalian erythrocytes PGLM, BPGP, and BPGM activities are determined by one and the same protein.[3]

## REFERENCES

1. Rosa, R., Gaillardon, J., and Rosa, J., Characterization of 2,3-diphosphoglycerate phosphatase activity: electrophoretic study, *Biochim. Biophys. Acta*, 293, 285, 1973.
2. Chen, S.-H., Anderson, J., Giblett, E. R., and Lewis, M., Phosphoglyceric acid mutase: rare genetic variants and tissue distribution, *Am. J. Hum. Genet.*, 26, 73, 1974.
3. Rosa, R., Audit, I., and Rosa, J., Evidence for three enzymatic activities in one electrophoretic band of 3-phosphoglycerate mutase from red cells, *Biochimie*, 57, 1059, 1975.

OTHER NAMES     Glucose phosphomutase

REACTION     α-D-Glucose 1-phosphate = α-D-glucose 6-phosphate (also see General Notes)

ENZYME SOURCE   Bacteria, green algae, fungi, plants, invertebrates, vertebrates

## METHOD 1

### Visualization Scheme

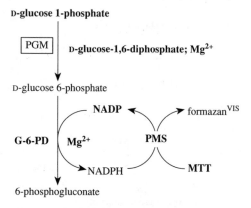

### Staining Solution[1] (modified)

A. 0.05 *M* Tris–HCl buffer, pH 8.2 — 25 ml
   Glucose 1-phosphate (Na$_2$ salt, 4H$_2$O; containing about 1% of glucose-1,6-diphosphate) — 100 mg
   MgCl$_2$ (6H$_2$O) — 40 mg
   NADP — 8 mg
   Glucose-6-phosphate dehydrogenase (G-6-PD; see *Notes*) — 6 units
   PMS — 1 mg
   MTT — 7 mg
B. 2% Agar solution (60°C) — 25 ml

### Procedure

Mix A and B components of the staining solution and pour the mixture over the gel surface. Incubate the gel in the dark at 37°C until dark blue bands appear. Fix stained gel in 50% ethanol.

*Notes:* The use of the NAD-dependent form of the linking enzyme G-6-PD (available from Sigma) is preferable because substitution of NAD for NADP in the staining solution results in a cost saving.

## METHOD 2

### Visualization Scheme

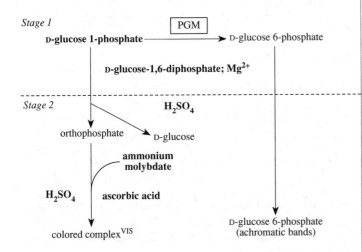

*Stage 1*

D-glucose 1-phosphate $\xrightarrow{\text{PGM}}$ D-glucose 6-phosphate

D-glucose-1,6-diphosphate; $Mg^{2+}$

*Stage 2* $\quad$ $H_2SO_4$

orthophosphate $\quad$ D-glucose

ammonium molybdate

$H_2SO_4$ $\quad$ ascorbic acid

colored complex$^{VIS}$ $\qquad$ D-glucose 6-phosphate (achromatic bands)

### Staining Solution[2]

A. 25 m$M$ Tris–2 m$M$ cysteine hydrochloride buffer, pH 8.0
   3 m$M$ D-Glucose 1-phosphate
   0.0147 m$M$ D-Glucose-1,6-diphosphate
   3 m$M$ MgCl$_2$
B. 2% Agar solution (60°C)
C. 1.25% Ammonium molybdate in 2 $N$ H$_2$SO$_4$ containing 50 mg/ml ascorbic acid

### Procedure

Mix equal volumes of A and B solutions and pour the mixture over the gel surface. Incubate the gel at 37°C for 2 h. Remove the agar overlay, mix equal volumes of B and C solutions, and pour the mixture over the gel surface. Achromatic bands of PGM activity appear on a blue gel background almost immediately or after 5 to 10 min of incubation at room temperature. Record or photograph zymogram because staining is not stable.

## GENERAL NOTES

The tetrazolium Method 1 gives better results. In the phosphate detection Method 2 the acid-labile phosphate tends to diffuse from the background into the clear areas of PGM activity.

Maximum PGM activity is only obtained in the presence of α-D-glucose-1,6-diphosphate. This diphosphate is an intermediate in the reaction, being formed by transfer of a phosphate residue from the enzyme to the substrate, but the dissociation of diphosphate from the enzyme complex is much slower than the overall isomerization.

The enzyme also, more slowly, catalyzes the interconversion of 1-phosphate and 6-phosphate isomers of many other α-D-hexoses, and the interconversion of α-D-ribose 1-phosphate and 5-phosphate. The last reaction is usually catalyzed by a separate enzyme, phosphopentomutase (see 5.4.2.7 — PPM). It was found, however, that some PGM isozymes exhibit strong phosphopentomutase activity.[2,3]

### REFERENCES

1. Spencer, N., Hopkinson, D. A., and Harris, H., Phosphoglucomutase polymorphism in man, *Nature*, 204, 742, 1964.
2. Quick, C. B., Fisher, R. A., and Harris, H., Differentiation of the PGM$_2$ locus isozymes from those of PGM$_1$ and PGM$_3$ in terms of phosphopentomutase activity, *Ann. Hum. Genet.*, 35, 445, 1972.
3. Quick, C. B., Fisher, R. A., and Harris, H., A kinetic study of the isozymes determined by the three human phosphoglucomutase loci PGM$_1$, PGM$_2$ and PGM$_3$, *Eur. J. Biochem.*, 42, 511, 1974.

OTHER NAMES    Diphosphoglycerate mutase, glycerate phosphomutase, bisphosphoglycerate syntase

REACTION    3-Phospho-D-glyceroyl phosphate = 2,3-bisphospho-D-glycerate (also see General Notes)

ENZYME SOURCE    Vertebrates

## METHOD

### Visualization Scheme

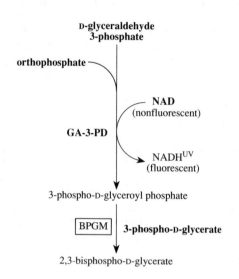

D-glyceraldehyde 3-phosphate

orthophosphate

NAD (nonfluorescent)

GA-3-PD

NADH$^{UV}$ (fluorescent)

3-phospho-D-glyceroyl phosphate

BPGM    **3-phospho-D-glycerate**

2,3-bisphospho-D-glycerate

### Staining Solution[1]
0.1 $M$ Tris–HCl buffer, pH 7.8
3.5 m$M$ D-Glyceraldehyde 3-phosphate
4 m$M$ 3-Phospho-D-glycerate
10 m$M$ $K_2HPO_4$
1.5 m$M$ NAD
1 U/ml Glyceraldehyde-3-phosphate dehydrogenase (GA-3-PD)

### Procedure
Apply the staining solution to the gel surface on a filter-paper overlay. After 20 to 30 min of incubation at 37°C monitor gel for fluorescent bands under long-wave UV light. Record the zymogram or photograph using a yellow filter.

*Notes:*    The method is based on removing the inhibitory effect of 3-phospho-D-glyceroyl phosphate on GA-3-PD activity via BPGM. As a result, NAD to NADH conversion is more pronounced in gel areas where BPGM activity is localized.

Arsenate may not be used as a substrate for GA-3-PD in place of $K_2HPO_4$ because of spontaneous arsenolysis of the product 3-phospho-D-glyceroyl arsenate and formation of free arsenate and 3-phospho-D-glycerate.

D-Glyceraldehyde-3-phosphate preparation may be obtained by 1 h of incubation at 37°C of the following mixture: aldolase — 10 units; fructose-1,6-diphosphate — 50 mg; 0.1 $M$ Tris–HCl buffer, pH 7.0 — 1 ml.

## OTHER METHODS

An alternative acid phosphomolybdate method for demonstration of BPGM which is based on bisphosphoglycerate phosphatase activity of the enzyme is also available (see 3.1.3.13 — BPGP, Method 2).

## GENERAL NOTES

The enzyme is phosphorylated by 3-phospho-D-glyceroyl phosphate to give phosphoenzyme and 3-phospho-D-glycerate. The latter is rephosphorylated by the enzyme to yield 2,3-bisphospho-D-glycerate, but this reaction is slowed by dissociation of 3-phospho-D-glycerate from the enzyme, which is therefore more active in the presence of added 3-phospho-D-glycerate.

The enzyme also catalyzes, slowly, the reaction of bisphosphoglycerate phosphatase (see 3.1.3.13 — BPGP) and phosphoglycerate mutase (see 5.4.2.1 — PGLM). Comparative electrophoretic studies showed that BPGM, BPGP, and PGLM activities in mammalian red cells are determined by one and the same protein.[2]

## REFERENCES
1. Chen, S.-H., Anderson, J. E., and Giblett, E. R., 2,3-Diphosphoglycerate mutase: its demonstration by electrophoresis and the detection of a genetic variant, *Biochem. Genet.*, 5, 481, 1971.
2. Rosa, R., Audit, I., and Rosa, J., Evidence for three enzymatic activities in one electrophoretic band of 3-phosphoglycerate mutase from red cells, *Biochimie*, 57, 1059, 1975.

## 5.4.2.7 — Phosphopentomutase; PPM

OTHER NAMES    Phosphodeoxyribomutase

REACTION    D-Ribose 1-phosphate = D-ribose 5-phosphate
(see also General Notes)

ENZYME SOURCE  Bacteria, invertebrates, vertebrates

## METHOD 1

### Visualization Scheme

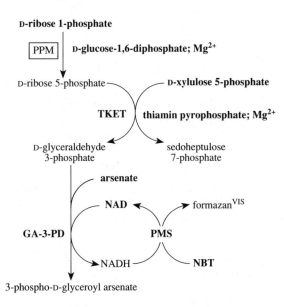

### Staining Solution[1]

A. 30 mM Tris–HCl buffer, pH 8.0
   3 mM D-Ribose 1-phosphate
   0.0147 mM D-Glucose-1,6-diphosphate
   12 mM MgCl$_2$
   2 mM D-Xylulose 5-phosphate (however, see Notes)
   0.01 U/ml Transketolase (TKET)
   0.2 U/ml Glyceraldehyde-3-phosphate dehydrogenase (GA-3-PD)
   2 mM Sodium arsenate
   0.2 mM Thiamin pyrophosphate
   1.5 mM NAD
   0.02 mg/ml PMS
   0.2 mg/ml NBT
B. 2% Agar solution (55°C)

### Procedure

Mix equal volumes of A and B components of the staining solution and pour the mixture over the gel surface. Incubate the gel in the dark at 37°C until dark blue bands appear. Fix stained gel in 50% ethanol.

*Notes:* In the original description of the method,[1] D-ribulose-5-phosphate is included in the staining solution as the second substrate for linking enzyme transketolase. However, this enzyme catalyzes the reaction D-ribose 5-phosphate + D-xylulose 5-phosphate = D-glyceraldehyde 3-phosphate + sedoheptulose 7-phosphate. Therefore, D-xylulose 5-phosphate is given in this version of the staining solution in place of D-ribulose 5-phosphate. D-Ribulose-5-phosphate can be used in place of D-xylulose 5-phosphate only in couple with ribulose-phosphate 3-epimerase (5.1.3.1 — RPE).

## METHOD 2

### Visualization Scheme

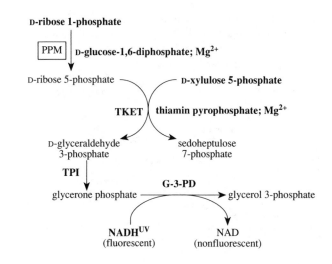

### Staining Solution[1]

A. 25 mM Tris–20 mM cysteine hydrochloride buffer, pH 8.0
   3 mM D-Ribose 1-phosphate
   0.0147 mM D-Glucose-1,6-diphosphate
   2 mM MgCl$_2$
   2 mM D-Xylulose 5-phosphate (however, see Method 1, *Notes*)
   0.01 U/ml Transketolase (TKET)
   0.2 U/ml Glycerol-3-phosphate dehydrogenase (G-3-PD)
   1 U/ml Triose-phosphate isomerase (TPI)
   0.2 mM Thiamin pyrophosphate
   1.5 mM NADH
B. 2% Agar solution (55°C)

### Procedure

Mix equal volumes of A and B solutions and pour the mixture over the gel surface. Incubate the gel at 37°C until dark (nonfluorescent) bands visible in long-wave UV light appear on a light (fluorescent) background. Record the zymogram or photograph using a yellow filter.

## METHOD 3

### Visualization Scheme

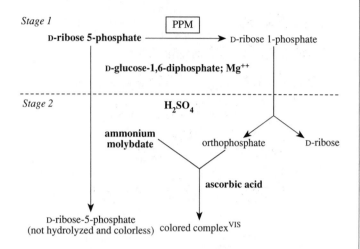

*Stage 1*

**D-ribose 5-phosphate** $\xrightarrow{\boxed{PPM}}$ D-ribose 1-phosphate

**D-glucose-1,6-diphosphate; Mg$^{++}$**

*Stage 2*

$H_2SO_4$

**ammonium molybdate** → orthophosphate, D-ribose

**ascorbic acid**

D-ribose-5-phosphate (not hydrolyzed and colorless), colored complex$^{VIS}$

### Staining Solution[1]

A. 2 m$M$ Cysteine hydrochloride buffer, pH 8.0
   3 m$M$ D-Ribose 5-phosphate
   2 m$M$ MgCl$_2$
   0.0147 m$M$ D-Glucose-1,6-diphosphate
B. 2% Agar solution (55°C)
C. 1.25% Ammonium molybdate in 2 $N$ H$_2$SO$_4$ containing 50 mg/ml ascorbic acid

### Procedure

Mix equal volumes of A and B solutions and pour the mixture over the gel surface. Incubate the gel at 37°C for 1 to 2 h. Remove the first agar overlay, mix equal volumes of B and C solutions, and pour the mixture over the gel surface. The labile phosphate from the product D-ribose 1-phosphate is hydrolyzed from the sugar moiety under the acid conditions. The free phosphate then forms a phosphomolybdate complex with the molybdate and this, in turn, is reduced by the ascorbic acid to form a blue compound in gel areas where PPM is localized. Record or photograph the zymogram because staining is not stable.

## METHOD 4

### Visualization Scheme

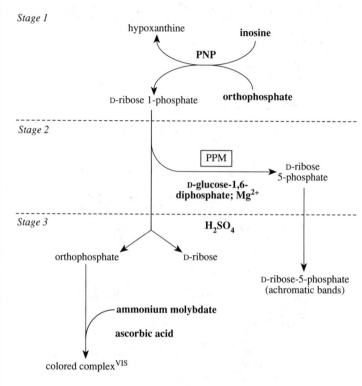

*Stage 1*

hypoxanthine, inosine
**PNP**
D-ribose 1-phosphate, **orthophosphate**

*Stage 2*

$\boxed{PPM}$ → D-ribose 5-phosphate

**D-glucose-1,6-diphosphate; Mg$^{2+}$**

*Stage 3*

$H_2SO_4$

orthophosphate, D-ribose, D-ribose-5-phosphate (achromatic bands)

**ammonium molybdate**
**ascorbic acid**

colored complex$^{VIS}$

### Staining Solution[1]

A. 20 m$M$ Tris–2 m$M$ cysteine hydrochloride buffer, pH 8.0
   2.5 m$M$ K$_2$HPO$_4$ (see *Notes*)
   0.024 U/ml Purine-nucleoside phosphorylase (PNP)
   3 m$M$ Inosine
   2 m$M$ MgCl$_2$
B. D-Glucose-1,6-diphosphate (see *Procedure*)
C. 2% Agar solution (55°C)
D. 1.25% Ammonium molybdate in 2 $N$ H$_2$SO$_4$ containing 50 mg/ml ascorbic acid

### Procedure

Prepare solution A and incubate at 37°C overnight. Then add component B (D-glucose-1,6-diphosphate) to solution A to give a final concentration of 0.0147 m$M$. Finally, add an equal volume of C and pour the resulting mixture over the gel surface. Incubate the gel at 37°C for 1 to 2 h. Remove the first agar overlay. Mix equal volumes of C and D solutions and pour the mixture over the gel surface again. White bands indicating PPM activity appear on a blue gel background. Record or photograph the zymogram because staining is labile.

*Notes:* If too much orthophosphate is added to solution A, the residual orthophosphate molecules can interact with ammonium molybdate in gel areas occupied by PPM and thus mask the development of achromatic PPM bands on a blue background.

## GENERAL NOTES

The enzyme also converts 2-deoxy-D-ribose 1-phosphate into 2-deoxy-D-ribose 5-phosphate. The enzyme requires D-ribose-1,5-diphosphate or 2-deoxy-D-ribose-1,5-diphosphate as cofactors. D-Glucose-1,6-diphosphate also acts as cofactor.

It was found that some isozymes of mammalian red cell phosphoglucomutase (see 5.4.2.2 — PGM) exhibit strong PPM activity.[1,2]

## REFERENCES

1. Quick, C. B., Fisher, R. A., and Harris, H., Differentiation of the PGM$_2$ locus isozymes from those of PGM$_1$ and PGM$_3$ in terms of phosphopentomutase activity, *Ann. Hum. Genet.*, 35, 445, 1972.
2. Quick, C. B., Fisher, R. A., and Harris, H., A kinetic study of the isozymes determined by the three human phosphoglucomutase loci PGM$_1$, PGM$_2$ and PGM$_3$, *Eur. J. Biochem.*, 42, 511, 1974.

OTHER NAMES     Chalcone–flavanone isomerase

REACTION     Chalcone = flavanone

ENZYME SOURCE   Plants

## METHOD

### Visualization Scheme

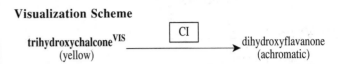

### Staining Solution[1]
0.25% 2′,4,4′-Trihydroxychalcone in 0.002 *N* NaOH

### Procedure
Spray electrophorized PAG with the staining solution and incubate at room temperature. Within 10 to 60 min the yellow color of the chalcone disappears from the areas where CI activity is located. Record the zymogram.

*Notes:* 2′,4,4′,6′-Tetrahydroxychalcone can also be used as colored CI substrate. The corresponding product of the CI reaction is a natural fluorochrome and can be observed under long-wave UV light.[2]

The enzyme from some sources (e.g., parsley) is inactive with chalcones lacking a 6′-hydroxyl group.

## REFERENCES

1. Hahlbrock, K., Wong, E., Schill, L., and Grisebach, H., Comparison of chalcone-flavanone isomerase heteroenzymes and isoenzymes, *Phytochemistry*, 9, 949, 1970.
2. Eigen, E., Blitz, M., and Gunsberg, E., The detection of some naturally occurring flavanone compounds on paper chromatography, *Arch. Biochem. Biophys.*, 68, 501, 1957.

OTHER NAMES    Tryptophanyl-tRNA synthetase

REACTION    ATP + L-tryptophan + tRNA$^{Trp}$ = AMP + pyrophosphate + L-tryptophanyl-tRNA$^{Trp}$ (see also *Notes*)

ENZYME SOURCE    Bacteria, fungi, plants, protozoa, invertebrates, vertebrates

## METHOD

### Visualization Scheme

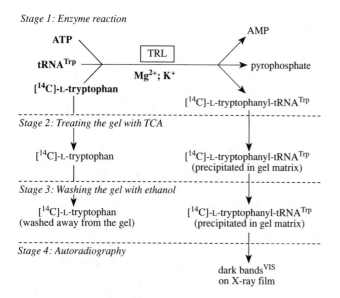

Stage 1: Enzyme reaction

Stage 2: Treating the gel with TCA

Stage 3: Washing the gel with ethanol

Stage 4: Autoradiography

### Staining Solution[1]

A.  50 m$M$ Tris–HCL buffer, pH 7.4
    10 m$M$ ATP
    40 m$M$ Magnesium acetate
    10 m$M$ Potassium chloride
    20 m$M$ 2-Mercaptoethanol
    1 mg/ml Bovine serum albumin
    $10^{-5}$ $M$ [$^{14}$C]-L-tryptophan
    1 mg/ml Crude yeast tRNA
B.  5% Trichloroacetic acid (TCA)
C.  95% Ethanol : 1 $M$ acetate buffer, pH 5.0 (9:1)

### Procedure

*Stage 1.*  Apply solution A (0.5 ml) by holding electrophorized acetate cellulose gel (7.8 by 15 cm) at one end with forceps and placing the gel, porous side down, into solution A placed in a plastic tray. Invert gel (porous side up) avoiding the formation of air bubbles between the gel and the tray. Blot excess liquid with filter paper. Moisten two strips of Whatman 3MM (4 by 8 cm) with 50 m$M$ tris–HCl buffer, pH 8.5, containing 20 m$M$ 2-mercaptoethanol and 15% glycerol and place lengthwise across both ends of the gel to prevent dessication. Place a tight-fitting cover on the tray and place the tray in a water bath at 37°C for 30 min.

*Stage 2.*  After 30 min of incubation flood the tray with 250 ml of cold solution B and expose for 10 min at 4°C with occasional agitation to stop the TRL reaction and precipitate tRNA in the gel matrix. Repeat this procedure twice.

*Stage 3.*  Discard solution B and wash the gel twice for 10 min with 250 ml of cold solution C.

*Stage 4.*  Dry the gel and mark the origin of each sample with red ink containing $^{35}$S ($2 \times 10^{6}$ dpm/ml). Place dry gel (porous side up) in contact with Kodak Blue Brand X-ray film and expose for a week at room temperature. Develop exposed film using Kodak D19 developer.

Dark bands on developed X-ray film indicate areas occupied by TRL on electrophoretic gel.

*Notes:*  There is strong evidence that an aminoacyl-tRNA ligase reaction proceeds in two steps: (1) an enzyme + an amino acid + ATP = an enzyme·aminoacyl-AMP + pyrophosphate; (2) an enzyme·aminoacyl-AMP + a tRNA = an enzyme + AMP + an aminoacyl-tRNA. It is obvious that the first-step reaction can be used to detect an aminoacyl-tRNA ligase activity in the absence of tRNA by the use of the product pyrophosphate.

## OTHER METHODS

A sensitive method for the localization in PAG of enzymes that produce pyrophosphate is available.[2] This method is based on the formation of white calcium pyrophosphate precipitate. It was successfully used to detect leucine-tRNA ligase (6.1.1.4 — LRL), valine-tRNA ligase (6.1.1.9 — VRL), and cysteine-tRNA ligase (6.1.1.16 — CRL) activities after PAG electrophoresis.[3] The calcium pyrophosphate method can also be applied to TRL. This method, however, requires control staining of an additional gel to identify ATPase (see 3.6.1.3 — ATPASE) activity bands, which can also develop on TRL zymograms.

### REFERENCES

1.  Denney, R. M. and Craig, I. W., Assignment of a gene for tryptophanyl–transfer ribonucleic acid synthetase (E.C. 6.1.1.2) to human chromosome 14, *Biochem. Genet.*, 14, 99, 1976.
2.  Nimmo, H. G. and Nimmo, G. A., A general method for the localization of enzymes that produce phosphate, pyrophosphate, or $CO_2$ after polyacrylamide gel electrophoresis, *Anal. Biochem.*, 121, 17, 1982.
3.  Chang, G.-G., Deng, R.-Y., and Pan, F., Direct localization and quantitation of aminoacyl-tRNA synthetase activity in polyacrylamide gel, *Anal. Biochem.*, 149, 474, 1985.

# 6.1.1.4 — Leucine-tRNA Ligase; LRL

OTHER NAMES    Leucyl-tRNA synthetase

REACTION    ATP + L-leucine + tRNA$^{Leu}$ = AMP + pyrophosphate + L-leucyl-tRNA$^{Leu}$ (see also *Notes*)

ENZYME SOURCE    Bacteria, fungi, plants, protozoa, invertebrates, vertebrates

## METHOD

### Visualization Scheme

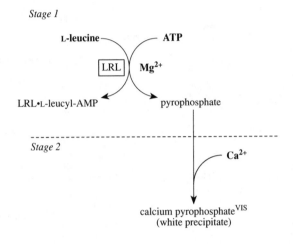

*Stage 1*

L-leucine — ATP

LRL   Mg$^{2+}$

LRL·L-leucyl-AMP     pyrophosphate

*Stage 2*

Ca$^{2+}$

calcium pyrophosphate$^{VIS}$ (white precipitate)

### Staining Solution[1]
A. 50 m$M$ Tris–HCL buffer, pH 7.7
   5 m$M$ Magnesium acetate
   5 m$M$ ATP
   5 m$M$ L-Leucine
B. 100 m$M$ CaCl$_2$ (pH 8.9)

### Procedure
Incubate electrophorized PAG in solution A at 37°C for 30 min and then in solution B at room temperature until white bands visible against a dark background appear. Store stained gel in 50 m$M$ glycine–KOH buffer, pH 10.0, containing 5 m$M$ CaCl$_2$ either at 5°C or at room temperature in the presence of an antibacterial agent (e.g., sodium azide).

*Notes:*   The reaction catalyzed by the aminoacyl-tRNA ligase proceeds in two steps: 1) enzyme + amino acid + ATP = enzyme·aminoacyl-AMP + pyrophosphate; (2) enzyme·aminoacyl-AMP + tRNA = enzyme + AMP + aminoacyl-tRNA.

The first reaction, which does not require tRNA$^{Leu}$, is used in the method described above.

The calcium pyrophosphate method is more simple than the autoradiographic method, which uses labeled ATP.[1] This method, however, requires control staining of an additional gel to identify ATPase (see 3.6.1.3 — ATPASE) activity bands, which can also develop on LRL zymograms. When using this method, a two-step procedure of gel staining is needed because of differences in pH-optimum of the enzyme and pH-optimum of the calcium pyrophosphate formation.

### REFERENCE
1. Chang, G.-G., Deng, R.-Y., and Pan, F., Direct localization and quantitation of aminoacyl-tRNA synthetase activity in polyacrylamide gel, *Anal. Biochem.*, 149, 474, 1985.

# 6.1.1.9 — Valine-tRNA Ligase; VRL

OTHER NAMES    Valyl-tRNA synthetase

REACTION    ATP + L-valine + tRNA$^{Val}$ = AMP + pyrophosphate + L-valyl-tRNA$^{Val}$ (see also *Notes*)

ENZYME SOURCE    Bacteria, fungi, plants, protozoa, invertebrates, vertebrates

## METHOD

### Visualization Scheme

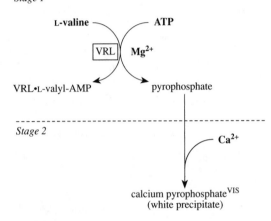

*Stage 1*

L-valine — ATP

VRL   Mg$^{2+}$

VRL·L-valyl-AMP     pyrophosphate

*Stage 2*

Ca$^{2+}$

calcium pyrophosphate$^{VIS}$ (white precipitate)

### Staining Solution[1]
A. 50 m$M$ Tris–HCL buffer, pH 7.7
   5 m$M$ Magnesium acetate
   5 m$M$ ATP
   5 m$M$ L-Valine
B. 100 m$M$ CaCl$_2$ (pH 8.9)

### Procedure
Incubate electrophorized PAG in solution A at 37°C for 30 min and then in solution B at room temperature until white bands visible against a dark background appear. Store stained gel in 50 m$M$ glycine–KOH buffer, pH 10.0, containing 5 m$M$ CaCl$_2$ either at 5°C or at room temperature in the presence of an antibacterial agent (e.g., sodium azide).

*Notes:*   The reaction catalyzed by the aminoacyl-tRNA ligase proceeds in two steps: (1) enzyme + amino acid + ATP = enzyme·aminoacyl-AMP + pyrophosphate; (2) enzyme·aminoacyl-AMP + tRNA = enzyme + AMP + aminoacyl-tRNA.

The first reaction which does not require tRNA$^{Val}$, is used in the method described above.

The calcium pyrophosphate method is simpler than the autoradiographic method, which uses labeled ATP.[1] This method, however, requires control staining of an additional gel to identify ATPase (see 3.6.1.3 — ATPASE) activity bands, which can also develop on VRL zymograms. When using this method, a two-step procedure of gel staining is needed because of differences in pH-optimum of the enzyme and pH-optimum of the calcium pyrophosphate formation.

### REFERENCE
1. Chang, G.-G., Deng, R.-Y., and Pan, F., Direct localization and quantitation of aminoacyl-tRNA synthetase activity in polyacrylamide gel, *Anal. Biochem.*, 149, 474, 1985.

## 6.1.1.16 — Cysteine-tRNA Ligase; CRL

OTHER NAMES    Cystenyl-tRNA synthetase

REACTION    ATP + L-cysteine + tRNA$^{Cys}$ = AMP + pyrophosphate + L-cystenyl-tRNA$^{Cys}$ (see also *Notes*)

ENZYME SOURCE    Bacteria, fungi, plants, protozoa, invertebrates, vertebrates

## METHOD

### Visualization Scheme

*Stage 1*

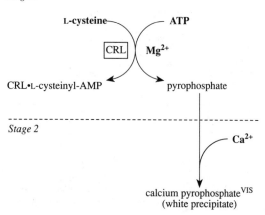

*Stage 2*

### Staining Solution[1]

A. 50 mM Tris–HCL buffer, pH 7.7
   5 mM Magnesium acetate
   5 mM ATP
   5 mM L-Cysteine
B. 100 mM CaCl$_2$ (pH 8.9)

### Procedure

Incubate electrophorized PAG in solution A at 37°C for 30 min and then in solution B at room temperature until white bands visible against a dark background appear. Store stained gel in 50 mM glycine–KOH buffer, pH 10.0, containing 5 mM CaCl$_2$ either at 5°C or at room temperature in the presence of an antibacterial agent (e.g., sodium azide).

*Notes:*  The reaction catalyzed by the aminoacyl-tRNA ligase proceeds in two steps: (1) enzyme + amino acid + ATP = enzyme·aminoacyl-AMP + pyrophosphate; (2) enzyme·aminoacyl-AMP + tRNA = enzyme + AMP + aminoacyl-tRNA.

The first reaction, which does not require tRNA$^{Cys}$, is used to detect CRL by the method described above.

The calcium pyrophosphate precipitation method is simpler than the autoradiographic method, which uses labeled ATP.[1] This method, however, requires control staining of an additional gel to identify ATPase (see 3.6.1.3 — ATPASE) activity bands which can also develop on CRL zymograms.

The two-step procedure of gel staining is needed because of differences in the pH-optimum of the enzyme and the pH-optimum of the calcium pyrophosphate formation.

### REFERENCE

1. Chang, G.-G., Deng, R.-Y., and Pan, F., Direct localization and quantitation of aminoacyl-tRNA synthetase activity in polyacrylamide gel, *Anal. Biochem.*, 149, 474, 1985.

## 6.2.1.3 — Long-Chain Fatty Acid-CoA Ligase; ACAS

OTHER NAMES    Acyl-CoA synthetase, fatty acid thiokinase (long chain), acyl-activating enzyme, long chain acyl-CoA synthetase, palmitoyl-CoA synthetase

REACTION    ATP + acid + CoA = AMP + pyrophosphate + acyl-CoA; acts on acids from C6 to C20

ENZYME SOURCE    Bacteria, vertebrates

## METHOD

### Visualization Scheme

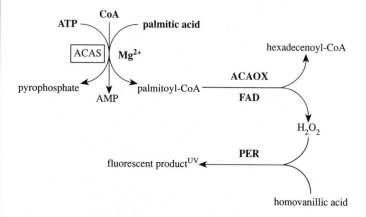

### Staining Solution[1] (adapted)

   0.01 M Tris–HCl buffer, pH 8.15
   20 mM ATP
   100 µM CoA
   50 µM Palmitic acid
   20 mM MgCl$_2$
   2.5 U/ml Acyl-CoA oxidase (ACAOX; Sigma)
   20 U/ml Horseradish peroxidase (PER)
   50 µM FAD
   1 mM Homovanillic acid

### Procedure

Apply the staining solution to the gel surface with filter paper or 1% agar overlay. Incubate the gel at 37°C and monitor under long-wave UV light for fluorescent bands. Record the zymogram or photograph using a yellow filter.

*Notes:*  In a coupled peroxidase reaction homovanillic acid reacts with hydrogen peroxide and a highly fluorescent dimer is formed which is excited at 313 nm and emits at 421 nm. Many other chromogenic substrates may be used in a coupled peroxidase reaction in place of homovanillic acid in order to generate products which are visible in daylight (see 1.11.1.7 — PER).

It is quite probable that the PMS/MTT system also works well coupled with FAD-dependent acyl-CoA oxidase as it does with other FAD-containing oxidases (e.g., see 1.1.3.4 — GO, Method 1; 1.1.3.22 — XOX, Method 1; 1.1.3.23 — TDH). If this is true, PMS and MTT (or NBT) may be included in the staining solution in place of peroxidase and homovanillic acid in order to generate blue formazan in gel areas where ACAS activity is localized.

## 6.2.1.3 — Long-Chain Fatty Acid-CoA Ligase; ACAS (continued)

### OTHER METHODS

A. Exogenous adenylate kinase may be used as a linking enzyme to produce ADP from ATP present in the staining solution (see above) and AMP produced by ACAS. Using two additional linked reactions catalyzed by exogenous pyruvate kinase and lactate dehydrogenase, areas of ADP generation may be detected in long-wave UV light as dark bands on the fluorescent background of the gel (for example, see 2.7.1.11 — PFK, Method 3). When using this method, it should be taken into account that ADP may be produced from ATP by ATPase, for which activity bands can also be detected by this method (see 3.6.1.3 — ATPASE, Method 2).

B. The calcium pyrophosphate method may be used to detect pyrophosphate produced by ACAS in transparent electrophoretic gels. This method is based on the formation of white calcium pyrophosphate precipitate in gel areas where a pyrophosphate-releasing enzyme is localized (for example, see 2.7.7.9 — UGPP, Method 3).

C. Auxiliary inorganic pyrophosphatase may be used to convert pyrophosphate produced by ACAS into orthophosphate, which can subsequently be detected by the acid molybdate method (see 3.6.1.1 — PP, Method 1), the enzymatic tetrazolium method, which involves two linked reactions catalyzed by auxiliary enzymes purine-nucleoside phosphorylase and xanthine oxidase (see 3.6.1.1 — PP, Method 2), the modified calcium phosphate method, suitable for detection of orthophosphate in opaque gels (see 3.1.3.1 — ALP, Method 7), or the acid molybdate–Malachite Green method (see 3.1.3.2 — ACP, Method 4), which results in a stabler colored product in comparison with the routine acid molybdate method and is ideal for use in the assay of detergent-solubilized membrane-associated enzymatic activity.

### REFERENCE

1. Lageweg, W., Steen, I., Tager, J. M., and Wanders, R. J. A., A fluorimetric assay for acyl-CoA synthetase activities, *Anal. Biochem.*, 197, 384, 1991.

## 6.2.1.X — Malonyl-CoA Synthase; MCAS

REACTION      ATP + malonate + CoA = malonyl-CoA + ADP + orthophosphate

ENZYME SOURCE   Bacteria, plants, vertebrates

### METHOD

#### Visualization Scheme

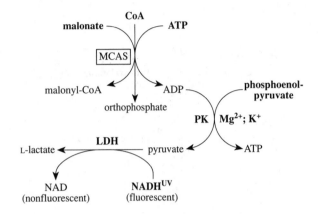

#### Staining Solution[1] (adapted)

A. 50 m$M$ Potassium phosphate buffer, pH 7.2
   10 m$M$ Sodium malonate
   5 m$M$ MgCl$_2$
   1 m$M$ Phosphoenolpyruvate
   0.2 m$M$ ATP
   0.2 m$M$ CoA
   0.1 m$M$ NADH
   3.5 U/ml Pyruvate kinase (PK)
   5 U/ml Lactate dehydrogenase (LDH)
B. 2% Agarose solution (60°C)

#### Procedure

Mix equal volumes of solutions A and B and pour the mixture over the gel surface. Incubate the gel at 37°C until dark (nonfluorescent) bands visible in long-wave UV light appear on a light (fluorescent) background. Record the zymogram or photograph using a yellow filter.

#### REFERENCE

1. Kim, Y. S. and Bang, S. K., Assays for malonyl-coenzyme A synthase, *Anal. Biochem.*, 170, 45, 1988.

OTHER NAMES   Glutamate–ammonia ligase (recommended name)

REACTION   ATP + L-glutamate + $NH_3$ = ADP + orthophosphate + L-glutamine

ENZYME SOURCE   Bacteria, fungi, plants, protozoa, vertebrates

## METHOD 1

### Visualization Scheme

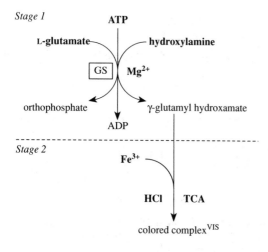

### Staining Solution[1]

A. 0.1 $M$ Tricine buffer, pH 7.8        100 ml
   L-Glutamic acid (Na salt)        1.4 g
   $MgSO_4$        250 mg
   ATP ($Na_3$; $2H_2O$)        500 mg
   Hydroxylamine hydrochloride        50 mg
   EDTA ($Na_4$; $3H_2O$)        50 mg
B. 2.5 $N$ HCl        100 ml
   Trichloroacetic acid (TCA)        5 g
   $FeCl_3$        10 g

### Procedure

Incubate the gel in freshly prepared solution A at 37°C for 15 min to 3 h (see *Notes*). Then wash gel in water and place in solution B. Greenish-brown bands appear in a few minutes. Wash stained gel in water and record or photograph zymogram immediately because the stain is ephemeral.

*Notes:*   Several slices from the same starch gel block should be used when assaying the enzyme for the first time. This is necessary to bracket the right incubation time in solution A, since the solution must be removed before one can see the stained bands.

## METHOD 2

### Visualization Scheme

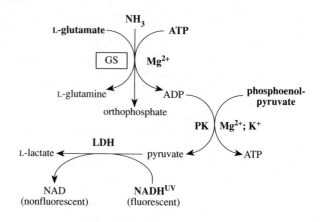

### Staining Solution[2] (adapted)

   0.1 $M$ Tris–HCl buffer, pH 7.5
   0.9 $M$ KCl
   50 m$M$ $MgCl_2$
   30 m$M$ L-Glutamate
   5 m$M$ ATP
   50 m$M$ $NH_4Cl$
   0.3 m$M$ NADH
   1 m$M$ Phosphoenolpyruvate
   1 U/ml Pyruvate kinase (PK)
   5 U/ml Lactate dehydrogenase (LDH)

### Procedure

Apply the staining solution to the gel surface on a filter-paper overlay and incubate the gel in a humid chamber at 37°C until dark (nonfluorescent) bands visible in long-wave UV light appear on a light (fluorescent) background. Record the zymogram or photograph using a yellow filter.

*Notes:*   When dark bands are clearly visible in UV light, treat the processed gel with the PMS/MTT solution to obtain a permanent negative zymogram (white bands on a blue background).

   In some organisms (e.g., mammals) additional bands caused by phosphoenolpyruvate phosphatase activity can also be developed by this method. Thus, an additional gel should be stained for activity of this phosphatase (see 3.1.3.18 — PGP, Method 2) as a control.

## OTHER METHODS

A. Using the reverse reaction, GS activity bands may be visualized by detecting the product ATP using two linking enzymes, hexokinase and glucose-6-phosphate dehydrogenase, in couple with the PMS/MTT system (see 2.7.1.1 — HK). This method, however, requires control staining of an additional gel for adenylate kinase (see 2.7.4.3 — AK), whose activity bands can also become apparent on GS zymograms.

B. The product of the reverse GS reaction, L-glutamate, may be detected using auxiliary glutamate dehydrogenase in couple with the PMS/MTT system (e.g., see 2.6.1.2 — GPT, Method 2).

## 6.3.1.2 — Glutamine Synthetase; GS (continued)

### GENERAL NOTES

The enzyme from a variety of sources varies greatly in its ability to catalyze the reverse reaction. Thus, that from bacteria catalyzes the reverse reaction very slowly or not at all. With mammalian enzyme, however, the forward rate relative to the reverse rate is about 1.

### REFERENCES

1. Barratt, D. H. P., Method for the detection of glutamine synthetase activity on starch gels, *Plant Sci. Lett.*, 18, 249, 1980.
2. Soliman, A. and Nordlund, S., Purification and partial characterization of glutamine synthetase from the photosynthetic bacterium *Rhodospirillum rubrum*, *Biochim. Biophys. Acta*, 994, 138, 1989.

## 6.3.2.2 — Glutamate–cysteine Ligase; GCL

OTHER NAMES     γ-Glutamylcysteine synthetase

REACTION     ATP + L-glutamate + L-cysteine = ADP + orthophosphate + γ-L-glutamyl-L-cysteine

ENZYME SOURCE   Bacteria, vertebrates

### METHOD

#### Visualization Scheme

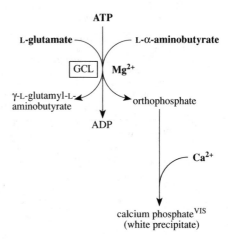

#### Staining Solution[1]
    0.14 $M$ Tris–HCl buffer, pH 8.0
    0.14 $M$ $MgCl_2$
    14 m$M$ L-Glutamate
    14 m$M$ L-α-Aminobutyrate
    14 m$M$ ATP
    38 m$M$ $CaCl_2$

#### Procedure

Incubate electrophorized PAG in the staining solution at 37°C until white bands of calcium phosphate precipitation appear. Store the stained gel in 50 m$M$ glycine–KOH buffer, pH 10.0, containing 5 m$M$ $Ca^{2+}$, either at 5°C or at room temperature in the presence of an antibacterial agent.

*Notes:* Calcium phosphate precipitate may be counterstained with Alizarin Red S. This does not increase the sensitivity of the staining method, although it would be of advantage when more opaque gels are used (e.g., starch or acetate cellulose).

    Some compounds, including L-α-aminobutyrate, can replace L-cysteine.

### OTHER METHODS

The product ADP can be detected by a negative fluorescent method using two linking enzymes, pyruvate kinase and lactate dehydrogenase (e.g., see 6.3.1.2 — GS, Method 2).

### REFERENCE

1. Seelig, G. F., Simondsen, R. P., and Meister, A., Reversible dissociation of γ-glutamylcysteine synthetase into two subunits, *J. Biol. Chem.*, 259, 9345, 1984.

## 6.3.4.5 — Argininosuccinate Synthase; AS

OTHER NAMES    Citrulline–aspartate ligase

REACTION    ATP + L-citrulline + L-aspartate = AMP + pyrophosphate + L-argininsuccinate

ENZYME SOURCE   Bacteria, plants, vertebrates

## METHOD

### Visualization Scheme

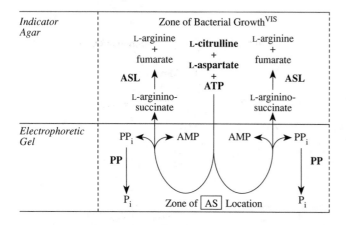

### Indicator Agar[1]

1.5% Indicator agar containing 100 µg/ml l-citrulline, 100 µg/ml L-aspartate, 100 µg/ml ATP, 1 U/ml argininosuccinate lyase (ASL), 0.5 U/ml inorganic pyrophosphatase (PP), $10^8$ bacteria/ml of *E. coli* 1115 (Arg G⁻) in minimal medium (see Appendix A-1) lacking L-arginine

### Procedure

Prepare indicator agar and pour it into a sterile plate. After the bacteria-seeded indicator agar solidifies, a slice of electrophoretic starch gel (cut surface down), cellulose acetate strip, or PAG is laid over the agar, avoiding the formation of air bubbles between indicator agar and electrophoretic gel. The bands of bacterial growth become visible in transmitted light after 6 to 12 h of incubation at 37°C.

*Notes:*   As a control for bacterial growth, L-arginine should be spotted at one corner of the indicator agar. The origin and slot locations should be marked on the indicator agar before it is removed.

     *P. cerevisiae* (ATCC 8081) with arginine biosynthesis defect can also be used in place of *E. coli*. In this case, however, citrate medium (see Appendix A-2) lacking L-arginine should be substituted for minimal medium in the indicator agar.

     Argininosuccinate lyase is used as a linking enzyme to produce L-arginine from L-argininosuccinate. Inorganic pyrophosphatase is used to remove pyrophosphate (PPi) which inhibits AS activity.

### REFERENCE

1. Naylor, S. L., Bioautographic visualization of enzymes, in *Isozymes: Current Topics in Biological and Medical Research, Vol. IV*, Rattazzi, M. C., Scandalios, J. G., and Whitt, G. S., Eds., Alan R. Liss, New York, 1980, 69.

## 6.4.1.1 — Pyruvate Carboxylase; PC

OTHER NAMES    Pyruvic carboxylase

REACTION    ATP + pyruvate + $HCO_3^-$ = ADP + orthophosphate + oxaloacetate

ENZYME SOURCE   Bacteria, fungi, vertebrates

## METHOD

### Visualization Scheme

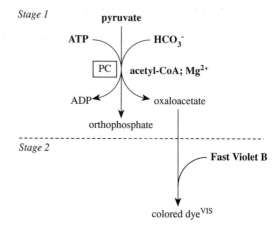

### Staining Solution[1]

A.   100 m$M$ Tris–HCl buffer, pH 7.8
     5 m$M$ Sodium pyruvate
     2 m$M$ ATP
     5 m$M$ MgCl$_2$
     50 m$M$ KHCO$_3$
     0.3 m$M$ Acetyl-CoA
B.   0.1% Fast Violet B

### Procedure

Incubate the gel in solution A for 20 to 30 min at room temperature, wash with distilled water, and place in solution B. Incubate the gel in the dark until red bands appear. Wash stained gel with water and fix in 5% acetic acid.

*Notes:*   Acetyl-CoA activates PC activity. Propionyl-CoA also may be used in some cases in place of acetyl-CoA. Fast Blue B and Fast Garnet GBC can be used instead of Fast Violet B.

## OTHER METHODS

A. The product pyruvate formed as a result of the reverse PC reaction can be detected by a negative fluorescent method using lactate dehydrogenase as a linking enzyme (e.g., see 2.7.1.40 — PK, Method 1).

B. Another product of the reverse PC reaction, the ATP, can be detected using two linking enzymes, hexokinase and NAD- or NADP-dependent glucose-6-phosphate dehydrogenase, coupled with the PMS/MTT system (e.g., see 2.7.1.40 — PK, Method 2).

C. There are several methods suitable for detection of orthophosphate produced by the forward PC reaction: the lead sulphide method (e.g., see 2.1.3.2 — ACT), the calcium phosphate method (e.g., see 3.1.3.2 — ACP, Method 5), the acid phosphomolybdate method (e.g., see 3.6.1.1 — PP, Method 1), and the tetrazolium enzymatic method (e.g., see 3.1.3.1 — ALP, Method 8). It should be taken into account that all these methods can also visualize the activity bands of acetyl-CoA carboxylase (see 6.4.1.2 — ACC) and propionyl-CoA carboxylase (when propionyl-CoA is used as PC activator). In contrast to PC, these bands can develop in staining solution lacking pyruvate. Control staining for ATPase (see 3.6.1.3 — ATPASE) is also needed.

D. Because PC is a biotinyl-protein, the biotin–streptavidin (or avidin) conjugation method can also be used to detect the enzyme protein molecules (e.g., see 6.4.1.2 — ACC). This method is not specific for PC and detects some other biotin-containing proteins.

## REFERENCE

1. Scrutton, M. C. and Fatebene, F., An assay system for localization of pyruvate and phosphoenolpyruvate carboxylase activity on polyacrylamide gels and its application to detection of these enzymes in tissue and cell extracts, *Anal. Biochem.*, 69, 247, 1975.

## 6.4.1.2 — Acetyl-CoA Carboxylase; ACC

REACTION — ATP + acetyl-CoA + $HCO_3^-$ = ADP + orthophosphate + malonyl-CoA

ENZYME SOURCE — Bacteria, plants, vertebrates

## METHOD

### Visualization Scheme (see *Notes*)

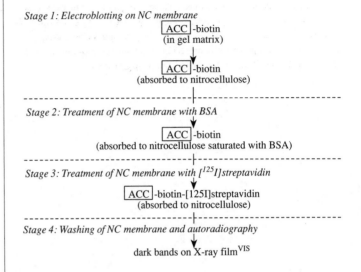

*Stage 1: Electroblotting on NC membrane*

ACC -biotin
(in gel matrix)

ACC -biotin
(absorbed to nitrocellulose)

- - - - - - - - - - - - - - - - - - - - - - - - - - - - - - - - - - - - -

*Stage 2: Treatment of NC membrane with BSA*

ACC -biotin
(absorbed to nitrocellulose saturated with BSA)

- - - - - - - - - - - - - - - - - - - - - - - - - - - - - - - - - - - - -

*Stage 3: Treatment of NC membrane with [$^{125}$I]streptavidin*

ACC -biotin-[125I]streptavidin
(absorbed to nitrocellulose)

- - - - - - - - - - - - - - - - - - - - - - - - - - - - - - - - - - - - -

*Stage 4: Washing of NC membrane and autoradiography*

dark bands on X-ray film$^{VIS}$

### Development by Autoradiography[1]

*Stage 1.* Transfer ACC molecules from electrophoretic gel to nitrocellulose membrane via electroblotting in 20 m$M$ tris–HCl (pH 8.3) buffer.

*Stage 2.* Incubate nitrocellulose membrane overnight in 10 m$M$ tris–HCl (pH 7.4), 0.9% NaCl, 3% BSA to saturate free protein-binding sites of nitrocellulose.

*Stage 3.* Place nitrocellulose membrane in 3% BSA solution containing 8·10$^5$ cpm [$^{125}$I]streptavidin for 2 h.

*Stage 4.* Wash nitrocellulose membrane in three changes of 10 m$M$ tris–HCl (pH 7.4), 0.9% NaCl to remove unbound [$^{125}$I]streptavidin. Dry nitrocellulose membrane and expose to X-ray film at –90°C.

Dark bands on developed X-ray film indicate areas of ACC localization in electrophoretic gel.

*Notes:* The method is based on specific conjugation of labeled streptavidin molecules with biotinyl-protein molecules of ACC. Labeled avidin may be used in place of streptavidin.

Streptavidin and avidin can also be labeled by peroxidase, β-galactosidase, or alkaline phosphatase. Such conjugates are now commercially available (e.g., from Sigma). After specific conjugation with biotin-containing ACC molecules, these enzymes may be detected by routine histochemical procedures (see 1.11.1.7 — PER; 3.2.1.23 — β-GAL; 3.1.3.1 — ALP).

In plants, ACC is the only known biotin-containing enzyme. In animals some other enzymes are known to be biotinyl-proteins: pyruvate carboxylase (see 6.4.1.1 — PC), propionyl-CoA carboxylase (EC 6.4.1.3), methyl-crotonoyl-CoA carboxylase (EC 6.4.1.4), and geranoyl-CoA carboxylase (EC 6.4.1.5). Thus, the biotin-streptavidin (or avidin) conjugation method is thought to be specific only for ACC from plant sources.

## OTHER METHODS

A. The product ADP can be detected by a negative fluorescent method using pyruvate kinase and lactate dehydrogenase as linking enzymes (e.g., see 2.7.1.35 — PNK).

B. The product orthophosphate can be detected by the lead sulfide method (e.g., see 2.1.3.2 — ACT), the calcium phosphate method (e.g., see 3.1.3.2 — ACP, Method 5), the acid phosphomolybdate method (e.g., see 3.6.1.1 — PP, Method 1), and the tetrazolium enzymatic method (e.g., see 3.1.3.1 — ALP, Method 8).

Both methods (A and B) can also detect ATPase activity bands. Thus, when these methods are used, a control staining of an additional gel for ATPase activity is needed (see 3.6.1.3 — ATPASE).

## REFERENCE

1. Nikolau, B. J., Wurtele, E. S., and Stumpf, P. K., Tissue distribution of acetyl-coenzyme A carboxylase in leaves, *Plant Physiol.*, 75, 895, 1984.

# Appendix A-1
# Minimal Medium for
# *Escherichia coli*[1,2]

## I. STOCK SOLUTIONS FOR MINIMAL MEDIUM

### A. Minimal salts

| | |
|---|---|
| $NH_4Cl$ | 20 g |
| $NH_4NO_3$ | 4 g |
| $Na_2SO_4$ (anhydrous) | 8 g |
| $K_2HPO_4$ ($3H_2O$) | 15.7 g |
| $KH_2PO_4$ | 4 g |
| $MgSO_4$ ($7H_2O$) | 0.4 g |

Dissolve salts in distilled water in the indicated order. Adjust pH to 7.2 with 1 *N* NaOH and bring total volume to 1000 ml with distilled water. Filtrate the solution through Whatman No. 1 filter paper and autoclave appropriate aliquots at 15 psi for 15 min.

### B. Nutrients

1. 0.2 g/ml Glucose
2. 2 mg/ml Amino acids
   0.1 mg/ml Vitamins
   2 mg/ml Purines and pyrimidines

Use amino acids, vitamins, purines, and pyrimidines required by particular *E. coli* mutant stocks. Prepare nutrient solutions using distilled water and sterilize by filtration through 0.22-μm Millipore filter.

## II. 2× STOCK MINIMAL MEDIUM (2× MM)

Mix 50 ml A, 2 ml B.1., and 2 ml B.2. stock solutions under aseptic conditions. Bring total volume to 100 ml with sterile water.

## III. MINIMAL MEDIUM (MM)

Add an equal volume of sterile water to 2× stock minimal medium.

*Notes:* Minimal medium (MM) containing all nutrients required by a particular *E. coli* mutant is used for the maintenance of stock cultures of *E. coli* mutant strains.

To prepare *E. coli* microbial reagent for bioautographic assay, transfer mutant *E. coli* from a stock culture into MM containing all required nutrients and aerate at 37°C for 4 to 6 h. Centrifuge bacteria at 5000 g for 10 min. Wash bacteria by centrifugation and resuspend in MM lacking the nutrient to be detected.

To prepare 1.5% indicator agar for bioautography, sterilize 3% Bacto agar (Difco) solution by autoclaving at 15 psi for 15 min. Cool melted 3% Bacto agar solution to 47°C and mix with an equal volume of 2× MM (47°C). Store agar-containing mixture at 47°C to prevent solidification. The substrate(s) for the enzyme to be detected, which have been prepared as 100x stocks and sterilized by filtration through a 0.22-μm membrane, are added to the agar-containing mixture at this point as well as washed bacteria ($10^8$ bacteria/ml final concentration). After this the mixture is poured into sterile trays of appropriate size.

## REFERENCES

1. Naylor, S. L. and Klebe, R. J., Bioautography: a general method for the visualization of isozymes, *Biochem. Genet.*, 15, 1193, 1977.
2. Naylor, S. L., Bioautographic visualization of enzymes, in *Isozymes: Current Topics in Biological and Medical Research, Vol. IV*, Rattazzi, M. C., Scandalios, J. G., and Whitt, G. S., Eds., Alan R. Liss, New York, 1980, 69.

# Appendix A-2
# Citrate Medium for
# *Pediococcus cerevisiae*[1,2]

## I. STOCK SOLUTIONS FOR CITRATE MEDIUM

### Glucose Buffer

| | |
|---|---|
| Glucose | 200 g |
| Trisodium citrate (2H$_2$O) | 200 g |
| Sodium acetate (3H$_2$O) | 30 g |
| KH$_2$PO$_4$ | 30 g |
| Ammonium sulfate | 30 g |
| NaCl | 10 g |

Dissolve in distilled water and bring total volume to 2 l with distilled water.

### Amino Acid Mixture I

| | |
|---|---|
| L-Isoleucine | 1.5 g |
| L-Leucine | 1.5 g |
| L-Valine | 1.5 g |
| L-Phenylalanine | 1.0 g |
| L-Proline | 1.0 g |

Dissolve in 250 ml distilled water.

### Amino Acid Mixture II

| | |
|---|---|
| L-Alanine | 1.5 g |
| L-Arginine hydrochloride | 5.0 g |
| L-Glutamate | 5.0 g |
| Glycine | 3.0 g |
| L-Histidine hydrochloride (H$_2$O) | 1.0 g |
| L-Serine | 1.0 g |
| L-Threonine | 1.0 g |

Dissolve in 400 ml distilled water. Adjust pH to 6.0 with 1 *N* NaOH and bring total volume to 500 ml with distilled water.

### Amino Acid Mixture III

| | |
|---|---|
| L-Asparagine | 2.0 g |
| L-Aspartate | 1.0 g |
| L-Cystine | 2.0 g |
| L-Tyrosine | 1.0 g |
| L-Tryptophan | 1.0 g |

Dissolve in 400 ml distilled water. Adjust pH to 11.0 with 1 *N* NaOH and bring total volume to 500 ml with distilled water.

### Amino Acid Mixture IV

| | |
|---|---|
| L-Lysine hydrochloride | 2.0 g |
| L-Methionine | 1.0 g |
| L-Cysteine hydrochloride | 2.0 g |

Dissolve in 150 ml distilled water. Adjust pH to 2.0 with concentrated HCl and bring total volume to 200 ml with distilled water.

### Purines and Pyrimidine Solution

| | |
|---|---|
| Adenine | 0.1 g |
| Guanine hydrochloride | 0.1 g |
| Uracil | 0.1 g |
| Xanthine | 0.1 g |

Suspend in 90 ml distilled water. Add 8 ml 1 *N* NaOH and dissolve by stirring. Bring total volume to 100 ml with distilled water.

### Vitamin Mixture I

| | |
|---|---|
| Thiamin hydrochloride | 10 mg |
| Niacin | 10 mg |
| Calcium pantothenane | 10 mg |
| Pyridoxine hydrochloride | 10 mg |
| Pyridoxamine | 10 mg |
| Pyridoxal dihydrochloride | 10 mg |
| Biotin (100 µg/ml in 50% EtOH) | 1.0 ml |

Dissolve dry components of the mixture in 80 ml distilled water. Add biotin solution. Bring total volume to 100 ml with distilled water.

### Vitamin mixture II

| | |
|---|---|
| Folic acid (0.1 mg/ml in 0.01 *N* NaOH) | 1.0 ml |
| Folinic acid (0.1 mg/ml solution) | 1.0 ml |

Bring total volume to 100 ml with distilled water.

### *p*-Aminobenzoic Acid Solution

| | |
|---|---|
| *p*-Aminobenzoic acid | 5 mg |

Dissolve in 10 ml of 10% acetic acid.

### Tween 80 and CaCl$_2$ Solution

| | |
|---|---|
| Tween 80 | 2.0 ml |
| CaCl$_2$ | 1.0 g |

Add Tween 80 to 90 ml warm distilled water. Add CaCl$_2$ and dissolve by stirring. Bring total volume to 100 ml with distilled water.

### Riboflavin Solution

| | |
|---|---|
| Riboflavin | 10 mg |

Add riboflavin to mixture of 10 ml distilled water, 0.5 ml glacial acetic acid, and 3 ml EtOH. Heat the mixture gently to dissolve riboflavin. Bring total volume to 100 ml with distilled water.

### Metal Salts Solution

| | |
|---|---|
| MgSO$_4$ (7H$_2$O) | 5.0 g |
| MnSO$_4$ (4H$_2$O) | 1.5 g |
| FeSO$_4$ | 0.5 g |

Dissolve metal salts in 100 ml of 0.03 *N* HCl.

*Note*:   All stock solutions are stable for several months when stored at –20°C. Precipitation can occur in some stock solutions (e.g., in amino acid mixtures). To dissolve precipitate, heat stock solution to 60°C.

## II. 2× STOCK CITRATE MEDIUM

| | |
|---|---|
| Glucose buffer | 2000 ml |
| Amino acid mixture I | 250 ml |
| Amino acid mixture II | 500 ml |
| Amino acid mixture III | 500 ml |
| Amino acid mixture IV | 200 ml |
| Purines and pyrimidine solution | 100 ml |
| Vitamin mixture I | 100 ml |
| Vitamin mixture II | 100 ml |
| *p*-Aminobenzoic acid solution | 10 ml |
| Tween 80 and CaCl$_2$ solution | 100 ml |
| Ascorbate | 10 g |

Add the stock solutions to 600 ml distilled water in the indicated order. Adjust pH to 6.8 with 12 *N* HCl and then add:

| | |
|---|---|
| Riboflavin solution | 100 ml |
| Metal salts solution | 100 ml |

Bring total volume to 5000 ml with distilled water. Sterilize 2× stock citrate medium by filtration through 0.22-μm Millipore filter and store at −20°C. It is stable for several months.

## III. CITRATE MEDIUM

Add an equal volume of sterile water to 2x stock citrate medium.

*Notes:* Citrate medium is a complete medium suitable for maintenance of *P. cerevisiae* stock culture.

To maintain exponentially growing *P. cerevisiae* culture, which may be used as a microbial reagent for bioautographic assay, transfer *P. cerevisiae* into complete citrate medium at a 1:20 dilution three times per day. Wash bacteria, 6 to 7 h after transfer, twice with citrate medium lacking the nutrient to be detected, by centrifugation at 5000 g for 10 min.

Preparation of 1.5% indicator agar for bioautographic assay using *P. cerevisiae* as a microbial reagent is essentially the same as described in Appendix A-1, except citrate medium is used in place of *E. coli* minimal medium.

## REFERENCES

1. Naylor, S. L. and Klebe, R. J., Bioautography: a general method for the visualization of isozymes, *Biochem. Genet.*, 15, 1193, 1977.
2. Naylor, S. L., Bioautographic visualization of enzymes, in *Isozymes: Current Topics in Biological and Medical Research, Vol. IV*, Rattazzi, M. C., Scandalios, J. G., and Whitt, G. S., Eds., Alan R. Liss, New York, 1980, 69.

# Appendix B
# Alphabetical List of Enzymes

This list is provided to enable the location of certain enzymes arranged in the Enzyme Sheets in Part III according to their numbers and not names. Therefore, the list includes the enzyme names and corresponding nomenclature numbers used in the Enzyme Sheets, but arranged alphabetically. As a rule, these are the enzyme names recommended by the Nomenclature Committee of the International Union of Biochemistry. In some cases, however, names other than the recommended ones were used in the Enzyme Sheets. Usually these are widely used routine enzyme names. All the enzyme names (recommended and routine) used as titles in the Enzyme Sheets are given in the list in bold letters. For example, **"Alcohol dehydrogenase 1.1.1.1"** (recommended name), **"Glutamic–oxaloacetic transaminase 2.6.1.1"** (widely used routine name). Recommended enzyme names are given in regular type for those enzymes for which routine names were used as titles in the Enzyme Sheets. For convenience and cross-reference purposes these recommended names are given with special references to the corresponding routine names. For example, "Aspartate aminotransferase, see **Glutamic–oxaloacetic transaminase**".

| | |
|---|---|
| **Acetylcholinesterase** | 3.1.1.7 |
| **Acetyl-CoA carboxylase** | 6.4.1.2 |
| **Acetyl-CoA hydrolase** | 3.1.2.1 |
| N-Acetyl-β-glucosaminidase, see **Hexosaminidase** | |
| **β-N-Acetylgalactosaminidase** | 3.2.1.53 |
| **N-Acetyllactosamine synthase** | 2.4.1.90 |
| **Acid phosphatase** | 3.1.3.2 |
| **Aconitase** | 4.2.1.3 |
| Aconitate hydratase, see **Aconitase** | |
| **Acrosin** | 3.4.21.10 |
| **Acyl-CoA dehydrogenase** | 1.3.99.3 |
| **Acylphosphatase** | 3.6.1.7 |
| **Adenine phosphoribosyltransferase** | 2.4.2.7 |
| **Adenosine deaminase** | 3.5.4.4 |
| **Adenosine kinase** | 2.7.1.20 |
| **Adenosinetriphosphatase** | 3.6.1.3 |
| **Adenosylhomocysteinase** | 3.3.1.1 |
| **Adenylate kinase** | 2.7.4.3 |
| **Alanine aminopeptidase** | 3.4.11.2 |
| Alanine aminotransferase, see **Glutamic–pyruvic transaminase** | |
| **Alanine dehydrogenase** | 1.4.1.1 |
| **Alanopine dehydrogenase** | 1.5.1.17 |
| **Alcohol dehydrogenase** | 1.1.1.1 |
| **Alcohol dehydrogenase (NADP)** | 1.1.1.2 |
| **Aldehyde dehydrogenase (NAD)** | 1.2.1.3 |
| **Aldehyde oxidase** | 1.2.3.1 |
| **Aldolase** | 4.1.2.13 |
| D-threo-Aldose dehydrogenase, see L-**Fucose dehydrogenase** | |
| **Aldose 1-epimerase** | 5.1.3.3 |
| **Alkaline phosphatase** | 3.1.3.1 |
| **Amine oxidase (copper-containing)** | 1.4.3.6 |
| Amine oxidase (flavin-containing), see **Monoamine oxidase** | |
| D-**Amino acid oxidase** | 1.4.3.3 |
| L-**Amino acid oxidase** | 1.4.3.2 |
| **Aminoacylase** | 3.5.1.14 |
| **4-Aminobutyrate aminotransferase** | 2.6.1.19 |
| **AMP deaminase** | 3.5.4.6 |
| **α-Amylase** | 3.2.1.1 |
| **Anthranilate synthase** | 4.1.3.27 |
| A-L-**Arabinofuranosidase** | 3.2.1.55 |
| **Arginase** | 3.5.3.1 |
| **Arginine aminopeptidase** | 3.4.11.6 |
| **Arginine kinase** | 2.7.3.3 |
| **Argininosuccinate lyase** | 4.3.2.1 |
| **Argininosuccinate synthase** | 6.3.4.5 |
| **Aromatic-L-amino acid decarboxylase** | 4.1.1.28 |
| **Aromatic α-keto acid reductase** | 1.1.1.96 |
| **Arylsulfatase** | 3.1.6.1 |
| L-**Ascorbate oxidase** | 1.10.3.3 |
| **Asparaginase** | 3.5.1.1 |
| Aspartate aminotransferase, see **Glutamic–oxaloacetic transaminase** | |
| **Aspartate carbamoyltransferase** | 2.1.3.2 |
| **Aspartate dehydrogenase** | 1.4.1.X |
| D-**Aspartate oxidase** | 1.4.3.1 |
| **Biliverdin reductase** | 1.3.1.24 |
| **Bisphosphoglycerate mutase** | 5.4.2.4 |
| **Bisphosphoglycerate phosphatase** | 3.1.3.13 |
| **Branched-chain amino acid aminotransferase** | 2.6.1.42 |
| **Butyryl-CoA dehydrogenase** | 1.3.99.2 |
| **Calf thymus ribonuclease H** | 3.1.26.4 |
| Carbonate dehydratase, see **Carbonic anhydrase** | |
| **Carbonic anhydrase** | 4.2.1.1 |
| **Carboxypeptidase A** | 3.4.17.1 |
| **Catalase** | 1.11.1.6 |
| **Catechol methyltransferase** | 2.1.1.6 |
| **Catechol oxidase** | 1.10.3.1 |
| **Cellulase** | 3.2.1.4 |
| **Cellulose 1,4-β-cellobiosidase** | 3.2.1.91 |
| **Ceruloplasmin** | 1.16.3.1 |
| **Chalcone isomerase** | 5.5.1.6 |
| **Chitin synthase** | 2.4.1.16 |
| **Choline dehydrogenase (NAD)** | 1.1.1.X |
| **Cholinesterase** | 3.1.1.8 |
| **Chorismate synthase** | 4.6.1.4 |
| **Chymotrypsin** | 3.4.21.1 |
| **Citrate lyase** | 4.1.3.6 |
| Citrate (pro-3S)-lyase, see **Citrate lyase** | |
| **Citrate synthase** | 4.1.3.7 |
| Citrate (si)-synthase, see **Citrate synthase** | |
| CMP-N-acylneuraminate phosphodiesterase, see **CMP–sialate hydrolase** | |
| **CMP–sialate hydrolase** | 3.1.4.40 |
| **Creatine kinase** | 2.7.3.2 |
| **Cyclic-CMP phosphodiesterase** | 3.1.4.37 |
| 2′,3′-Cyclic-nucleotide 3′-phosphodiesterase, see **Cyclic-CMP phosphodiesterase** | |
| **3′,5′-Cyclic-nucleotide phosphodiesterase** | 3.1.4.17 |
| Cystathionine β-synthase, see **Serine sulfhydrase** | |
| **Cysteine-conjugate β-lyase** | 4.4.1.13 |
| **Cysteine-tRNA ligase** | 6.1.1.16 |
| **Cystyl-aminopeptidase** | 3.4.11.3 |
| **Cytidine deaminase** | 3.5.4.5 |
| **Cytochrome c oxidase** | 1.9.3.1 |
| Cytosol aminopeptidase, see **Leucine aminopeptidase** | |
| **3-Dehydroquinate synthase** | 4.6.1.3 |
| **Deoxyadenosine kinase** | 2.7.1.76 |
| **Deoxycytidine kinase** | 2.7.1.74 |

| | | | |
|---|---|---|---|
| Deoxyguanosine kinase | 2.7.1.113 | Glutamine synthetase | 6.3.1.2 |
| Deoxyribonuclease I | 3.1.21.1 | Glutamine transaminase K | 2.6.1.64 |
| Dextranase | 3.2.1.11 | γ-Glutamylcyclotransferase | 2.3.2.4 |
| Dextransucrase | 2.4.1.5 | γ-Glutamyltransferase, see **Glutamyl transpeptidase** | |
| α-Dextrin endo-1,6-α-glucosidase | 3.2.1.41 | Glutamyl transpeptidase | 2.3.2.2 |
| Diaminopimelate decarboxylase | 4.1.1.20 | Glutathione peroxidase | 1.11.1.9 |
| Dihydrofolate reductase | 1.5.1.3 | Glutathione reductase | 1.6.4.2 |
| Dihydrolipoamide dehydrogenase, see **NADH diaphorase** | | Glutathione reductase (NAD(P)H), see **Glutathione reductase** | |
| Dihydroorotate dehydrogenase | 1.3.1.14 | Glutathione transferase | 2.5.1.18 |
| Dihydrouracil dehydrogenase (NADP) | 1.3.1.2 | Glyceraldehyde-3-phosphate dehydrogenase | 1.2.1.12 |
| Dihydroxy-acid dehydratase | 4.2.1.9 | Glyceraldehyde-3-phosphate dehydrogenase (NADP) | 1.2.1.13 |
| Diiodophenylpyruvate reductase, see **Aromatic α-keto acid reductase** | | Glycerate dehydrogenase | 1.1.1.29 |
| DNA (cytosine-5)-methyltransferase | 2.1.1.37 | Glycerol dehydrogenase (NADP) | 1.1.1.72 |
| DNA-directed DNA polymerase | 2.7.7.7 | Glycerol kinase | 2.7.1.30 |
| DNA-directed RNA polymerase | 2.7.7.6 | Glycerol-3-phosphate dehydrogenase | 1.1.1.8 |
| dTDPglucose 4,6-dehydratase | 4.2.1.46 | Glycerol-3-phosphate dehydrogenase (FAD) | 1.1.99.5 |
| Elastase | 3.4.21.36 | Glycolate oxidase | 1.1.3.15 |
| Endo-1,3(4)-β-glucanase | 3.2.1.6 | Glyoxalase I | 4.4.1.5 |
| Endo-1,4-β-xylanase | 3.2.1.8 | Guanine deaminase | 3.5.4.3 |
| Enolase | 4.2.1.11 | Guanylate kinase | 2.7.4.8 |
| Esterases | 3.1.1... | L-Gulonate dehydrogenase | 1.1.1.45 |
| Esteroprotease | 3.4.21.40 | Hexokinase | 2.7.1.1 |
| Fatty acid synthase | 2.3.1.85 | Hexosaminidase | 3.2.1.30 |
| Ferroxidase, see **Ceruloplasmin** | | Histidinol dehydrogenase | 1.1.1.23 |
| Formaldehyde dehydrogenase (glutathione) | 1.2.1.1 | Homoserine dehydrogenase | 1.1.1.3 |
| Formate dehydrogenase | 1.2.1.2 | Hyaluronoglucosaminidase | 3.2.1.35 |
| S-Formylglutathione hydrolase | 3.1.2.12 | L-2-Hydroxy-acid oxidase, see **Glycolate oxidase** | |
| β-Fructofuranosidase | 3.2.1.26 | 3-Hydroxyacyl-CoA dehydrogenase | 1.1.1.35 |
| Fructokinase | 2.7.1.4 | Hydroxyacylglutathione hydrolase | 3.1.2.6 |
| Fructose bisphosphatase | 3.1.3.11 | 3-Hydroxybutyrate dehydrogenase | 1.1.1.30 |
| Fructose-bisphosphate aldolase, see **Aldolase** | | (R)-20-Hydroxysteroid dehydrogenase | 1.1.1.53 |
| L-Fucose dehydrogenase | 1.1.1.122 | 3β-Hydroxy-Δ⁵-steroid dehydrogenase | 1.1.1.145 |
| α-L-Fucosidase | 3.2.1.51 | Hypoxanthine phosphoribosyltransferase | 2.4.2.8 |
| Fumarate hydratase | 4.2.1.2 | L-Iditol dehydrogenase, see **Sorbitol dehydrogenase** | |
| Galactokinase | 2.7.1.6 | IMP dehydrogenase | 1.1.1.205 |
| Galactose dehydrogenase | 1.1.1.48 | Indoleacetaldehyde dehydrogenase | 1.2.1.X |
| Galactose-1-phosphate uridyl transferase | 2.7.7.12 | Inorganic pyrophosphatase | 3.6.1.1 |
| α-Galactosidase | 3.2.1.22 | Isocitrate dehydrogenase (NAD) | 1.1.1.41 |
| β-Galactosidase | 3.2.1.23 | Isocitrate dehydrogenase (NADP) | 1.1.1.42 |
| Galacturan 1,4-α-galacturonidase | 3.2.1.67 | Isocitrate lyase | 4.1.3.1 |
| Glucan endo-1,3-β-glucosidase | 3.2.1.39 | Isopropanol dehydrogenase (NADP) | 1.1.1.80 |
| Gluconate 5-dehydrogenase | 1.1.1.69 | Kanamycin kinase | 2.7.1.95 |
| Glucose dehydrogenase | 1.1.1.47 | β-Lactamase, see **Penicillinase** | |
| Glucose oxidase | 1.1.3.4 | L-Lactate dehydrogenase | 1.1.1.27 |
| Glucose-6-phosphatase | 3.1.3.9 | Lactoylglutathione lyase, see **Glyoxalase I** | |
| Glucose-6-phosphate dehydrogenase | 1.1.1.49 | Leucine aminopeptidase | 3.4.11.1 |
| Glucose-6-phosphate isomerase | 5.3.1.9 | Leucine dehydrogenase | 1.4.1.9 |
| α-Glucosidase | 3.2.1.20 | Leucine-tRNA ligase | 6.1.1.4 |
| β-Glucosidase | 3.2.1.21 | Lipoxygenase | 1.13.11.12 |
| Glucuronate reductase | 1.1.1.19 | Long-chain fatty acid-CoA ligase | 6.2.1.3 |
| β-Glucuronidase | 3.2.1.31 | Lysine dehydrogenase | 1.4.1.15 |
| Glutamate–ammonia ligase, see **Glutamine synthetase** | | L-Lysine-lactamase | 3.5.2.11 |
| Glutamate–cysteine ligase | 6.3.2.2 | Lysozyme | 3.2.1.17 |
| Glutamate decarboxylase | 4.1.1.15 | Malate dehydrogenase | 1.1.1.37 |
| Glutamate dehydrogenase (NAD(P)) | 1.4.1.2-4 | Malate dehydrogenase (NADP) | 1.1.1.40 |
| Glutamic–oxaloacetic transaminase | 2.6.1.1 | Malate synthase | 4.1.3.2 |
| Glutamic–pyruvic transaminase | 2.6.1.2 | Malonyl-CoA synthase | 6.2.1.X |
| Glutaminase | 3.5.1.2 | Mannitol dehydrogenase | 1.1.1.67 |
| Glutamine–phenylpyruvate aminotransferase, see **Glutamine transaminase K** | | Mannitol dehydrogenase (NADP) | 1.1.1.138 |
| | | Mannitol-1-phosphate dehydrogenase | 1.1.1.17 |
| | | Mannokinase | 2.7.1.7 |
| Glutamine–pyruvate aminotransferase | 2.6.1.15 | Mannose-6-phosphate isomerase | 5.3.1.8 |

α-Mannosidase — 3.2.1.24

Microsomal aminopeptidase,
    see **Alanine aminopeptidase**

Monoamine oxidase — 1.4.3.4

NAD ADP–ribosyltransferase — 2.4.2.30

NADH diaphorase — 1.8.1.4

NADPH dehydrogenase, see **NADPH diaphorase**

NAD(P)H dehydrogenase (quinone) — 1.6.99.2

NADPH diaphorase — 1.6.99.1

NAD(P) nucleosidase — 3.2.2.6

Nitrate reductase — 1.7.99.4

Nitrate reductase (NAD(P)H) — 1.6.6.2

Nitrite reductase — 1.7.99.3

Nonspecific phosphodiesterase — 3.1.4.X

"Nothing dehydrogenase" — 1.X.X.X

Nucleoside-diphosphate kinase — 2.7.4.6

Nucleoside-diphosphosugar pyrophosphatase — 3.6.1.X

Nucleoside-phosphate kinase — 2.7.4.4

Nucleoside-triphosphate-adenylate kinase — 2.7.4.10

Nucleoside-triphosphate pyrophosphatase — 3.6.1.19

3′-Nucleotidase — 3.1.3.6

5′-Nucleotidase — 3.1.3.5

Octanol dehydrogenase — 1.1.1.73

D-Octopine dehydrogenase — 1.5.1.11

Oligo-1,6-glucosidase — 3.2.1.10

Ornithine carbamoyltransferase — 2.1.3.3

Ornithine-oxoacid aminotransferase — 2.6.1.13

Orotate reductase (NADH),
    see **Dihydroorotate dehydrogenase**

Oxoglutarate dehydrogenase — 1.2.4.2

5-Oxoprolyl-peptidase — 3.4.19.3

Pancreatic elastase, see **Elastase**

Pancreatic ribonuclease, see **Ribonuclease I**

**Pantetheinase** — 3.5.1.X

Pectate lyase, see **Polygalacturonate lyase**

**Pectinesterase** — 3.1.1.11

**Penicillinase** — 3.5.2.6

**Pepsin(ogen)s** — 3.4.23.1-3

**Peptidases** — 3.4.11 or 13...

**Peroxidase** — 1.11.1.7

**Phospho-2-dehydro-3-deoxyheptonate aldolase** — 4.1.2.15

**Phosphodiesterase I** — 3.1.4.1

**Phosphoenolpyruvate carboxylase** — 4.1.1.31

**6-Phosphofructokinase** — 2.7.1.11

**6-Phosphofructo-2-kinase** — 2.7.1.105

**Phosphoglucomutase** — 5.4.2.2

**Phosphogluconate dehydrogenase** — 1.1.1.44

**Phosphoglycerate kinase** — 2.7.2.3

**Phosphoglycerate mutase** — 5.4.2.1

**Phosphoglycolate phosphatase** — 3.1.3.18

**Phospholipase C** — 3.1.4.3

**Phosphopentomutase** — 5.4.2.7

**Phosphorylase** — 2.4.1.1

**Phosphoserine phosphatase** — 3.1.3.3

3-Phosphoshikimate 1-carboxyvinyltransferase,
    see **3-*enol*-Pyruvoylshikimate-5-phosphate synthase**

**Plasma kallikrein** — 3.4.21.34

**Plasminogen activator, see Urokinase**

**Polygalacturonase** — 3.2.1.15

**Polygalacturonate lyase** — 4.2.2.2

**Polyribonucleotide nucleotidyltransferase** — 2.7.7.8

Porphobilinogen deaminase,
    see **Uroporphyrinogen-I synthase**

**Porphobilinogen synthase** — 4.2.1.24

**Proline dipeptidase** — 3.4.13.9

**Proteinases** — 3.4.21 to 24...

**Protein–glutamine γ-glutamyltransferase** — 2.3.2.13

**Protein kinase** — 2.7.1.37

**Protein–tyrosine kinase** — 2.7.1.112

**Purine-nucleoside phosphorylase** — 2.4.2.1

Pyridoxal kinase, see **Pyridoxine kinase**

**Pyridoxine kinase** — 2.7.1.35

**Pyrophosphate-fructose-6-phosphate
    1-phosphotransferase** — 2.7.1.90

**1-Pyrroline-5-carboxylate dehydrogenase** — 1.5.1.12

**Pyruvate carboxylase** — 6.4.1.1

**Pyruvate decarboxylase** — 4.1.1.1

**Pyruvate kinase** — 2.7.1.40

**3-*enol*-Pyruvoylshikimate-5-phosphate synthase** — 2.5.1.19

**Retinol dehydrogenase** — 1.1.1.105

**Ribonuclease I** — 3.1.27.5

**Ribonuclease III** — 3.1.26.3

**Ribose-5-phosphate isomerase** — 5.3.1.6

**Ribose-phosphate pyrophosphokinase** — 2.7.6.1

**Ribulose-phosphate 3-epimerase** — 5.1.3.1

**RNA-directed RNA polymerase** — 2.7.7.48

**Saccharopine dehydrogenase (NAD, L-lysine–forming)** — 1.5.1.7

**Sarcosine oxidase** — 1.5.3.1

**Serine carboxypeptidase** — 3.4.16.1

**L-Serine dehydratase** — 4.2.1.13

**Serine sulfhydrase** — 4.2.1.22

**Shikimate dehydrogenase** — 1.1.1.25

**Sialidase** — 3.2.1.18

**Sorbitol dehydrogenase** — 1.1.1.14

**Spleen exonuclease** — 3.1.16.1

**Strombine dehydrogenase** — 1.5.1.X

Submandibular proteinase A, see **Esteroprotease**

**Succinate dehydrogenase** — 1.3.99.1

**Succinate-semialdehyde dehydrogenase** — 1.2.1.16

**Sucrose α-glucosidase** — 3.2.1.48

**Sucrose phosphorylase** — 2.4.1.7

**Sulfate adenylyltransferase** — 2.7.7.4

**Sulfite oxidase** — 1.8.3.1

**Superoxide dismutase** — 1.15.1.1

**Thiamin dehydrogenase** — 1.1.3.23

Thiamin oxidase, see **Thiamin dehydrogenase**

**Thioglucosidase** — 3.2.3.1

**Thiosulfate sulfurtransferase** — 2.8.1.1

**Thiosulfate-thiol sulfurtransferase** — 2.8.1.3

**Threonine dehydratase** — 4.2.1.16

**L-Threonine 3-dehydrogenase** — 1.1.1.103

**Thrombin** — 3.4.21.5

**Thymidine kinase** — 2.7.1.21

**Transaldolase** — 2.2.1.2

**Transketolase** — 2.2.1.1

**α,α-Trehalase** — 3.2.1.28

**Triacylglycerol lipase** — 3.1.1.3

**Trimethylamine-*N*-oxide reductase** — 1.6.6.9

**Triokinase** — 2.7.1.28

**Triose-phosphate isomerase** — 5.3.1.1

**Trypsin** — 3.4.21.4

**Tryptophan synthase** — 4.2.1.20

**Tryptophan-tRNA ligase** — 6.1.1.2

**Tyrosine aminotransferase** — 2.6.1.5

**UDPglucose dehydrogenase** — 1.1.1.22